EKG Plain and Simple

Second Edition

Karen M. Ellis, RN

Touro Infirmary and Delgado Community College, New Orleans

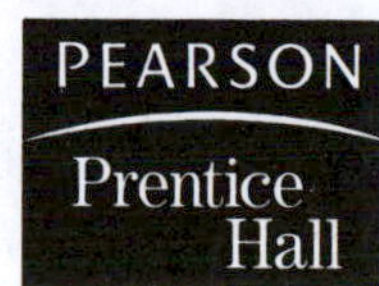

Upper Saddle River, New Jersey 07458

Library of Congress Cataloging-in-Publication Data

Ellis, Karen.
EKG plain and simple / Karen M.
Ellis. – 2nd ed.
p. ; cm.
Includes index.
ISBN 0-13-170814-7
1. Electrocardiography. I. Title.
[DNLM: 1. Electrocardiography. WG 140 E465e 2007]
RC683.5.E5E442 2007
616.1'207547–dc22

2006001613

Publisher: Julie Levin Alexander
Executive Assistant & Supervisor: Regina Bruno
Executive Editor: Mark Cohen
Associate Editor: Melissa Kerian
Media Editor: John J. Jordan
Director of Production and Manufacturing: Bruce Johnson
Director of Marketing: Karen Allman
Manager of Media Production: Amy Peltier
New Media Project Manager: Stephen J. Hartner
Managing Production Editor: Patrick Walsh
Production Liaison: Christina Zingone
Production Management/Composition: Pine Tree Composition/Laserwords Private Limited
Production Editor: Christine Furry
Manufacturing Manager: Ilene Sanford
Manufacturing Buyer: Pat Brown
Design Coordinator: Maria Guglielmo
Senior Marketing Manager: Harper Coles
Printer/Binder: Banta Company, Harrisonburg, VA
Cover Printer: Phoenix Color Corp.
Cover Design: Kevin Kall
Cover Image: Getty Images Inc.–Image Bank

Notice: The author and the publisher of this book have taken care to make certain that the equipment and schedules of treatment are correct and compatible with the standards generally accepted at the time of publication. Nevertheless, as new information becomes available, changes in treatment and in the use of equipment and procedures become necessary. The reader is advised to consult carefully the instruction and information material included in each piece of equipment or device before administration. Students are warned that the use of any techniques must be authorized by their medical advisor, where appropriate, in accordance with local laws and regulations. The publisher disclaims any liability, loss, injury, or damage incurred as a consequence, directly or indirectly, of the use and application of any of the contents of this book.

Pearson Education Ltd., *London*
Pearson Education Australia Pty. Limited, *Sydney*
Pearson Education Singapore, Pte. Ltd.
Pearson Education North Asia Ltd., *Hong Kong*
Pearson Education Canada, Ltd., *Toronto*
Pearson Educación de Mexico, S.A. de C.V.
Pearson Education—Japan, *Tokyo*
Pearson Education Malaysia, Pte. Ltd.
Pearson Education, Upper Saddle River, New Jersey

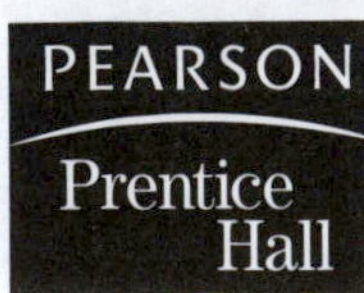

10 9 8 7 6 5 4
ISBN 0-13-170814-7

Contents

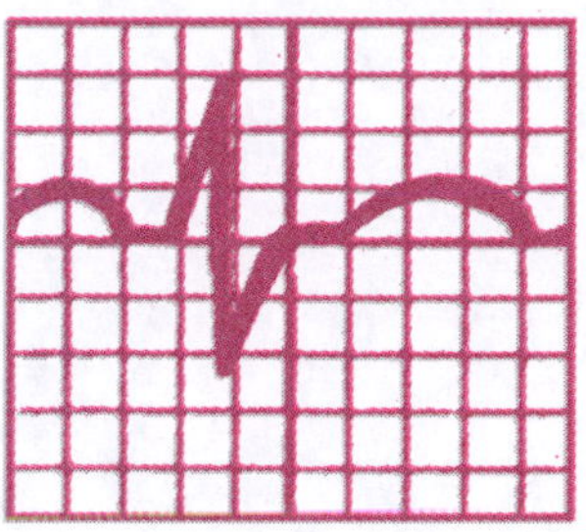

PART II ADVANCED CONCEPTS

Introduction

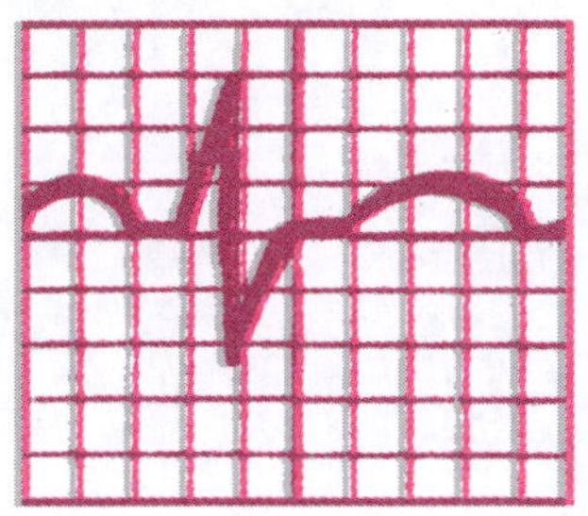

Welcome to the second edition of *EKG Plain and Simple*. There have been many changes from the first edition:

Fewer chapters. Condensed from 31 chapters to 19, this edition simplifies EKG even more, so you have less material to read through to "get to the point."

More practice strips. More strips in each rhythms chapter and 250 in chapter 12 make learning rhythm interpretation easier.

Critical Thinking Exercises. Each chapter has exercises that might include case scenarios, diagrams to label, or other exercises that challenge you to put what you learned into practice. Additionally, the book's final chapter is an entire chapter of scenarios that requires you to analyze the situation and decide on the rhythm or EKG, the normal treatment, and the expected outcome of that treatment. These exercises put "the real world" into your learning experience. Let's face it, what's the point of studying EKG if you don't know how to apply it?

Accompanying Student CD-ROM. This is an exciting addition. The student CD-ROM includes videos, animations, diagrams, The Rhythm Randomizer, and practice tests–all certain to help you fine-tune your understanding of the book's material. The Rhythm Randomizer comes courtesy of Basic Arrhythmias, 6th edition by Gail Walraven.

Instructor Resource Manual. A separate Instructor's Resource Manual contains chapter synopses, outlines, objectives, frequently asked questions and suggested class activities.

Instructor's Resource CD-ROM. The Instructor's Resource CD-ROM packaged along with the Instructor's Resource Manual includes the complete test bank which allows instructors to generate customized exams and quizzes. It also includes a comprehensive, turn-key lecture package in PowerPoint format.

This is a more "user-friendly" guide to EKG, from the basics (you're pretty sure you have a heart, but other than that you know nothing about it) to the advanced (you know rhythms and now want to learn 12-lead interpretation). A lot of extraneous material has been excised and what's left is lean and informative.

The book starts, as before, with the basics in Part I. First is a little coronary anatomy and physiology, then EKG waves and complexes, lead morphology, and rhythms. You'll learn what the rhythm is, how to calculate the heart rate, and what the adverse effects and treatments are. There are critical thinking exercises and lots of practice strips to perfect your interpretation skills.

Part II covers 12-lead EKG interpretation. You'll learn what is normal on a 12-lead and what is pathological. Axis, hypertrophy, bundle branch blocks, myocardial infarction, and pacemakers are just a few topics covered in Part II. Again there are lots of critical thinking exercises and an entire chapter of 12-leads for practice.

This second edition of *EKG Plain and Simple* is written in the same conversational style as the first edition. And in places, there is even humor. Think of your favorite instructors from the past. Didn't they crack you up sometimes? And I'll bet you still remember what they taught you. Humor can be a great teaching aid.

So sit back and relax. This is going to be a piece of cake.

Happy learning!

Karen Ellis

Acknowledgments

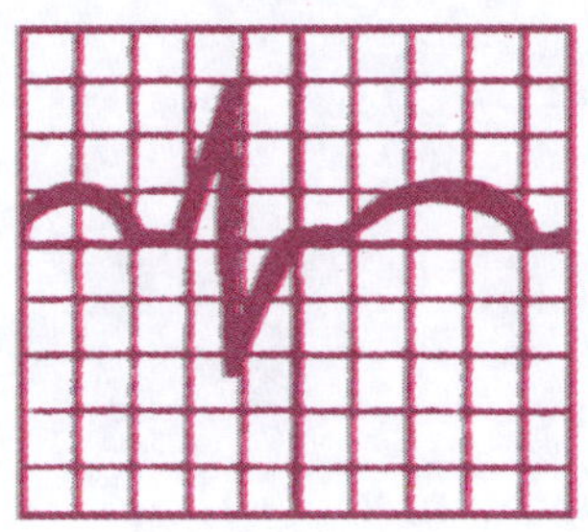

The following people have been instrumental in their contributions to this effort and I'd like to thank them all:

Lehman Ellis, my husband, who almost constantly has had to put up with my wheedling, "Can you help me on the computer?" as I worked on this edition. So far he's never said no to me, though he does give me that "so you can't figure this out, huh" look while he smirks at me with that darned twinkle in his eye. Lee is good at everything–a constant source of pride and just a little annoyance to me. Why I had to be so normal and him so perfect is something I'm determined to find out, even if it takes 28 **more** years of marriage.

My sons Jason, Mark, and Matthew, and my new daughter-in-law Lauren, for being my comic relief and for showing me, in my moments of stress, what's really important in life.

Theresa Hollins, telemetry tech at Touro Infirmary, who once again provided me with countless rhythm strips to peruse. And who still comes to me to ask my interpretation of a rhythm when she knows what it is all along. I personally think she does that just so I feel needed . . . .

The staff in ICU, ER, and telemetry for challenging me to prove **why** that rhythm is what I say it is. That's helped this book tremendously. The last thing that's needed is the philosophy that "this is what it is because I said so." The "why" question is what drove many changes in this edition.

My editor Melissa Kerian, whose suggestions were always intelligent and insightful. Melissa kept me to task on this edition–constantly pushing me to make improvements–and her influence is seen in every page.

My other editor Mark Cohen, who had great ideas for new additions to the book.

Thank you all.

Karen

Reviewers

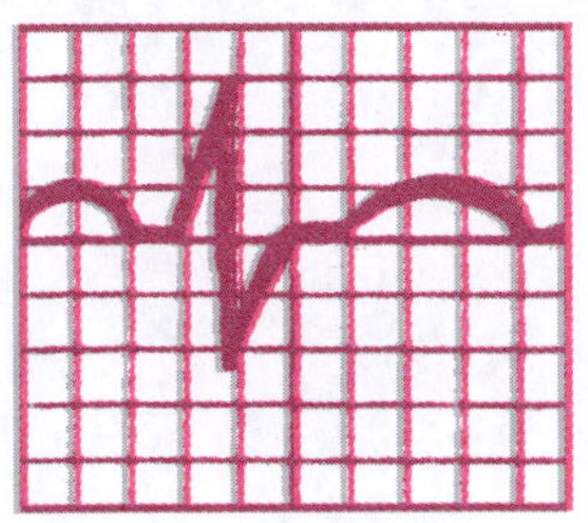

John Beckman, FF/PM
EMS Assistant Instructor
Addison Fire Protection District
Good Samaritan Hospital EMS
Addison, Illinois

Gloria Carr, RN, MSN
Instructor
Department of Nursing
University of Memphis
Memphis, Tennessee

David J. Derrico, MSN
Assistant Clinical Professor
College of Nursing
University of Florida
Gainesville, Florida

Diane A. Hawley, RN, PhD, CCNS
Lecturer
Harris School of Nursing
Texas Christian University
Fort Worth, Texas

Regina Kukulski, MSN, RN, APRN, BC
Course Coordinator
School of Nursing
Capital Health System
Trenton, New Jersey

Patty Leary, MSN
Instructor
School of Nursing
Ferris State University
Big Rapids, Michigan

Jeff Mitchell, NREMT-P, RN
Program Director
EMS
Calhoun Community College
Decatur, Alabama

Linda Nicholson, RN, MSN
Instructor
School of Nursing
Houston Community College
Houston, Texas

Sharon Rana, PhD
Assistant Professor
School of Recreation and Sport Sciences
Ohio University
Athens, Ohio

Gail Saxowsky, RNC, BSN, MPH
Clinical Coordinator
EMT Program
Chemeketa Community College
Salem, Oregon

Sheila M. Williams, AA, CMA, CET, CCT
MDCA Instructor
Coleman Health Science Center
Houston, Texas

PART **ONE**

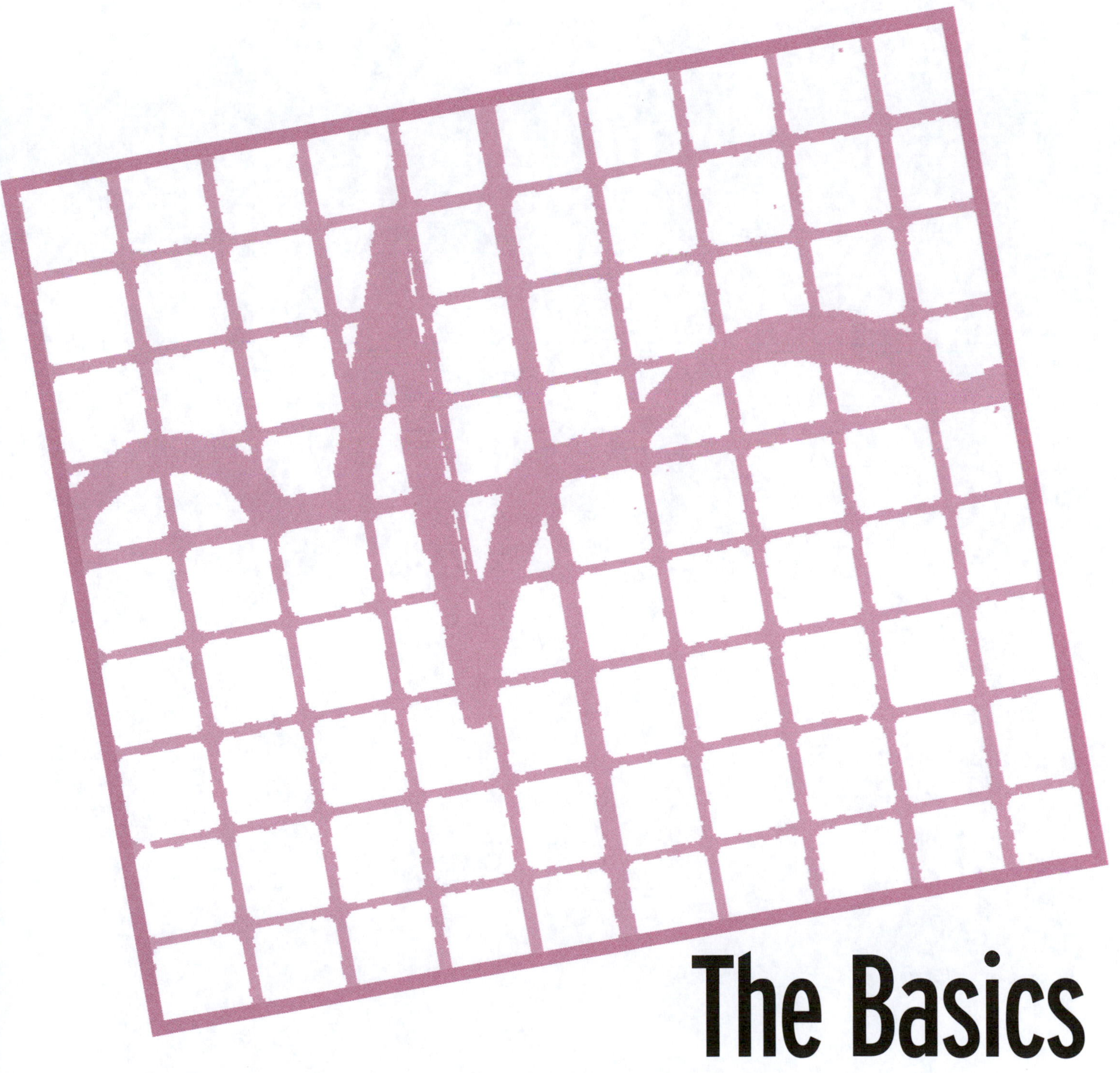

The Basics

CHAPTER **1**

Coronary Anatomy and Physiology

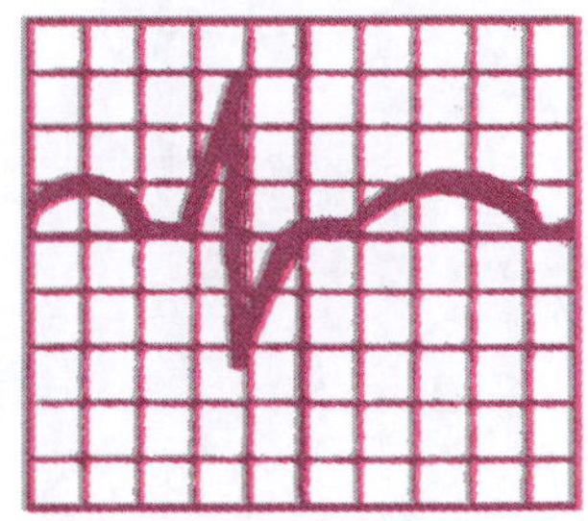

Chapter 1 Objectives

Upon completion of this chapter, the student will be able to:

- State the location of the heart and its normal size.
- Name the walls and layers of the heart.
- Name all the structures of the heart.
- Track the flow of blood through the heart.
- State the oxygen saturation of the heart's chambers.
- Describe the function and location of the heart valves.
- Describe the relationship of the valves to heart sounds.
- List the great vessels and the chamber into which they empty or from which they arise.
- State what occurs in each phase of the cardiac cycle.
- Relate the effects of diastole and systole to the EKG.
- Name and describe the function of the coronary arteries
- Differentiate between the two kinds of cardiac cells.
- Describe the sympathetic and parasympathetic nervous system.
- Describe the *fight-or-flight* and *rest-and-digest* responses.

Introduction

The function of the heart, a muscular organ about the size of a man's closed fist, is to pump enough blood to meet the body's metabolic needs. To accomplish this, the heart beats 60 to 100 times per minute and circulates 4 to 8 liters of blood per minute. Thus each day the average person's heart beats approximately 90,000 times and pumps out about 6,000 liters of blood. With stress, exertion, or certain pathological conditions, these numbers can quadruple.

The heart is located in the **thoracic (chest) cavity,** between the lungs in a cavity called the **mediastinum,** above the diaphragm, behind the **sternum** (breastbone), and in front of the spine. It is entirely surrounded by bony structures for protection. This bony cage also serves as a means to revive the stricken heart, as the external chest compressions of CPR compress the heart between the sternum and spine and squeeze blood out until the heart's function can be restored.

The top of the heart is the **base,** where the great vessels emerge. The bottom of the heart is the **apex,** the pointy part that rests on the diaphragm. The heart lies at an angle in the chest, with the bottom pointing to the left.

Layers of the Heart

The heart has three layers:

I. **Epicardium.** Outermost layer of the heart. The coronary arteries run along this layer.

II. **Myocardium.** The middle and thickest layer. The myocardium is made of pure muscle and does the work of contracting. It is the part that's damaged during a heart attack.

III. **Endocardium.** The thin innermost layer that lines the heart's chambers and folds back onto itself to form the heart valves. The endocardium is watertight to prevent leakage of blood out into the other layers. The cardiac conduction system is found in this layer.

Surrounding the heart is the **pericardium,** a double-walled sac that encloses the heart. Think of it as the film on a hard-boiled egg. The pericardium serves as support and protection and anchors the heart to the diaphragm and great vessels. A small amount of fluid is found between the layers of the pericardium. This **pericardial fluid** minimizes friction of these layers as they rub against each other with every heartbeat. See Figure 1-1.

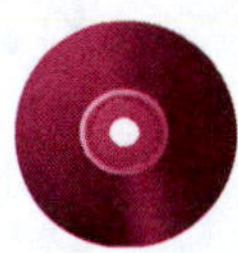

Heart Chambers

The heart has four chambers (see CD-ROM for animations showing the heart layers and heart chambers):

- **Right atrium.** A receiving chamber for deoxygenated blood (blood that's had some oxygen removed by the body's tissues) returning to the heart from the body, the right atrium has an oxygen (O_2) saturation of only 60% to 75%. The blood in this chamber has so little oxygen, its color is bluish black. Carbon dioxide (CO_2) concentration is high.
- **Right ventricle.** The right ventricle pumps the blood to the lungs for a fresh supply of oxygen. O_2 saturation is 60% to 75%. Again, the blood is bluish black in color. CO_2 concentration is high.
- **Left atrium.** This is a receiving chamber for the blood returning to the heart from the lungs. O_2 saturation is now about 100%. The blood is full of oxygen and is now bright red in color. CO_2 concentration is extremely low, as it was removed by the lungs.

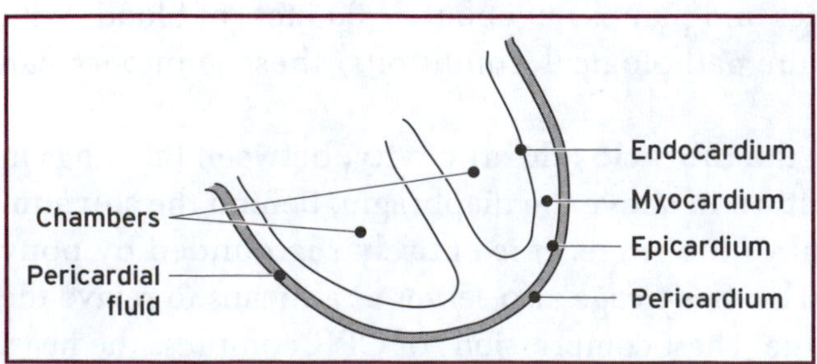

Figure 1-1 Layers of the heart.

- **Left ventricle.** The left ventricle's job is to pump blood out to the entire body. It is the major pumping chamber of the heart. O_2 saturation is about 100%. Again, the blood is bright red in color. CO_2 concentration is minimal.

The atria's job is to deliver blood to the ventricles that lie directly below them. Since this is a very short trip and minimal contraction is needed to transport this blood to the ventricles, the atria are thin-walled, low-pressure chambers.

The ventricles, on the other hand, are higher pressure chambers because they must contract more forcefully to deliver their blood into the pulmonary system and the systemic circulation. Since the trip from the right ventricle to the lungs is a short trip and pulmonary pressures are normally low, the right ventricle's pressure is relatively low (though higher than the atrial pressures), and its muscle bulk is relatively thin. The left ventricle generates the highest pressures, as it not only must pump the blood the farthest (throughout the entire body), it also must pump against great resistance–the blood pressure. For this reason, the left ventricle has three times the muscle bulk of the right ventricle and plays the prominent role in the heart's function.

The heart is divided into right and left sides by the **septum,** a muscular band of tissue. The septum separating the atria is called the **interatrial septum.** The septum separating the ventricles is called the **interventricular septum.** See Figure 1-2.

Heart Valves

The heart has four valves to prevent backflow of blood. Two are semilunar valves and two are AV valves:

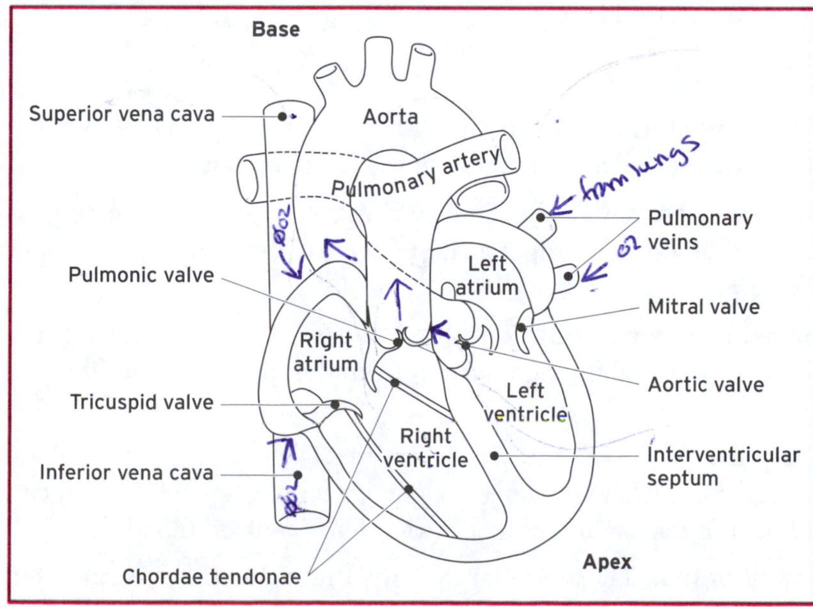

Figure 1-2 Anatomy of the heart.

Semilunar valves separate a ventricle from an artery and have three half-moon-shaped cusps. The term *semilunar* means half-moon. There are two *semilunar* valves:

- **Pulmonic.** This valve is located between the right ventricle and the pulmonary artery.
- **Aortic.** The aortic valve is located between the left ventricle and the aorta.

Atrioventricular (AV) valves are located between an atrium and a ventricle. They are supported by **chordae tendoneae** (tendonous cords), which are attached to **papillary muscles** (muscles that outpouch from the ventricular wall) and anchor the valve cusps to keep the closed AV valves from flopping backward and allowing backflow of blood. There are two AV valves:

- **Tricuspid.** This valve, located between the right atrium and ventricle, has three cusps.
- **Mitral.** The mitral valve, also called the *bicuspid valve,* is located between the left atrium and ventricle. It has two cusps.

Valves work based purely on changes in pressure. For example, the tricuspid and mitral valves open when the atrium's pressure is higher than the ventricle's. Blood then flows down from atrium to ventricle. The aortic and pulmonic valves open when the pressure in the ventricles exceeds that in the aorta and pulmonary artery. Blood then flows up into those arteries.

Valve closure is responsible for the sounds made by the beating heart. The normal lub-dub of the heart is made not by blood flowing through the heart, but by the closing of the heart's valves. S_1, the first heart sound, reflects closure of the mitral and tricuspid valves. S_2, the second heart sound, reflects closure of the aortic and pulmonic valves. Between S_1 and S_2, the heart beats and expels its blood (called **systole**). Between S_2 and the next S_1, the heart rests and fills with blood (called **diastole**). Each heartbeat has an S_1 and S_2. Note the valves on Figure 1-2.

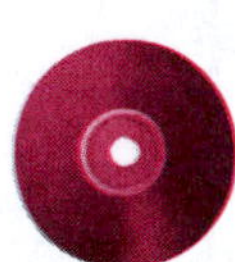

Great Vessels

Attached to the heart at its base are the five great vessels (see CD-ROM for a virtual tour of the heart and an animation of the heart vessels):

- **Superior vena cava (SVC).** The SVC is the large vein that returns deoxygenated blood to the right atrium from the head, neck, and upper chest and arms.
- **Inferior vena cava (IVC).** The IVC is the large vein that returns deoxygenated blood to the right atrium from the lower chest, abdomen, and legs.
- **Pulmonary artery.** This is the large artery that takes deoxygenated blood from the right ventricle to the lungs to load up on oxygen and unload carbon dioxide. It is the *only* artery that carries deoxygenated blood.
- **Pulmonary veins.** These are large veins that return the oxygenated blood from the lungs to the left atrium. They are the *only* veins that carry oxygenated blood.

- **Aorta.** The largest artery in the body, the aorta takes oxygenated blood from the left ventricle to the systemic circulation to feed all the organs of the body.

Note the great vessels on Figure 1-2.

Blood Flow through the Heart

Now let's track a single blood cell as it travels through the heart:

Superior or inferior vena cava →→ right atrium →→ tricuspid valve →→ right ventricle

↓↓

left atrium ←← pulmonary veins ←← lungs ←← pulmonary artery ←← pulmonic valve

↓↓

mitral valve →→ left ventricle →→ aortic valve →→ aorta →→ body (systemic circulation)

- The blood cell enters the heart via either the **superior** or **inferior vena cava.**
- It then enters the **right atrium.**
- Next it travels through the **tricuspid valve** into the **right ventricle.**
- Then it passes through the **pulmonic valve** into the **pulmonary artery,** then into the **lungs** for oxygen/carbon dioxide exchange.
- It is then sent through the **pulmonary veins** to the **left atrium.**
- Then it travels through the **mitral valve** into the **left ventricle.**
- It passes through the **aortic valve** into the **aorta** and out to the **body (systemic circulation).**

This blood flow is accomplished by way of the cardiac cycle. Let's look at that in depth.

The Cardiac Cycle

The **cardiac cycle** refers to the mechanical events that occur to pump blood. There are two phases to the cardiac cycle–**systole** and **diastole.** During systole the ventricles contract and expel their blood. During diastole the ventricles relax and fill. Each of these phases has several phases of its own. See Figures 1-3 and 1-4.

Diastole

- **Rapid-filling phase.** This is the first phase of diastole. The atria, having received blood from the superior and inferior venae cavae as well as the coronary sinus, are full of blood and therefore have high pressure. The ventricles, having just expelled their blood into the pulmonary artery and the aorta, are essentially empty and have lower pressure. This difference in pressure causes the AV valves to pop open and the atrial blood to flow down to the ventricles. (Fluid moves from high pressure to low pressure.) Imagine the atria as a sponge. When the sponge is saturated with water, the water pours out in a steady stream at first.

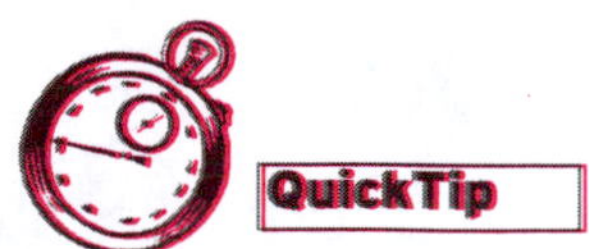

Rapid-filling phase = atria dumping blood into ventricles.
Diastasis = slowing blood flow.
Atrial kick = atria contracting to squeeze remainder of blood into ventricles.

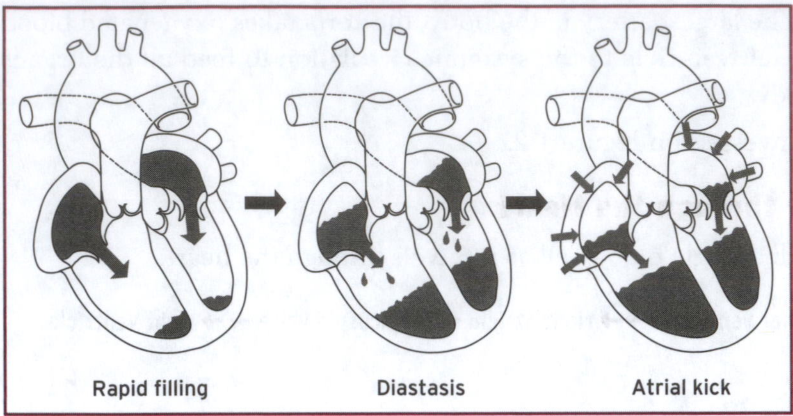

Figure 1-3 Phases of diastole.

- **Diastasis.** In the second phase of diastole, the pressure in the atria and ventricles starts to equalize as the ventricles fill and the atria empty, so blood flow slows. As the sponge becomes emptier, the flow slows to a trickle.

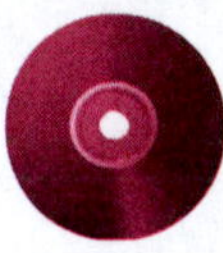

- **Atrial kick** (see CD-ROM for animations showing atrial contraction and the atrial cycle). This is the last phase of diastole. The atria are essentially empty, but there is still a little blood to deliver to the ventricle. Since the sponge is almost empty of water, what must be done to get the last little bit of water out of it? Right, the sponge must be squeezed. The atria therefore contract, squeezing in on themselves and

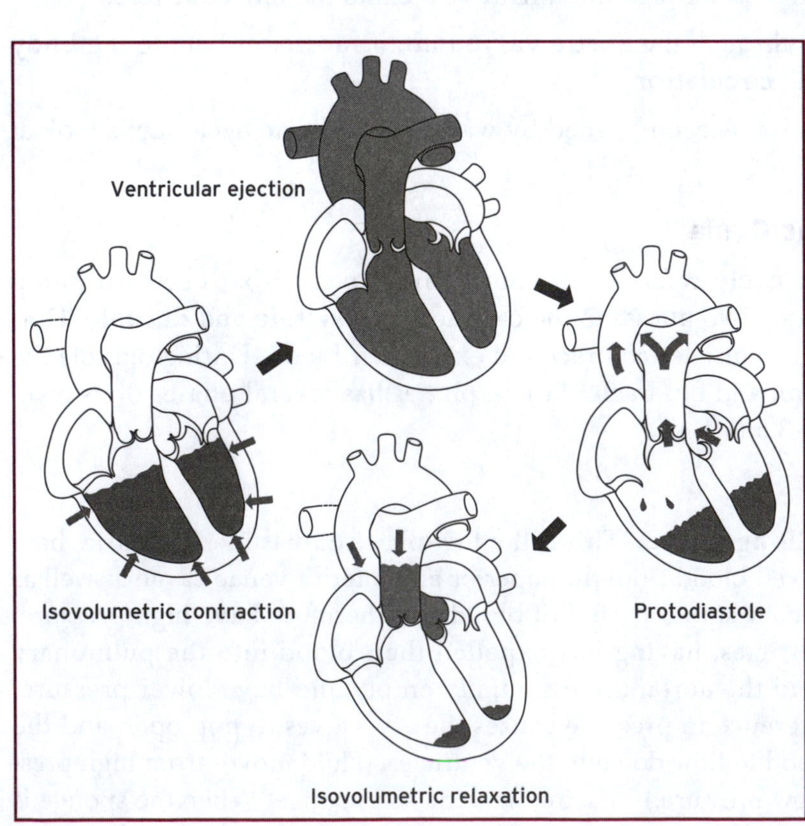

Figure 1-4 Phases of systole.

propelling the remainder of blood into the ventricles. The pressure in the ventricles at the end of this phase is high, as the ventricles are now full. Atrial pressure is low, as the atria are essentially empty. The AV valve leaflets, which have been hanging down in the ventricle in their open position, are pushed upward by the higher ventricular volume and its sharply rising pressure until they slam shut, ending diastole. S_1 is heard at this time. Atrial kick provides 15% to 30% of ventricular filling and is a very important phase.

Some heart rhythm abnormalities cause a loss of the atrial kick by causing the atria to fibrillate (wiggle) instead of contract. This causes an automatic decrease in cardiac output.

Effects of Diastole on the EKG

The first two phases of diastole are not manifested on the EKG. The final phase, atrial kick, is. Atrial contraction occurs as a result of **atrial depolarization** (the delivery of an electrical stimulus to the atria). In order for atrial kick to occur, the atria must first have been depolarized. No tissue in the heart will contract until it has been depolarized. On the EKG, this atrial depolarization is seen as a **P wave.** Chapter 2 covers this electrophysiology in depth. The EKG reflects only the heart's electrical activity, not its mechanical functioning.

Systole

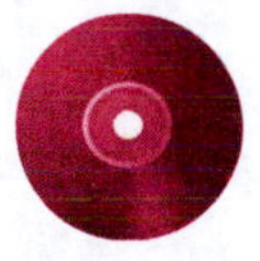

- **Isovolumetric contraction** (see CD-ROM for animations showing ventricular contractions and the cardiac cycle). This is the first phase of systole. The ventricles are full, but the pressure in them is not high enough to exceed the blood pressure and pop the semilunar valves open. Since the ventricles cannot increase their pressure by adding more volume (they're as full as they're going to get), they squeeze down on themselves, forcing their muscular walls inward, thereby putting pressure on the blood inside and causing the ventricular pressure to rise sharply. No blood flow occurs during this phase because all the valves are closed. This phase results in the greatest consumption of myocardial oxygen.
- **Ventricular ejection.** The second phase of systole. With the ventricular pressures now high enough, the semilunar valves pop open and blood pours out of the ventricles into the pulmonary artery and the aorta. Half the blood empties quickly and the rest a little slower.
- **Protodiastole.** The third phase of systole. Ventricular contraction continues, but blood flow slows as the ventricular pressure drops (since the ventricle is becoming empty) and the aortic and pulmonary arterial pressures rise (because they are filling with blood from the ventricles). Pressures are equalizing between the ventricles and the aorta and pulmonary artery.
- **Isovolumetric relaxation.** The final phase of systole. Ventricular pressure is low because the blood has essentially been pumped out. The ventricles relax, causing the pressure to drop further. The aorta and pulmonary artery have higher pressures now, as they are full of blood.

Isovolumetric contraction = ventricles squeezing but not pumping.
Ventricular ejection = pumping vigorously.
Protodiastole = pumping less.
Isovolumetric relaxation = relaxing, valves closing to end systole.

Since there is no longer any forward pressure from the ventricles to propel this blood further into the aorta and pulmonary artery, some of the blood in these arteries starts to flow back toward the aortic and pulmonic valves. This back pressure causes the valve leaflets, which had been pushed up into the aorta and pulmonary arteries in their open position, to slam shut, ending systole. S_2 is heard now.

When the ventricles are expelling their blood out, the atria are filling with blood. And when the *atria are expelling* their blood out, the ventricles are filling. The chambers are either filling or expelling continuously.

Effects of Systole on the EKG

Once the atria have delivered their blood to the ventricles, the ventricles are depolarized and a **QRS complex** is written on the EKG. Ventricular contraction then follows. Remember, depolarization is necessary before any heart tissue can contract.

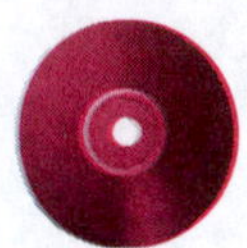

Blood Flow through the Systemic Circulation

Now let's track the blood's course throughout the systemic circulation (see CD-ROM for animation describing blood pressure):

Aorta → → arteries → → arterioles → → capillaries → → venules → → veins → → vena cava

- Oxygenated blood leaves the **aorta** and enters **arteries,** which narrow into **arterioles** and empty into each organ's **capillary bed,** where nutrient and oxygen extraction occurs.
- Then, on the other side of the capillary bed, this now-deoxygenated blood enters narrow **venules,** which widen into **veins,** and then return to the **vena cava** for transport back to the heart. Then the cycle repeats.

See Figure 1-5.

Coronary Arteries

The heart must not only meet the needs of the body, it has its own needs. Since the heart is primarily made of muscle, it requires considerable nourishment, and with the endocardium being watertight, none of the blood in the chambers can get to the myocardium to nourish it. So it has its own circulation–the **coronary arteries**–to do that. Coronary arteries arise from the base of

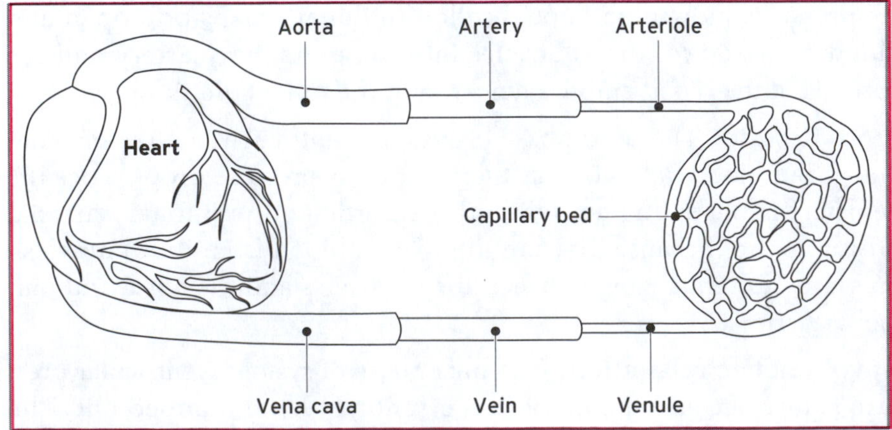

Figure 1-5 Systemic circulation.

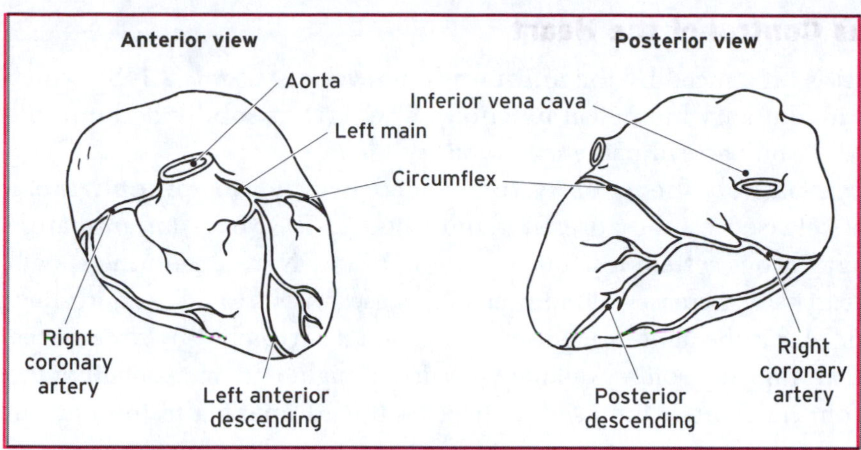

Figure 1-6 Coronary arteries.

the aorta and course along the epicardial surface of the heart, then dive into the myocardium to provide its blood supply. Unlike the rest of the body, however, the myocardium does not receive its blood supply during systole. Only in diastole is the heart able to feed itself. Why is that? Blood cannot enter the coronary arteries during systole because the heart muscle is contracting and essentially squeezing the coronary arteries shut. During diastole, the heart muscle stops contracting and the blood can then enter the coronary arteries and feed the myocardium. Let's look at the three main coronary arteries (see Figure 1-6):

- **Left anterior descending (LAD).** The LAD is a branch off the **left main coronary artery.** The LAD supplies blood to the anterior wall of the left ventricle.
- **Circumflex.** The circumflex, also a branch of the left main coronary artery, feeds the lateral wall of the left ventricle. Since the LAD and the circumflex coronary arteries are branches off the left main coronary artery, blockage of the left main itself would knock out flow to both these branches. That produces a huge heart attack sometimes referred to as the *widow-maker.*
- **Right coronary artery (RCA).** The RCA feeds the right ventricle and the inferior wall of the left ventricle.

Once the myocardium has been fed by the coronary arteries, the deoxygenated blood is returned to the right atrium by **coronary veins.**

Heart Cells

The heart has two kinds of cells:

- **Contractile cells** cause the heart muscle to contract, resulting in a heartbeat.
- **Conduction system cells** create and conduct electrical signals to tell the heart when to beat. Without these electrical signals, the contractile cells would *never* contract.

Nervous Control of the Heart

The heart is influenced by the **autonomic nervous system (ANS),** which controls involuntary biological functions. The ANS is subdivided into the sympathetic and parasympathetic nervous systems.

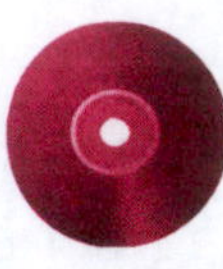

The **sympathetic nervous system** is mediated by **norepinephrine,** a chemical released by the adrenal gland (see CD-ROM for an animation regarding nervous system influence with the heart). Norepinephrine speeds up the heart rate, increases blood pressure, causes pupils to dilate, and slows digestion. This is the fight-or-flight response, and it's triggered by stress, exertion, or fear. Imagine you're walking your dog at night and an assailant puts a gun to your head. Your intense fear triggers the adrenal gland to pour out norepinephrine. Your heart rate and blood pressure shoot up. Your pupils dilate to let in more light so you can see the danger and the escape path better. Digestion slows down as the body shunts blood away from nonvital areas. (Is it essential to be digesting your pizza when your life is at stake? The pizza can wait.) So the body puts digestion on hold and shunts blood to vital organs, such as the brain, to help you think more clearly and to the muscles to help you fight or flee.

The **parasympathetic nervous system** is mediated by **acetylcholine,** a chemical secreted as a result of stimulation of the **vagus nerve,** a nerve that travels from the brain to the heart, stomach, and other areas. It slows the heart rate, decreases blood pressure, and enhances digestion. This is the rest-and-digest response. Parasympathetic stimulation can be caused by any action that closes the **glottis,** the flap over the top of the **trachea** (the windpipe). Breath-holding and straining to have a bowel movement are two actions that can cause the heart rate to slow down. It is not uncommon for paramedics to be summoned to the scene of a person found unconscious in the bathroom. Straining at stool causes vagal stimulation, which causes the heart rate to slow down. If the heart rate slows enough, **syncope** (fainting) can result. In extreme cases, the heart can stop, requiring resuscitation. Though the heart is influenced by the autonomic nervous system, it can also, in certain extreme circumstances, function for a time without any input from this system. For example, a heart that is removed from a donor in preparation for transplant is no longer in communication with the body, yet it continues to beat on its own for a while. This is possible because of the heart's conduction system cells, which create and conduct electrical impulses to tell the heart to beat.

In a nutshell, the sympathetic nervous system is the accelerator and the parasympathetic nervous system is the brakes.

Practice Quiz

1. The function of the heart is to ______________________________

____

2. Name the four layers of the heart. ______________________________

____

____

____

3. Name the four chambers of the heart. ____

____

____

4. Name the four heart valves. ____

____

5. The purpose of the heart valves is to ______________________.
6. Name the five great vessels of the heart. ______________________

____

7. List the phases of diastole. ______________________________

____

____

8. List the phases of systole. ______________________________

____

____

9. Once the atria have delivered blood to the ventricles, the ventricles depolarize and a ______________ is written on the EKG.
10. The atrial kick is represented on the EKG as a ______________.

Putting It All Together—Critical Thinking Exercises

These exercises may consist of diagrams to label, scenarios to analyze, brain-stumping questions to ponder, or other challenging exercises to boost your understanding of the chapter material.

1. Label the heart diagram.

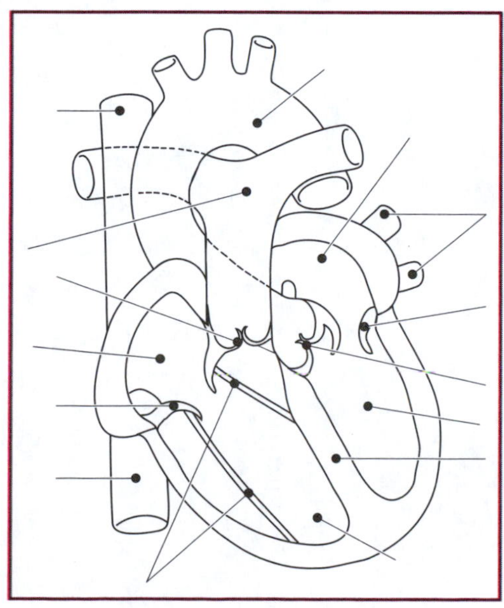

2. Number the following structures 1–14 in order of blood flow through the heart:

_____ superior and inferior vena cava

_____ tricuspid valve

_____ mitral valve

_____ aortic valve

_____ pulmonic valve

_____ body

_____ aorta

_____ pulmonary artery

_____ lungs

_____ pulmonary veins

_____ right atrium

_____ left atrium

_____ right ventricle

_____ left ventricle

3. What would happen to the tricuspid and mitral valves if their chordae tendonae "snapped" loose?

CHAPTER **2**

Electrophysiology

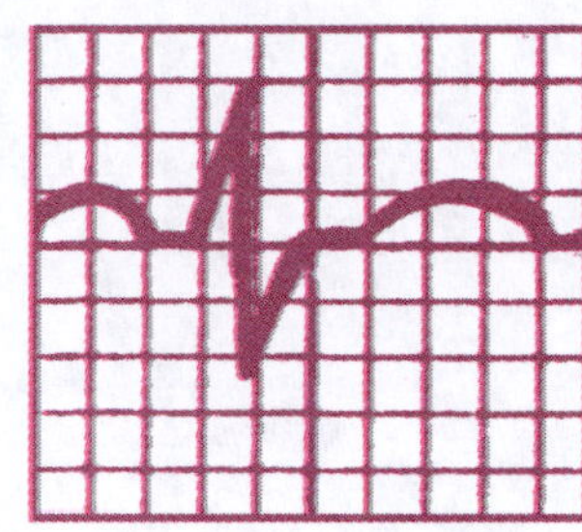

Chapter 2 Objectives

Upon completion of this chapter, the student will be able to:

- Define the terms *polarized*, *depolarization*, and *repolarization* and relate them to contraction and relaxation.
- Describe and label the phases of the action potential.
- Define *transmembrane potential.*
- Draw and explain the P wave, QRS complex, T wave, and U wave.
- Explain where the PR and ST segments are.
- Define the *absolute* and *relative refractory periods* and the implications of each.
- Be able to label, on a rhythm strip, all the waves and complexes.
- Explain the delineations of EKG paper. How many seconds in a small block and big block? How many small blocks in one minute? How many big blocks in a minute?
- On a rhythm strip, determine if the PR, QRS, and QT intervals are normal or abnormal.
- Name the waves in a variety of QRS complexes.
- Define *pacemaker.*
- List the different pacemakers of the heart and their inherent rates.
- Track the cardiac impulse from the sinus node through the conduction system.
- Define the four characteristics of cardiac cells.
- Describe the difference between *escape* and *usurpation.*
- Label a rhythm strip as being representative of either escape or usurpation.
- Define *arrhythmia.*
- Tell what happens in each of the following scenarios:

  When the sinus node fails
  When the sinus node and atria both fail
  When the sinus node, atria, and AV node all fail

Introduction

Cardiac cells at rest are electrically negative on the inside as compared with the outside. Movement of charged particles (**ions**) of sodium and potassium into and out of the cell cause changes that can be picked up by sensors on the skin and printed out as an EKG.

Depolarization and Repolarization

The negatively charged resting cardiac cell is called **polarized.** There are sodium ions primarily outside the cell and potassium ions primarily inside the cell. Though both these ions carry a positive electrical charge, the sodium has a stronger positive charge than the potassium. Thus the inside of the cell is electrically negative compared with the outside. The polarized state is a state of readiness–the cardiac cell is ready for electrical action. When the cardiac cell is stimulated by an electrical impulse, a large amount of sodium rushes into the cell and a small amount of potassium leaks out, causing a discharge of electricity. The cell becomes positively charged. This is called **depolarization.** An electrical wave then courses from cell to cell, spreading this electrical charge throughout the heart. During cell recovery, sodium and potassium ions are shifted back to their original places by way of the **sodium-potassium pump,** an active transport system that returns the cell to its negative charge. This is called **repolarization.** See Figure 2-1.

Depolarization and repolarization are electrical events. Contraction and relaxation are mechanical events. Depolarization should result in muscle contraction. Repolarization should result in muscle relaxation. *Electrical precedes mechanical.* There can be no heartbeat (a mechanical event) without first having had depolarization (the electrical stimulus). This is like a vacuum cleaner. Its job is to suck up dirt, but it cannot do its job without being plugged into an electrical source first.

Does plugging in that vacuum cleaner guarantee it will work? No. It could have a mechanical malfunction that prevents it from working. So can the heart. The electrical and mechanical systems are two separate systems. Either one (or both) can malfunction. Electrical malfunctions show up on the EKG. Mechanical malfunctions show up clinically.

Are you lost? Imagine this scenario: A man has a heart attack that damages a large portion of his myocardium. If his heart's electrical system has not been damaged, it sends out its impulses as usual. The muscle cells, however,

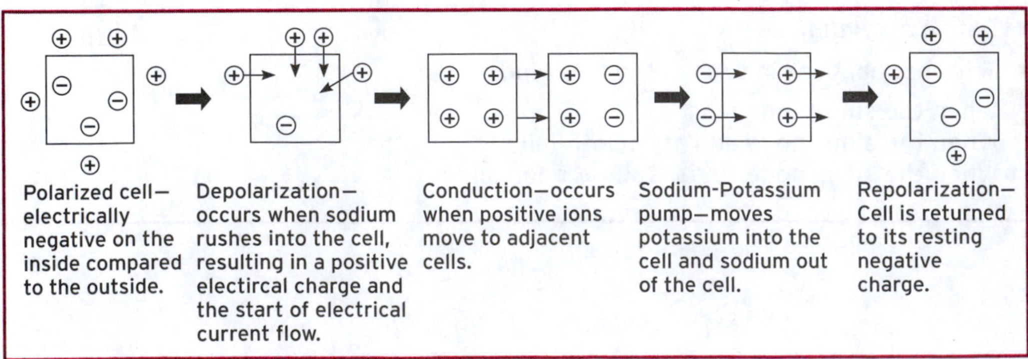

Polarized cell—electrically negative on the inside compared to the outside.
Depolarization—occurs when sodium rushes into the cell, resulting in a positive electircal charge and the start of electrical current flow.
Conduction—occurs when positive ions move to adjacent cells.
Sodium-Potassium pump—moves potassium into the cell and sodium out of the cell.
Repolarization—Cell is returned to its resting negative charge.

Figure 2-1 Depolarization and repolarization.

have been so damaged that they are unable to respond to those impulses by contracting. Consequently, the EKG shows the electrical system is still working, but the patient is clinically dead–no pulse, no breathing, nothing. The vacuum cleaner was plugged in, but it was broken and couldn't do its job.

Depolarization **should** result in muscle contraction. Repolarization **should** result in muscle relaxation.

The Action Potential

Let's look at what happens to a ventricular muscle cell when it's stimulated. See Figure 2-2. There are four phases to the action potential:

- In **phase 4,** the cardiac cell is at rest. It is negatively charged with a resting **transmembrane potential** (the electrical charge at the cell membrane) of −90 millivolts. Electrically, nothing is happening. (Note phase 4 is a flat line. *Flat lines indicate electrical silence*).
- In **Phase 0,** the cardiac cell is stimulated. Sodium rushes into the cell, potassium leaks out, and this results in a positive charge within the cell. This is called **depolarization.** You can see that at the top of phase 0, the cell's charge is above the zero mark and is thus positively charged. Phase 0 corresponds with the **QRS complex** on the EKG. The QRS complex is a spiked waveform on the EKG that represents depolarization of the ventricular myocardium.
- **Phases** 1 and 2 are **early repolarization.** Calcium is released in these two phases, resulting in ventricular contraction. Phases 1 and 2 correspond with the **ST segment** of the EKG. The ST segment is a flat line on the EKG that follows the QRS complex and represents a period of electrical silence. But the heart is not physically at rest–it is contracting. Phase 2 is called the **plateau phase,** because the waveform levels off here.
- **Phase** 3 is **rapid repolarization.** Sodium and potassium return to their normal places via the sodium-potassium pump, thus returning the cell to its resting negative charge. Phase 3 corresponds with the **T wave** of the EKG. The T wave is a broad rounded wave that follows the ST segment and represents ventricular repolarization. The cardiac cell then relaxes.

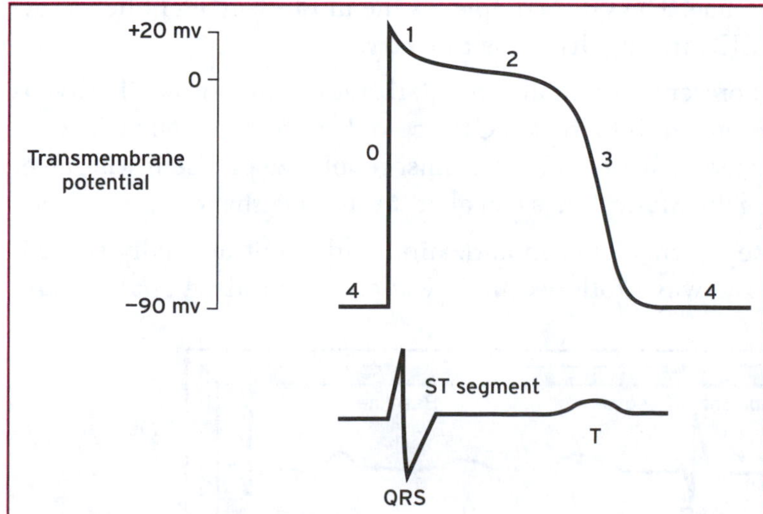

Figure 2-2 Action potential.

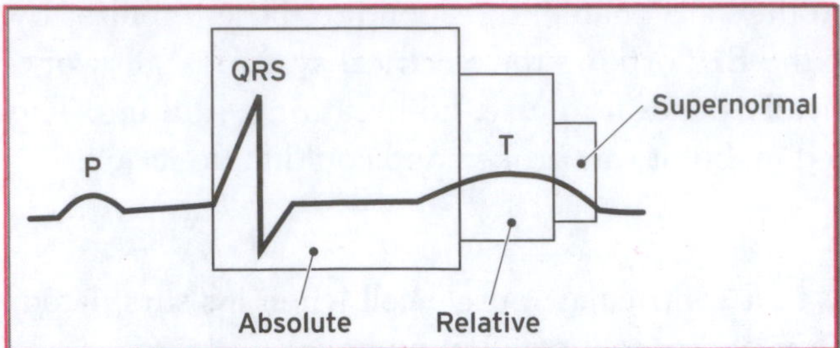

Figure 2-3 Refractory periods.

Refractory Periods

The word **refractory** means "resistant to." Let's look at the periods when the cardiac cell resists responding to an impulse. See Figure 2-3.

- **Absolute.** The cell cannot accept another impulse because it's still dealing with the last one. Absolutely no stimulus, no matter how strong, will result in another depolarization during this time.
- **Relative.** A strong stimulus will result in depolarization.
- **Supernormal period.** Even a weak stimulus will cause depolarization. The cardiac cell during this period is "hyper," and it doesn't take much to set it off and running. In fact, stimulation at this time often results in very fast, dangerous rhythms.

EKG Waves and Complexes

Depolarization and repolarization of the atria and ventricles result in waves and complexes on the EKG paper. Let's examine these waveforms. See Figure 2-4.

- **P wave.** Represents atrial depolarization. The normal P is small, rounded, and upright, but many things can alter the P wave shape.
- **T_a wave.** Represents atrial repolarization–usually not seen, as it occurs at the same time as the QRS complex.
- **QRS complex.** Represents ventricular depolarization. The normal QRS is spiked in appearance, consisting of one or more deflections from the baseline. The QRS complex is the most easily identified structure on the EKG tracing. Its shape can vary.
- **T wave.** Represents ventricular repolarization. The normal T wave is broad and rounded. If there is a QRS complex, there *must* be a T wave after it. Any tissue that depolarizes must repolarize or else it will never depolarize again. Many things can alter the T wave shape.
- **U wave.** Represents late repolarization and is not normally seen. If present, the U wave follows the T wave. It should be shallow and

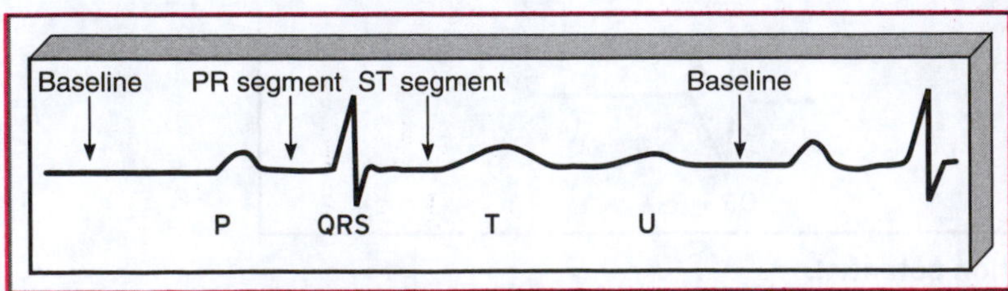

Figure 2-4 EKG waves and complexes.

rounded, the same deflection as the T wave (i.e., if the T wave is upright, the U wave should be also).

Each P-QRS-T sequence is one heartbeat. The flat lines between the P wave and the QRS and between the QRS and T wave are called the **PR segment** and the **ST segment,** respectively. During these segments, no electrical activity is occurring. Remember, flat lines indicate electrical silence. The flat line between the T wave of one beat and the P wave of the next beat is called the **baseline** or **isoelectric line.** The baseline is the line from which the waves and complexes take off.

Atrial contraction occurs during the P wave and the PR segment. Ventricular contraction occurs during the QRS and the ST segment. It's like this: The atria depolarize and a P wave is written on the EKG paper. Following this, the atria contract, filling the ventricles with blood. Then the ventricles depolarize, causing a QRS complex on the EKG paper. The ventricles then contract. The EKG waves and complexes tell us something electrical is happening. Flat lines indicate that no electrical activity is occurring.

Waves and Complexes Identification Practice

Following are strips on which to practice identifying P waves, QRS complexes, and T waves. You'll recall that P waves are normally upright, but they can also be inverted (upside down) or biphasic (up *and* down). P waves usually precede the QRS complex, so find the QRS and then look for the P wave. Some rhythms have more than one P wave and others have no P at all. Write the letter *P* over each P wave you see.

The QRS complex is the most easily identified structure on the strip because of its spiked appearance. Write *QRS* over each QRS complex.

T waves are normally upright, but can also be inverted or biphasic. Wherever there is a QRS complex, there must be a T wave. Write a *T* over each T wave.

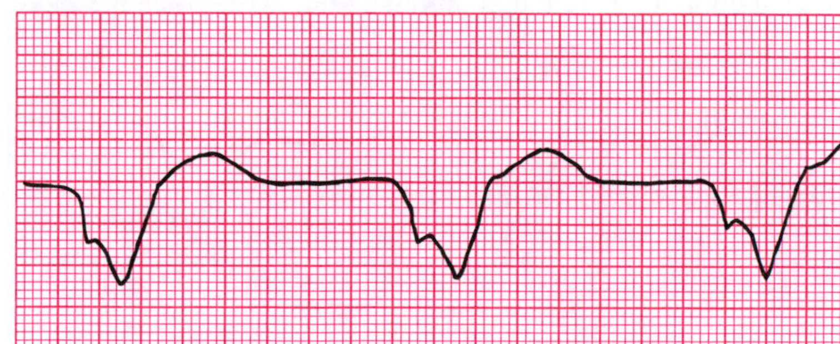

1.

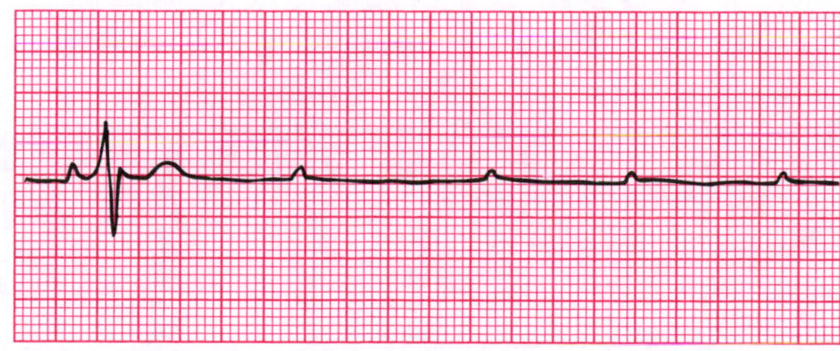

2.

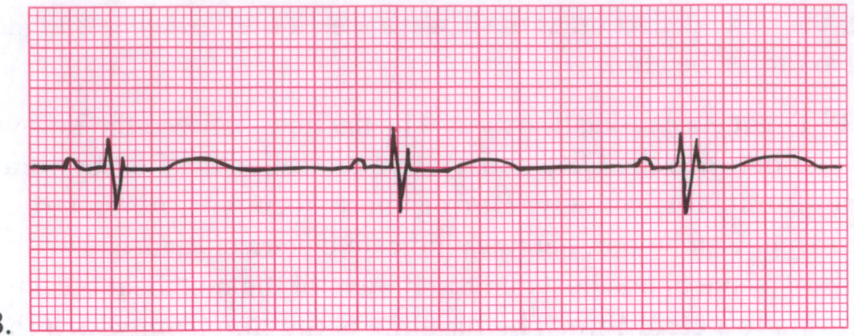
3.

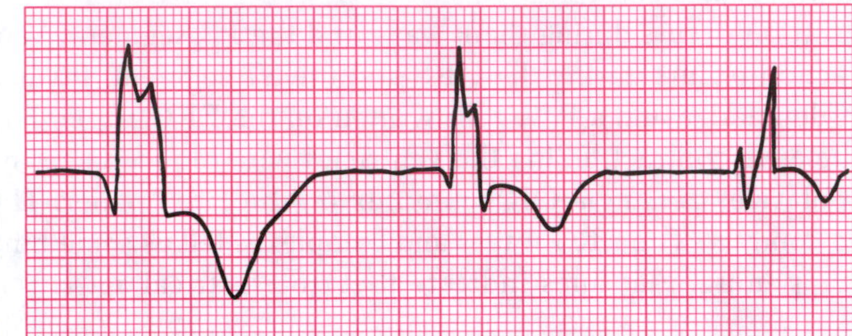
4.

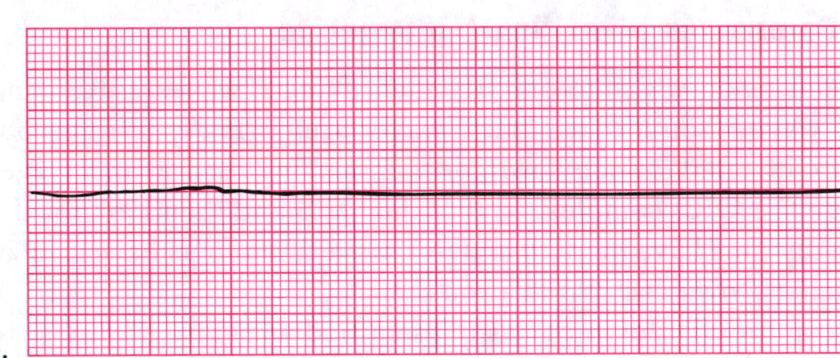
5.

Answers to Waves and Complexes Practice

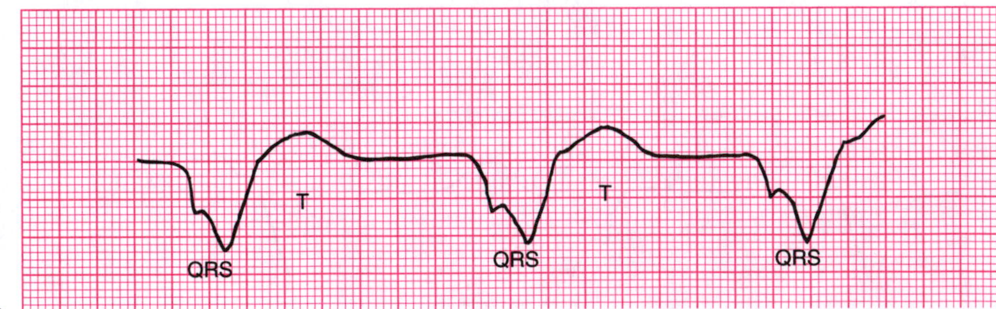

1.

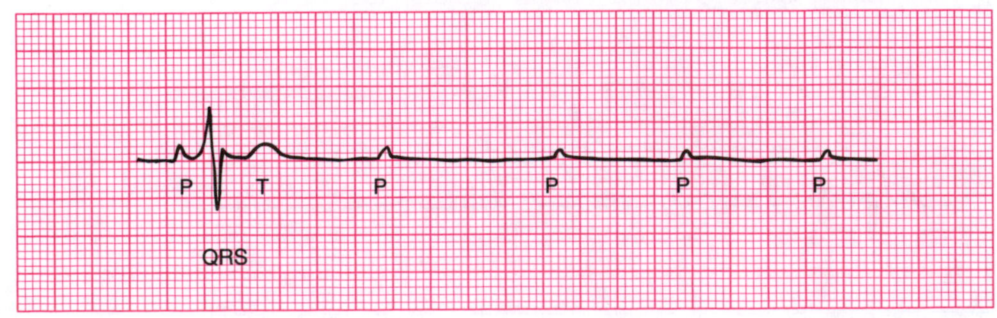

2.

3. 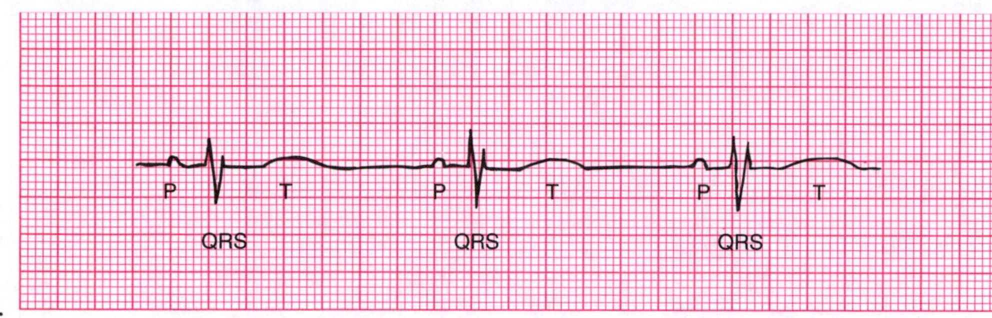

4. 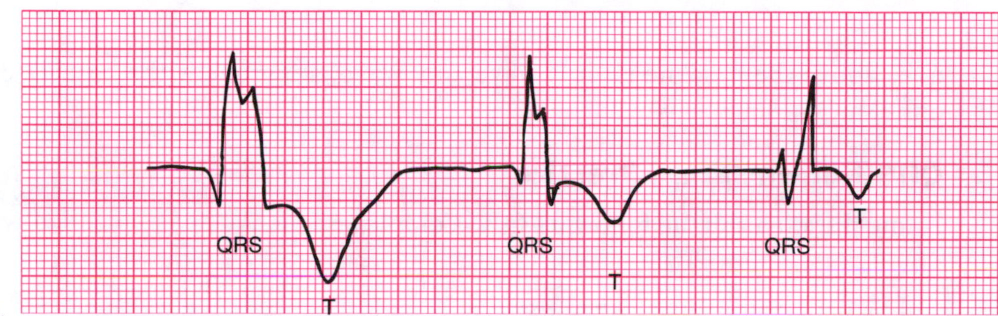

5. 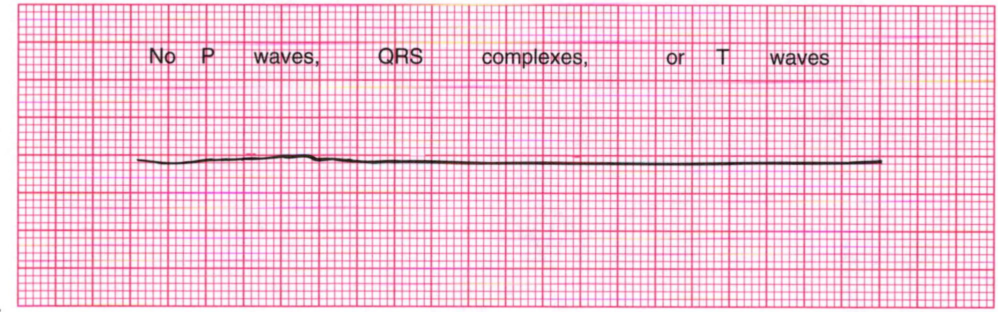

QRS Nomenclature

Now that we know basically what a QRS complex looks like, let's fine-tune that a bit. The QRS complex is composed of waves that have different names–Q, R, and S–but no matter what waves it's composed of, it's still referred to as the **QRS complex.** Think of it like this: There are many kinds of dogs–collies, boxers, terriers, and so forth–but they're still dogs. Likewise, the QRS complex can have different names, but it's still a QRS complex. Let's look at the waves that can make up the QRS complex.

- A **Q wave** is a negative deflection that occurs before a positive deflection. There can be only one Q wave, and it must be the first wave of the QRS complex.
- An **R wave** is any positive deflection. There can be more than one R wave. A second R wave is called **R prime,** written R′.
- An **S wave** is a negative deflection that follows an R wave.
- A **QS wave** is a negative deflection with no positive deflection at all.

As in the alphabet, Q comes before R and S comes after R. See Figure 2-5. The dotted line indicates the baseline. Any wave in the QRS complex that

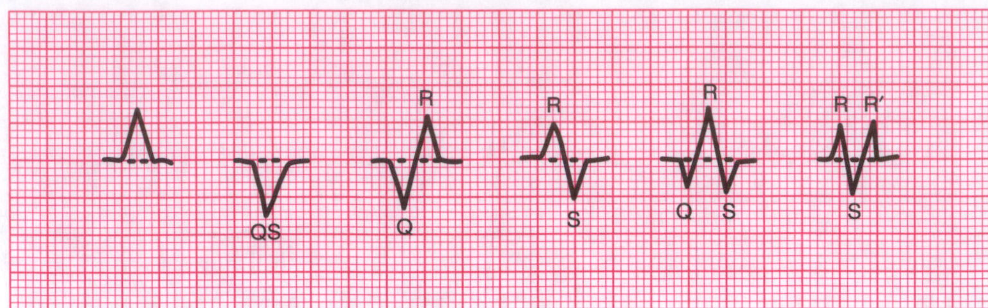

Figure 2-5 Examples of QRS complexes.

goes above the baseline is an R wave; any wave going below the baseline is either a Q or an S wave.

QRS Nomenclature Practice

Name the waves in the following QRS complexes:

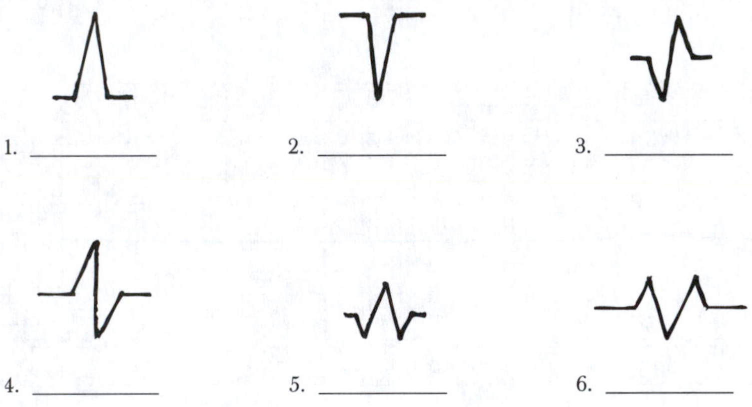

Now draw the following:

1. RSR′
2. QRS
3. QS
4. QR
5. RS
6. R

Answers to QRS Nomenclature Practice

Answers to "Name the waves"

1. R.
2. QS. This cannot be called a Q or an S because there is no R wave to precede or follow, so the QRS complex that is completely negative is called QS.
3. QR.

4. RS.
5. QRS.
6. RSR′.

Answers to "Draw the QRS complexes"

1. 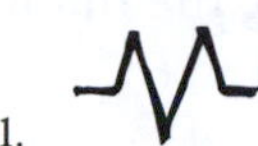

2. 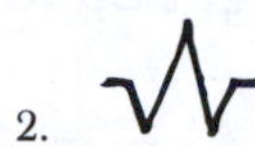

3. 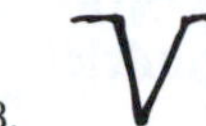

4. 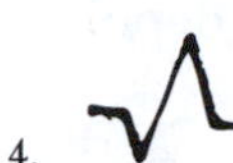

5. 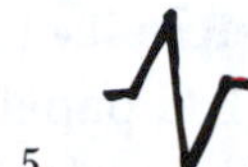

6.

Cardiac Conduction System

The conduction system is a pathway of specialized cells whose job is to create and conduct the electrical impulses that tell the heart when to pump. The area of the conduction system that initiates the impulses is called the **pacemaker.** See Figure 2-6.

Conduction Pathway

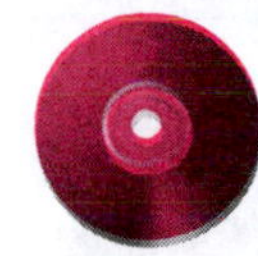

Let's look at the conduction pathway through the heart (see CD-ROM for an animation of the conduction system):

Sinus node ➔➔ interatrial tracts ➔➔ atrium ➔➔ internodal tracts ➔➔ AV node

ventricle ⬅⬅ Purkinje fibers ⬅⬅ bundle branches ⬅⬅ bundle of His

- The impulse originates in the **sinus node,** located in the upper right atrium just beneath the opening of the superior vena cava. The sinus node is the heart's normal pacemaker.
- From here it travels through the **interatrial tracts.** These special conductive highways carry the impulses through the atria to the **atrial tissue.** The atria then depolarize, and a P wave is written on the EKG.

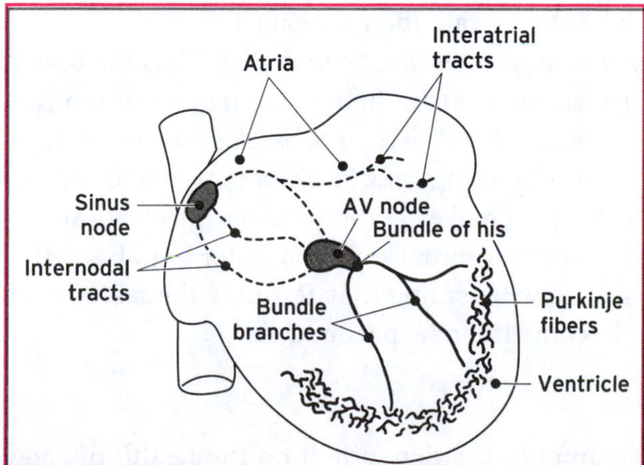

Figure 2-6 Cardiac conduction system.

- The impulse travels through the **internodal tracts** to the **AV node,** a specialized group of cells located just to the right of the septum in the lower right atrium. The AV node slows impulse transmission a little, allowing the newly depolarized atria to propel their blood into the ventricles.
- Then the impulse travels through the **bundle of His,** located just beneath the AV node, to the **left** and **right bundle branches,** the main highways to the ventricles.
- Then the impulse is propelled through the **Purkinje fibers.**
- Finally, the impulse arrives at the **ventricle** itself, causing it to depolarize. A QRS complex is written on the EKG paper.

Cardiac Cells

Cardiac cells have several characteristics:

- **Automaticity.** The ability to create an impulse without outside stimulation.
- **Conductivity.** The ability to pass this impulse along to neighboring cells.
- **Excitability.** The ability to respond to this stimulus by depolarizing.
- **Contractility.** The ability to contract and do work.

The first three characteristics are electrical. The last is mechanical.

Though the sinus node is the normal pacemaker of the heart, other cardiac cells can become the pacemaker if the sinus node fails. Let's look at that a little closer. (See CD-ROM for an animation showing the heart inherent rates.)

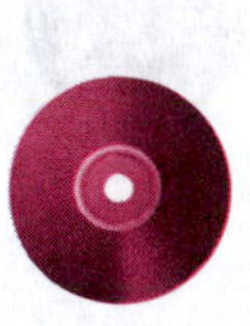

Inherent (Escape) Rates of the Pacemaker Cells

Unlike the sinus node and the ventricle, the AV node itself has no pacemaker cells. The tissue between the atria and the AV node, however–an area called the **AV junction**–does have pacemaking capabilities. Thus the term AV node is an anatomical term and AV junction refers to a pacemaking area.

- Sinus node: 60 to 100 beats per minute
- AV junction: 40 to 60 beats per minute
- Ventricle: 20 to 40 beats per minute

The sinus node, you'll note, has the fastest inherent rate of all the potential pacemaker cells. This means that, barring any outside stimuli that speed it up or slow it down, the sinus node will fire at its rate of 60 to 100 beats per minute. The lower pacemakers (AV junction and ventricle) have slower inherent rates, each one having a slower rate than the one above it.

The fastest pacemaker at any given moment is the one in control. Thus the lower pacemakers are inhibited, or restrained, from firing as long as some other pacemaker is faster. The lower pacemakers serve as a backup in case of conduction failure from above. The only thing that inhibits those pacemakers from **escaping** (taking over as the pacemaker at their slower inherent rate) is if they have been depolarized by a faster impulse. If that faster impulse never arrives, the next pacemaker in line will assume that *it* is now the fastest and should escape its restraints to become the new pacemaker.

Conduction Variations

Normal conduction of cardiac impulses is dependent on the health of each part of the conduction system. Failure of any part of the system necessitates a

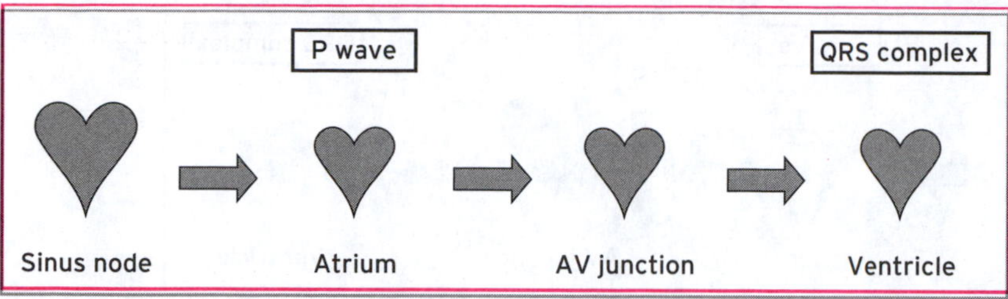

Figure 2-7 Normal conduction.

variation in conduction. Let's look at several conductive possibilities. In the following figures, the large heart represents the pacemaker in control. See Figure 2-7.

In Figure 2-7, the sinus node fires out its impulse. When the impulse depolarizes the atrium, a P wave is written. The impulse then travels to the AV node, and on to the ventricle. A QRS is written when the ventricle is depolarized.

If the sinus node fails, however, one of the lower pacemakers will escape its restraints and take over at its slower inherent rate, thus becoming the heart's new pacemaker. If the AV junction escapes, it will fire at a rate of 40 to 60. If the ventricle takes over, the rate will be 20 to 40. Needless to say, if the ventricle has to kick in as the pacemaker, it is a grave situation, since it means that all the pacemakers above it have failed. Remember–no pacemaker can escape unless it's the fastest at that particular time.

In Figure 2-8, the sinus node has failed. The AV junction is now the fastest escape pacemaker. It creates an impulse and sends it forward toward the ventricle and backward toward the atria, providing the P and the QRS.

In Figure 2-9, the sinus node and AV junction have both failed. The only remaining pacemaker is the ventricle, so it takes over as the pacemaker, providing the QRS. There is no P wave when the ventricle escapes.

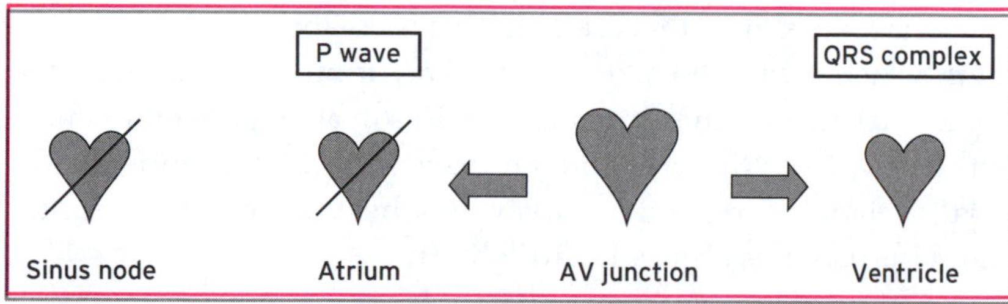

Figure 2-8 Sinus fails. AV junction escapes.

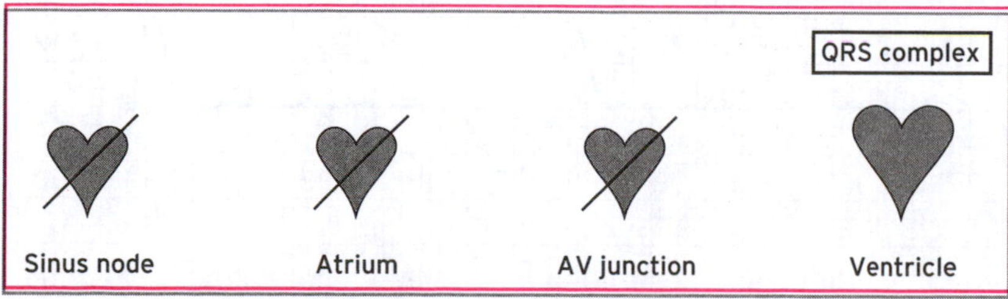

Figure 2-9 All higher pacemakers fail. Ventricle escapes.

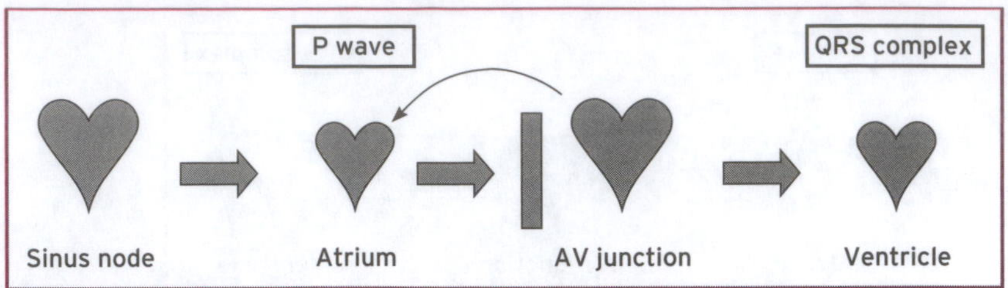

Figure 2-10 Block in conduction. AV junction escapes.

What if the sinus node fires its impulse out but the impulse is blocked at some point along the conduction pathway? The first pacemaker below the block should escape and become the new pacemaker.

In Figure 2-10, the sinus node fires out its impulse, which depolarizes the atrium and writes a P wave. The impulse is then blocked between the atrium and the AV node. Since the faster sinus impulse never reaches the AV node, the AV junction assumes the sinus node has failed. So it escapes, creates its own new impulse, and becomes the new pacemaker, sending the impulse down to the ventricle and backward to the atria. (Backward conduction can work even when forward conduction is blocked.) If the impulse were blocked between the AV node and the ventricle, the ventricle would become the new pacemaker.

Each of the pacemakers can fire at rates faster or slower than their inherent rates if there are outside stimuli. We've talked briefly about escape. Let's look at an example of escape compared with usurpation.

Escape occurs when the predominant pacemaker slows dramatically (or fails completely) and a lower pacemaker takes over at its inherent rate, providing a new rhythm that is slower than the previous rhythm. *An escape beat is any beat that comes in after a pause that's longer than the normal heartbeat-to-heartbeat cycle **(R-R interval)**.* Escape beats are lifesavers.

In Figure 2-11, the normal pacemaker stops suddenly and there is a long pause, at the end of which is a beat from a lower pacemaker and then a new rhythm with a heart rate slower than before. This is escape.

Usurpation, which means "to take control away from," occurs when one of the lower pacemakers becomes irritable and fires in at an accelerated rate, stealing control away from the predominant pacemaker. Usurpation results in a faster rhythm than before, and it starts with a beat that comes in earlier than expected. Usurpation is also called irritability.

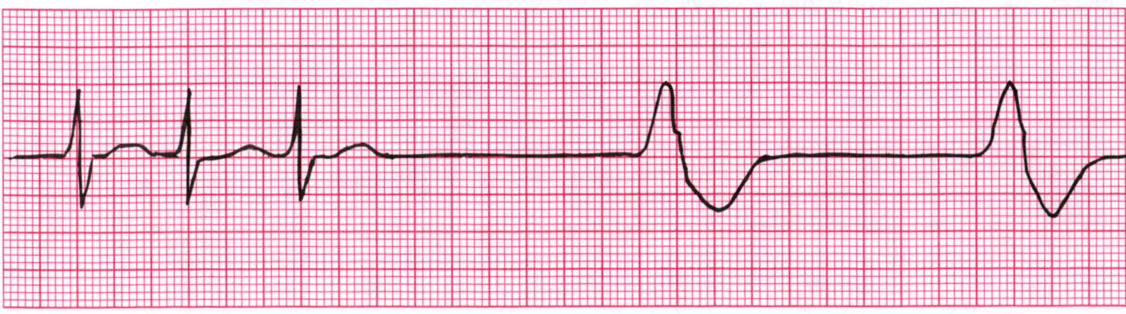

Figure 2-11 Escape.

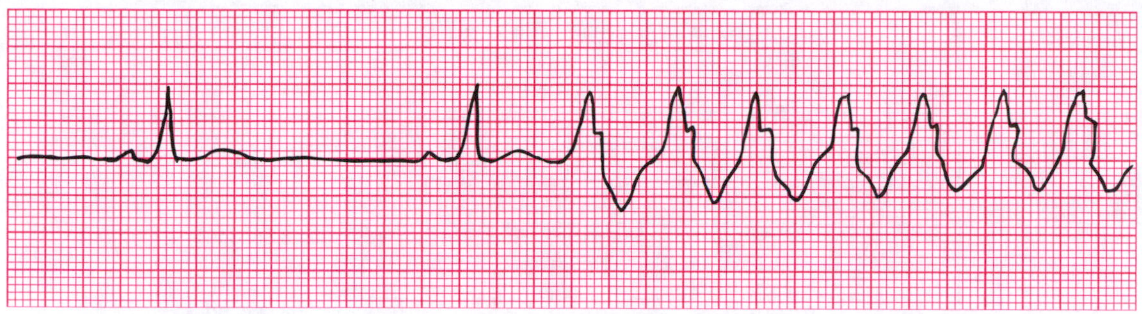

Figure 2-12 Usurpation.

In Figure 2-12, the controlling pacemaker is cruising along and suddenly an impulse from a lower pacemaker fires in early, takes control, and is off and running with a new, faster rhythm. This is usurpation.

Proper function of the conduction system results in a **heart rhythm,** a pattern of successive heart beats, that originates in the sinus node. Abnormalities of the conduction system can produce **dysrhythmias,** abnormal heart rhythms. Though most often these conduction system problems are related to heart disease, there are also specific diseases that affect the conduction system outright. Whatever the cause, conduction system abnormalities can prove harmful or fatal if not treated appropriately.

EKG Paper

Before we go any further, let's look at EKG paper. EKG paper is simply graph paper divided into small blocks that are 1 millimeter (mm) in height and width. Dark lines are present every fifth block to further subdivide the paper both vertically and horizontally. Measurements of the EKG waves and complexes are done by counting these blocks. Counting horizontally measures time, or **intervals.** Intervals are measured in seconds. Counting vertically measures **amplitude,** or the height of the complexes. Amplitude is measured in millimeters.

A **12-lead EKG** is a printout of the heart's electrical activity viewed from twelve different angles as seen in twelve different leads. A **lead** is simply an electrocardiographic picture of the heart's electrical activity. A 12-lead EKG is typically done on special 8 × 11 inch paper, using a **three-channel recorder** that prints a simultaneous view of three leads at a time in sequence until all 12 leads are recorded.

A **rhythm strip** is a printout of only one or two leads at a time and is done to assess the patient's heart rhythm. Rhythm strips are recorded on small rolls of special paper about 3–5 inches wide and several hundred feet in length. A 6- to 12-second strip is usually obtained, and the paper is cut to the desired length afterward. Rhythm strip paper often has lines at the top of the paper at 1- to 3-second intervals. Rhythm strips are run on **single-or double-channel recorders,** which print out only one or two leads at a time.

Let's look at the EKG paper delineations:

- Each small block on the EKG paper measures 0.04 second (from one small line to the next).
- Five small blocks equals one big block.

Figure 2-13 EKG paper.

- One big block equals 0.20 second.
- 25 small blocks equals 1 second.
- Five big blocks equals 1 second.
- 1,500 small blocks equals 1 minute.
- 300 big blocks equals 1 minute.
- One small block in amplitude is a millimeter.

No matter whether the EKG paper is 12-lead size or rhythm strip size, the delineations will be the same.

Figure 2-13 is an example of EKG paper. **Identifying data,** such as name, date, time, and room number, and **interpretive data,** such as heart rate, are printed at the top of the paper. Figure 2-14 shows single-and double-lead

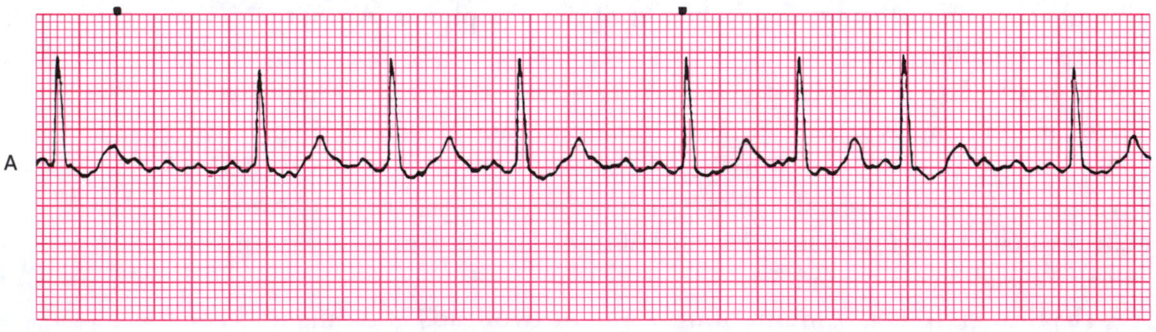

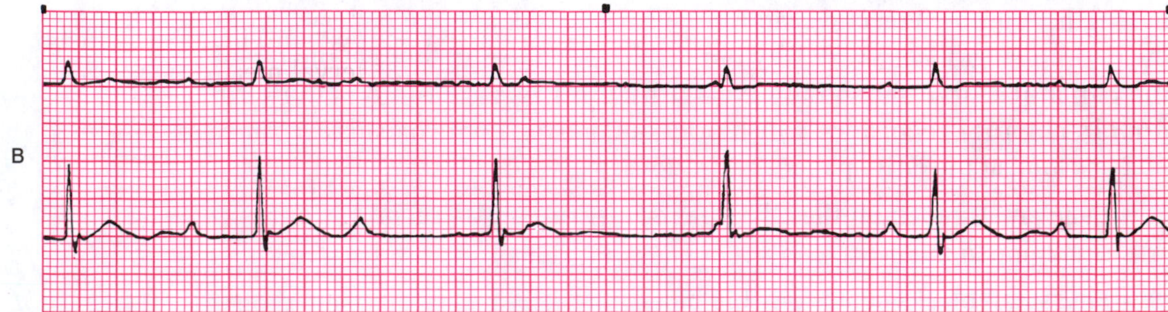

Figure 2-14 (A) Single- and (B) double-lead rhythm strips.

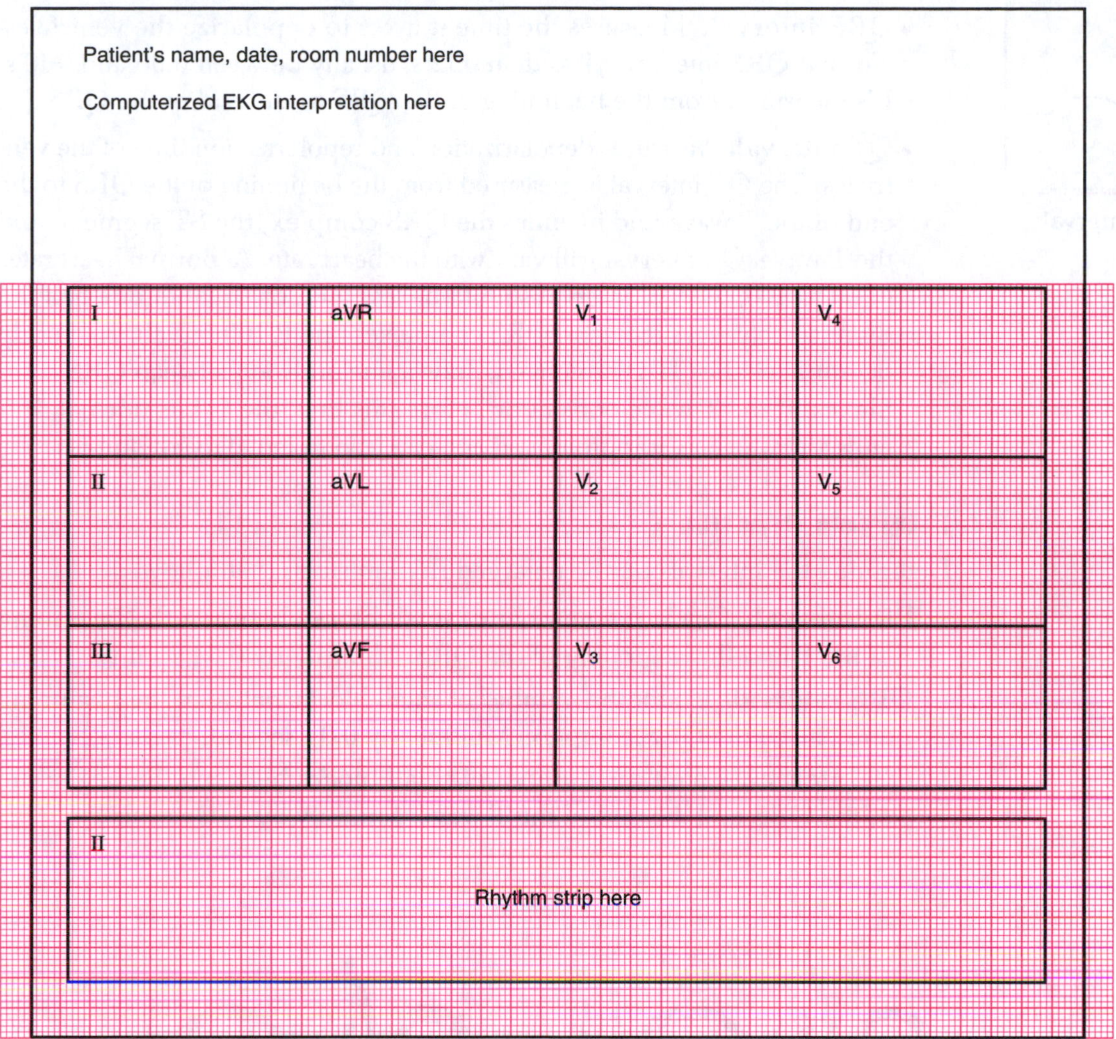

Figure 2-15 12-lead EKG.

rhythm strips. Note that on the double-lead strip, one lead's waves and complexes show up much more clearly than on the other lead. This is typical.

See Figure 2-15 for a 12-lead EKG. Note the lead markings. Leads are arranged in four columns of three leads. Leads I, II, and III are in the first column, then aVR, aVL, and aVF in the second column, V_1 to V_3 in the third column, and V_4 to V_6 in the last column. At the very bottom of the paper is a page-wide rhythm strip, usually of either lead II or V_1.

Intervals

Now let's look at **intervals,** the measurement of time between the P-QRS-T waves and complexes. The heart's current normally starts in the right atrium, then spreads through both atria and down to the ventricles. Interval measurements enable a determination of the heart's efficiency at transmitting its impulses down the pathway. See Figure 2-16.

- **PR interval.** Measures the time it takes for the impulse to get from the atria to the ventricles. Normal PR interval is 0.12 to 0.20 s. It's measured from the beginning of the P wave to the beginning of the QRS and includes the P wave and the PR segment. The P wave itself should measure no more than 0.10 seconds in width and 2.5 mm in height.

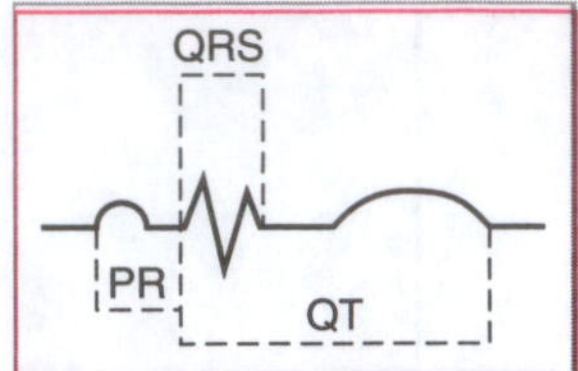

Figure 2-16 Intervals.

- **QRS interval.** Measures the time it takes to depolarize the ventricles. Normal QRS interval is less than 0.12 s, usually between 0.06 and 0.10 s. It's measured from the beginning of the QRS to the end of the QRS.
- **QT interval.** Measures depolarization and repolarization time of the ventricles. The QT interval is measured from the beginning of the QRS to the end of the T wave and includes the QRS complex, the ST segment, and the T wave. QT interval will vary with the heart rate. At normal heart rates of 60 to 100, the QT interval should be less than or equal to one-half the distance between successive QRS complexes (the R-R interval). To quickly determine if the QT is prolonged, draw a line midway between QRS complexes. If the T wave ends at or before this line, the QT is normal. If it ends after the line, it is prolonged and can lead to lethal dysrhythmias.

Intervals Practice

Determine the intervals on the enlarged rhythm strips that follow.

PR interval. Count the number of small blocks between the beginning of the P and the beginning of the QRS. Multiply by 0.04 second.

QRS interval. Count the number of small blocks between the beginning and end of the QRS complex. Multiply by 0.04 second.

QT interval. Count the number of small blocks between the beginning of the QRS and the end of the T wave. Multiply by 0.04 second.

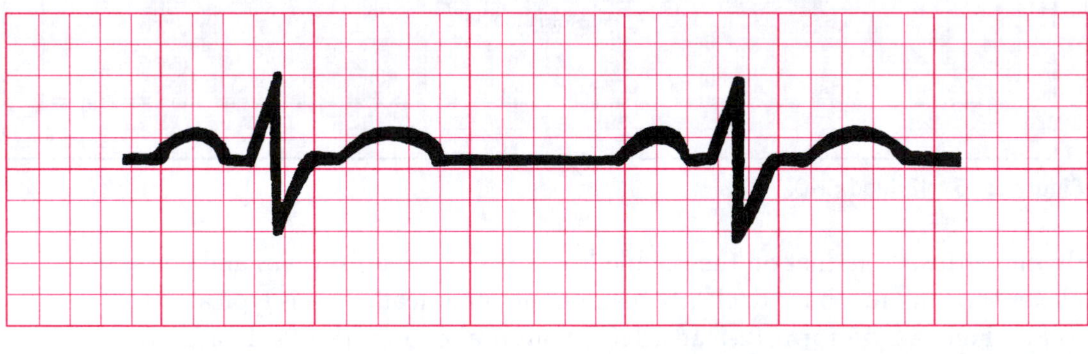

1. PR ____________ QRS ____________ QT ____________

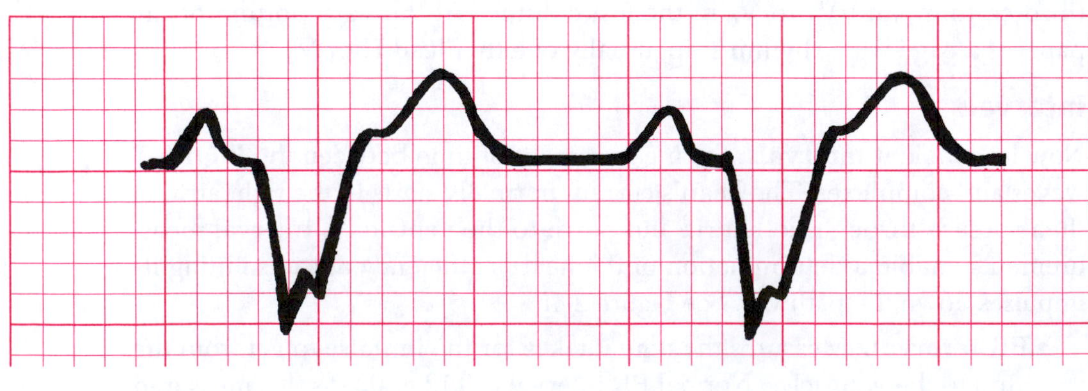

2. PR ____________ QRS ____________ QT ____________

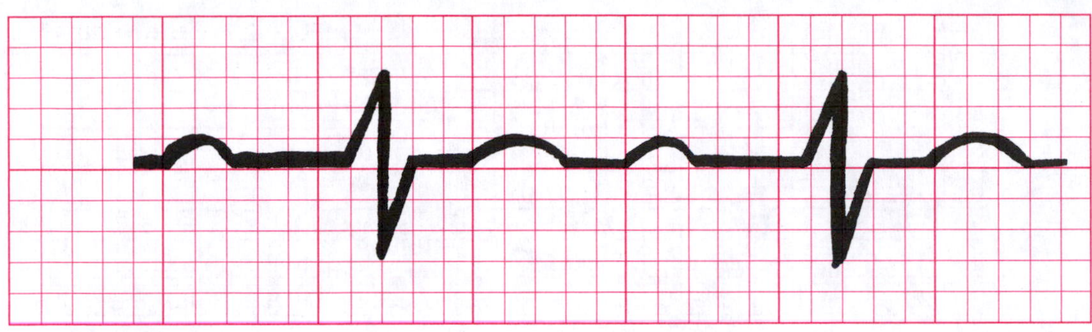

3. PR ______________ QRS ______________ QT ______________

Answers

1. PR 0.12, QRS 0.08, QT 0.24.
2. PR 0.12, QRS 0.14, QT 0.32.
3. PR 0.24, QRS 0.08, QT 0.28.

Now let's practice intervals on normal-size EKG paper.

Intervals Practice

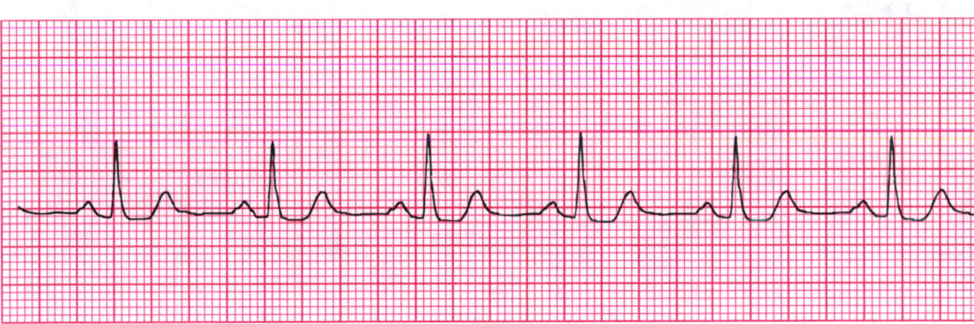

1. PR ______________ QRS ______________ QT ______________

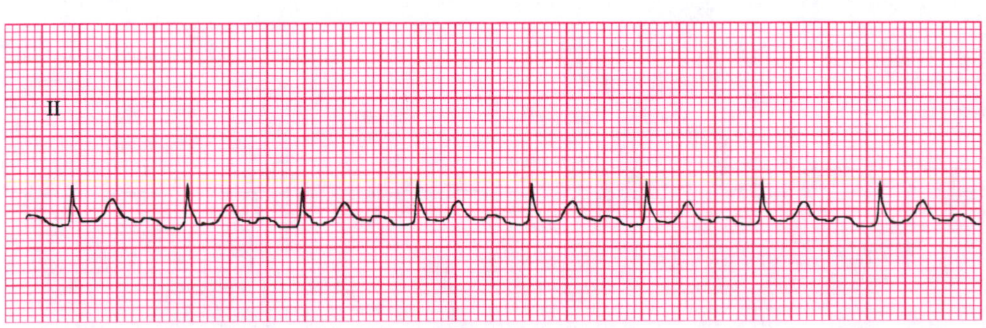

2. PR ______________ QRS ______________ QT ______________

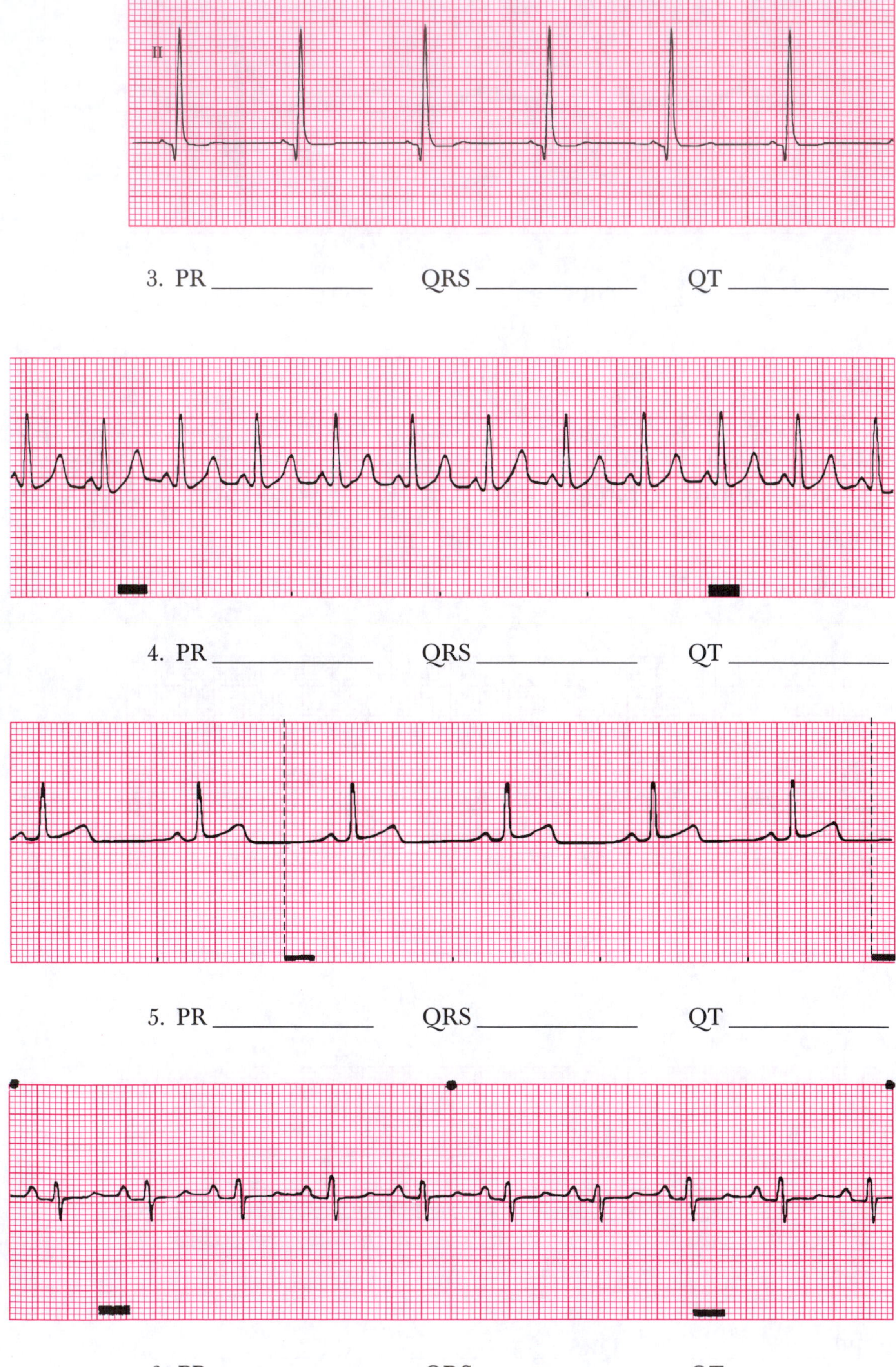

3. PR ______________ QRS ______________ QT ______________

4. PR ______________ QRS ______________ QT ______________

5. PR ______________ QRS ______________ QT ______________

6. PR ______________ QRS ______________ QT ______________

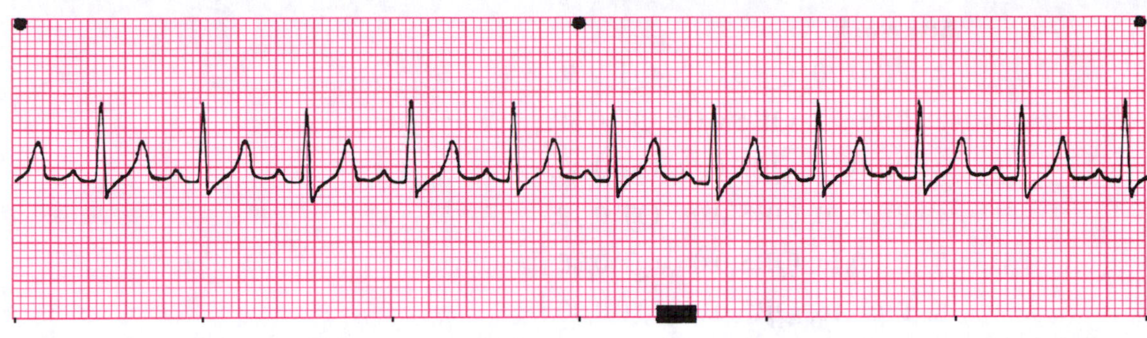

7. PR ______________ QRS ______________ QT ______________

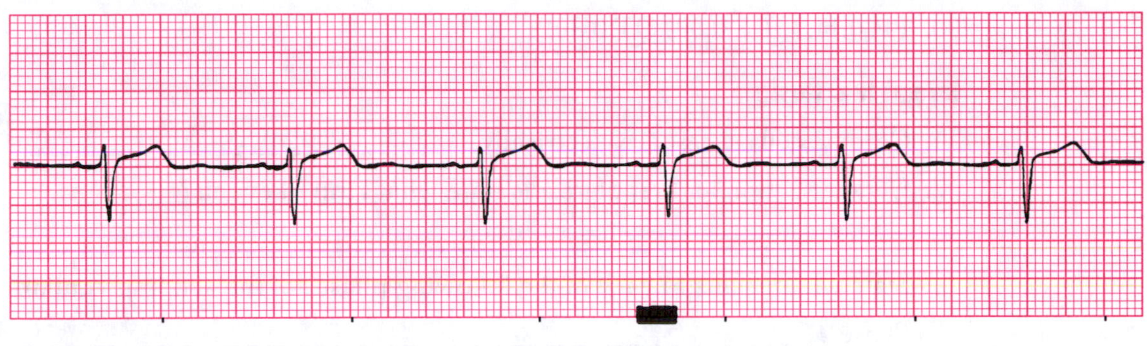

8. PR ______________ QRS ______________ QT ______________

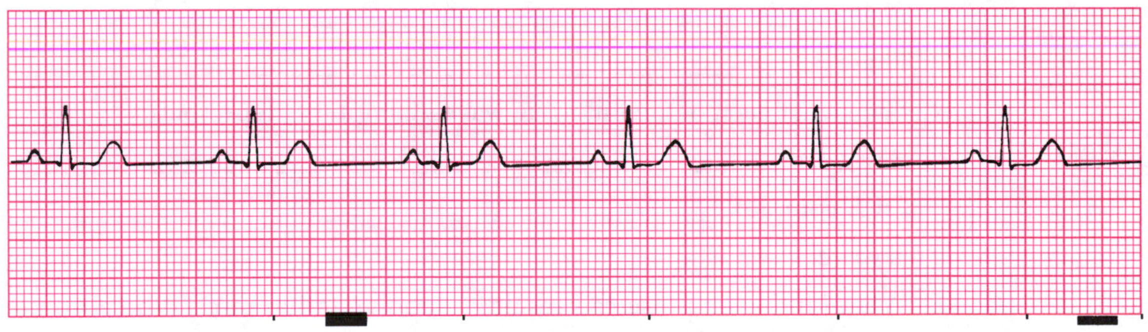

9. PR ______________ QRS ______________ QT ______________

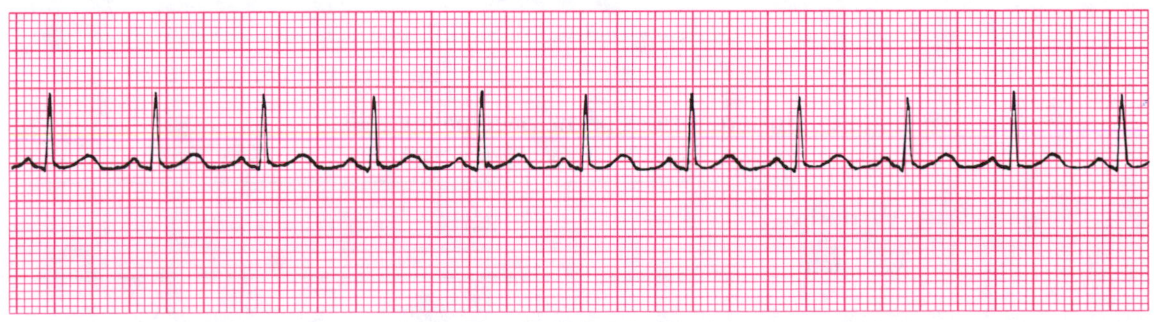

10. PR ______________ QRS ______________ QT ______________

Answers

1. PR 0.20, QRS 0.08, QT 0.36.
2. PR 0.22, QRS 0.08, QT 0.32.
3. PR 0.08, QRS 0.12, QT 0.36.
4. PR 0.10, QRS 0.08, QT 0.32.
5. PR 0.16, QRS 0.06, QT 0.36
6. PR 0.16, QRS 0.08, QT 0.30.
7. PR 0.16, QRS 0.08, QT 0.30.
8. PR 0.14, QRS 0.09, QT 0.38.
9. PR 0.16, QRS 0.10, QT 0.37.
10. PR 0.14, QRS 0.08, QT 0.30.

Practice Quiz

1. Cardiac cells at rest are electrically ______________________
2. Depolarization and repolarization are what kind of events?

   ____
3. State what occurs in each of the following phases of the action potential.

   Phase 4. ______________________

   Phase 0. ______________________

   Phase 1. ______________________

   Phase 2. ______________________

   Phase 3. ______________________
4. State what each of the following waves/complexes represents.

   P wave. ______________________

   QRS complex. ______________________

   T wave. ______________________
5. What kind of impulse can result in depolarization during the absolute refractory period? ______________________

   ____
6. List the four characteristics of heart cells. ______________________

   ____

   ____
7. State the inherent rates of the pacemaker cells.

   Sinus junction ______________________

   AV node ______________________

   Ventricle ______________________

   ____

8. List, in order of conduction, the structures of the conduction pathway through the heart.

____

____

9. Define *escape.* ________________________________

____

10. Define *usurpation.* ____________________________

Putting It All Together–Critical Thinking Exercises

These exercises may consist of diagrams to label, scenarios to analyze, brain-stumping questions to ponder, or other challenging exercises to boost your knowledge of the chapter material.

1. If the sinus node is firing at a rate of 65 and the AV node kicks in at a rate of 70, what will happen? Which pacemaker will be in control? Explain your answer.

2. Your patient's PR interval last night was 0.16 seconds. This morning it is 0.22. Which part of the conduction system is responsible for this delay in impulse transmission?

3. Explain how it is possible for the heart's pumping ability to fail but its electrical conduction ability to remain intact.

4. Label the parts of the conduction system on the diagram.

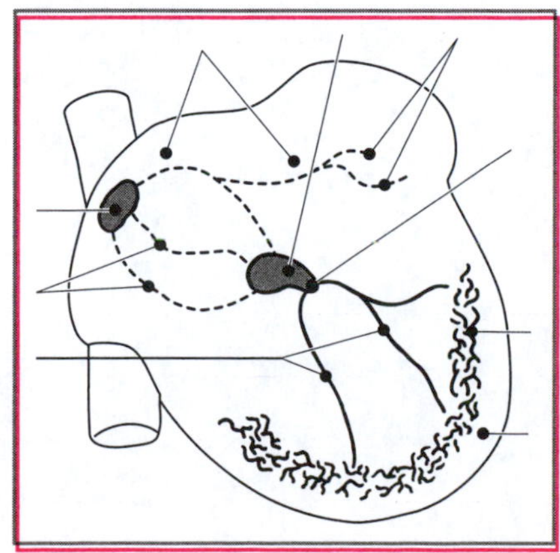

CHAPTER 3

Lead Morphology and Placement

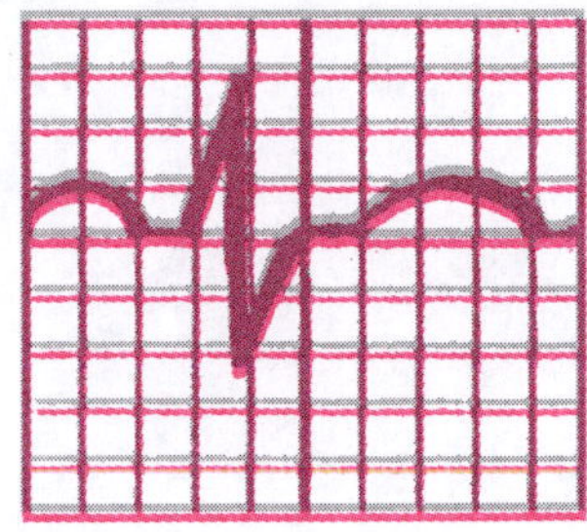

Chapter 3 Objectives

Upon completion of this chapter, the student will be able to:

- Define *electrode.*
- Describe the difference between an electrocardiograph and an electrocardiogram.
- Name the bipolar leads and state the limbs that compose them.
- Name the unipolar augmented leads.
- Explain what augmentation does to the EKG.
- Explain Einthoven's law.
- Draw and label Einthoven's triangle.
- Name the leads composing the hexiaxial diagram.
- Describe the location of the precordial leads.
- Name the two leads most commonly used for continuous monitoring in the hospital.
- Explain the electrocardiographic truths.
- Describe the normal QRS complex deflections in each of the 12 leads on an EKG.

Introduction

Electrocardiography is the recording of the heart's electrical impulses by way of sensors, called **electrodes,** placed at various locations on the body. Willem Einthoven, inventor of the EKG machine and the "father of electrocardiography," postulated that the heart is in the center of the electrical field that it generates. He put electrodes on the arms and legs, far away from the heart. The right-leg electrode was used as a ground electrode to minimize the hazard of electric shock to the patient and to stabilize the EKG. The electrodes on the other limbs were used to create leads. A **lead** is simply an electrocardiographic picture of the heart. A 12-lead EKG provides 12 different views of the heart's electrical activity.

Why is it necessary to have 12 leads? The more leads, the better the chance of interpreting the heart's electrical activity. Have you ever waved to someone you saw from a distance, then realized when you got a better look that it wasn't who you thought it was? The more views you have, the better your chance of recognizing this person, right? Same thing with the heart.

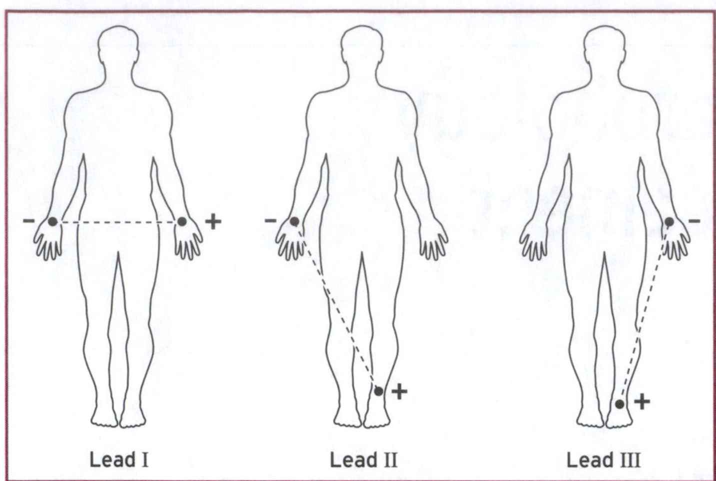

Figure 3-1 The bipolar leads.

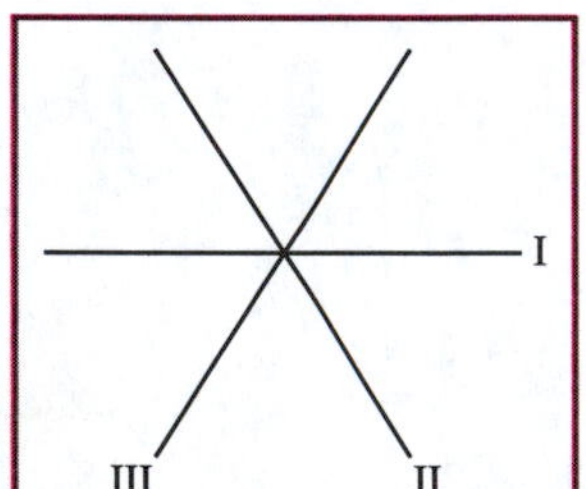

Figure 3-2 The triaxial diagram.

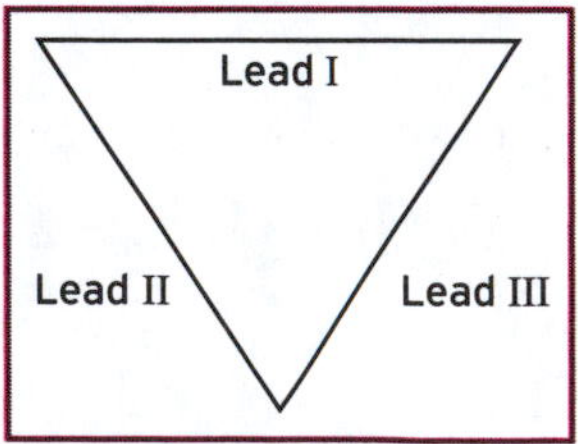

Figure 3-3 Einthoven's triangle.

The more views of the heart's electrical activity, the better the chance of recognizing its abnormalities. So we have leads that view the heart from the side, the front, the bottom, and anterior to posterior (front to back).

The printed EKG is called an **electrocardiogram.**

Bipolar Leads

Bipolar leads are so named because they require a positive pole and a negative pole. Think of the positive electrode as the one that actually "sees" the current.

- **Lead I.** Measures the current traveling between the right and left arms. The right arm is negative and the left arm is positive.
- **Lead II.** Measures the current traveling between the right arm and the left leg. The right arm is negative and the left leg is positive.
- **Lead III.** Measures the current traveling between the left arm and the left leg. The left arm is negative and the left leg is positive.

In Figure 3-1, you'll notice that in the bipolar leads the right arm is always negative and the left leg is always positive. Also note that the left arm can be positive or negative depending on which lead it is a part of. If you join leads I, II, and III at the middle, you get the **triaxial diagram** seen in Figure 3-2.

If you join Leads I, II, and III at their ends, you get a triangle called **Einthoven's triangle,** seen in Figure 3-3.

Einthoven stated that lead I + lead III = lead II. This is called **Einthoven's law.** It means that the height of the QRS in lead I added to the height of the QRS in lead III will equal the height of the QRS in lead II. In other words, lead II should have the tallest QRS of the bipolar leads. Einthoven's law can help determine if an EKG is truly abnormal or if the leads were inadvertently placed on the incorrect limb. See Figure 3-4.

Augmented Leads

- aVR. Measures the current traveling toward the right arm. This is a positive electrode. The electrode is on the right arm.
- aVL. Measures the current traveling toward the left arm. This is a positive electrode. The electrode is on the left arm.

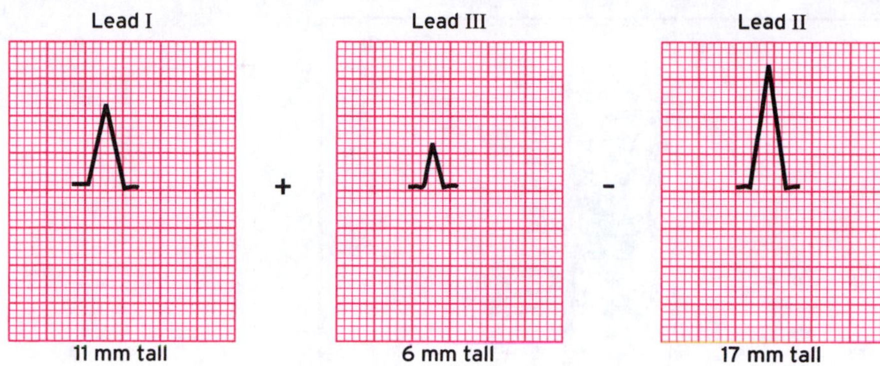

Figure 3-4 Einthoven's law.

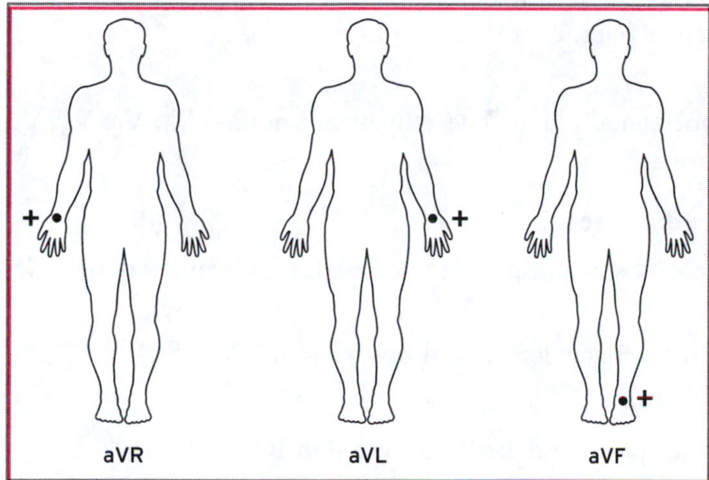

Figure 3-5 The augmented leads.

- aVF. Measures the current traveling toward the left foot (or leg). This is a positive electrode. The electrode is on the left leg.

See Figure 3-5. These are called **augmented leads** because they generate such small waveforms on the EKG paper that the EKG machine must augment (increase) the size of the waveforms so they'll show up on the EKG paper. These leads are also **unipolar,** meaning they require only one electrode to make the leads. In order for the EKG machine to augment the leads, it uses a midway point between the other two limbs as a negative reference point.

Both the bipolar and augmented leads are also called **frontal leads** because they look at the heart from only the front of the body.

If you join leads aVR, aVL, and aVF in the middle, you get the triaxial diagram shown in Figure 3-6.

If all the frontal leads–I, II, III, aVR, aVL, and aVF–are joined at the center, the result looks like Figure 3-7. This **hexiaxial diagram** is used to help determine the direction of current flow in the heart.

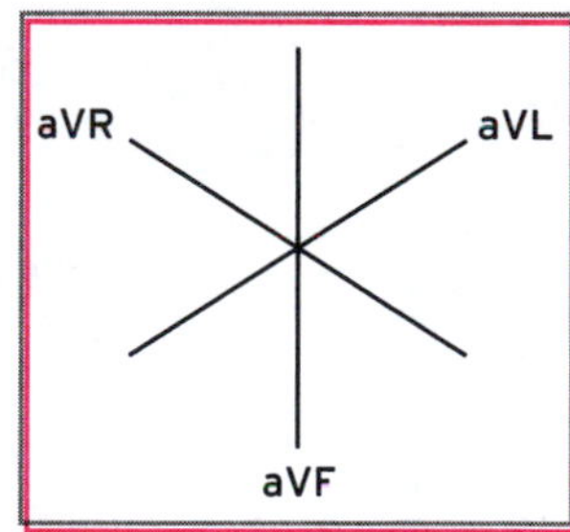

Figure 3-6 Triaxial diagram with augmented leads.

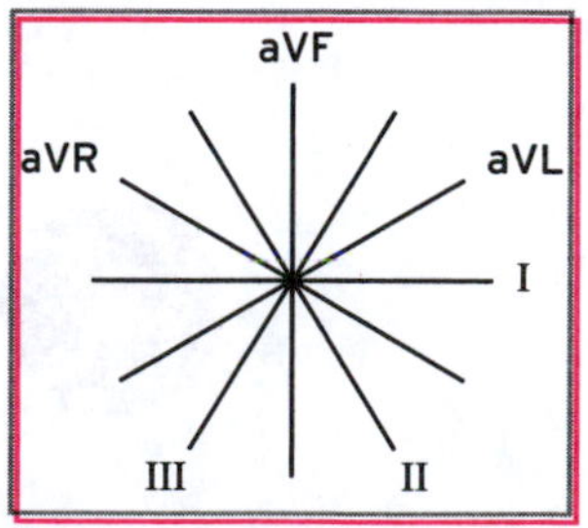

Figure 3-7 The hexiaxial diagram.

Precordial (Chest) Leads

These leads are located on the chest. They are also unipolar leads, and each one is a positive electrode. The precordial leads see a wraparound view of

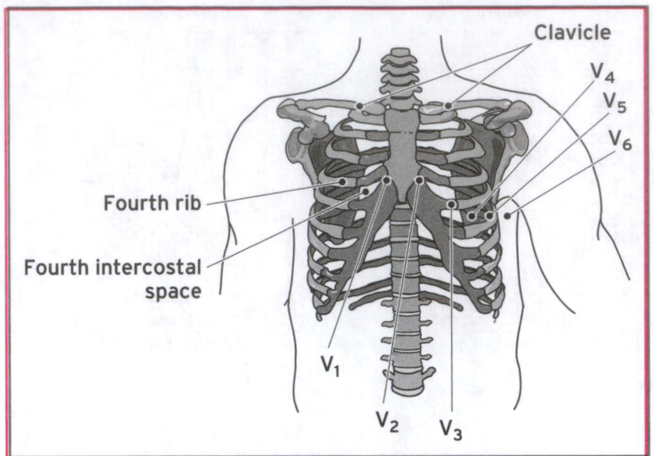

Figure 3-8 The precordial leads.

the heart from the horizontal plane. These leads are named V_1, V_2, V_3, V_4, V_5, and V_6. See Figure 3-8.

Location of the precordial leads

- V_1 Fourth intercostal space, right sternal border (abbreviated 4th ICS, RSB)
- V_2 Fourth intercostal space, left sternal border (4th ICS, LSB)
- V_3 Between V_2 and V_4
- V_4 Fifth intercostal space, midclavicular line (5th ICS, MCL)
- V_5 Fifth intercostal space, anterior axillary line (5th ICS, AAL)
- V_6 Fifth intercostal space, midaxillary line (5th ICS, MAL)

Intercostal spaces are the spaces between the ribs. The fourth intercostal space is the space below the fourth rib; the fifth intercostal space is below the fifth rib, and so on. The **midclavicular line** is a line down from the middle of the clavicle (collarbone). The **anterior axillary line** is a line down from the front of the axilla (armpit). The **midaxillary line** is down from the middle of the axilla.

Continuous Monitoring

For patients in the hospital, continuous EKG monitoring may be needed. These patients are attached to either a 3-lead or a 5-lead cable, which is then attached to a remote receiver/transmitter (called **telemetry**) or to a monitor at the bedside (see Figure 3-9). Both of these setups send the EKG display to a central terminal where the rhythms are observed and identified (see CD-ROM for an animation showing 12-lead EKG placement and video showing electrode placement for EKG and cardiac monitoring and the electrocardiogram).

Since these patients may be on the monitor for days or longer, it is necessary to alter the placement of lead electrodes to allow for freedom of movement and to minimize artifact.

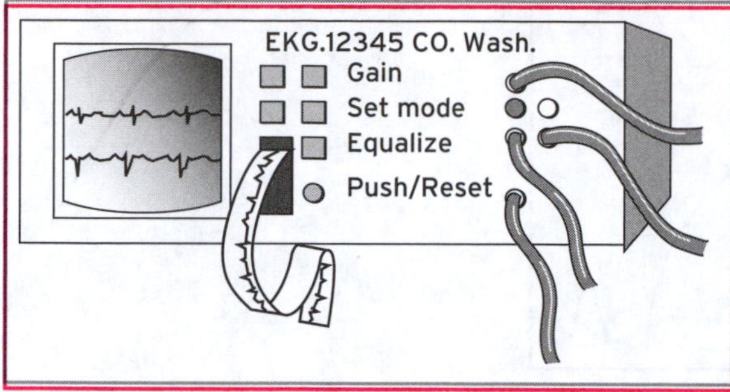

Figure 3-9 Bedside monitor.

Figure 3-10 shows the two most commonly used leads for continuous monitoring. Note lead placement is on the subclavicle (collarbone) area and the chest or lower abdomen instead of on the arms, legs, and chest. Also note the ground electrode may be located somewhere other than the right leg.

Electrocardiographic Truths

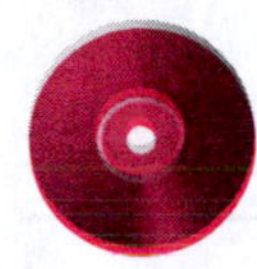

- An impulse traveling toward (or parallel to) a positive electrode writes a positive complex on the EKG paper (see CD-ROM for an animation showing the rule of electrical flow).
- An impulse traveling away from a positive electrode writes a negative complex.
- An impulse traveling perpendicularly to the positive electrode writes an **isoelectric** complex (one that is as much positive as it is negative).
- If there is no impulse at all, there will be no complex–just a flat line.

See Figure 3-11.

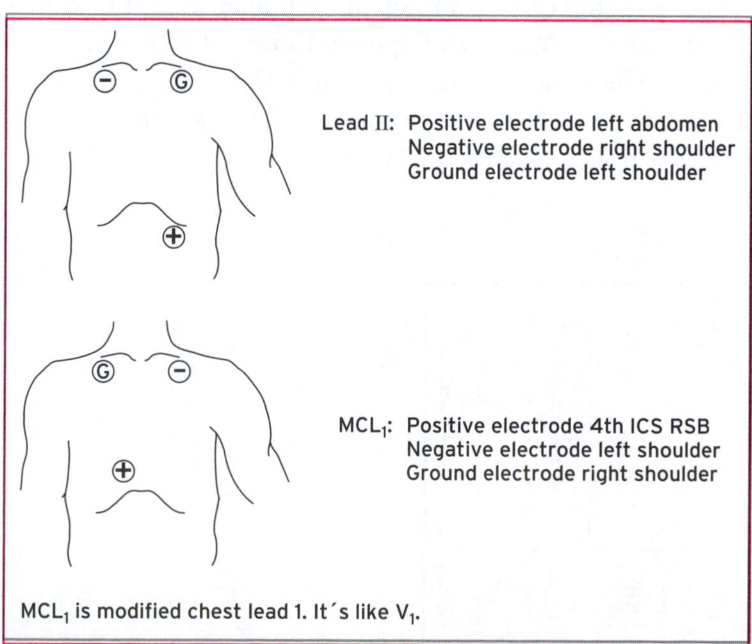

Lead II: Positive electrode left abdomen
Negative electrode right shoulder
Ground electrode left shoulder
MCL$_1$: Positive electrode 4th ICS RSB
Negative electrode left shoulder
Ground electrode right shoulder
MCL$_1$ is modified chest lead 1. It´s like V$_1$.

Figure 3-10 Lead placement for continuous monitoring.

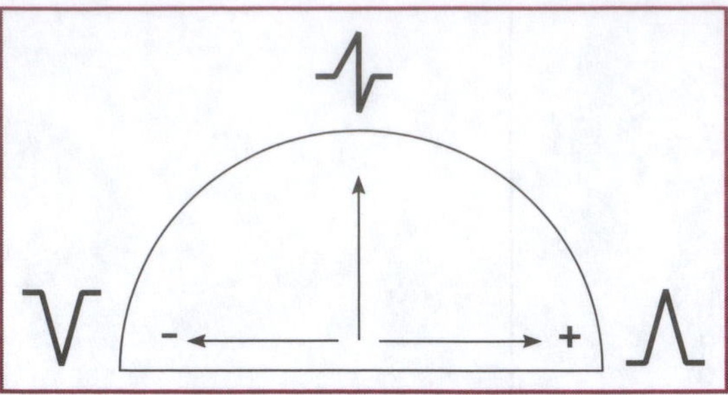

Figure 3-11 Electrocardiographic truths.

Normal QRS Deflections

How should the QRS complexes in the normal EKG look? Let's look at the frontal leads:

Lead I Should be positive.

Lead II Should be positive.

Lead III Should be small but mostly positive.

aVR Should be negative.

aVL Should be positive.

aVF Should be positive.

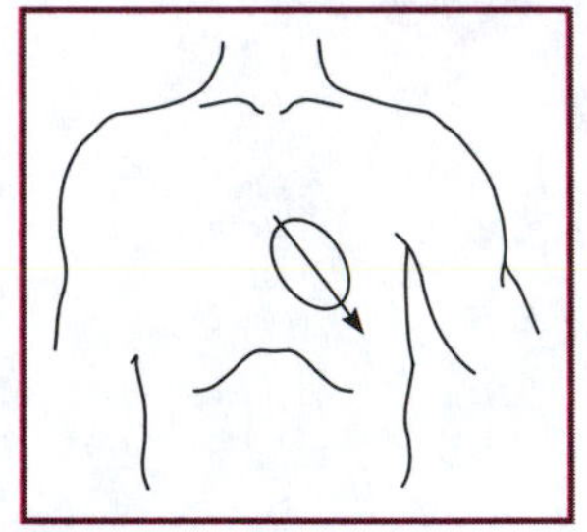

Figure 3-12 Normal vector.

Normal vector forces of the heart flow top to bottom, right to left. A **vector** is an arrow that points out the general direction of current flow. The current of the heart normally starts in the sinus node, which is in the right atrium, and terminates in the left ventricle. Figure 3-12 shows what the vector representing normal heart current looks like.

We've already said what the QRS complex in each lead should look like. Let's look at that a little more closely. In Figure 3-13 we have lead I, which joins right and left arms. The positive electrode is on the left arm. Normal current of the heart flows right to left, traveling toward the left side, where lead I's positive electrode is. This results in a positive (upward) complex in lead I.

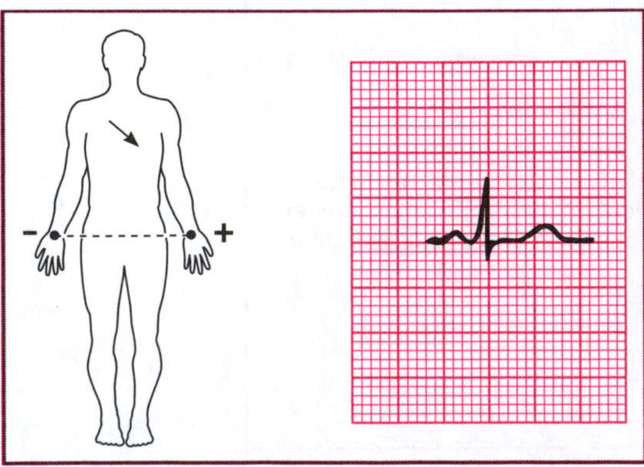

Figure 3-13 Normal QRS deflection in lead I.

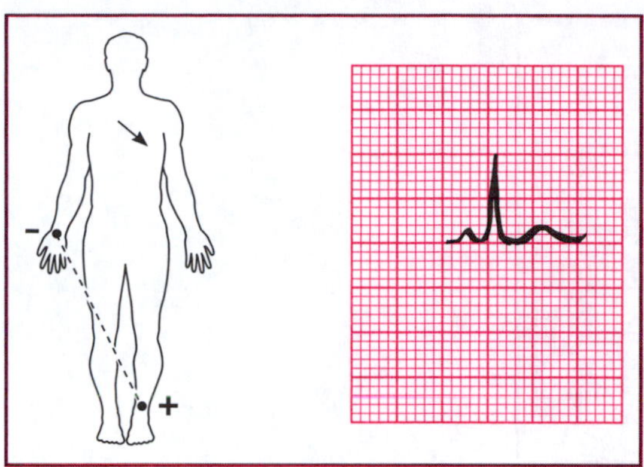

Figure 3-14 Normal QRS deflection in lead II.

In Figure 3-14, we have lead II, which connects the right arm and left leg. Recall the left leg is positive. Normal heart current flows top to bottom, right to left, parallel to lead II. Therefore lead II should be strongly positive.

Next is lead III, which joins left arm and left foot. The positive electrode is on the left leg. Normal current flows toward this electrode, producing a positive complex. The complex in lead III is very often small. See Figure 3-15.

In aVR, the positive electrode is on the right arm. Normal current flows right to left, away from this electrode, and aVR should therefore be negative. See Figure 3-16.

In aVL, the positive electrode is on the left arm. Normal current flows toward the left, producing a positive complex. See Figure 3-17.

In aVF, the positive electrode is on the left leg. Normal current flows toward the left leg, so aVF should have a positive complex. See Figure 3-18.

Now let's look at the precordial leads:

V_1 Should be negative.

V_2 Should be negative.

V_3 Should be about half up, half down.

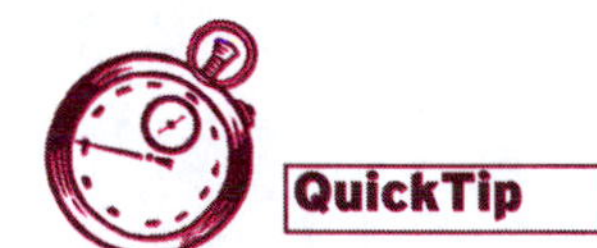

In the frontal leads all QRS complexes should be upright (except aVR).

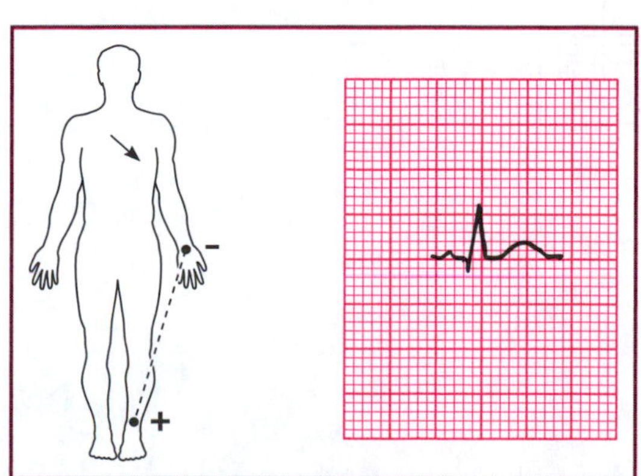

Figure 3-15 Normal QRS deflection in lead III.

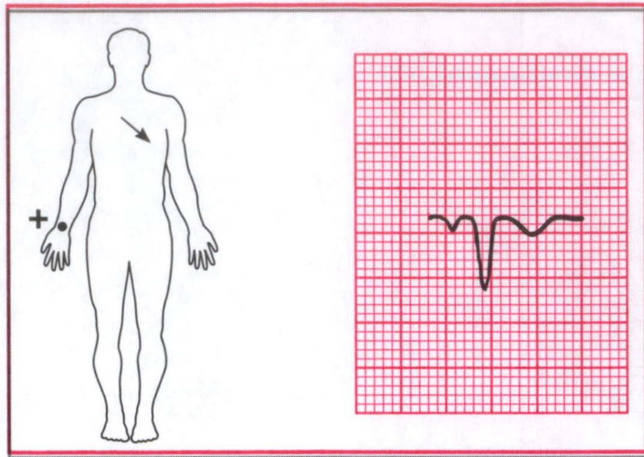

Figure 3-16 Normal QRS deflection in aVR.

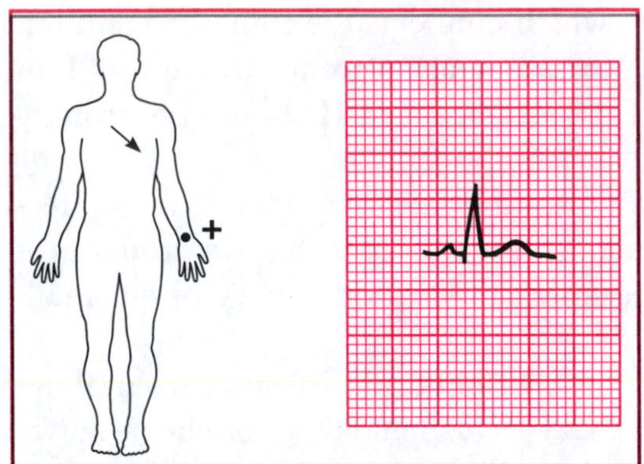

Figure 3-17 Normal QRS deflection in aVL.

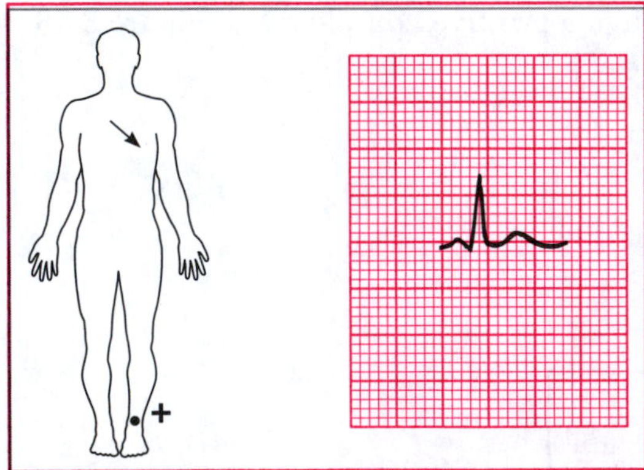

Figure 3-18 Normal QRS deflection in aVF.

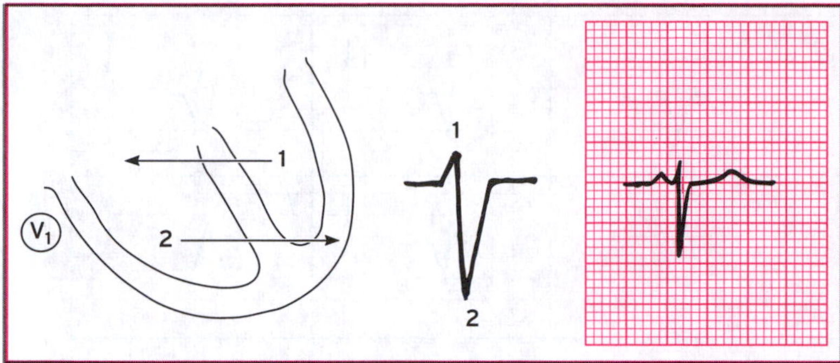

Figure 3-19 Normal QRS deflection in V_1.

V_4 Should be about half up, half down.

V_5 Should be positive.

V_6 Should be positive.

The precordial leads start out negative, then go through a transition zone where they become half-and-half, then they become positive. For the precordial leads we look at current flow in the **horizontal plane.** The septum depolarizes from left to right and the ventricles from right to left.

See Figure 3-19. In V_1, septal and right ventricular depolarization send the current toward the positive electrode, resulting in an initial positive deflection. Then the current travels away from the positive electrode as it heads toward the left ventricle. Thus, V_1 should have a small R wave and a deep S wave. The complex is mostly negative, since most of the heart's current is traveling toward the left ventricle, away from the V_1 electrode.

In V_6, just the opposite occurs. Initially, the impulse is heading away from the positive electrode during septal and right ventricular depolarization, then it travels toward it during left ventricular activation. See Figure 3-20.

The other leads in between show a gradual transition from negative to positive complexes.

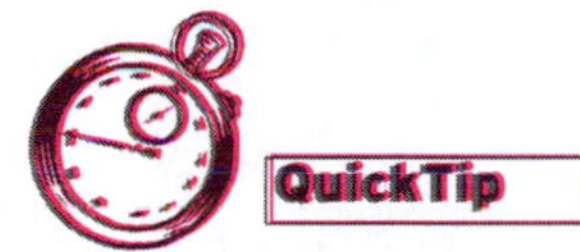

In the precordial leads, V_1 and V_2's QRS should be negative, V_3 and/or V_4 isoelectric, and V_5 and V_6 positive.

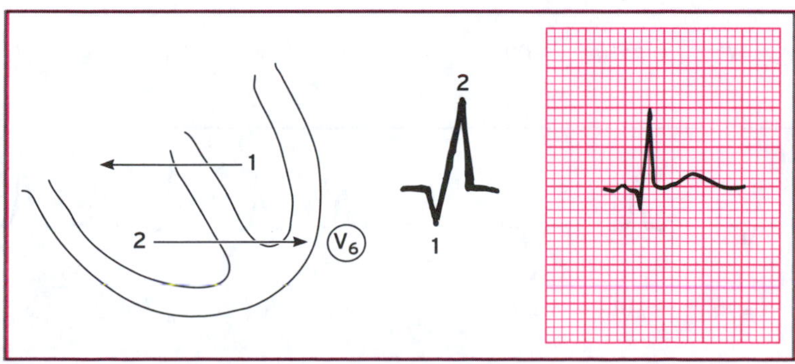

Figure 3-20 Normal QRS deflection in V_6.

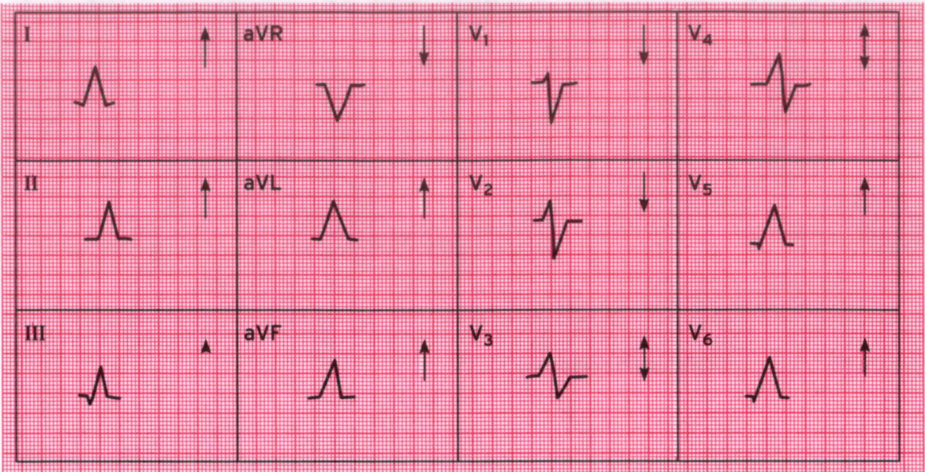

Normal 12-Lead EKG The arrows indicate the correct deflection of the QRS complexes.

Lead Morphology Practice

Determine if the following QRS morphologies are normal. If not, tell what the abnormality is.

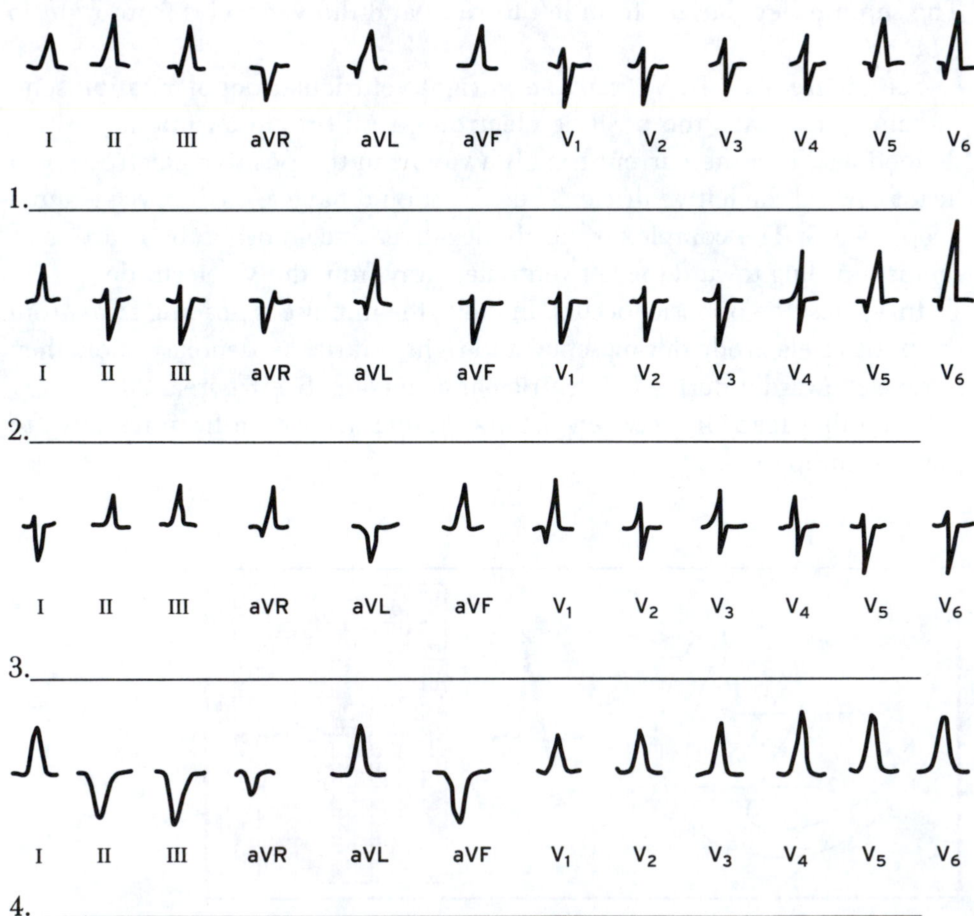

Answers to Lead Morphology Practice

1. **Normal morphology.**
2. **Abnormal morphology.** Let's go lead by lead. Lead I is normal. Leads II and III are negative deflections and they should be positive; aVR is OK, as is aVL; aVF is negative and it should be positive. The precordial leads are OK.
3. **Abnormal morphology.** Lead I is negative and it should be positive. Leads II and III are OK; aVR is positive and it should *always* be negative; aVL is negative and should be positive; aVF is OK. V_1 is positive, but should be negative. V_2 is OK, more negative than positive. V_3 is positive, but should be isoelectric. V_4 is isoelectric when it should be getting more positive. V_5 and V_6 are negative when they should be positive.
4. **Abnormal morphology.** Lead I is positive, as it should be. Leads II and III are negative, but should be positive; aVR and aVL are OK; aVF is negative but should be positive. The precordial leads are all positive–this is completely abnormal.

Just by analyzing the morphology of each lead, we can get an idea of whether there is any pathology on the EKG. Three of the preceding four EKGs were abnormal in some way. As we continue further along in this text, we will learn the implications of this abnormality, and we'll learn more ways to analyze EKGs.

Practice Quiz

1. Who is Willem Einthoven? ______________________________
2. List the three bipolar leads and the limbs they connect.

   ____

   ____

   ____
3. List the three augmented leads and the location of their positive pole.

   ____

   ____

   ____
4. The hexiaxial diagram consists of six leads joined at the center. List those six leads.

   ____
5. The precordial leads see the heart from what plane? ______________
6. List the six precordial leads and state their location. ______________

   ____

   ____

   ____

____

____

____

7. Name the two leads most commonly used for continuous monitoring.
____

8. An impulse traveling toward a positive electrode writes a _____ complex on the EKG.

9. Should aVR have a positive QRS complex or a negative one?
____

10. The QRS complexes in the precordial lead start out primarily
____

Putting It All Together–Critical Thinking Exercises

These exercises may consist of diagrams to label, scenarios to analyze, brain-stumping questions to ponder, or other challenging exercises to boost your understanding of the chapter material.

1. What can it imply if Lead I + Lead III do not equal Lead II? ________
____
____

2. If the QR complex in lead III is isoelectric, in what direction is the heart's current traveling? ______________________
____
____

3. If your patient has a heart rhythm in which the current starts in the left ventricle and travels upward toward the sinus node, what would you expect the frontal leads to look like? (i.e., indicate lead by lead whether the QRS complex in those leads would be positive or negative). ________
____
____

CHAPTER 4

Technical Aspects of the EKG

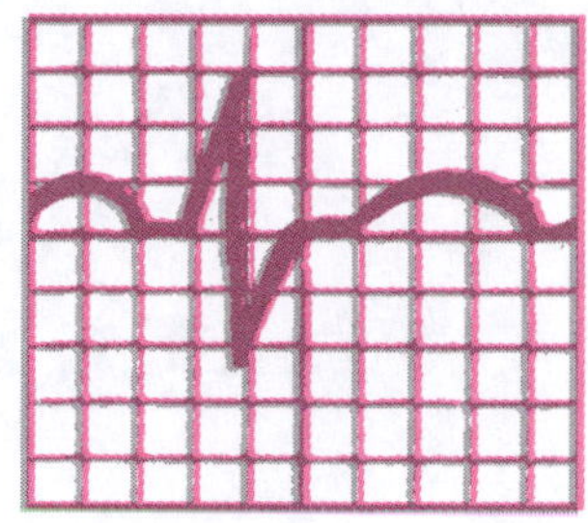

Chapter 4 Objectives

Upon completion of this chapter, the student will be able to:

- Identify the control features of an EKG machine and describe the functions of each.
- Describe what a galvanometer does.
- Differentiate between *macroshock* and *microshock*.
- Describe and identify on a rhythm strip the different kinds of artifact.
- Correctly tell how to troubleshoot artifact.
- Name the rhythms that can be mimicked by artifact.
- Tell how to differentiate between artifact and the real thing.
- Correctly identify artifact versus rhythm.
- Explain the purpose of telemetry monitoring.

Introduction

The heart, electrically speaking, is a transmitter, and the EKG machine is a receiver. Let's look at how the EKG machine works.

The electrical impulses sent out by the heart course not only through the conduction system but also throughout the body. **Electrodes,** small adhesive patches with conductive gel on the skin side, are applied to the skin and pick up these impulses, sending them through **lead wires** to a cable into the EKG machine. There an **amplifier** magnifies the signal and a **galvanometer** converts the electrical activity into mechanical energy, which in turn causes the **stylus** to record the EKG. See Figure 4-1.

Control Features

EKG machines have various control features:

- **Chart speed.** This regulates the speed at which the paper prints out. Normal speed is 25 mm/s. Changing the speed to 50 mm/s doubles the width of the waves and complexes.
- **Sensitivity control.** This regulates the height of the complexes. Normal setting is 1. Changing to 2 doubles the height of the complexes. Changing to 1/2 shrinks it.

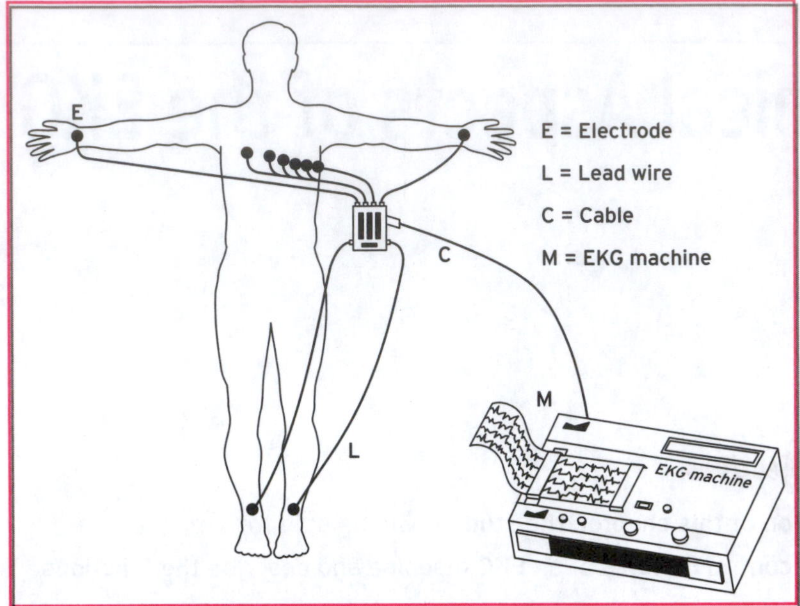

Figure 4-1 Man attached to EKG machine.

- **Standardization.** This checks the machine's calibration. Throwing 1 millivolt of electricity into the EKG machine should cause the stylus (the pen) to print out a square wave 10 mm high on the EKG paper. Incorrect standardization reveals a square wave that is too tall, too short, or slurred at the top or bottom. Do not use a machine that's not calibrated properly. Its printout may not be accurate. See Figure 4-2.
- **Position control.** This allows the baseline to be moved up or down on the paper.
- **Frequency response.** This filters out extraneous noise and artifact to provide a smoother tracing.
- **Stylus heat control.** This allows the stylus to write darker (hotter stylus) or lighter (cooler stylus).

Whenever any setting is changed from the norm, document this change at the top of the EKG printout. For example, if the sensitivity control is increased to 2 instead of set at the usual 1, note this: Documentation prevents misinterpretation of any EKG changes that might result from changes to the control features.

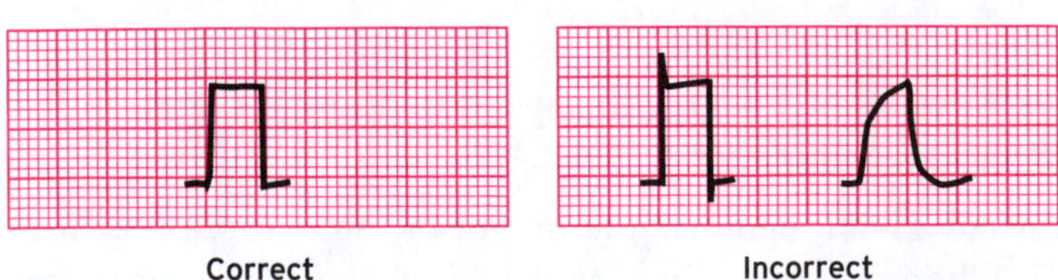

Figure 4-2 Calibration waves.

Electrical Safety

There are two kinds of electrical shock the patient can sustain from faulty equipment:

- **Macroshock.** This is a high-voltage shock that results from inadequate grounding of electrical equipment. If there is a frayed or broken wire or cord, electrical outlet damage, or other electrical malfunction, the 110 volts of electricity running through the power line can go directly to the patient, causing burns, neurologic damage, or fatal heart rhythm disturbances. The patient's dry, intact skin will offer some resistance to the electricity, but not enough to prevent injury.
- **Microshock.** This is a subtle hazard, but one that could have equally disastrous results for the patient. Microshock involves a direct path to the heart by means of a device inside or attached to it, such as a pacemaker. A small voltage exists on the outside of the metal pacemaker because of the proximity of the electrical components inside to the surrounding case. Normally a small **leakage current** is produced and carried harmlessly away by the ground wire attaching the patient's bed to the electrical socket in the room. If the ground wire is frayed, however, a small amount of current could travel into the heart and shock it from the inside. Since the inside of the body is a wet environment, there is less protection against shock. Even a small shock directed into the heart can cause injury or death.

Precaution: Check for frayed wires or components before doing an EKG.

Artifact

Artifact is unwanted interference or jitter on the EKG tracing. This makes reading the EKG difficult. There are four kinds of artifact:

- **Somatic tremors.** The word *somatic* means "body." This is a jittery pattern caused by the patient's tremors or by shaking wires. Try to help the patient relax. Cover him if he's cold. Make sure the wires are not tangled or loose. Sometimes this artifact cannot be corrected, such as in a patient with constant tremors from Parkinson's disease. In that case, make a few attempts at a readable tracing and keep the best one. At the top of the EKG, write "best effort times three attempts" or something to that effect so the physician will know this was not simply a poor tracing done by an inattentive technician. Note the shakiness of the tracing in Figure 4-3. Sometimes you can pick out the QRS complexes and sometimes not. Redo the EKG until the tracing is more easily readable.
- **Baseline sway.** This is where the baseline moves up and down on the EKG paper. It's often caused by lotion or sweat on the skin interfering with the signal reaching the machine. Sometimes it's associated with the breathing pattern. Wipe off any lotion or sweat with a towel and put a little alcohol at the electrode site to defat the skin and help the patches stick better. On Figure 4-4, note the baseline swaying upward

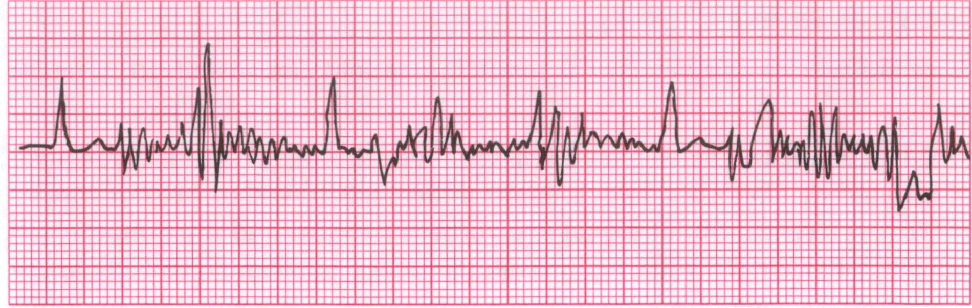

Figure 4-3 Somatic tremors artifact.

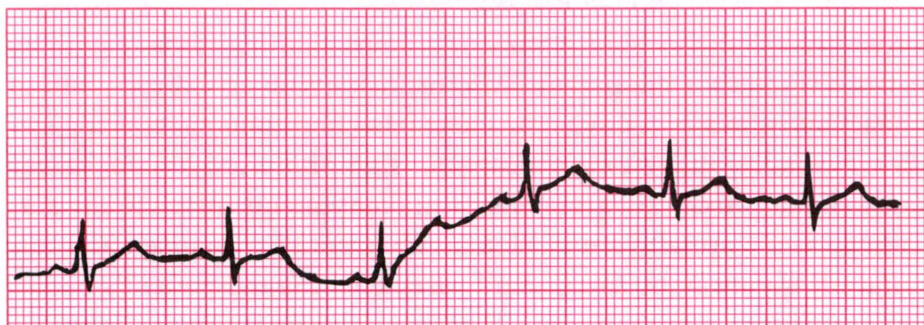

Figure 4-4 Baseline sway.

as if someone had snagged a finger under it and pulled it upward. It's not a big problem, because the waves and complexes are all still clear.

- **60-cycle interference.** This results in a thick-looking pattern on the paper. It's caused by too many electrical things plugged in close by. Unplug as many machines as you safely can until you finish doing the EKG. Don't forget portable phones and pagers–they can cause interference also. In Figure 4-5, see how the baseline is very thick-looking? It's as if someone used a thick highlighter to write this baseline. Normally the baseline is much finer.
- **Broken recording.** This can be caused by a frayed or fractured wire or by a loose electrode patch or cable. Check first for loose electrodes or cables. If those are OK, the artifact may be from a fractured wire. If so, use a different EKG machine. Never do an EKG with a faulty machine. In Figure 4-6, note that at first the QRS complexes are easily visible, then the stylus is all over the place, going up and down trying to find the signal.

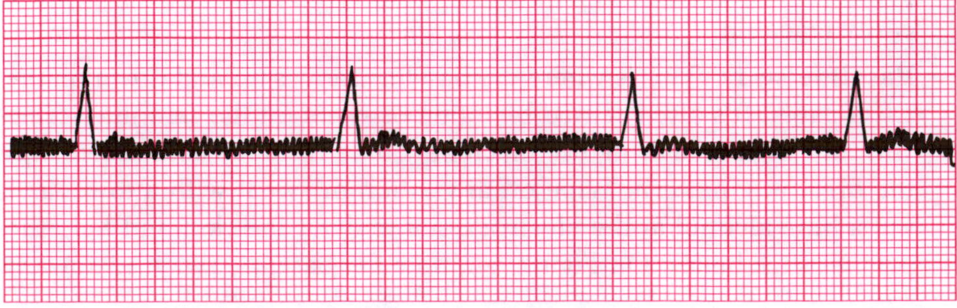

Figure 4-5 60-cycle interference.

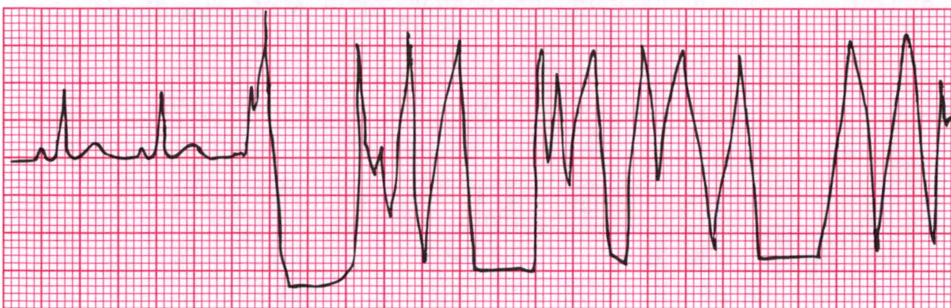

Figure 4-6 Broken recording.

Troubleshooting

Troubleshooting involves determining and alleviating the cause of artifact and recording errors. For example, what if you only saw baseline sway in leads I, II, and aVR? Lead I connects the right and left arms, lead II is right arm and left foot, and aVR is right arm. The common lead is on the right arm. Change that electrode, and the problem should be corrected. Always note what leads the problem is in and find the common limb. Direct your corrective efforts there.

How do you know if the electrodes are properly placed? Remember the normal configuration of the leads. All the frontal leads except aVR should be positive, and the precordial leads start out negative, then eventually become positive. Say you do an EKG and the complexes are all screwed up—I is negative, aVR is positive, and the precordial leads start out positive and become negative. Obviously the lead placement is wrong. Redo the EKG with the leads correctly placed. A big clue to incorrect lead placement or lead reversal is a negative P-QRS-T in lead I. That is completely wrong unless the patient's heart is on the right side (a rare occurrence). So if you find that your lead I is completely negative, check your lead placement. The right and left arm leads were probably accidentally reversed.

Artifact Troubleshooting Practice

On these EKGs, state in which leads the artifact is found, and the necessary corrective action.

1.

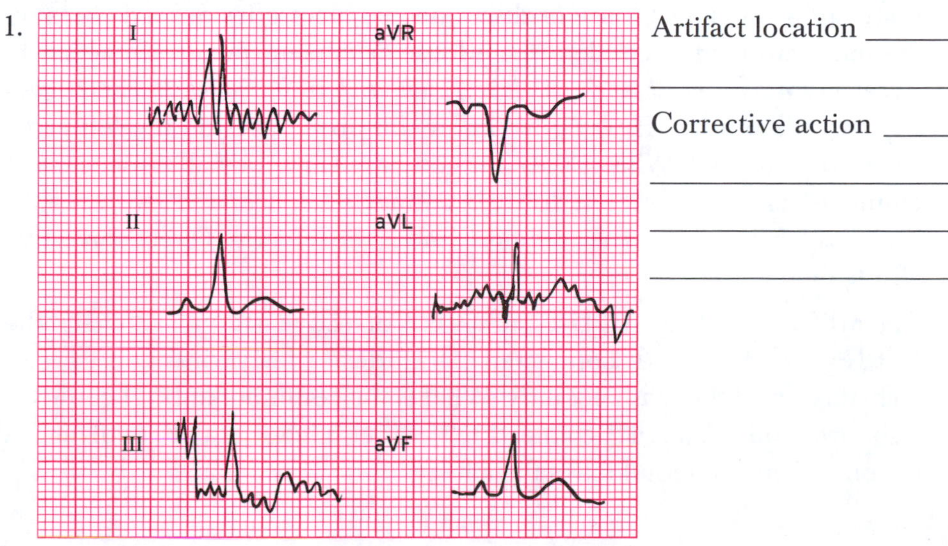

Artifact location ______

____

Corrective action _____

____

____

____

2.

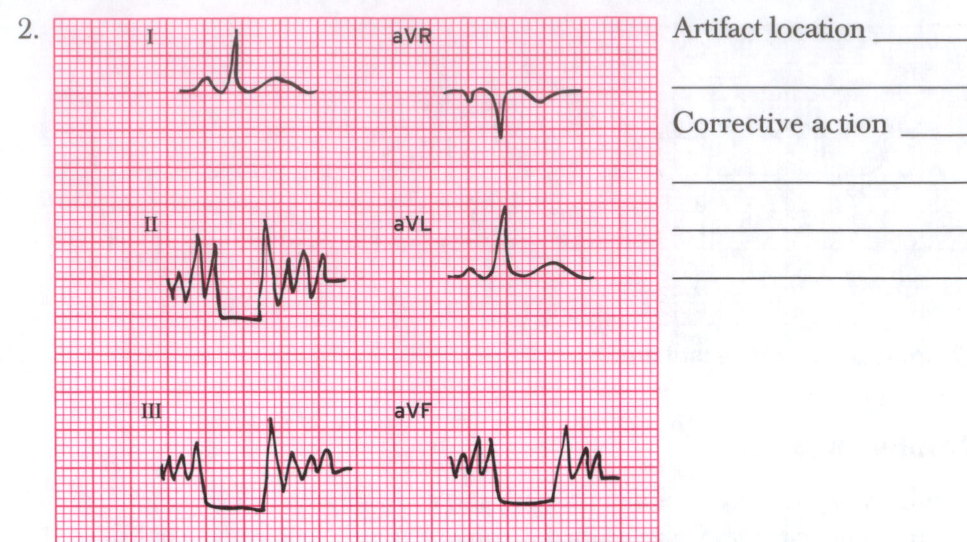

Artifact location ______

______

Corrective action ______

______

______

______

3.

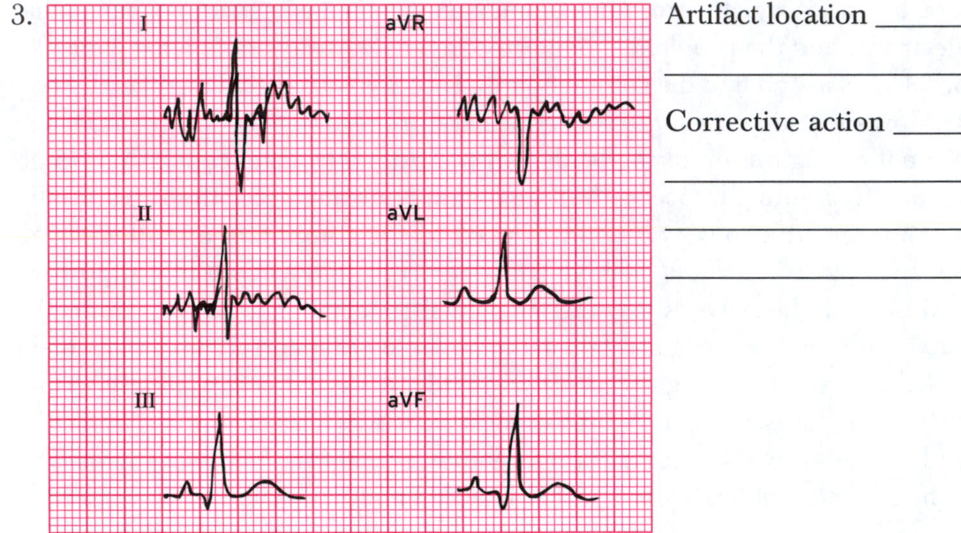

Artifact location ______

______

Corrective action ______

______

______

______

Answers to Artifact Troubleshooting Practice

1. The artifact is in leads **I, III,** and **aVL.** Corrective action is to check for and reattach or reconnect loose or disconnected electrodes or lead wires on the **left arm.** If an electrode patch is loose or missing, put on a new patch. *Never put a used patch back on. It will not stick well enough to ensure good impulse transmission.* How do we know the problem is on the left arm? Refer to Figure 4-7. What is the common limb shared by all these leads? I connects right arm and left arm. III connects left arm and left leg. aVL involves left arm only. The common limb is the left arm. Direct corrective efforts there.
2. The artifact is in leads **II, III,** and **aVF.** Corrective action is to check the **left leg** for loose or disconnected electrodes or lead wires and to reattach/reconnect them as necessary. What is the common limb? II connects right arm and left leg. III connects left arm and left leg. aVF involves left leg only. The common limb is the left leg.

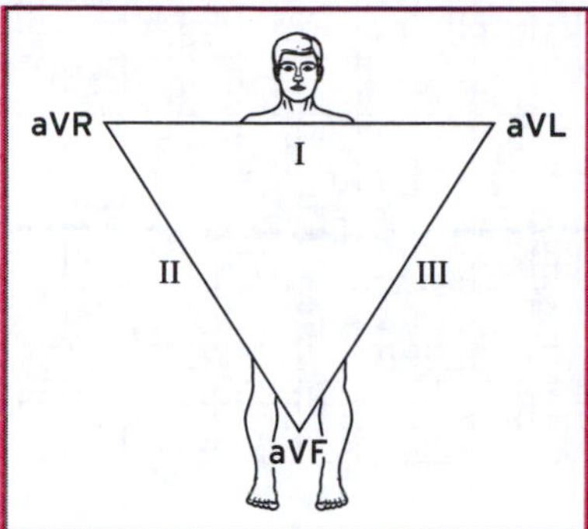

Figure 4-7 Leads.

3. The artifact is in leads **I, II,** and **aVR.** Corrective action is to check the **right arm** for loose or disconnected electrodes or lead wires and to reattach/reconnect them as necessary. What is the common limb? I connects right arm and left arm. II connects right arm and left leg. III involves right arm only. The common limb is the right arm.

Artifact Masquerading as Rhythms

Artifact can mimic rhythms quite convincingly, so much so that emergency teams are sometimes summoned to deal with patients with "life-threatening" rhythms that are later discovered to be nothing but artifact. The scenarios that follow will emphasize the importance of assessing the patient who has a change in rhythm. In other words, *do not always believe what you see on the rhythm strip. Check your patient.*

Artifact Masquerading as Asystole

Figure 4-8 is from an elderly man who'd had an MI two days prior. He was on the telemetry floor wearing a portable heart monitor. The nurse at the monitoring station saw this rhythm on the screen and ran into the patient's room. The patient was awake and feeling fine, but his rhythm indicated that his heart had completely stopped beating. Since this obviously was not the case, the nurse checked the man's monitor patches and wires and discovered several were loose or disconnected. She reconnected them and his rhythm pattern then returned to normal. Thus the rhythm in Figure 4-8 was *not* really a rhythm, but rather was **artifact** masquerading as a rhythm.

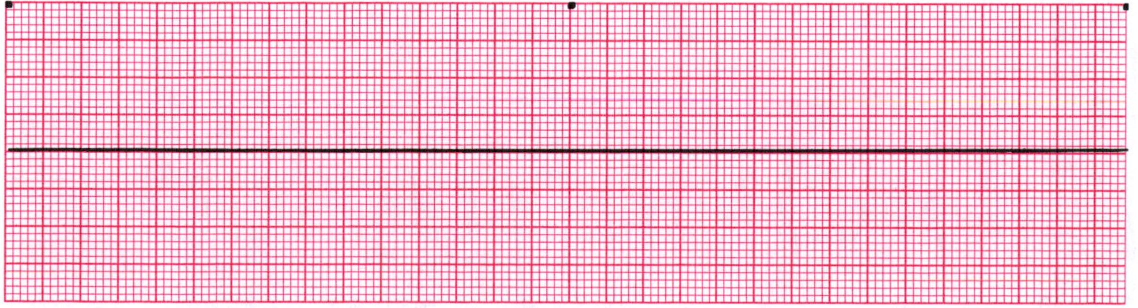

Figure 4-8 Artifact masquerading as asystole (flat-line).

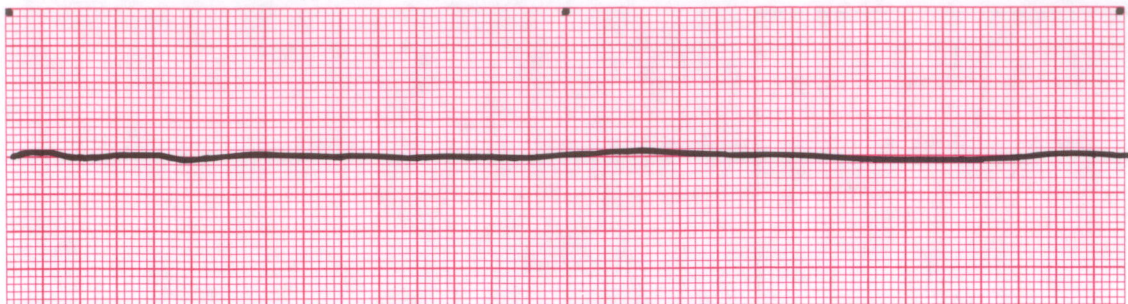

Figure 4-9 True asystole.

Now look at Figure 4-9. This is a strip of a heart that has indeed stopped beating. Notice the similarity between this strip and Figure 4-8.

"Toothbrush Tachycardia"

Mr. Johnson was brushing his teeth when the strip in Figure 4-10 printed out at the nurses's station, along with an auditory alarm that indicated the patient was experiencing a potentially fatal arrhythmia. The nurse, thinking Mr. Johnson was in a lethal rhythm, yelled for help and ran into Mr. Johnson's room to find him brushing his teeth and in no distress. The repetitive arm movements of his tooth brushing jiggled the EKG lead wires and caused a common type of artifact that healthcare workers sometimes refer to as "toothbrush tachycardia." When he stopped brushing his teeth, Mr. Johnson's rhythm strip returned to normal.

Now see Figure 4-11, this time of a patient in true lethal rhythm . Note the similarity.

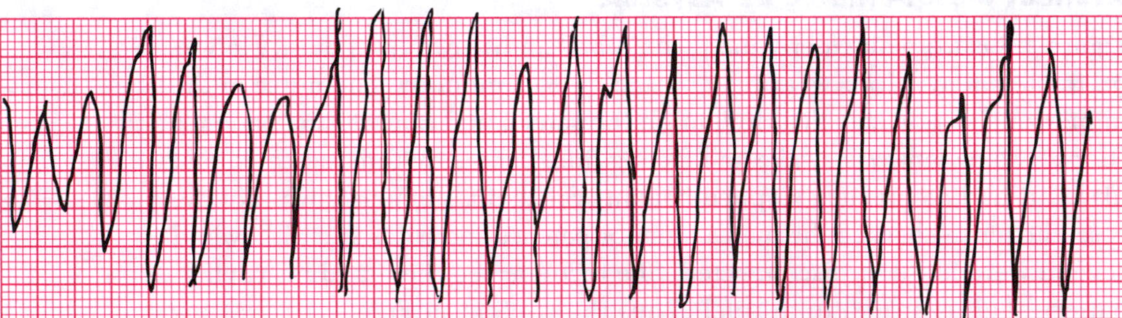

Figure 4-10 "Toothbrush tachycardia" masquerading as a rhythm.

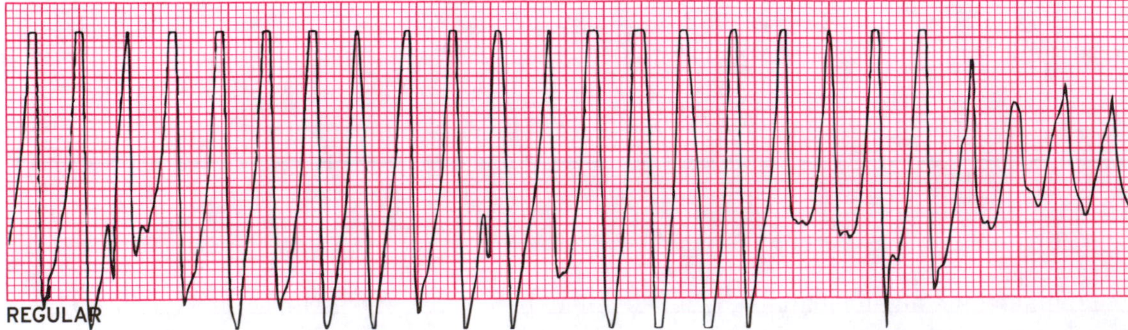

Figure 4-11 Ventricular tachycardia.

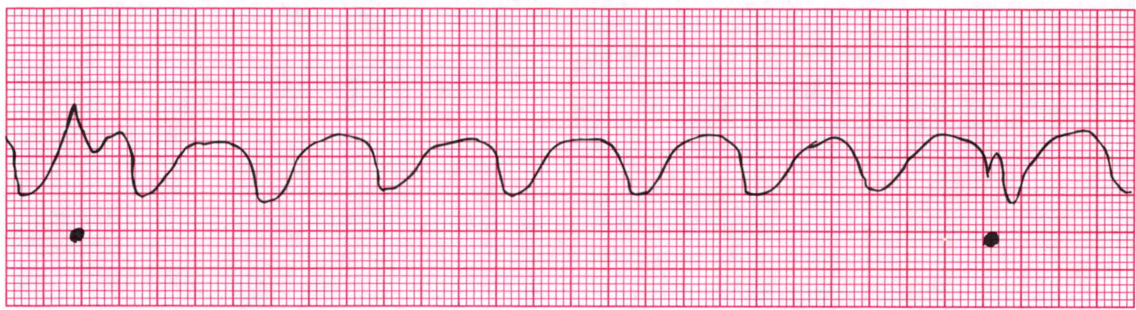

Figure 4-12 CPR artifact.

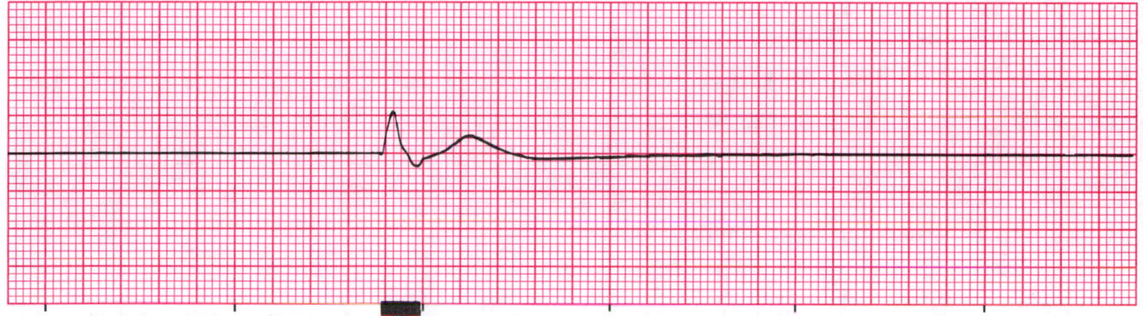

Figure 4-13 Rhythm without CPR artifact.

CPR Artifact

Artifact is seen frequently during resuscitation efforts. The external chest compressions of CPR produce artifact that can resemble rhythms. See Figure 4-12, in which the pattern resembles a rhythm with abnormally wide QRS complexes. But look closer. See the dots? Look above them. See how the pattern gets a bit spiked here? Those are the patient's own QRS complexes popping out. Now look at Figure 4-13. Here CPR was stopped momentarily to allow evaluation of the rhythm without CPR artifact.

In Figure 4-13, there is one QRS complex and then flatline. This is the patient's true rhythm. The two QRS complexes in the first strip were obviously the rhythm of a dying heart. The rest of the pattern in the first strip were simply pseudo-QRS complexes produced by CPR.

Artifact in Three Leads Monitored Simultaneously

Figure 4-14 is a beautiful example of artifact masquerading as a rhythm. This patient was being monitored simultaneously in three different leads—V_1, lead II, and lead I. *Since the three are recorded simultaneously, all three are the same rhythm, just seen in different leads.* Note that leads II and I look alike, with multiple spiked waves scattered between the QRS complexes. But V_1 looks different, with the normal P waves preceding each QRS complex. How can that be? The strips all have to be the same rhythm. Think about this for a moment. Consider the location of the electrodes composing each lead.

The answer is simple. The true rhythm is seen in V_1. Leads II and I have artifact that obscures the P waves and provides what looks like spiked waves. You'll recall that leads II and I are limb leads and are therefore subject to artifact from muscle movement. Since V_1 is a precordial lead and is located

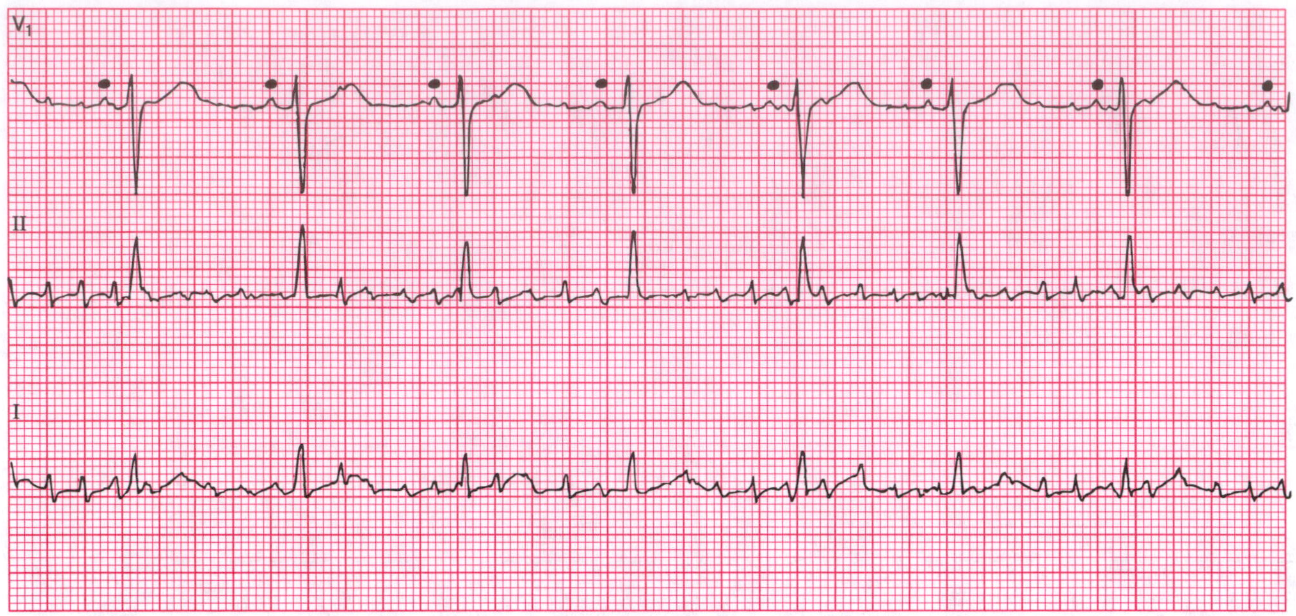

Figure 4-14 Artifact in three leads monitored simultaneously.

on the chest, it picks up less artifact. This patient, it turns out, had tremors from Parkinson's disease. That's what was causing the spiked artifact.

As you've seen, artifact can be very deceptive. Experts can pore over rhythm strips for quite a while trying to determine the legitimacy of the rhythm. *So how do you know if the rhythm you see is real or artifact?*

- If the rhythm you see is different from the patient's previous rhythm, *go check your patient.* Ask how he or she feels and check vital signs (respiratory rate, heart rate, and blood pressure). This is especially important if the rhythm appears to be life-threatening. Patients with life-threatening arrhythmias will exhibit symptoms of low cardiac output (not enough blood flow to meet the body's needs) and/or cardiovascular collapse. Artifact will not produce such symptoms.
- Observe the rhythm in another lead, preferably a lead such as V_1 or MCL_1, which has minimal muscle artifact.
- Check to be sure the "rhythm" meets all its normal criteria. If it doesn't, be suspicious and check another lead.
- Check the patient's monitor wires and patches to see if they are loose or detached.
- See if the patient is having any muscle activity that could cause artifact mimicking a rhythm.
- The bottom line is this: *Always check your patient, not just the monitor!*

QuickTip

Do not try to interpret a strip or EKG obscured by artifact! Redo the strip or EKG until you get a readable tracing. Remember the patient's treatment depends on accurate interpretation.

Telemetry Monitoring

Most hospitals have a floor dedicated to the care of patients on telemetry, which you recall is remote cardiac monitoring. Most or all of the patients on this floor are on telemetry, and the nurse or technician monitoring the telemetry desk is responsible for watching those patients' rhythms.

Patients on telemetry are often *ambulatory,* meaning they are able to get out of bed and walk around. As a result, artifact is not uncommon. The altered lead placement helps–you'll recall the 3-lead or 5-lead wires used in telemetry monitoring are all on the chest or abdomen instead of the arms and legs as with a 12-lead EKG–but artifact still occurs. Troubleshoot artifact the same way as with a 12-lead EKG.

Rhythm strips become part of the patient's permanent medical record, as do 12-lead EKGs. Unlike 12-lead EKGs, however, rhythm strips are small and must be mounted onto a standard-size page for inclusion in the record. The **telemetry monitoring sheet** is a special form for mounting and interpreting these rhythm strips. See a sample telemetry sheet, Figure 4-15. At the top of the form is a space for the patient's name and other identifying information.

Rhythm strips are mounted onto their slots on the form, usually by taping them from behind with double-sided tape. If tape touches the front of the strip, the rhythm beneath the tape will fade and become unreadable.

Telemetry Monitoring Analysis

Date ______

Rate ______

PR ______

QRS ______

QT ______

Analysis ______________________ Signature ______________

Date ______

Rate ______

PR ______

QRS ______

QT ______

Analysis ______________________ Signature ______________

Date ______

Rate ______

PR ______

QRS ______

QT ______

Analysis ______________________ Signature ______________

Figure 4-15 Sample telemetry monitoring sheet.

Each rhythm strip is examined for heart rate, intervals, and rhythm identification. If there are alarm limits set to alert the technician that the heart rate or rhythm has violated those settings, those alarm limits are documented as well. Most monitors are equipped with alarm limits that can be set by the technician.

Rhythm strips are obtained at intervals that vary from institution to institution, but are typically once every four to eight hours, and also in between if rhythm or rate changes occur. The goal is to provide a representative sample of the patient's rhythms throughout the day. This will enable the physician to assess the effect of treatment and to diagnose arrhythmias (rhythm abnormalities). For example, say a patient is being treated with medication to slow down her very rapid heart rate. Yesterday, when the medication was started, her heart rate was 145. Today, four doses later, her heart rate is 122. Telemetry has documented that the treatment is working.

Practice Quiz

1. What is the function of the EKG machine? ______________________
____
2. Normal chart speed for running a 12-lead EKG is ________ millimeters per second.
3. What does the sensitivity control do? ______________________
____
4. How much should the stylus be deflected when 1 millivolt of electricity is thrown into the system? ______________________
____
5. Define *macroshock*. ______________________
____
6. Define *microshock*. ______________________
____
7. The first anatomic landmark to look for when placing electrodes is the ____
____
8. Name the four kinds of artifact. ______________________
____
____
____
9. If there is artifact in leads I, aVR, and II, toward which limb would you direct your troubleshooting efforts? ______________________
10. List three ways to determine if a rhythm is real or artifact. __________
____

Putting It All Together–Critical Thinking Exercises

1. Your patient, who is on telemetry monitoring, is noted to have two electrodes that have fallen off–the right arm and left foot. In what leads would you expect to see artifact? ______________________________
____
____

2. Explainhow you would know that your patient is having artifact and not a life-threatening dysrhythmia (abnormal heart rhythm)? ______________
____
____
____

Calculating Heart Rate

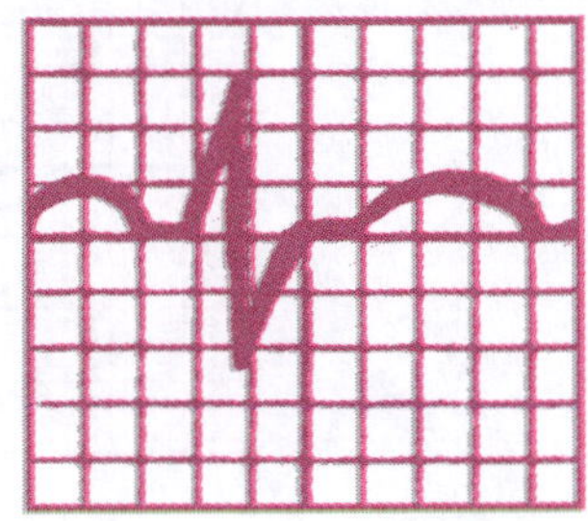

Chapter 5 Objectives

Upon completion of this chapter, the student will be able to:

- Define *heart rate.*
- Calculate the heart rate on a variety of strips, using the different methods.
- Differentiate between the three types of rhythm regularity.
- Tell what kind of heart rate to calculate for the different kinds of rhythm regularity.

Introduction

Calculating heart rate involves counting the number of QRS complexes in one minute and is recorded in **beats per minute.** Heart rate is the same as **ventricular rate.** We can also determine the **atrial rate** by counting P waves, but the bottom line is this: When we calculate heart rate, we count QRS complexes. Though the most accurate way to determine the heart rate would be to run a minute-long rhythm strip and count every QRS complex, this is extremely time-consuming and impractical. Imagine calculating the heart rate of 40 patients on a telemetry floor. It would take close to an hour–obviously not the most practical use of time. So we use other methods to calculate heart rate, and these methods all use a 6- or 12-second rhythm strip and the following premise: If the heart rate stays for the full minute as it is right now, at the end of that minute the heart rate will be so-and-so. That's a big leap of faith, since the second we print out our rhythm strip, the heart rate could change drastically. Nevertheless, the following methods have been used for years and are the next best thing to counting the whole minute's worth of QRS complexes.

Methods for Calculating Heart Rate

- **The 6-second strip method.** This is the least accurate of all the methods. Though it is considered by many experts to be the method of choice for irregular rhythms, it does not give much information and can be misleading. Using this method, count the number of QRS complexes on a 6-second rhythm strip and multiply by 10. This tells the **mean rate,** or average rate. If there are 3 QRS complexes on a 6-second strip, for example, the rate would be 30 beats per minute. (If there are 3 QRS complexes in 6 seconds, there would be 30 in 60 seconds, or 1 minute.) See Figure 5-1.

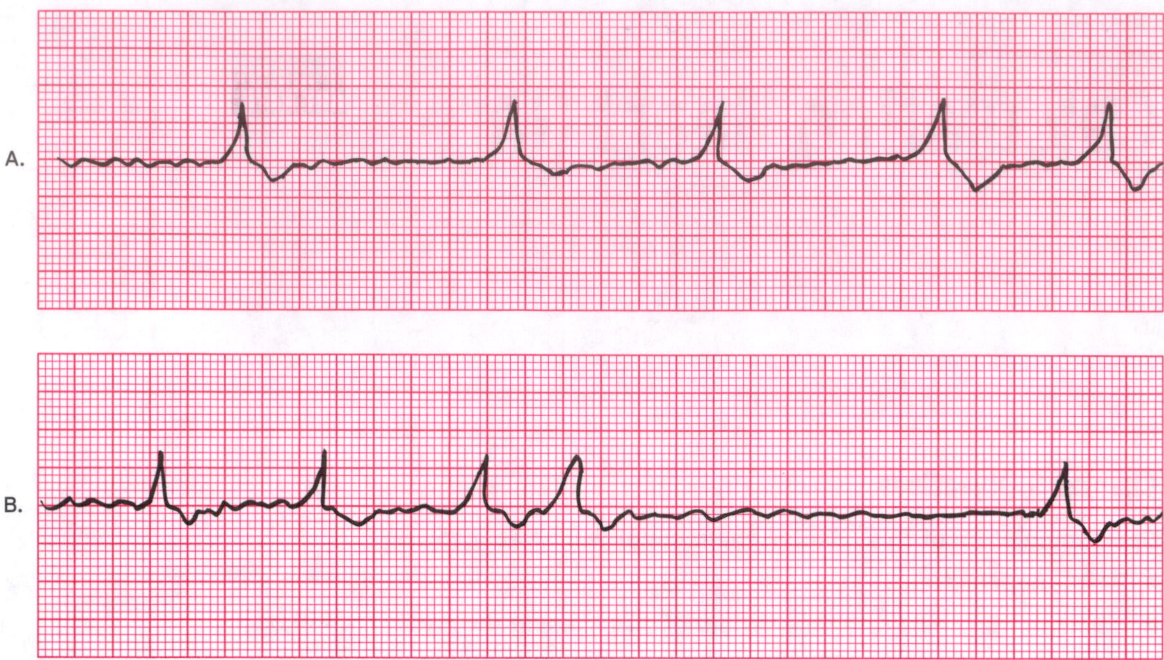

Figure 5-1 Two rhythms, both with mean rate of 50.

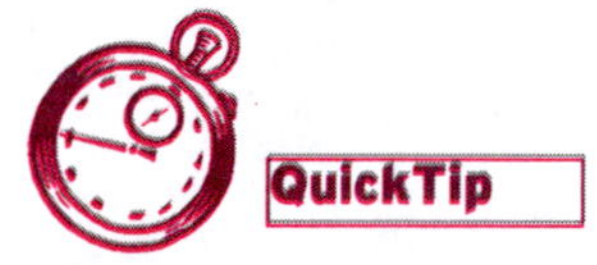

Do not use the 6-second strip method by itself to calculate heart rate! Use the memory method or the little-block method.

In Figure 5-1, both strips have 5 QRS complexes in 6 seconds, so both have a mean rate of 50. Though both rhythms are irregular, with QRS complexes unevenly spaced throughout the strip, strip B is much more irregular than strip A. In fact, the heart rate in strip A varies only from a rate of 40 to a rate of 68 beats per minute (you'll learn that soon), whereas strip B varies from a rate of 23 to 137 beats per minute. Obviously, strip B has wild heart rate swings. Saying the mean rate is 50 doesn't really provide adequate information. Since treatment for rhythm disturbances depends in large part on the heart rate, it makes more sense to provide a *range* of heart rates from the slowest to the fastest, in addition to the mean rate. If a person is being treated with medication to slow down a fast heart rate, for example, it is important to know how slow and how fast the heart rate is in order to determine the effectiveness of treatment. A mean rate alone simply does not provide this information–the heart rate range does. The heart rate range is calculated using one of the other methods. Bottom line: The mean heart rate, as determined using the 6-second strip method, should only be used along with the heart rate range. It is not adequate by itself.

- **The memory method.** This is the fastest method and is widely used in hospitals. See Table 5-1. The number of big blocks between QRS complexes is divided into 300 to arrive at the answer. Since there are 300 big blocks every minute, if you count the number of big blocks between consecutive QRS complexes and divide that number into 300, you end up with the sequence below.

Memorize the sequence 300–150–100–75–60–50–43–37–33–30. Using this memory method, what would the heart rate be if there were five big blocks between QRS complexes? One big block would be 300, two would be 150, three would be 100, four would be 75, and five would be 60. So the

Table 5-1 Memory Method of Calculating Heart Rate

NUMBER OF BIG BLOCKS BETWEEN QRS	HEART RATE	NUMBER OF BIG BLOCKS BETWEEN QRS	HEART RATE
1	300	6	50
2	150	7	43
3	100	8	37
4	75	9	33
5	60	10	30

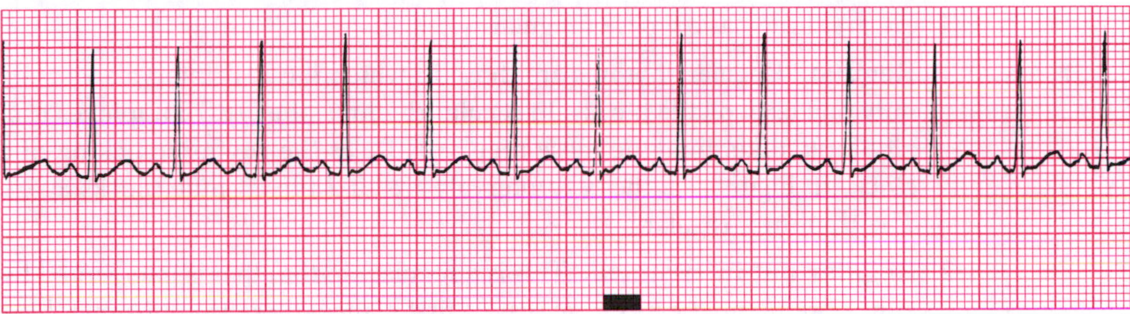

Figure 5-2 Little block method of calculating heart rate.

heart rate would be 60. *Memorize this sequence of numbers!* It will save you lots of time.

- **The little block method.** In this method, count the number of little blocks between QRS complexes and divide into 1,500, since there are 1,500 little blocks in one minute. By now you're thinking, "You've got to be kidding! Count those tiny blocks?!" (You may well be in bifocals by the end of this chapter.) Actually, it's not that bad. Remember each big block is made up of five little blocks. Simply count each big block as five and the leftover little blocks as one. See Figure 5-2.

In Figure 5-2, there are 11 little blocks between QRS complexes, so the calculation is 1,500 ÷ 11 = 137. You can also use this method to calculate the heart rate range in irregular rhythms. Just find the two consecutive QRS complexes that are the farthest apart from each other and calculate that heart rate there–that's the slowest rate. Then find the two consecutive QRS complexes that are the closest together and calculate the heart rate there–that's the fastest rate.

Regularity-Based Heart Rate Calculation

Heart rate calculation is regularity-based. The kind of heart rate you calculate will depend on the rhythm's regularity. **Rhythm regularity** is concerned with the constancy of the QRS complexes. Though we can also determine **atrial regularity** by examining constancy of P waves, this chapter focuses on regularity of the QRS complexes. To determine the regularity of a rhythm, compare the **R-R intervals** (the distance between consecutive QRS complexes). To compare R-Rs, count the number of little blocks between QRS complexes.

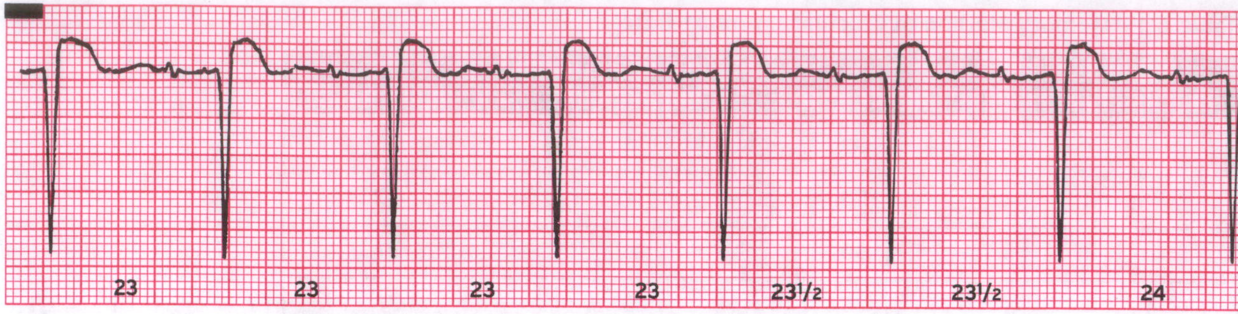

Figure 5-3 Regular rhythm.

Regularity Types

There are three basic types of regularity.

1. **Regular.** Regular rhythms are those in which the R-R intervals vary by only one or two little blocks. In regular rhythms, the QRS complexes usually look alike. Imagine these regular R-Rs as the rhythmic ticking of a clock. In Figure 5-3, the R-R intervals are all 23 to 24 little blocks apart. The rhythm is regular.

2. **Regular but interrupted.** This is a regular rhythm that is interrupted by either premature beats or pauses. At first glance, these rhythms may look irregular, but closer inspection reveals that only one or two beats, or a burst of several beats, make them look irregular, and that the rest of the R-R intervals are constant. The beats that interrupt this otherwise regular rhythm may look the same as the surrounding regular beats or may look quite different. Some texts would say that a rhythm that is interrupted by premature beats or pauses is indeed not regular and must therefore be called irregular. This text, however, makes the distinction between a rhythm that is regular except for an occasional "hiccup" and rhythms that are "all over the place" in their irregularity.

   In Figure 5-4, the rhythm is regular until the sixth QRS pops in prematurely. *Premature beats* are those that arrive early, before the next normal beat is due. Typically, after a premature beat, there is a short pause, then the regular rhythm resumes. That's what happened on this strip. The R-R intervals are 15 to 16 little blocks apart except where beat number 6 popped in. Think of premature beats as hiccups. Imagine you're breathing normally and suddenly you hiccup. This hiccup pops in between your normal breaths and temporarily disturbs the regularity of

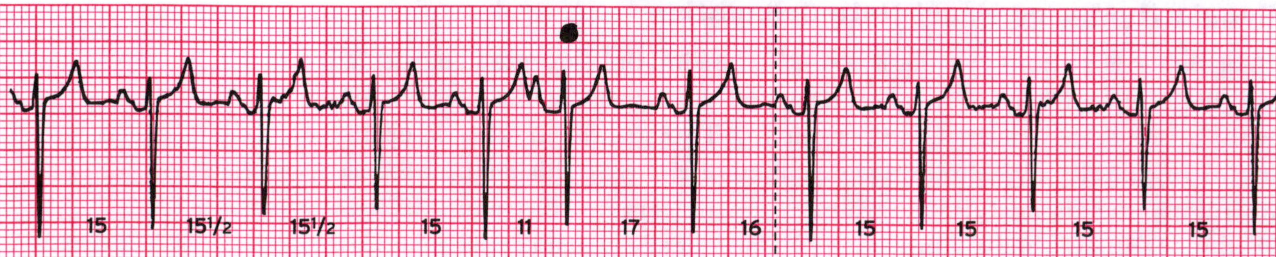

Figure 5-4 Regular rhythm interrupted by a premature beat.

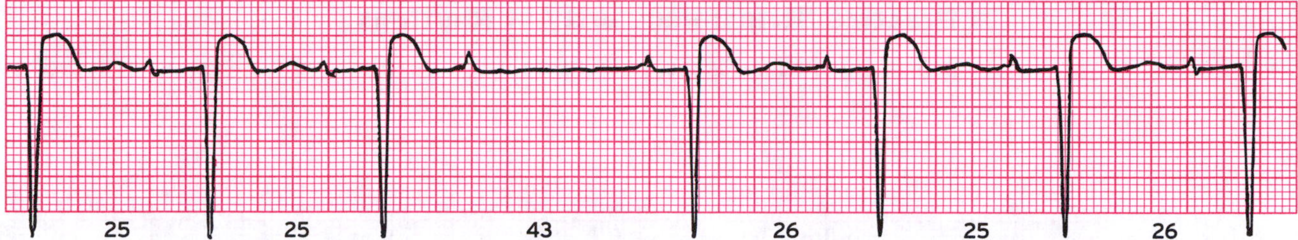

Figure 5-5 Regular rhythm interrupted by a pause.

your breathing pattern. Afterward, your breathing returns to normal. You wouldn't characterize your breathing pattern as irregular just because of one hiccup.

In Figure 5-5, the rhythm is regular until a sudden pause temporarily disturbs the regularity of the rhythm. Before and after the pause, the R-R intervals are constant–25 to 26 little blocks apart. During the pause, the R-R is 43 little blocks. Imagine these pauses are like a sudden power outage. Say you've got an electric clock ticking regularly, and suddenly, the power goes out for a few seconds, then comes back on. The outage temporarily disturbs the clock's otherwise normal, regular ticking pattern.

3. **Irregular.** Irregular rhythms are those in which the R-R intervals vary, not just because of premature beats or pauses, but because the rhythm is intrinsically chaotic. R-R intervals will vary throughout the strip. Imagine these varying R-Rs as the interval of time between rain showers. Maybe it rains once a week for two weeks in a row, then it rains again in three weeks, then after a month passes, then after a week and a half, then two months. The pattern is one of unpredictability–it happens when it happens.

In Figure 5-6, the R-R intervals are all over the place. Some QRS complexes are close together, others are farther apart. There is no sudden change, no regular pattern interrupted by a premature beat or pause. From beat to beat, the R-Rs vary. This is an intrinsically irregular rhythm. Do you see the difference between this rhythm and the strips of the regular but interrupted rhythms? *Whenever you see a rhythm that looks irregular, look closely to make sure it's not a regular but interrupted rhythm.* Let's practice a few.

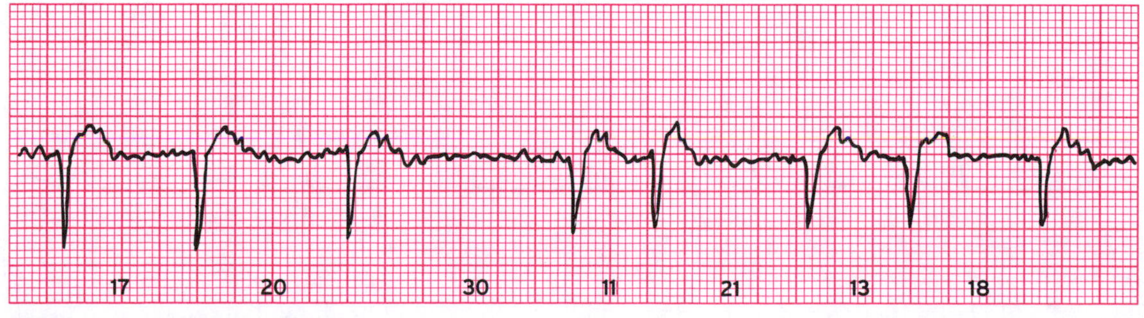

Figure 5-6 Irregular rhythm.

Practice Strips: Regularity of Rhythms

For each of these strips, determine if it is regular, regular but interrupted, or irregular.

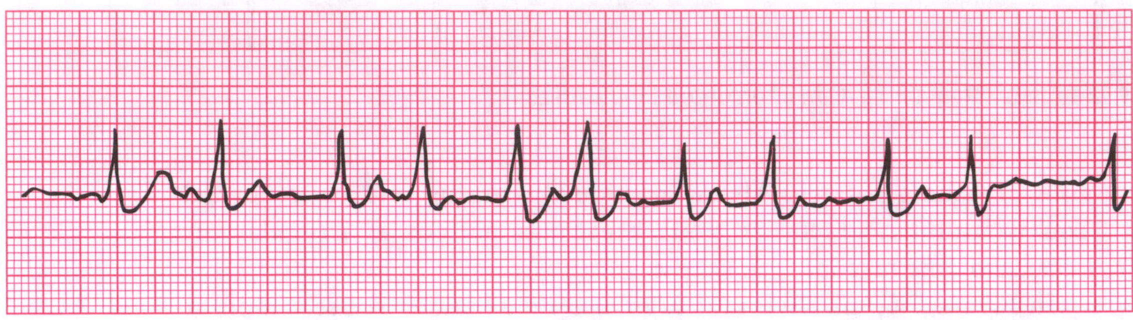

1. Answer ______________________

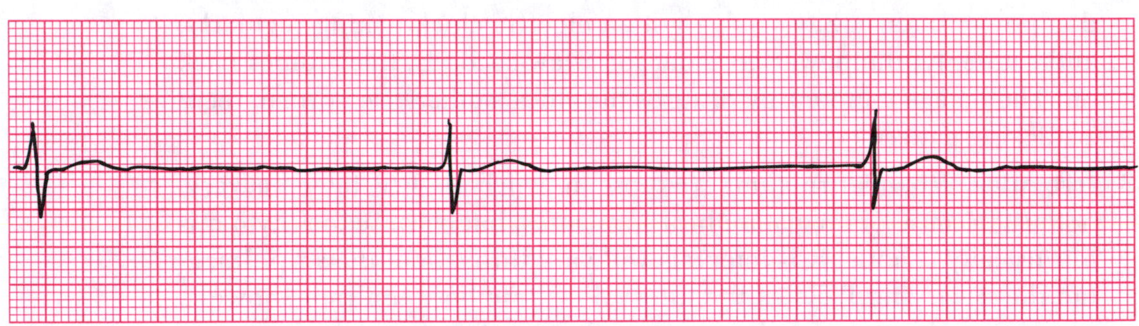

2. Answer ______________________

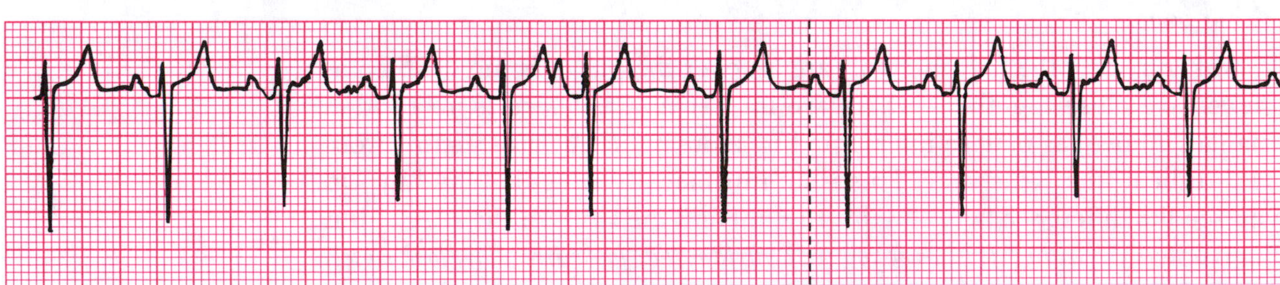

3. Answer ______________________

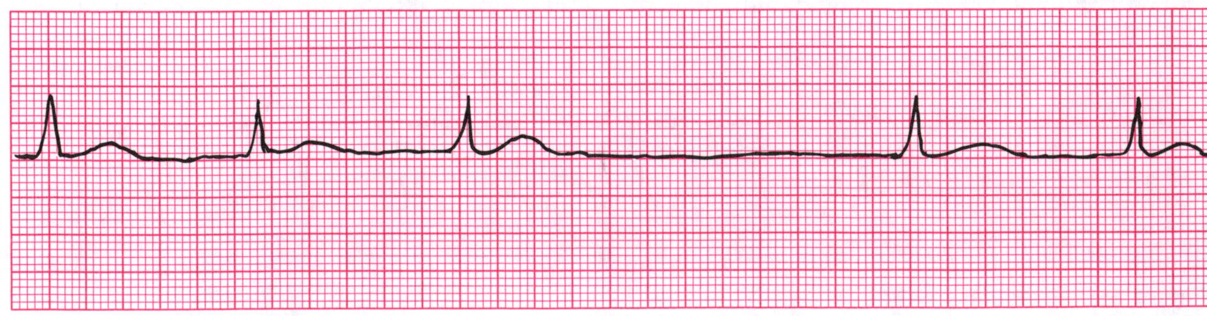

4. Answer ______________________

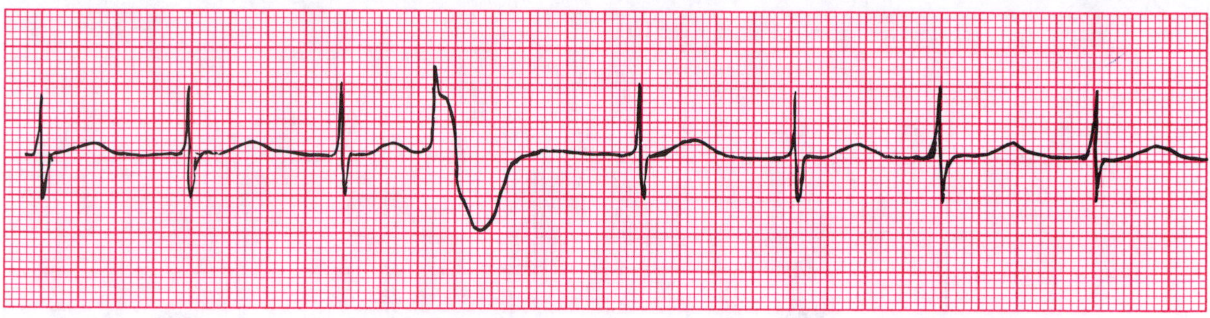

5. Answer ____

Answers to Regularity Practice Strips

1. **Irregular.** The R-R intervals are all over the place, with no hint of regularity.
2. **Regular.** The R-R intervals are all about 56 little blocks.
3. **Regular but interrupted.** This is the strip shown a few pages ago as an example of regular but interrupted rhythms. Look back if you don't recognize it.
4. **Regular but interrupted.** The R-R intervals are all 28 to 29 blocks except for the long pause that interrupts this otherwise regular rhythm.
5. **Regular but interrupted.** Again, the R-R intervals are regular before and after the premature beat (and the expected short pause after it).

Kind of Heart Rate to Calculate for Different Types of Regularity

- **For regular rhythms,** calculate the heart rate by choosing any two successive QRS complexes and using the little block method.
- **For irregular rhythms,** calculate the mean rate by using the 6-second strip method, then calculate the heart rate range using the little block method.
- **For rhythms that are regular but interrupted by premature beats,** ignore the premature beats and calculate the heart rate, using the little block method, on an uninterrupted part of the strip. Premature beats do not impact the heart rate much, as they are typically followed by a short pause that at least partially, if not completely, makes up for the prematurity of the beat. See Figure 5-7. In Figure 5-7, the fifth QRS is a premature beat. Ignore this premature beat for purposes of heart rate calculation. The heart rate is 100.

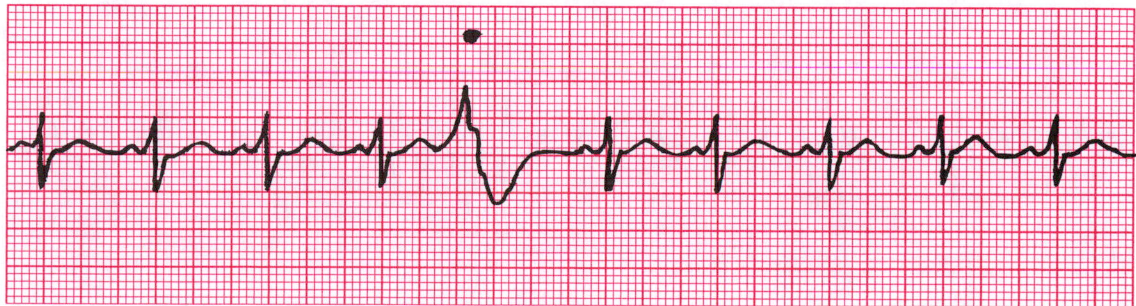

Figure 5-7 Regular rhythm interrupted by a premature beat.

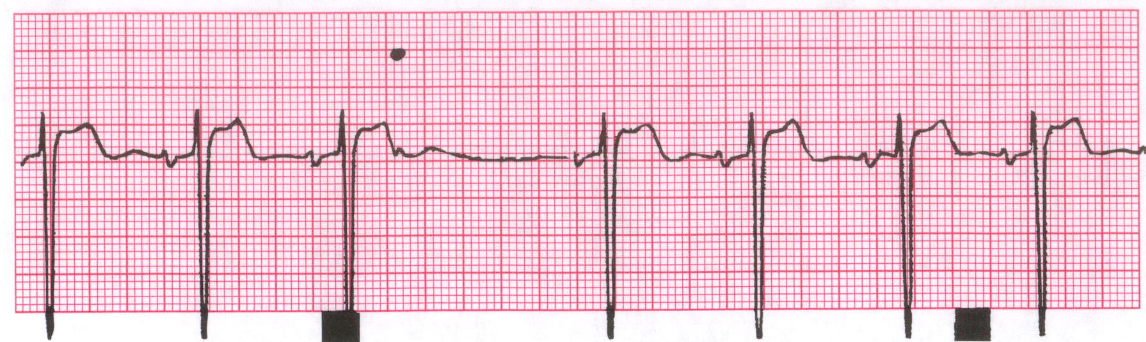

Figure 5-8 Regular rhythm interrupted by a pause.

Table 5-2 Kind of Heart Rate to Calculate for Different Types of Regularity

RHYTHM REGULARITY	KIND OF HEART RATE TO CALCULATE
Regular	One heart rate
Irregular	Range slowest to fastest, plus mean rate
Regular but interrupted by premature beats	One heart rate (ignoring premature beats)
Regular but interrupted by pauses	Range slowest to fastest, plus mean rate

- **For rhythms that are regular but interrupted by pauses,** calculate the heart rate range slowest to fastest, along with the mean rate. Since pauses can be very lengthy, they can greatly impact the heart rate, so it's important to take them into account when calculating heart rate. See Figure 5-8.

In Figure 5-8, the regular rhythm is interrupted by a pause. Here the mean rate is 70, since there are 7 QRS complexes on this 6-second strip. There are 34 little blocks between the third and fourth QRS complexes, giving a rate of 44. There are 20 little blocks between the remainder of QRS complexes, for a heart rate of 75. The heart rate range is 44 to 75.

To sum up, see Table 5-2.

Calculating heart rate is a basic skill you will use throughout this book, and indeed throughout your work with EKGs. With practice, you will become expert at it. Now let's get to the practice.

Practice Strips: Calculating Heart Rate

Calculate the heart rate on these strips.

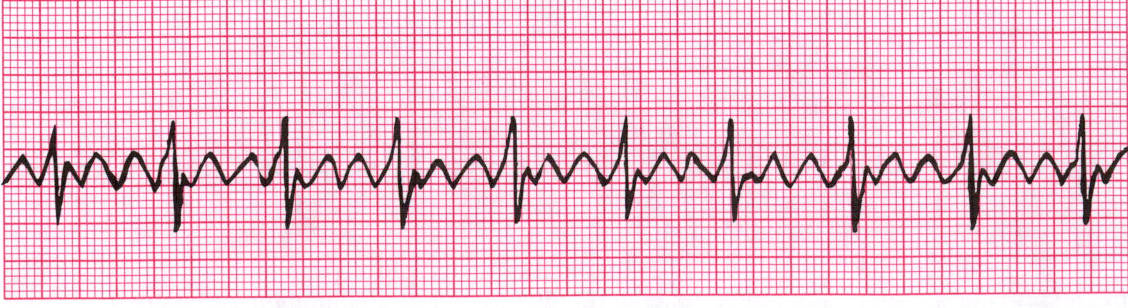

1. Heart rate ______________________________

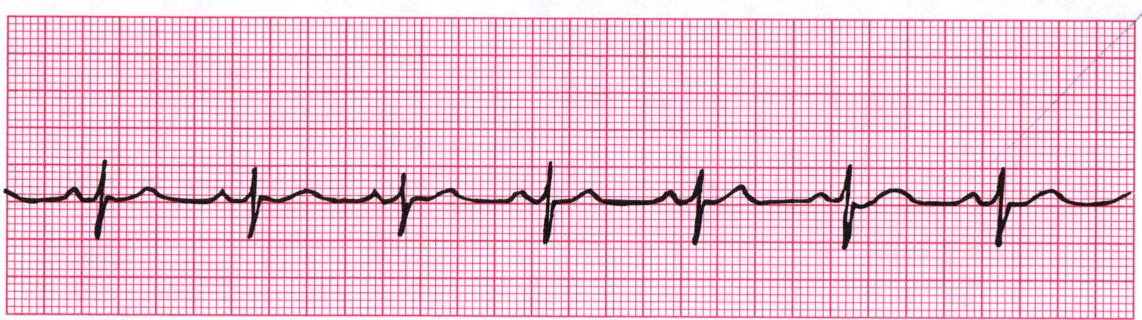

2. Heart rate ______________________________

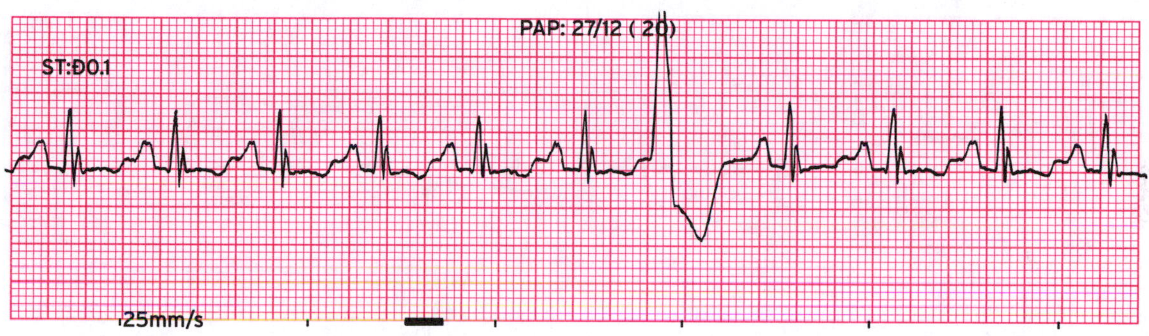

3. Heart rate ______________________________

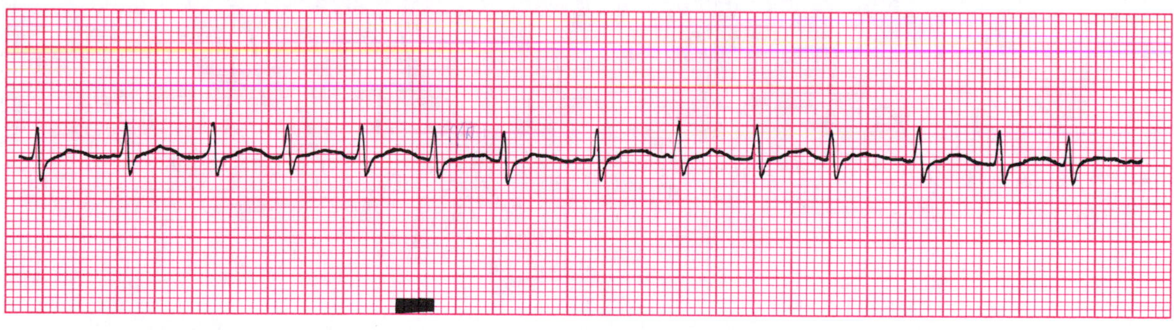

4. Heart rate ______________________________

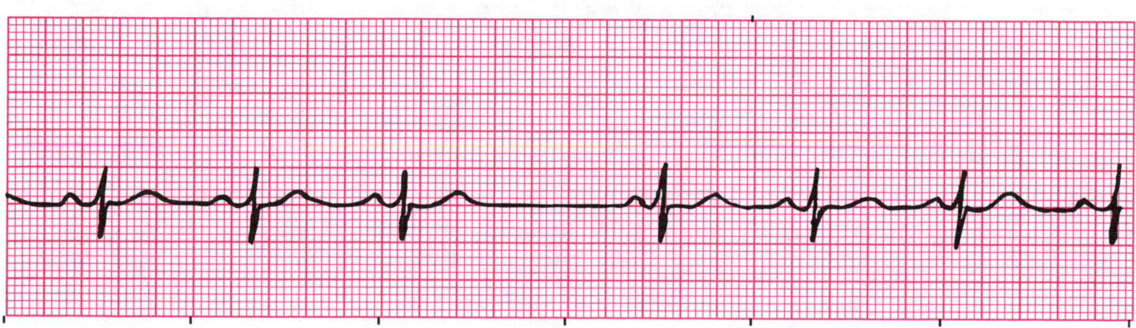

5. Heart rate ______________________________

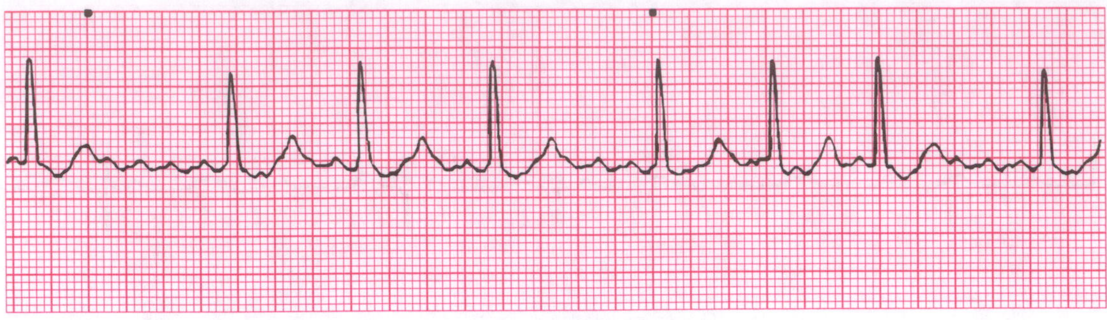

6. Heart rate ______________________________

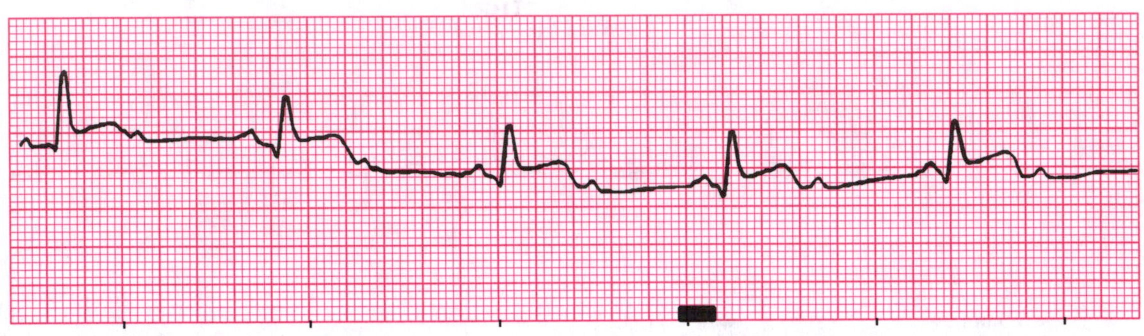

7. Heart rate ______________________________

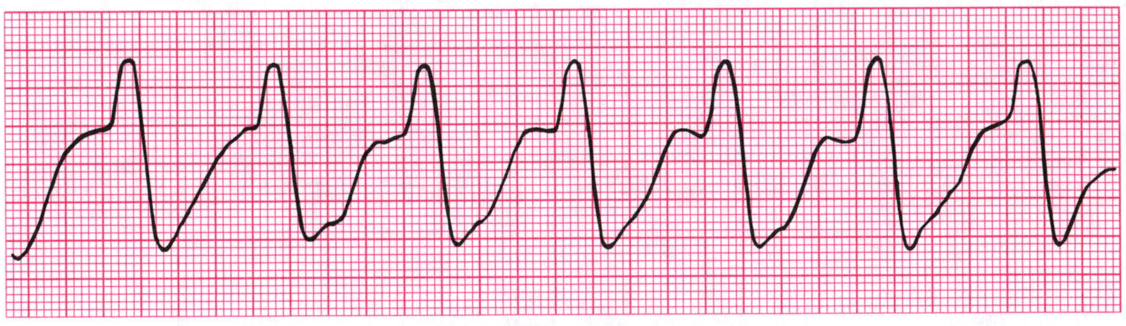

8. Heart rate ______________________________

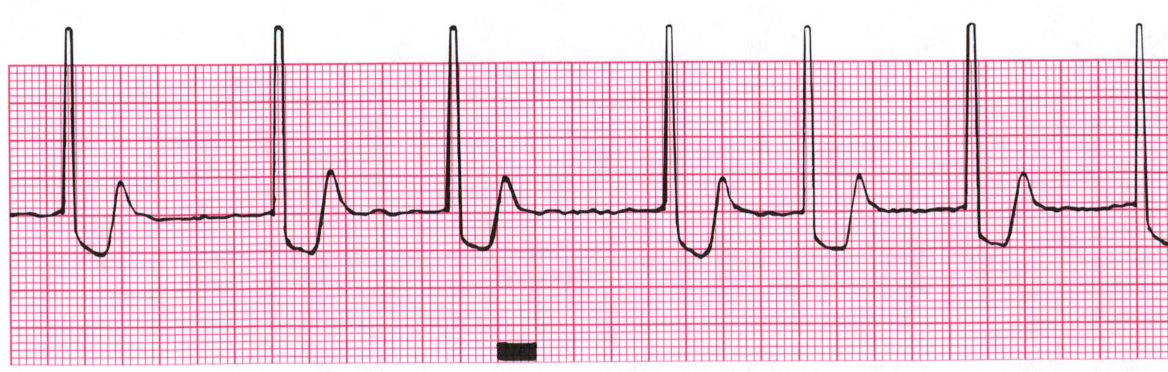

9. Heart rate ______________________________

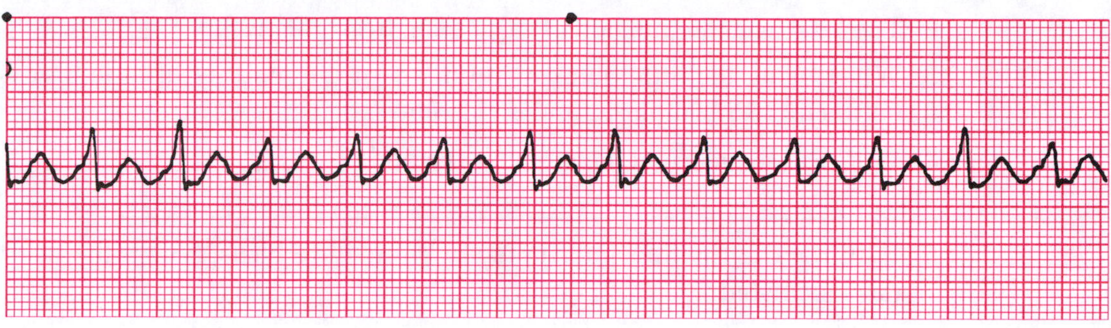

10. Heart rate ____________________

Answers to Calculating Heart Rate Practice

1. This is a regular rhythm, so choose any two consecutive QRS complexes and calculate the heart rate there. There are 15 little blocks between QRSs. Divide 1,500 ÷ 15 for the little block method. The heart rate is **100.**
2. Another regular rhythm. The heart rate is **75.**
3. This is a regular rhythm interrupted by a premature beat. We therefore ignore the premature beat for the purposes of heart rate calculation. The heart rate is **107,** as there are 14 little blocks between QRS complexes.
4. Though at first glance this rhythm appears regular, closer examination reveals that the R-R intervals vary from 91/2 to 121/2 little blocks apart. Since it is an irregular rhythm, we need the heart rate range along with the mean rate. The range is **about 120 to 155, with a mean rate of 140.**
5. This is a regular rhythm interrupted by a pause, so we calculate the range and the mean rate. There are 35 little blocks during the pause, and 20 little blocks between the regular QRS complexes. The heart rate range is therefore **43 to 75, with a mean rate of 70.**
6. This is an irregular rhythm. The **mean heart rate is 80 and the range is 56 to 107.** The first two QRS complexes are the farthest apart on the strip and thus represent the slowest heart rate (56). The 6th and 7th QRS complexes are the closest together and represent the fastest heart rate on the strip (107).
7. Here the rhythm is regular. Heart rate is **50.**
8. The QRS complexes are HUGE on this strip, but the rhythm is regular. Heart rate is **75.**
9. The rhythm is irregular. Heart rate **range is 52 to 81, with a mean rate of 70.**
10. The rhythm is regular. Heart rate is **130.**

Practice Quiz

1. Name the three methods for calculating heart rate. ____________________

____

____

____

2. The least accurate method of calculating heart rate is the ____________
3. When using the little block method, count the number of little blocks between QRS complexes and divide into ____________
4. Write the sequence of the memory method. ____________

   ____
5. With regular rhythms interrupted by premature beats, how is the heart rate calculated? ____________

   ____
6. Name the three types of regularity. ____________

   ____

   ____
7. A rhythm with R-R intervals that vary throughout the____________ strip is a rhythm.
8. A rhythm that is regular except for premature beats or pauses is a ____________ rhythm.
9. A rhythm in which the R-R intervals vary by only one or two little blocks is a ____________ rhythm.
10. Define R-R interval. ____________

    ____

Putting It All Together—Critical Thinking Exercises

These exercises may consist of diagrams to label, scenarios to analyze, brain-stumping questions to ponder, or other challenging exercises to boost your understanding of the chapter material.

1. A rhythm whose R-R intervals are 23, 24, 23, 23, 12, 24, 23, 24, 23, 23 would be considered what kind of regularity? ____________. What's the heart rate? ____________
2. A rhythm with R-R intervals of 12, 17, 22, 45, 10, and 18 would be considered what type of regularity? ____________. What's the heart rate? ____________
3. A rhythm with R-R intervals of 22, 23, 22, 22, 23, 22, 22, 22 would be considered what kind of regularity? ____________ What's the heart rate? ____________

CHAPTER **6**

How to Interpret a Rhythm Strip

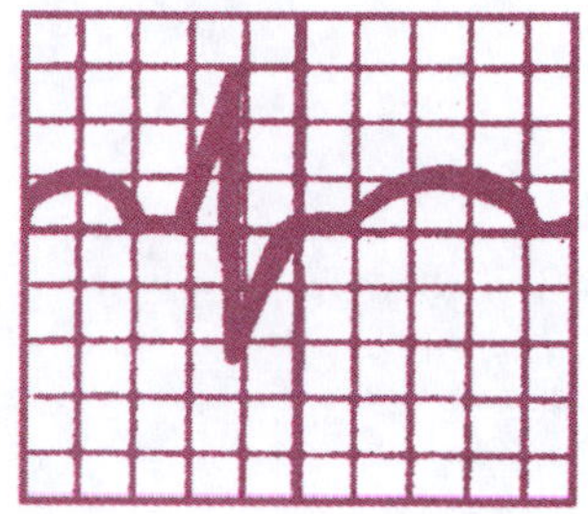

Chapter 6 Objectives

Upon completion of this chapter, the student will be able to:

- Use the five steps to interpret a variety of rhythms.

Introduction

When we analyze a rhythm strip, we are looking for pathology in the form of dysrhythmias (abnormal rhythms). Dysrhythmias can originate in any of the heart's pacemakers. Some of these rhythms are benign, causing no problem, and others are lethal, killing almost instantly. It's important to know not just what rhythm the patient is in now, but what rhythm preceded it and what's normal for this particular patient. Every patient is an individual, and what is "normal" for one person may not be what the textbooks say is normal. Even so-called "normal" rhythms or heart rates can be cause for concern. For example, if a patient has a heart rate of 110 (abnormally fast) for two consecutive days, and it suddenly drops to 66, which is normal, it may be a sign of trouble–the heart rate may be at 66 on its way to 0. *Always look at the trend.* Only so much information can be obtained from a single rhythm strip. Comparing the present rhythm strip to previous ones paints a better picture of the patient's condition.

It's important to *treat the patient, not just the rhythm.* As a rule, any significant change in rhythm or heart rate should prompt an immediate assessment of the patient's condition. Two patients can have the same rhythm and heart rate, but differ drastically in their tolerance of it. If the patient has a rhythm you cannot immediately identify, but it's a change from previously, *check on the patient and come back to the strip later.* The patient's life may well depend on your prompt action.

The Five Steps to Rhythm Interpretation

It's important to have a "plan of attack" in analyzing EKG rhythms. In the previous chapters you learned how to identify the waves and complexes on rhythm strips, and how to calculate the heart rate and measure intervals. Let's put all that together now. Asking the following questions for each rhythm strip will help to identify the rhythm (see CD-ROM for a video showing dysrhythmia):

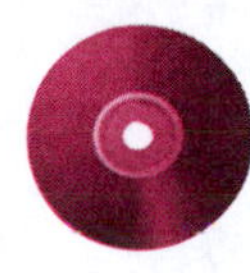

1. Are there QRS complexes? There are a few rhythms that have no QRS complexes at all, so look for the QRS complexes first. It can save you some time and trouble.
    - If yes, are they the same shape, or does the shape vary?
    - If no, skip to question 4.
2. Is the rhythm regular, regular but interrupted, or irregular?
    - Compare the R-R intervals.

3. What is the heart rate?
   - If the heart rate is greater than 100, the patient is said to have a **tachycardia.**
   - If the heart rate is less than 60, the patient has a **bradycardia.**
4. Are there P waves?
   - If so, what is their relationship to the QRS? In other words, are the Ps always in the same place relative to the QRS, or are the Ps in different places with each beat?
   - Are any Ps not followed by a QRS?
   - Are the Ps all the same shape, or does the shape vary?
   - Is the **P-P interval** (the distance between consecutive P waves) regular?
5. What are the PR and QRS intervals?
   - Are the intervals within normal limits, or are they too short or too long?
   - Are the intervals constant on the strip, or do they vary from beat to beat?

What Is Normal?

You'll recall that the heart's normal pacemaker is the sinus node. The normal rhythm originating from the sinus node is called **sinus rhythm.** Normal sinus rhythms have the following:

- Narrow QRS complexes of uniform shape.
- Regularly spaced QRS complexes.
- Heart rate between 60 and 100.
- Upright, rounded, matching P waves "married to" the QRS complexes (in the same place preceding each QRS).
- PR interval between 0.12 to 0.20 seconds, constant from beat to beat.
- QRS interval less than 0.12 seconds.

Dysrhythmias, on the other hand, will exhibit some combination of the following:

- QRS complexes that are absent or abnormally shaped.
- P waves that are absent, multiple in number, or abnormally shaped.
- Abnormally prolonged or abnormally short PR intervals.
- Abnormally prolonged QRS intervals.
- Heart rate that is abnormally slow or abnormally fast.
- Irregular rhythm or a rhythm that has interruptions by premature beats or pauses.

The Five Steps Practice

Let's practice the five steps on the five rhythm strips that follow:

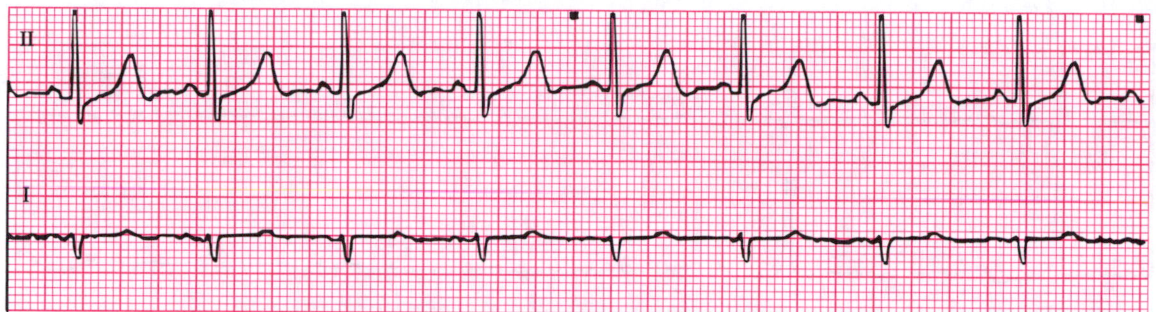

1. Note this is a double-lead strip. The top strip is labeled lead II, and the bottom is lead I. Use either lead (whichever one is clearer to you) to gather your data about the strips. **QRS complexes:** There are QRS complexes on the strip. They are all shaped the same (in each lead). **Regularity:** The rhythm is regular, as evidenced by the R-R intervals all measuring about 18 small blocks. **Heart rate:** Since the rhythm is regular we choose any two successive QRS complexes and calculate the heart rate there. 1500 divided by 18 equals a heart rate of 83. **P waves:** There are upright matching P waves preceding each QRS. P waves are "married" to the QRS complexes–they are in the same place relative to the QRS. All P waves are followed by a QRS. P-P interval is regular, meaning the P waves are regularly spaced. **PR interval:** PR interval is about 0.12 seconds (normal) and is constant from beat to beat **QRS interval:** QRS interval is about 0.08 seconds (normal, constant beat to beat).

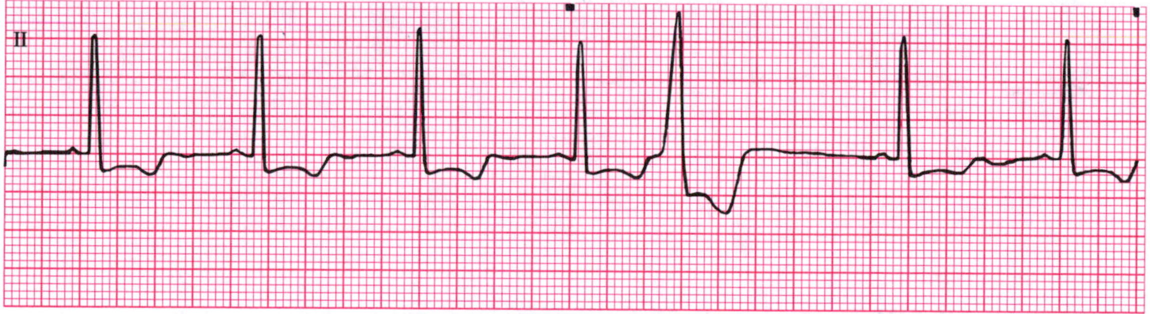

2. **QRS complexes:** There are QRS complexes, all but one of which is narrow and shaped the same. The fifth QRS is taller and wider than the others. **Regularity:** regular but interrupted by a premature beat. The R-R intervals are 21, 21 1/2, 21, 13 (the premature beat), 30 (the normal pause following a premature beat), and 21. **Heart rate:** 1,500 divided by 21 equals 71. **P waves:** upright and matching preceding all but the fifth QRS. That QRS has no P wave. The P waves are married to the QRS–they are in the same place relative to their QRS complexes. P-P interval is constant except

for the wide-QRS beat that has no P wave. **PR interval:** 0.12 seconds (normal), constant from beat to beat. **QRS interval:** 0.06 (normal) on the narrow beats, 0.12 (abnormally wide) on the wide beat.

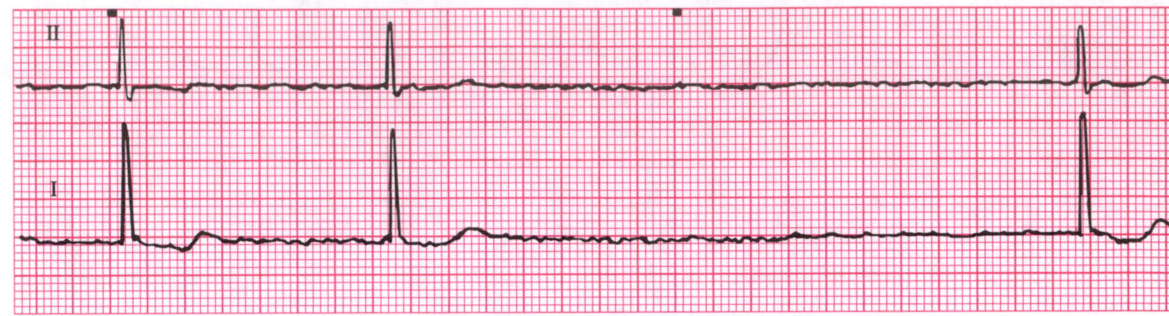

3. **QRS complexes:** There are only three QRS complexes in each lead of this double-lead strip. They are narrow and of uniform shape. **Regularity:** irregular. (It would be nice to have had a longer strip to see if this is a regular rhythm interrupted by a pause, but since this is all we have, we must call it irregular). R-R intervals are 34 and 91. **Heart rate:** mean rate of 30, range is 16 to 44. **P waves:** There are no P waves. There are undulations (waviness) of the baseline between QRS complexes. Cannot assess P-P interval since there are no P waves. Absence of P waves is abnormal. **PR interval:** Since there are no P waves there can be no PR interval. **QRS interval:** 0.08 (normal), constant from beat to beat.

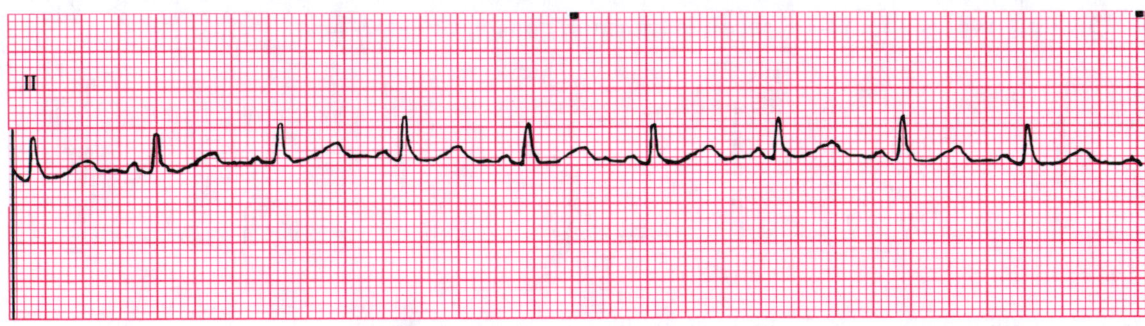

4. **QRS complexes:** All QRS complexes are narrow and of uniform shape. **Regularity:** regular, as evidenced by the R-R intervals of about 16 small blocks. **Heart rate:** 1,500 divided by 16 equals 94. **P waves:** upright and matching preceding each QRS. P waves are married to the QRS. P-P interval is regular. **PR interval:** 0.12 seconds (normal), constant. **QRS interval:** 0.08 seconds (normal), constant.

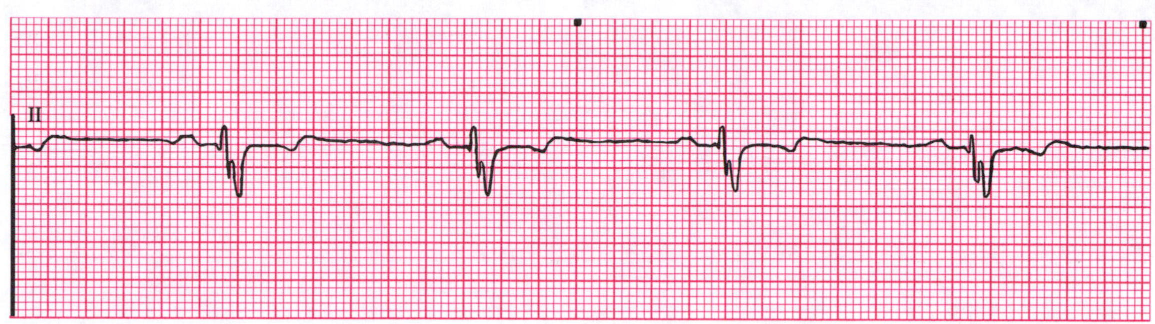

5. **QRS complexes:** All QRS complexes are wide and of uniform shape. **Regularity:** regular, as evidenced by the R-R intervals of about 33 small blocks. **Heart rate:** 1,500 divided by 33 equals 45. **P waves:** P waves are upright, matching, and married to the QRS complexes. P-P interval is regular. **PR interval:** 0.20 seconds (abnormally long). **QRS interval:** 0.16 seconds (abnormally long).

You now should have a feel for what to look for on rhythm strips. In Chapters 7–11 you'll learn about the different rhythms themselves. Let's get to it.

Practice Quiz

1. A heart rate that is greater than 100 is said to be a ________________.
2. A heart rate less than 60 is a ________________.
3. A drop in heart rate from a tachycardia to a normal heart rate (is/is not) cause for concern.
4. Dysrhythmia means ________________.
5. The five steps to rhythm interpretation are ________________ ________________.

CHAPTER 7

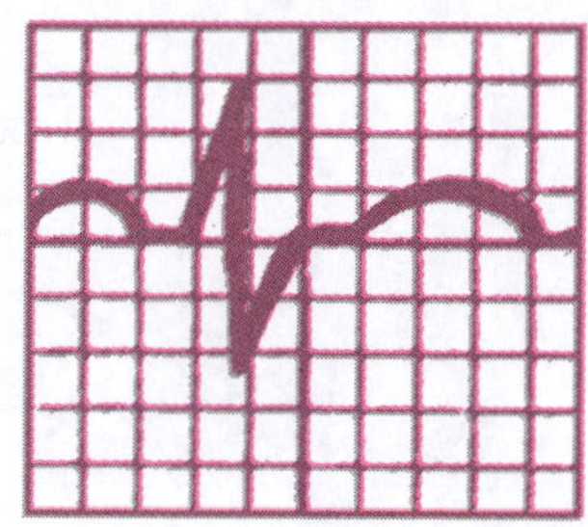

Rhythms Originating in the Sinus Node

Chapter 7 Objectives

Upon completion of this chapter, the student will be able to:

- State the criteria for each of the sinus rhythms.
- Using the five steps, correctly interpret a variety of sinus rhythms on single- and double-lead strips.
- State the adverse effects for each of the sinus rhythms.
- State the possible treatment for the sinus rhythms.

Introduction

Sinus rhythms originate in the sinus node, travel through the atria to depolarize them, then head down the normal conduction pathway to depolarize the ventricles. Most rhythms from the sinus node are regular rhythms, but as you will see, this is not always the case. You'll recall the sinus node is the normal pacemaker of the heart. See Figure 7-1.

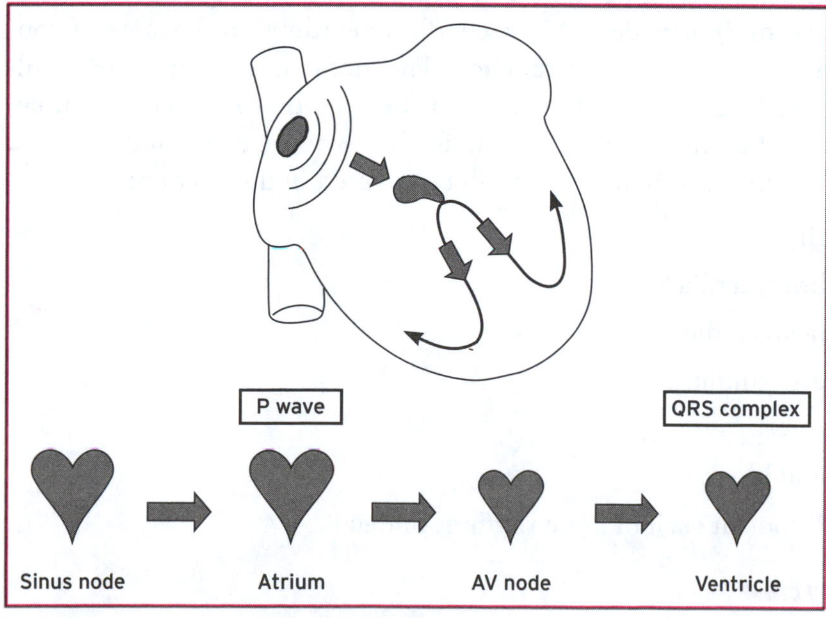

Figure 7-1 Conduction in sinus rhythms.

The Word on Sinus Rhythms

The sinus node is the acknowledged king of the conduction system's pacemaker cells. And there are only two ways for the sinus node king to relinquish its throne:

1. By illness or death, requiring a lower pacemaker to step in for it (escape)
2. By being overthrown by a lower pacemaker (usurpation)

Though they can be irregular at times, sinus rhythms are, for the most part, notoriously regular. They're like the ticking of a clock–predictable and expected. You'll recall the inherent rate of the sinus node is 60 to 100. But also remember that this rate can go higher or lower if the sinus node is acted on by the sympathetic or parasympathetic nervous system. The individual's tolerance of these rhythms will depend in large part on the heart rate. Heart rates that are too fast or too slow can cause symptoms of decreased cardiac output.

Treatment is not needed unless symptoms develop. At that time, the goal is to return the heart rate to normal levels.

Sinus rhythms are the standard against which all other rhythms are compared. Since most of the rhythms you will see in real life will be sinus rhythms, you'll need a thorough understanding of them. Let's look at the criteria for sinus rhythms. *All these criteria must be met for the rhythm to be sinus in origin.*

- Upright matching P waves followed by a QRS *and*
- PR intervals constant *and*
- Heart rate less than or equal to 160 at rest

All matching upright P waves in lead II are considered sinus P waves until proven otherwise. The width and deflection of the QRS complex is irrelevant in determining whether a rhythm is sinus. The QRS may be narrow (<0.12 second) or wide (≥0.12 second), depending on the state of conduction through the bundle branches. The deflection of the QRS will depend on the lead in which the patient is being monitored. For example, the QRS in lead II would be upright but in aVR would be inverted.

The following sinus rhythms that will be covered in this section:

- Sinus rhythm
- Sinus bradycardia
- Sinus tachycardia
- Sinus arrhythmia
- Sinus arrest
- Sinus exit block

Now let's look at each of these rhythms in detail.

Sinus Rhythm

What is it? Sinus rhythm is *the* normal rhythm. The impulse is born in the sinus node and heads down the conduction pathway to the ventricle. Every

P wave is married to a QRS complex, and the heart rate is the normal 60 to 100.

Rate	60 to 100.
Regularity	Regular.
P waves	Upright in most leads, though may be normally inverted in V_1; one P to each QRS; all P waves have the same shape. *All matching, upright P waves are sinus P waves until proven otherwise* (this is the most crucial criterion to identifying rhythms originating in the sinus node); P-P interval is regular.
PR	0.12 to 0.20 second; PR interval is constant from beat to beat.
QRS	<0.12 second (can be ≥ 0.12 s if conduction through the ventricle is abnormal, as in a bundle branch block [BBB]).
Cause	Normal.
Adverse effects	None.
Treatment	None.

In Figure 7-2, there are QRS complexes, and they are all shaped the same. The rhythm is regular. Heart rate is 88. P waves are present, one before each QRS complex, and they are all matching and upright. *Remember—all matching upright P waves are sinus P waves until proven otherwise.* P-P interval is regular. PR interval is 0.20, QRS interval is 0.10, both normal. Interpretation: sinus rhythm.

Sinus Bradycardia

What is it? In sinus bradycardia, the sinus node fires at a heart rate slower than normal. The impulse originates in the sinus node and travels the conduction system normally.

Rate	Less than 60.
Regularity	Regular.
P waves	Upright in most leads, though may be inverted in V_1; one P to each QRS; P waves shaped the same; P-P interval regular.

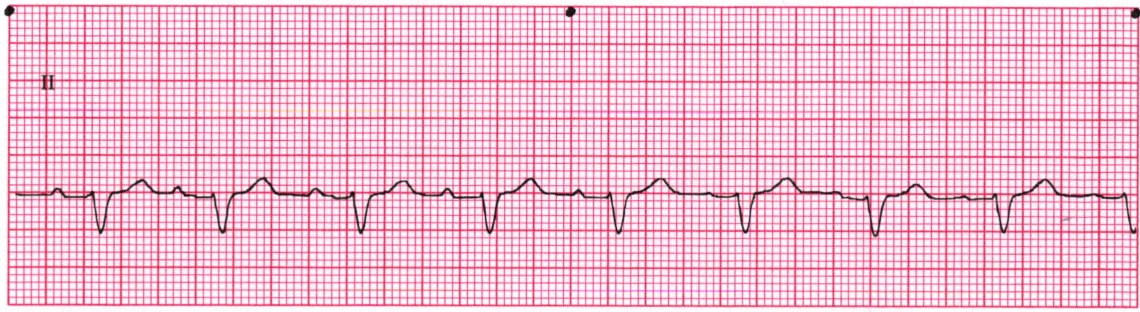

Figure 7-2 Sinus rhythm.

PR	0.12 to 0.20 second, constant from beat to beat.
QRS	<0.12 second (will be ≥0.12 s if BBB present).
Cause	Vagal stimulation such as vomiting or straining to have a bowel movement, myocardial infarction (MI), **hypoxia** (low blood oxygen level), digitalis toxicity (an overabundance of the medication digitalis in the bloodstream), and other medication side effects. Sinus bradycardia is common in athletes because their well-conditioned heart pumps more blood out with each beat and therefore doesn't need to beat as often.
Adverse effects	Too slow a heart rate can cause dizziness, weakness, syncope, **diaphoresis** (cold sweat), pallor, and hypotension, all of which are signs of decreased cardiac output. Many individuals, however, tolerate a slow heart rate and do not require treatment.
Treatment	None unless the patient is symptomatic. A medication called *atropine* can be used if needed to speed up the heart rate. Atropine speeds up the rate at which the sinus node propagates (creates) its impulses and also speeds up impulse conduction through the AV node. Thus, it causes an increase in heart rate. If atropine is unsuccessful, an electronic pacemaker can be utilized, although that is not usually necessary for sinus bradycardia unless the individual is in shock. Other medications such as epinephrine, dopamine, and isoproterenol can also be used to increase the heart rate, but, as with the pacemaker, are usually not necessary for sinus bradycardia. Consider starting oxygen. If the heart does not receive adequate oxygen, conduction system cells become ischemic (oxygen-starved) and may respond by firing at rates above or below their norm. Providing supplemental oxygen can help these stricken cells return to more normal functioning and a more normal heart rate.

In Figure 7-3, there are QRS complexes and they are all shaped the same. The rhythm is regular. Heart rate is 54. P waves are present, one before each

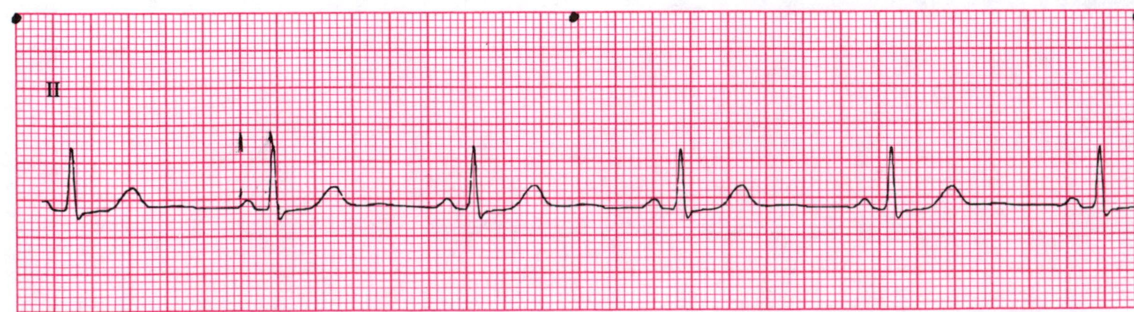

Figure 7-3 Sinus bradycardia.

QRS complex, and they are upright and matching. P-P interval is regular. PR interval is 0.16, QRS interval is 0.09, both normal. Interpretation: sinus bradycardia. *The only difference between sinus rhythm and sinus bradycardia is the heart rate—the other interpretation criteria are the same.*

Sinus Tachycardia

What is it? Sinus tachycardia is a rhythm in which the sinus node fires at a heart rate faster than normal. The impulse originates in the sinus node and travels down the conduction pathway normally.

Rate	101 to 160. According to most experts, the sinus node does not fire at a rate above 160 in supine resting adults. Though this is somewhat controversial, we will adopt this as the upper limit of the sinus node. *All strips in this text are from supine resting adults unless otherwise specified.*
Regularity	Regular.
P waves	Upright in most leads, though may be inverted in V_1; one P to each QRS; P waves shaped the same; P-P interval regular.
PR	0.12 to 0.20 second, constant from beat to beat.
QRS	<0.12 second (≥0.12 s if BBB present).
Cause	Medications such as atropine; emotional upset, **pulmonary embolus** (blood clot in the lung), MI, congestive heart failure (**CHF**), fever, inhibition of the vagus nerve, hypoxia, and **thyrotoxicosis** (thyroid storm—an emergent medical condition in which the thyroid gland so overproduces thyroid hormones that the heart rate, blood pressure, and temperature all rise to dangerously high levels).
Adverse effects	Increased heart rate causes increased cardiac workload. The faster a muscle works, the more blood and oxygen it requires. This can stress an already weakened heart. Cardiac output can drop. This is especially true in the patient with an acute MI, as the increased blood and oxygen demand cannot easily be met by the damaged heart muscle.
Treatment	Treat the cause. For example, if the patient in sinus tachycardia has a fever, give medications such as acetaminophen or ibuprofen to decrease the fever. If the tachycardia is caused by anxiety, consider sedation. For cardiac patients with persistent sinus tachycardia, a class of medications called **beta-blockers** may be used to slow the heart rate. Consider starting oxygen to decrease the heart's workload.

Every one degree increase in body temperature causes the heart rate to rise by about 10 beats per minute.

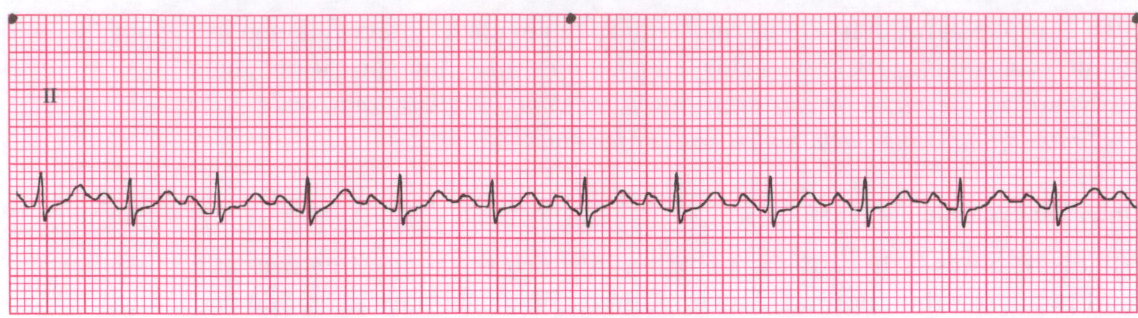

Figure 7-4 Sinus tachycardia.

In Figure 7-4, there are QRS complexes, all shaped the same. The rhythm is regular. Heart rate is about 125. P waves are present, one before each QRS, and they are all upright and matching. P-P interval is regular. PR interval is 0.14, QRS interval is 0.06, both within normal limits. Interpretation: sinus tachycardia. *Just as in sinus rhythm and sinus bradycardia, all the criteria for interpretation are the same for sinus tachycardia–the only difference is the heart rate.*

Sinus Arrhythmia

What is it? Sinus arrhythmia is the only **irregular** rhythm from the sinus node, and it has a pattern that is cyclic and usually corresponds with the breathing pattern.

Rate	Varies with respiratory pattern–faster with inspiration, slower with expiration. The negative pressure in the chest during inspiration sucks up blood from the lower extremities, causing an increase in blood returning to the right atrium. The heart rate speeds up to circulate this extra blood. Sinus arrhythmia is especially common during sleep, especially among those with **sleep apnea** (a temporary, often repetitive cessation of breathing during sleep).
Regularity	Irregular in a repetitive pattern; longest R-R cycle exceeds the shortest by ≥0.16 second (four or more little blocks).
P waves	Upright in most leads, though may be inverted in V_1; P waves shaped the same; one P to each QRS; P-P interval is irregular.
PR	0.12 to 0.20 second, constant from beat to beat.
QRS	<0.12 second (≥0.12 s if BBB present).
Cause	Usually caused by the breathing pattern, but can also be caused by heart disease.
Adverse effects	Usually no ill effects.
Treatment	Usually none required.

In Figure 7-5, there are QRS complexes, all shaped the same. The rhythm is irregular. Heart rate is 62 to 88, with a mean rate of 80. The longest R-R

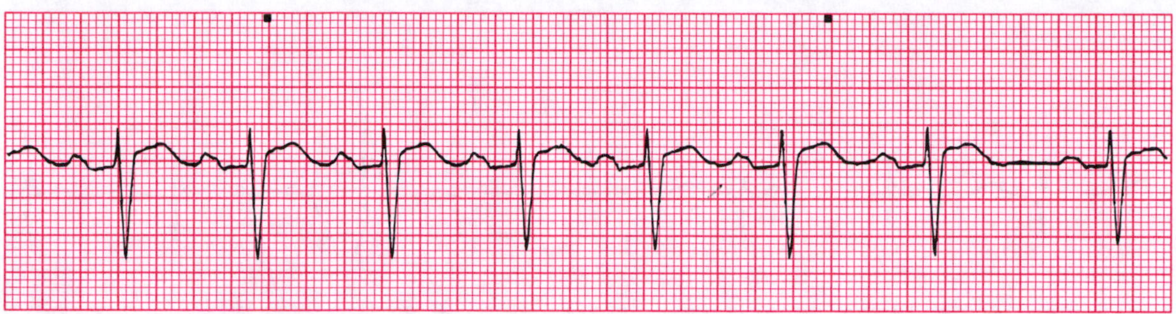

Figure 7-5 Sinus arrhythmia.

interval (24 little blocks) exceeds the shortest (17 blocks) by four little blocks or more. P waves are present, one before each QRS, and all are upright and shaped the same. P-P interval varies. PR interval is 0.24 seconds (abnormally long), QRS interval is 0.10 (normal). Interpretation: sinus arrhythmia with an abnormally prolonged PR interval.

Sinus Arrest

What is it? A sinus arrest is a pause that occurs when the regularly firing sinus node suddenly stops firing for a brief period. One or more P-QRS-T sequences will be missing. An escape beat from a lower pacemaker may then take over for one or more beats. The sinus node may resume functioning after missing one or more beats, or the lower pacemaker may continue as the pacemaker, creating a new rhythm.

Rate	Can occur at any heart rate.
Regularity	Regular but interrupted (by a pause). In any rhythm with a pause, always measure the length of the pause in seconds.
P waves	Normal sinus P waves before the pause, normal or different-shaped Ps (if even present) on the beat ending the pause. P-P interval is usually regular before the pause and may vary after the pause, depending on whether the sinus node regains pacemaking control.
PR	0.12 to 0.20 second before the pause, may be shorter or absent after the pause.
QRS	On the sinus beats, the QRS interval will be <0.12 second (≥ 0.12 s if BBB present). On the escape beat(s), the QRS will be narrow (<0.12 s) if the AV junction escapes as the pacemaker (called a **junctional escape beat**), and wide (>0.12 s) if the ventricle escapes as the pacemaker (called a **ventricular escape beat**).
Cause	Sinus node ischemia, hypoxia, **digitalis toxicity,** excessive vagal tone, other medication side effects.
Adverse effects	Frequent or very long sinus arrests can cause decreased cardiac output.

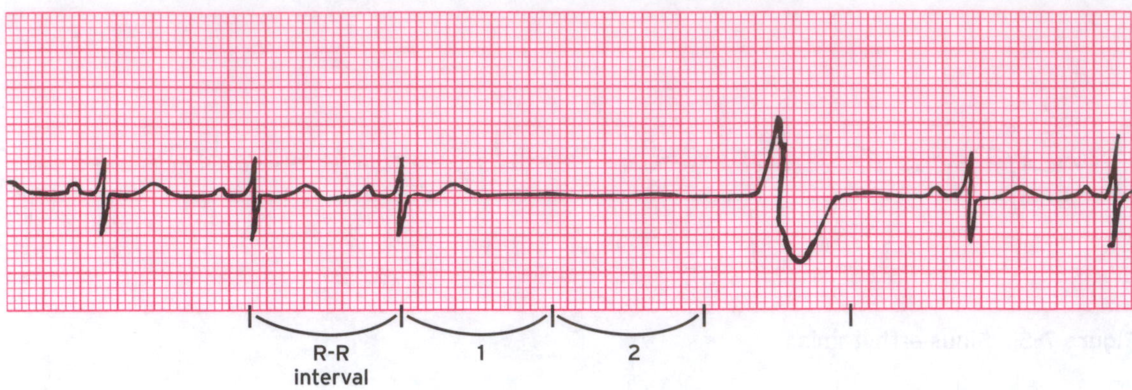

Figure 7-6 Sinus arrest.

Treatment	Occasional sinus arrests may not cause a problem—the patient has no ill effects. Frequent sinus arrests may require that the medication causing it be stopped and can require atropine and/or a pacemaker to speed up the heart rate. Consider starting oxygen.

In Figure 7-6, the first three beats are sinus beats firing along regularly. Suddenly there is a long pause, at the end of which is a beat from a lower pacemaker. How do we know the beat that ends the pause (the escape beat) is not a sinus beat? Sinus beats all have matching upright P waves. This beat has no P wave at all, plus its QRS complex is huge, completely unlike the other QRS complexes. Going through our steps now: There are QRS complexes, all but one having the same shape. Regularity is regular but interrupted. Heart rate is 30 to 75, with a mean rate of 60. P waves are upright, matching, one before all QRS complexes except the escape beat. PR interval is 0.16, QRS interval is 0.08 on the sinus beats and 0.14 on the escape beat. Interpretation: sinus rhythm interrupted by a 2-second sinus arrest (You'll recall every 5 big blocks equals 1 second. There are 10 big blocks between these QRS complexes) and a ventricular escape beat. Note the sinus node resumes functioning after one ventricular escape beat.

Sinus Block (also Called Sinus Exit Block)

What is it? A sinus block is a pause that occurs when the sinus node fires its impulse on time, but the impulse's exit from the sinus node to the atrial tissue is blocked. *In other words, the beat that the sinus node propagated is not conducted anywhere.* This results in one or more P-QRS-T sequences being missing, creating a pause, the length of which will depend on how many sinus beats are blocked. When conduction of the regularly firing sinus impulses resumes, the sinus beats return on time at the end of the pause. The pause will be a multiple of the previous R-R intervals–that is, exactly two or more R-R cycles will fit into the pause.

Rate	Can occur at any heart rate.
Regularity	Regular but interrupted (by a pause).
P waves	Normal sinus Ps both before and after the pause; P waves shaped the same.

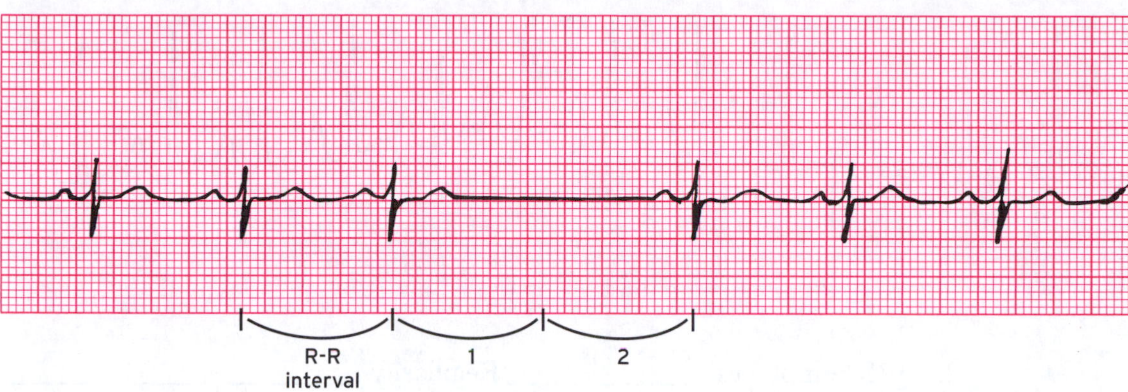

Figure 7-7 Sinus block.

PR	0.12 to 0.20 second.
QRS	<0.12 second (≥0.12 s if BBB present).
Cause	Medication side effects, hypoxia, or strong vagal stimulation.
Adverse effects	Same as sinus arrest.
Treatment	Same as sinus arrest.

In Figure 7-7, there is a pause that lasts exactly eight big blocks. This is exactly twice the R-R interval of the sinus beats that precede and follow the pause. The pause is therefore a multiple of the R-R intervals. The pause ends with a sinus beat. Going through our steps: There are QRS complexes, all shaped the same. Regularity is regular but interrupted. Heart rate is 37 to 75, with a mean rate of 60. P waves are upright, matching, one before each QRS complex. PR interval is 0.16, QRS interval is 0.08. Interpretation: sinus rhythm with a 1.6-second sinus block.

Practice Strips: Sinus Rhythms

Following are 20 rhythm strips, the first ten on single-lead strips, the remainder on double-lead strips.

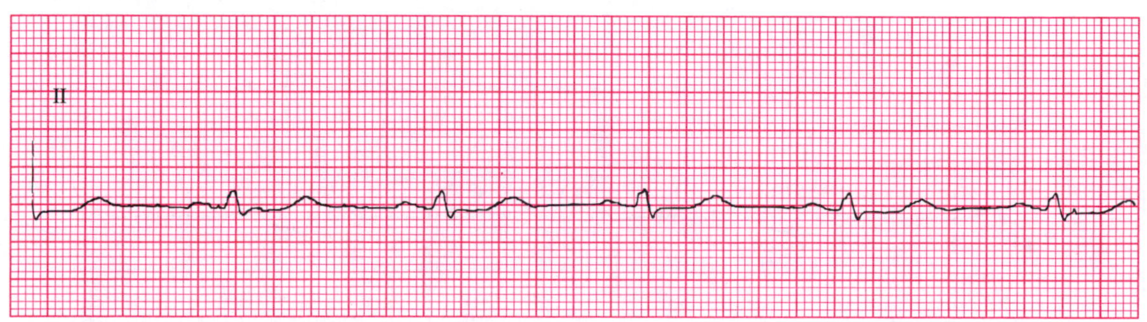

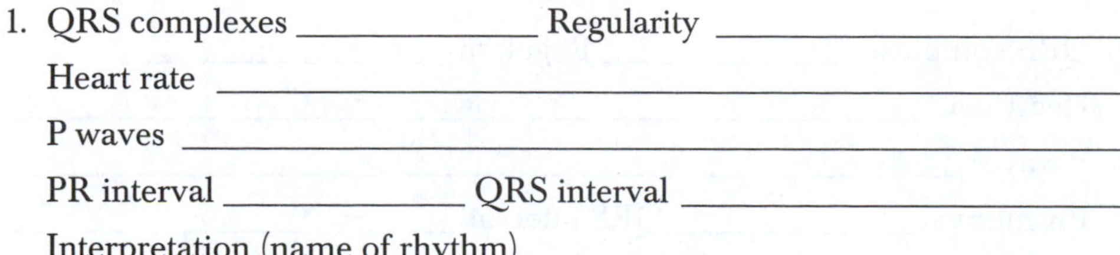

1. QRS complexes ____________ Regularity ____________________
   Heart rate ____
   P waves ____
   PR interval ____________ QRS interval ____________________
   Interpretation (name of rhythm) ____________________________

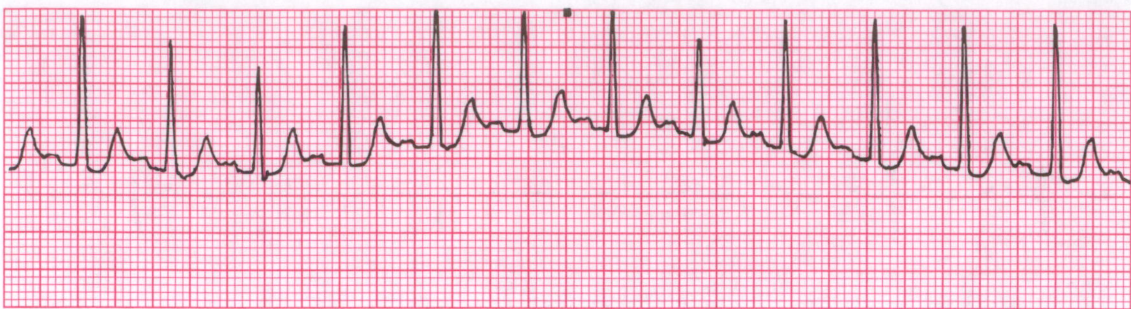

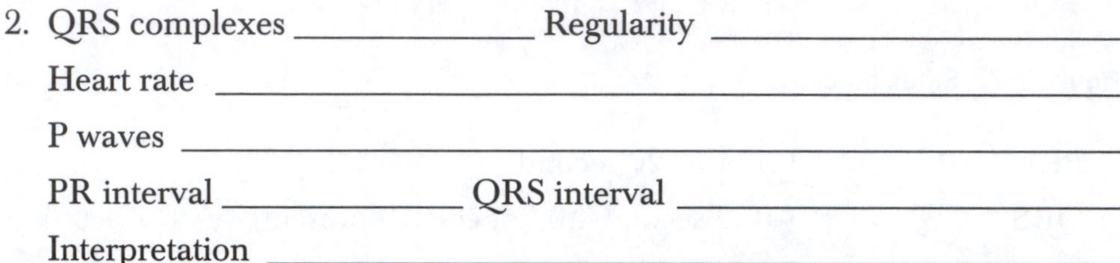

2. QRS complexes ______________ Regularity ______________________
   Heart rate ____
   P waves ____
   PR interval ______________ QRS interval ______________________
   Interpretation ____

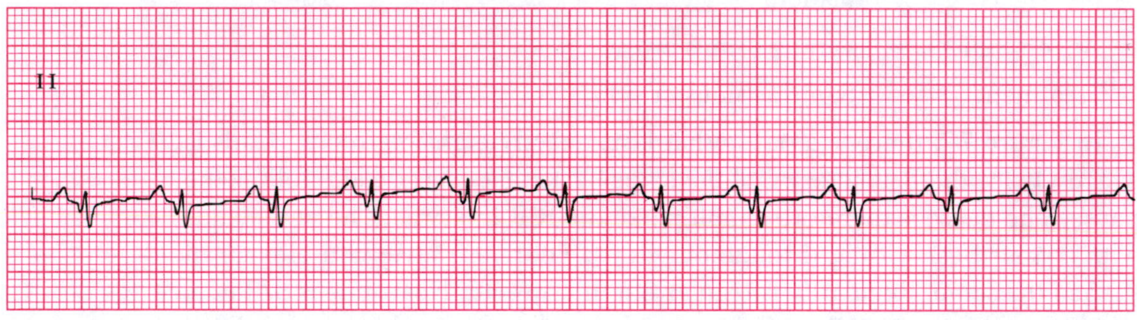

3. QRS complexes ______________ Regularity ______________________
   Heart rate ____
   P waves ____
   PR interval ______________ QRS interval ______________________
   Interpretation ____

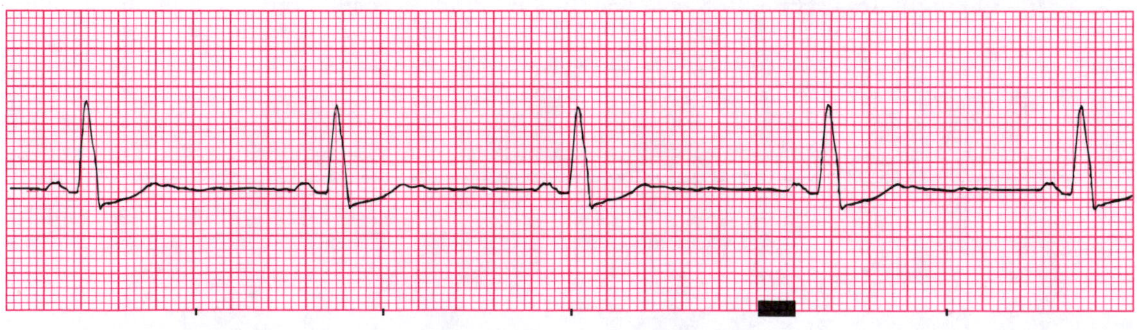

4. QRS complexes ______________ Regularity ______________________
   Heart rate ____
   P waves ____
   PR interval ______________ QRS interval ______________________
   Interpretation ____

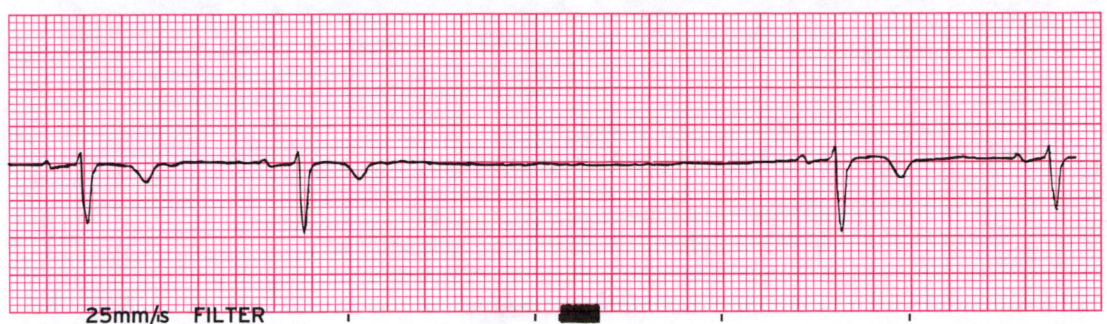

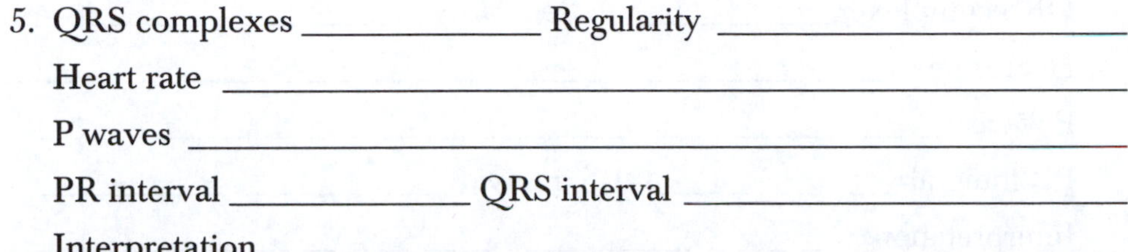

5. QRS complexes ______________ Regularity ________________________
   Heart rate ____
   P waves ____
   PR interval ______________ QRS interval __________________________
   Interpretation ____

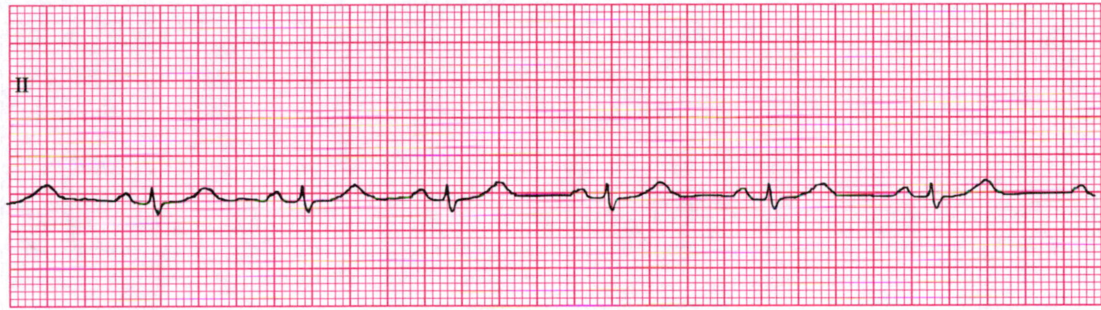

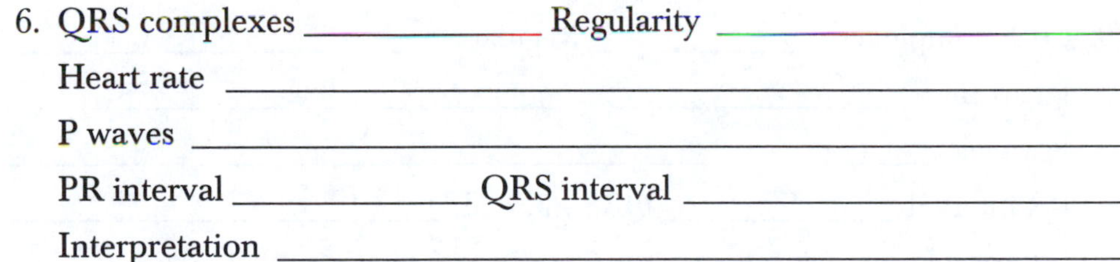

6. QRS complexes ______________ Regularity ________________________
   Heart rate ____
   P waves ____
   PR interval ______________ QRS interval __________________________
   Interpretation ____

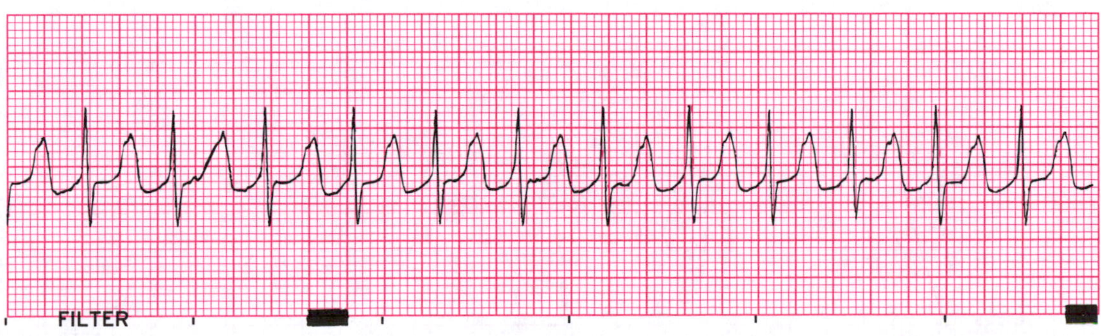

7. QRS complexes ______________ Regularity ________________________
   Heart rate ____
   P waves ____
   PR interval ______________ QRS interval __________________________
   Interpretation ____

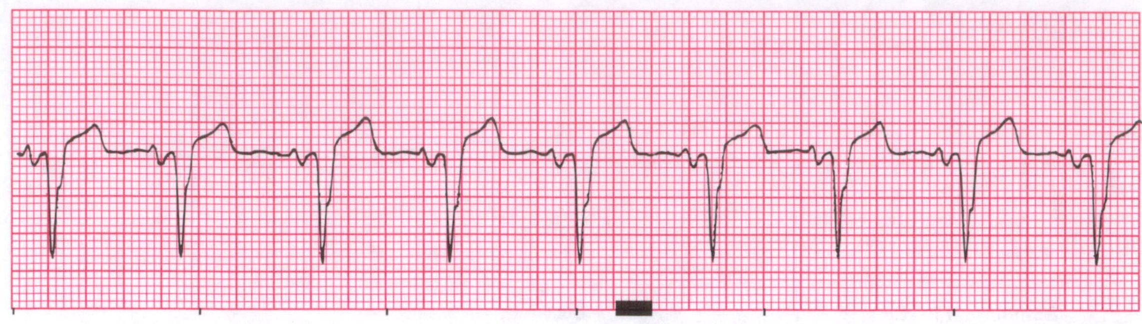

8. QRS complexes ____________ Regularity ____________
   Heart rate ____________
   P waves ____________
   PR interval ____________ QRS interval ____________
   Interpretation ____________

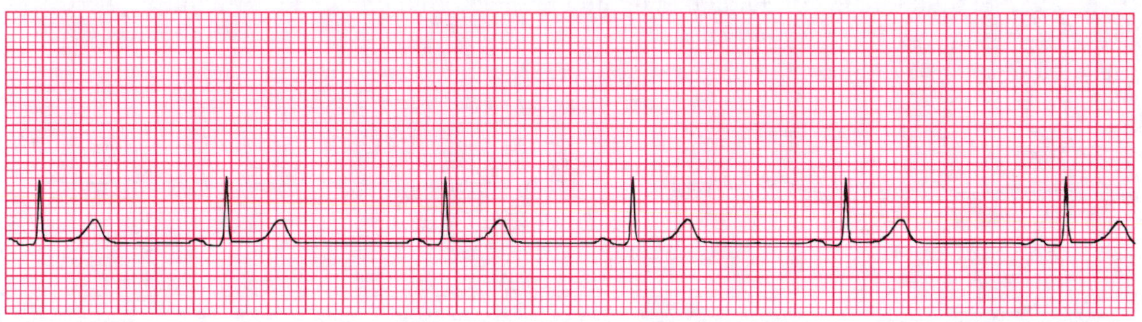

9. QRS complexes ____________ Regularity ____________
   Heart rate ____________
   P waves ____________
   PR interval ____________ QRS interval ____________
   Interpretation ____________

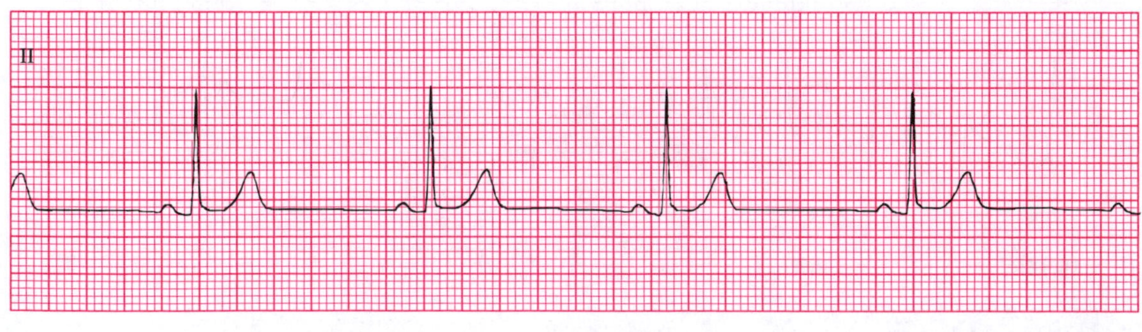

10. QRS complexes ____________ Regularity ____________
    Heart rate ____________

P waves ______________________________

PR interval ____________ QRS interval ______________

Interpretation ______________________________

Practice strips 11-20 are double-lead strips. On each strip, choose the lead that has the biggest and/or most clear waves and complexes and use that lead for interpretation. **Remember–both leads are the same patient at the same time, so both leads should have the same rhythm and intervals.**

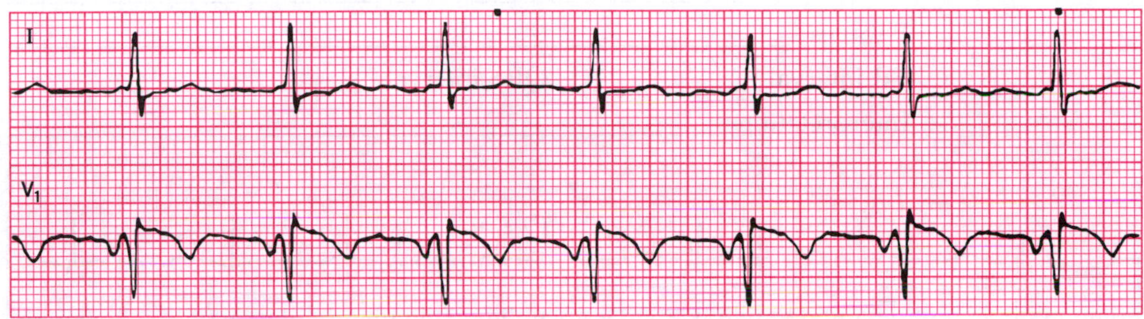

11. QRS complexes ____________ Regularity ______________

Heart rate ______________________________

P waves ______________________________

PR interval ____________ QRS interval ______________

Interpretation (name of rhythm) ______________

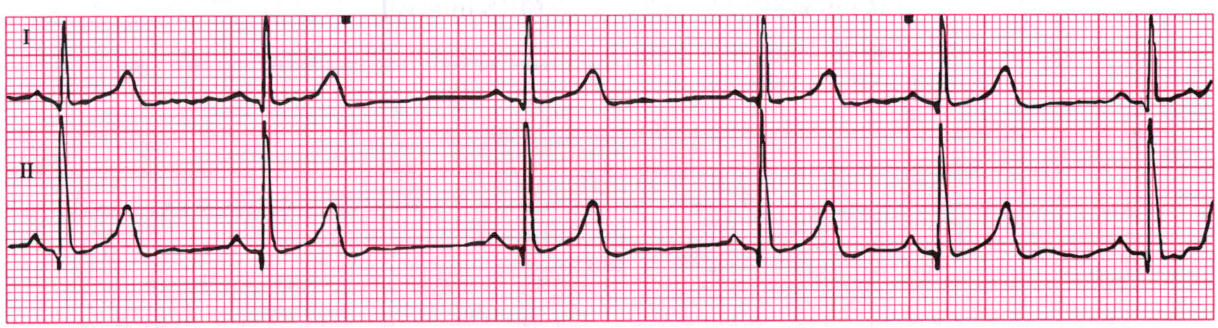

12. QRS complexes ____________ Regularity ______________

Heart rate ______________________________

P waves ______________________________

PR interval ____________ QRS interval ______________

Interpretation ______________________________

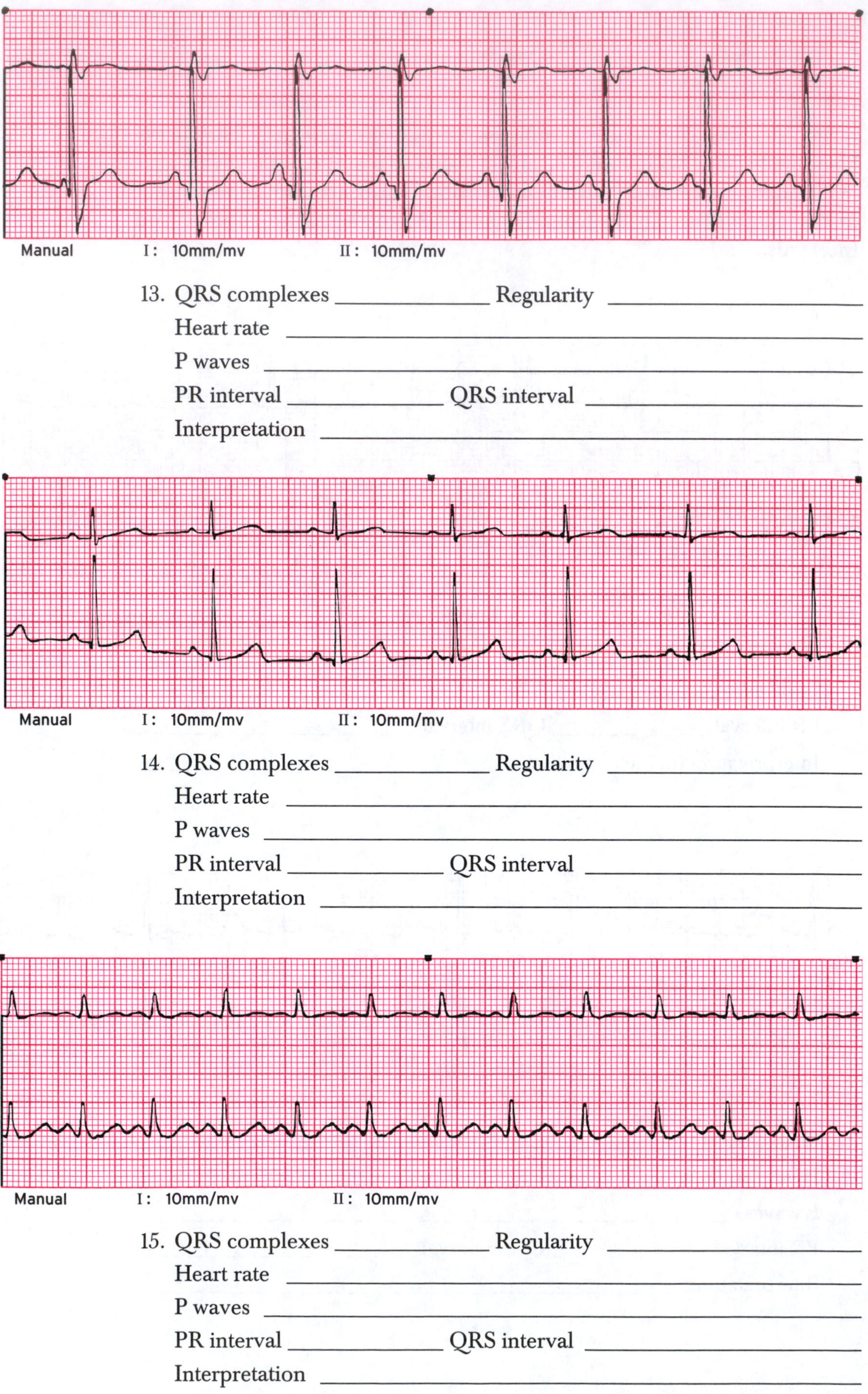

13. QRS complexes ______________ Regularity ______________________
    Heart rate ____
    P waves ____
    PR interval ______________ QRS interval ______________________
    Interpretation ____

14. QRS complexes ______________ Regularity ______________________
    Heart rate ____
    P waves ____
    PR interval ______________ QRS interval ______________________
    Interpretation ____

15. QRS complexes ______________ Regularity ______________________
    Heart rate ____
    P waves ____
    PR interval ______________ QRS interval ______________________
    Interpretation ____

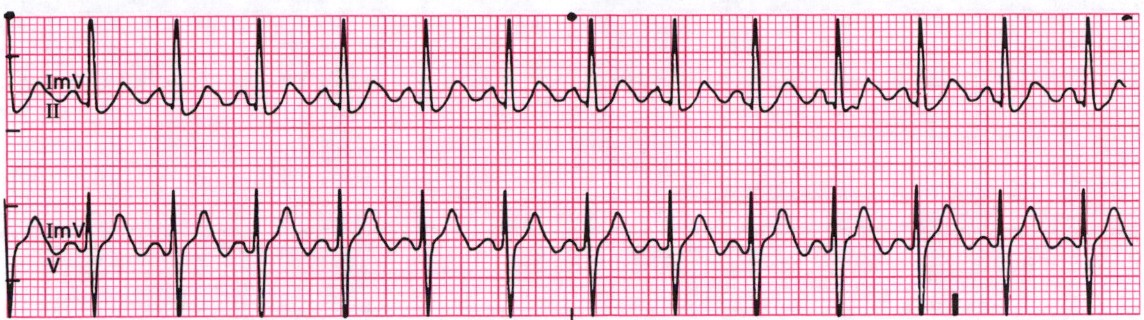

16. QRS complexes ______________ Regularity ______________
Heart rate ______________
P waves ______________
PR interval ______________ QRS interval ______________
Interpretation ______________

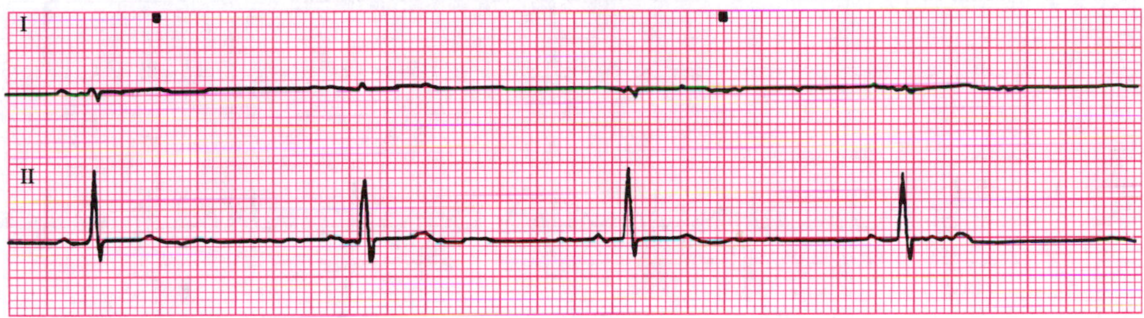

17. QRS complexes ______________ Regularity ______________
Heart rate ______________
P waves ______________
PR interval ______________ QRS interval ______________
Interpretation ______________

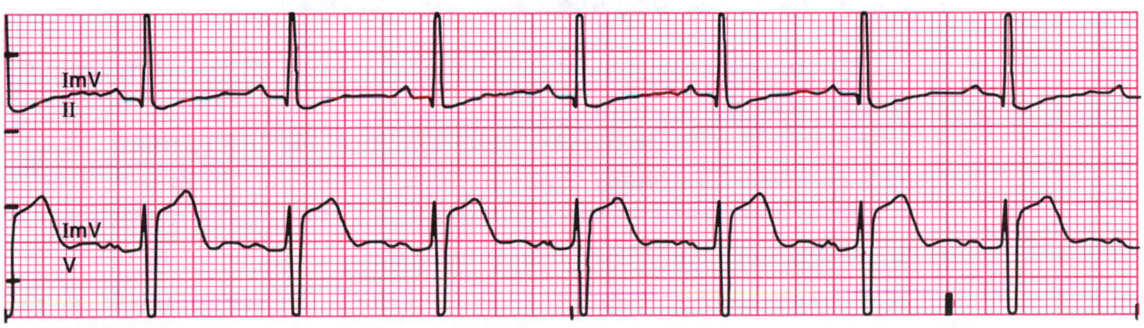

18. QRS complexes ______________ Regularity ______________
Heart rate ______________
P waves ______________
PR interval ______________ QRS interval ______________
Interpretation ______________

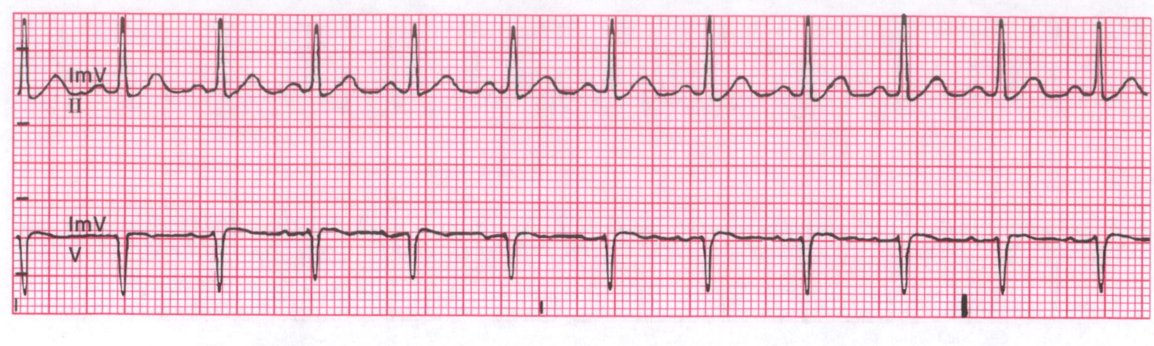

19. QRS complexes ____________ Regularity ____________
Heart rate ____________
P waves ____________
PR interval ____________ QRS interval ____________
Interpretation ____________

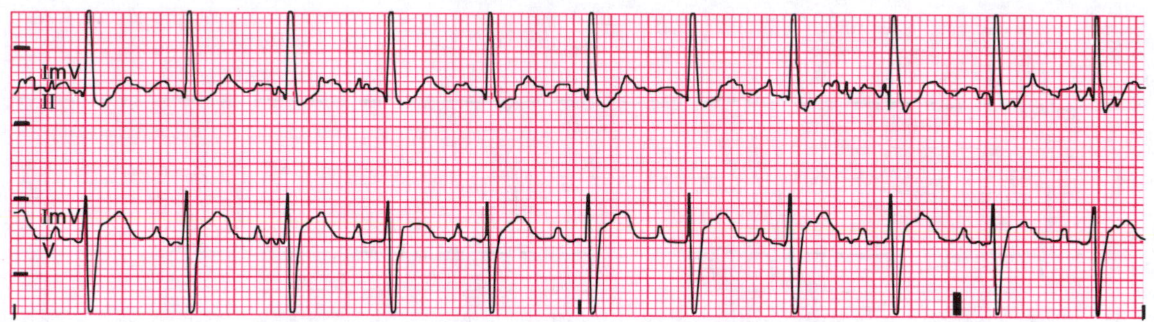

20. QRS complexes ____________ Regularity ____________
Heart rate ____________
P waves ____________
PR interval ____________ QRS interval ____________
Interpretation ____________

Answers to Sinus Rhythms Practice Strips

1. **QRS complexes:** present, all shaped the same. **Regularity:** regular. **Heart rate:** 56. **P waves:** upright, matching, one per QRS; P-P interval regular. **PR:** 0.18. **QRS:** 0.12 (wider than normal) **Interpretation:** sinus bradycardia with bundle branch block (BBB). Bundle Branch Block is indicated because the QRS interval is 0.12 seconds wide or greater. *If any rhythm from the sinus node has a QRS of 0.12 or wider, there is a BBB.*
2. **QRS complexes:** present, all shaped the same. **Regularity:** regular. **Heart rate:** 125. **P waves:** upright, matching, one per QRS; P-P interval regular. **PR:** 0.14. **QRS:** 0.08. **Interpretation:** sinus tachycardia.
3. **QRS complexes:** present, all shaped the same. **Regularity:** regular. **Heart rate:** 115. **P waves:** upright, matching, one per QRS; P-P interval regular. **PR:** 0.12. **QRS:** 0.10. **Interpretation:** sinus tachycardia.

4. **QRS complexes:** present, all shaped the same. **Regularity:** regular. **Heart rate:** 45. **P waves:** upright, matching, one per QRS; P-P interval regular. **PR:** 0.16. **QRS:** 0.14 (wider than normal). **Interpretation:** sinus bradycardia with BBB.
5. **QRS complexes:** present, all shaped the same. **Regularity:** regular but interrupted (by a pause). **Heart rate:** 21 to 54, with a mean rate of 40. **P waves:** upright, matching, one per QRS; P-P interval irregular due to the pause. **PR:** 0.18. **QRS:** 0.10. **Interpretation:** sinus bradycardia with a 3.08-second sinus arrest.
6. **QRS complexes:** present, all shaped the same. **Regularity:** regular (R-R intervals vary by only two small blocks). **Heart rate:** about 68. **P waves:** upright, matching, one per QRS; P-P interval regular. **PR:** 0.16. **QRS:** 0.08. **Interpretation:** sinus rhythm.
7. **QRS complexes:** present, all shaped the same. **Regularity:** regular. **Heart rate:** about 130. **P waves:** upright and matching, one per QRS. The heart rate is so fast that the T waves and P waves merge together. Do you see the notch at the top of the T wave? That's the P wave popping out. P-P interval regular. **PR:** cannot measure. **QRS:** 0.08. **Interpretation:** sinus tachycardia.
8. **QRS complexes:** present, all shaped the same. **Regularity:** regular. **Heart rate:** 88. **P waves:** biphasic (counts as upright), matching, one per QRS; P-P interval regular. **PR:** 0.12. **QRS:** 0.10. **Interpretation:** sinus rhythm.
9. **QRS complexes:** present, all shaped the same. **Regularity:** irregular; the R-R intervals vary from 25 to 29 small blocks. **Heart rate:** 52 to 60, with a mean rate of 60. **P waves:** upright, matching, one per QRS; P-P interval irregular. **PR:** 0.16. **QRS:** 0.06. **Interpretation:** sinus arrhythmia.
10. **QRS complexes:** present, all shaped the same. **Regularity:** regular. **Heart rate:** about 47. **P waves:** upright, matching, one preceding each QRS; P-P interval regular. **PR:** 0.16. **QRS:** 0.08. **Interpretation:** sinus bradycardia.
11. **QRS complexes:** present, all shaped the same within each lead. **Regularity:** regular. **Heart rate:** 75. **P waves:** upright in lead I and inverted in V_1 (you'll recall this is OK for this lead), matching, one per QRS; P-P interval regular. **PR:** 0.10 (unusually short). **QRS:** 0.10. **Interpretation:** sinus rhythm.
12. **QRS complexes:** present, all shaped the same within each lead. **Regularity:** irregular. **Heart rate:** 43 to 63, with a mean rate of 60. **P waves:** upright and matching, one per QRS. P-P interval irregular. **PR:** 0.16 **QRS:** 0.12. **Interpretation:** sinus arrhythmia with BBB.
13. **QRS complexes:** present, all shaped the same within each lead. **Regularity:** regular. **Heart rate:** 83. **P waves:** upright, matching, one per QRS; P-P interval regular. **PR:** 0.14. **QRS:** 0.14. **Interpretation:** sinus rhythm with BBB.

14. **QRS complexes:** present, all shaped the same within each lead. **Regularity:** regular. **Heart rate:** 71. **P waves:** upright, matching, one per QRS; P-P interval regular. **PR:** 0.16. **QRS:** 0.76. **Interpretation:** sinus rhythm.
15. **QRS complexes:** present, all shaped the same within each lead. **Regularity:** regular. **Heart rate:** 125. **P waves:** upright, matching, one preceding each QRS; P-P interval regular. **PR:** 0.12. **QRS:** 0.08. **Interpretation:** sinus tachycardia.
16. **QRS complexes:** present, all shaped the same within each lead. **Regularity:** regular. **Heart rate:** 136. **P waves:** upright, matching, one per QRS; P-P interval regular. **PR:** 0.12. **QRS:** 0.08. **Interpretation:** sinus tachycardia.
17. **QRS complexes:** present, all shaped the same within each lead. **Regularity:** regular. **Heart rate:** 42. **P waves:** upright and matching, one per QRS. P-P interval regular. **PR:** 0.16 **QRS:** 0.08. **Interpretation:** sinus bradycardia. Thank goodness this is a double-lead strip because if we only had the top strip we'd be hard-pressed to interpret it.
18. **QRS complexes:** present, all shaped the same within each lead. **Regularity:** regular. **Heart rate:** 79. **P waves:** upright, matching, one per QRS; P-P interval regular. **PR:** 0.20. **QRS:** 0.10. **Interpretation:** sinus rhythm.
19. **QRS complexes:** present, all shaped the same within each lead. **Regularity:** regular. **Heart rate:** 115. **P waves:** upright, matching, one per QRS; P-P interval regular. **PR:** 0.14. **QRS:** 0.06. **Interpretation:** sinus tachycardia.
20. **QRS complexes:** present, all shaped the same within each lead. **Regularity:** regular. **Heart rate:** 115. **P waves:** upright and matching, one per QRS. P-P interval regular. **PR:** 0.16. **QRS:** 0.12. **Interpretation:** sinus tachycardia.

Practice Quiz

1. True or false: All rhythms from the sinus node are irregular.
2. The only difference between sinus rhythm, sinus bradycardia, and sinus tachycardia is ______________________________

   ____
3. Sinus arrhythmia is typically caused by ______________________________
4. In what way does a sinus exit block differ from a sinus arrest? __________

   ____
5. True or false: Atropine is a medication that is useful in treating sinus tachycardia.
6. What rhythm would be expected in an individual with a fever of 103°F?

   ____

7. A regular rhythm from the sinus node that has a heart rate of 155 is called ____
8. True or false: All rhythms originating in the sinus node have matching P waves that are upright in most leads.
9. What effect does atropine have on the heart rate? ________________
10. True or false: Anyone with a heart rate of 45 should be given Atropine, whether or not he/she is symptomatic. ______________________

Putting It All Together—Critical Thinking Exercises

These exercises may consist of diagrams to label, scenarios to analyze, brain-stumping questions to ponder, or other challenging exercises to boost your understanding of the chapter material.

Let's play with sinus rhythms a bit. The following scenario will provide you with information about a fictional patient and ask you to analyze the situation, answer questions, and decide on appropriate actions.

Mr. Cavernum, age 62, is admitted to your telemetry floor with a diagnosis of pneumonia. He has a past medical history of sleep apnea and an "irregular heartbeat." On admission, his vital signs are as follows: Blood pressure (BP) normal at 132/84, heart rate 94 (normal), temperature 98.9 degrees (essentially normal), respirations normal at 20. His rhythm strip is below in Figure 7-8.

1. What is this rhythm? _________________________________

   At 3 A.M. Mr. Cavernum calls his nurse, saying he feels awful. The nurse notes his skin to be very hot and his face flushed. His vitals are as follows: BP 140/90 (slightly high), respirations 26 (rapid), temp 101.1 degrees (high). See his rhythm strip below in Figure 7-9.

2. What is the rhythm and heart rate? __________________________
3. What do you suspect is causing this change in heart rate? ____________.

   Your coworker brings three medications—atropine, a beta-blocker called diltiazem, and acetaminophen (Tylenol)—into Mr. Cavernum's room.

4. Which of the three medications is indicated in this situation? __________

   After receiving his medication, Mr. Cavernum falls asleep and within two hours his rhythm is below. See Figure 7-10.

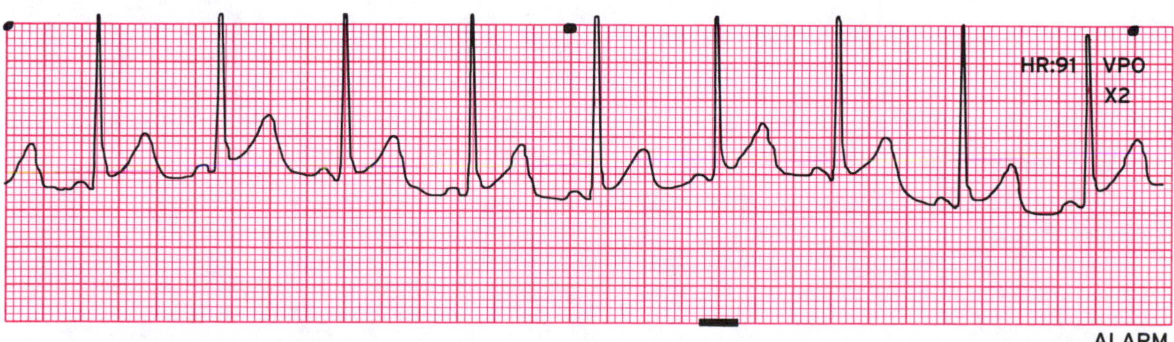

Figure 7-8 Admission rhythm strip.

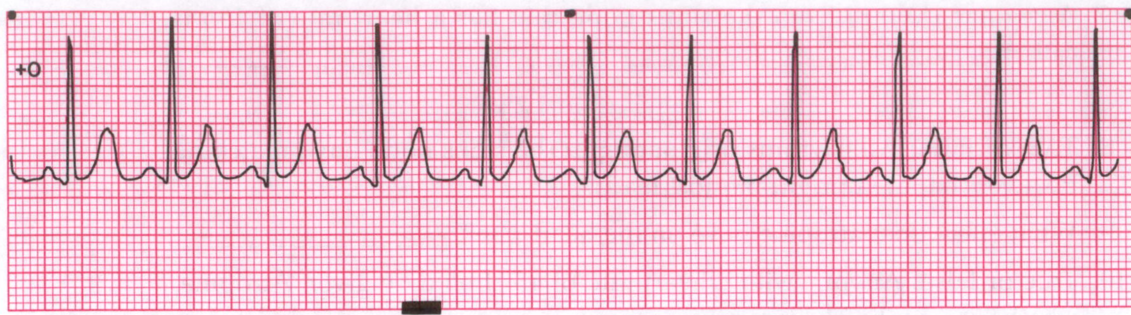

Figure 7-9 Second rhythm strip.

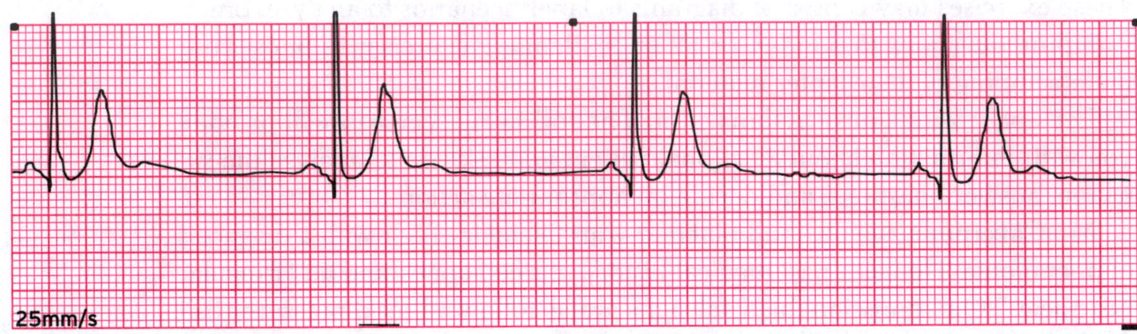

Figure 7-10 Final rhythm.

5. What is this rhythm? ______________________________.
6. Does this rhythm require emergency treatment? ____________
7. What in Mr. Cavernum's past medical history is a possible cause of this rhythm? ______________________________

CHAPTER 8

Rhythms Originating in the Atria

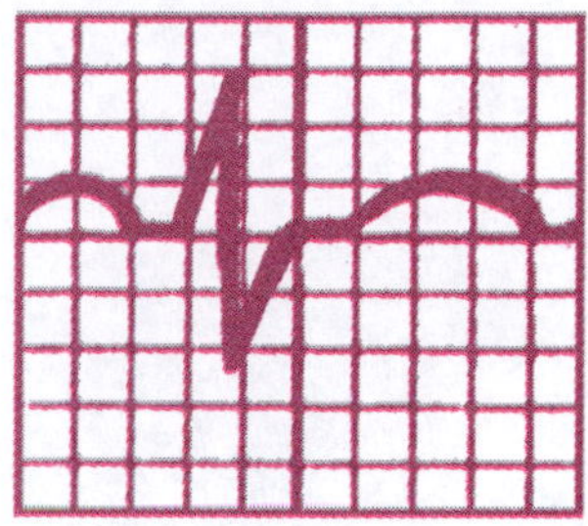

Chapter 8 Objectives

Upon completion of this chapter, the student will be able to:

- State the criteria for each of the atrial rhythms.
- Using the criteria and other rhythm analysis tools, correctly interpret a variety of atrial rhythms.
- State the adverse effects for each rhythm.
- State the possible treatment for each rhythm.

Introduction

Atrial rhythms originate in one or more irritable **foci** (locations) in the atria, then depolarize the atria and head down the conduction pathway to the ventricles. Atrial rhythms, and indeed all rhythms that originate in a pacemaker other than the sinus node, are called **ectopic rhythms.** See Figures 8-1 and 8-2.

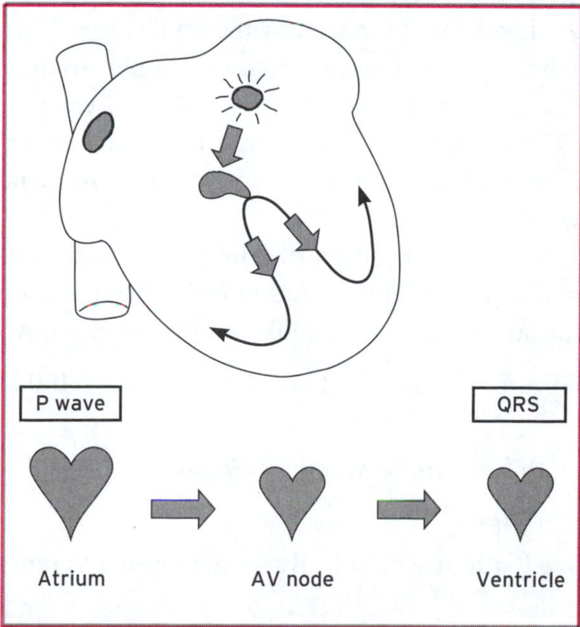

Figure 8-1 Conduction of a single atrial focus.

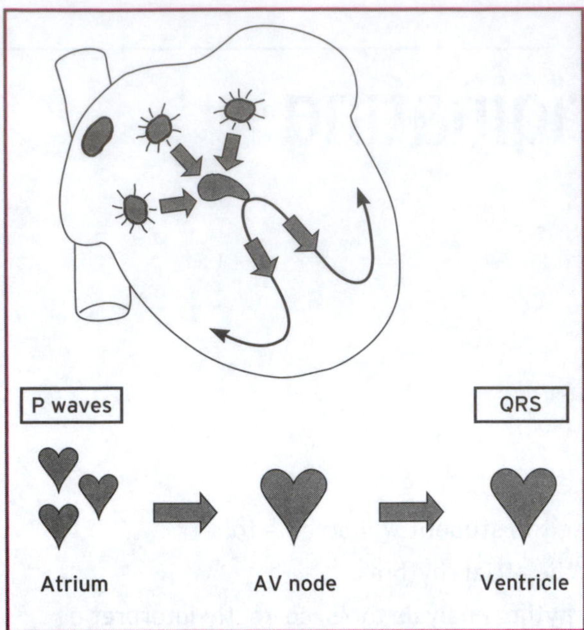

Figure 8-2 Conduction of multiple atrial foci.

The Word on Atrial Rhythms

Though the atrium is not considered an inherent pacemaker like the sinus node, AV junction, and ventricle (it is highly unusual for the atrium to fire in an escape capacity), the atrium is indeed another pacemaker of the heart. It is best known for usurping the underlying sinus rhythm and producing rhythms with very rapid heart rates. Because of these rapid heart rates, patients are often symptomatic. Every now and then the atrium will fire more slowly and produce rhythms with rates less than 100.

Treatment is aimed at converting the rhythm back to sinus rhythm, or, if that is not possible, returning the heart rate to more normal levels.

Atrial rhythms are extremely variable in their presentation. Some rhythms have obvious P waves. Others have no Ps at all–instead, they have a wavy or fluttery baseline between the QRS complexes. Some atrial rhythms are regular and others are completely irregular, even chaotic. Though most atrial rhythms are rapid, a few are slower.

Unlike sinus rhythms, which have a common set of criteria, atrial rhythms have multiple and variable possible criteria. If the rhythm or beat in question meets *any* of these criteria, it is atrial in origin. Let's look at these criteria now.

- Matching upright Ps, atrial rate (the heart rate of the P waves) >160 at rest *or*
- No Ps at all; wavy or sawtooth baseline between QRSs present instead *or*
- P waves of ≥ three different shapes *or*
- Premature abnormal P wave (with or without QRS) interrupting another rhythm, *or*
- Heart rate ≥ 130, rhythm regular, P waves not discernible (may be present, but can't be sure)

The atrial rhythms that will be covered in this section are the following:

- Wandering atrial pacemaker
- Premature atrial complexes (PACs)
- Paroxysmal atrial tachycardia
- Atrial flutter
- Atrial fibrillation
- Supraventricular tachycardia (SVT)

Let's look at each of these rhythms in detail.

Wandering Atrial Pacemaker

What is it? Wandering atrial pacemaker (WAP) occurs when the pacemaking impulses originate from at least three different foci in the atria. One of these atrial foci may be the sinus node or the AV node, as you'll recall both are located in the atria. Each different focus produces its own unique P wave, resulting in a rhythm with at least three different shapes of P waves. WAP is an example of a slow atrial arrhythmia.

A wandering atrial pacemaker with a mean heart rate greater than 100 is called Multifocal Atrial Tachycardia or MAT. It is usually associated with chronic lung disease.

Rate	<100, usually 50s to 60s.
Regularity	Irregular.
P waves	At least three different shapes. Some beats may have no visible P waves at all.
PR	Varies.
QRS	<0.12 second (≥0.12 s if BBB present).
Cause	Medication side effects, hypoxia, vagal stimulation, or MI.
Adverse effects	Usually no ill effects.
Treatment	Usually none needed.

In Figure 8-3, there are QRS complexes, all shaped the same. Regularity is irregular. Heart rate is 50 to 60, with a mean rate of 50. At least three different shapes of P waves precede the QRS complexes. P-P interval varies. PR interval varies from 0.24 to 0.32. QRS interval is 0.08. Interpretation: wandering atrial pacemaker.

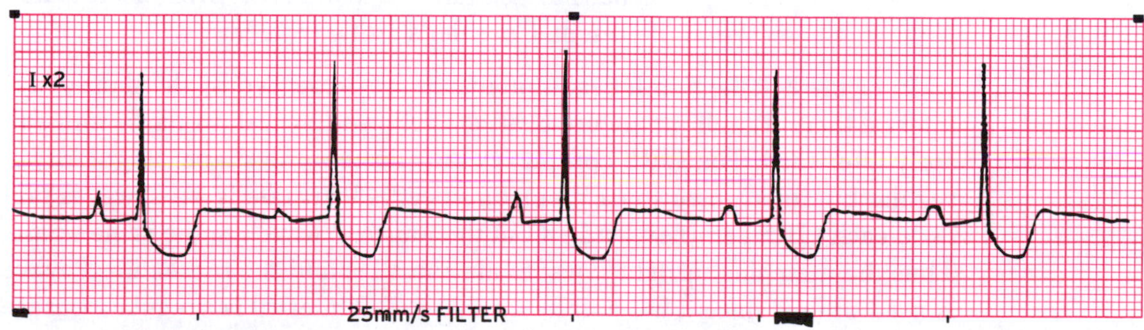

Figure 8-3 Wandering atrial pacemaker.

Premature Atrial Complexes (PACs)

What are they? PACs are premature beats that are fired out by irritable atrial tissue before the next sinus beat is due. The premature P wave may or may not be followed by a QRS, depending on how premature the PAC is. If the PAC is very premature, it will not be conducted to the ventricle because it will arrive during the ventricle's refractory period.

Rate	Can occur at any rate.
Regularity	Regular but interrupted (by the PACs).
P waves	Shaped differently from sinus P waves. The premature P waves of PACs may be hidden in the T wave of the preceding beat, and if so, will deform the shape of that T wave. Always be suspicious when a T wave suddenly changes shape. If the QRS complexes look the same, then the T waves that belong to them should also look the same. If one T wave is different, there's probably a P wave hiding in it. If the PAC's P wave is inverted, the PR interval should be 0.12 to 0.20 s.
PR	0.12 to 0.20 second.
QRS	<0.12 second (≥0.12 s if BBB present). QRS will be absent after a nonconducted PAC. The most common cause of an unexplained pause is a nonconducted PAC. If you see a pause and you're tempted to call it a sinus arrest or sinus block, make sure there's no P hiding in the T wave inside the pause. It might just be a nonconducted PAC.
Cause	The atria become hyper and fire early, before the next sinus beat is due. This can be caused by medications (stimulants, caffeine), tobacco, hypoxia, or heart disease. Occasional PACs are normal.
Adverse effects	Frequent PACs can be an early sign of impending heart failure or impending atrial tachycardia or atrial fibrillation. Patients usually have no ill effects from occasional PACs.
Treatment	Omit caffeine, tobacco, and other stimulants. Give digitalis or quinidine to treat PACs. Treat heart failure if present. Consider starting oxygen.

In Figure 8-4, the fourth beat is premature, as evidenced by the shorter R-R interval there. Recall premature beats are followed by a short pause immediately afterward. The QRS complexes are all the same shape. Regularity is regular but interrupted (by a premature beat). Heart rate is 54. P waves precede each QRS complex, and all but the fourth P wave are the same shape. Thus the matching upright P waves are sinus Ps, and the premature P wave is *not* a sinus P since it has a different shape. P-P interval is irregular because of the premature P wave. PR interval is 0.16. QRS interval is 0.08. Interpretation: sinus bradycardia with a PAC.

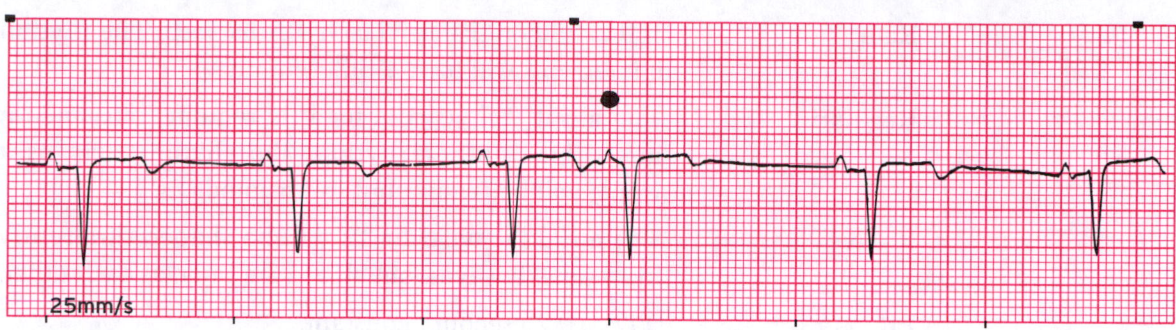

Figure 8-4 PAC.

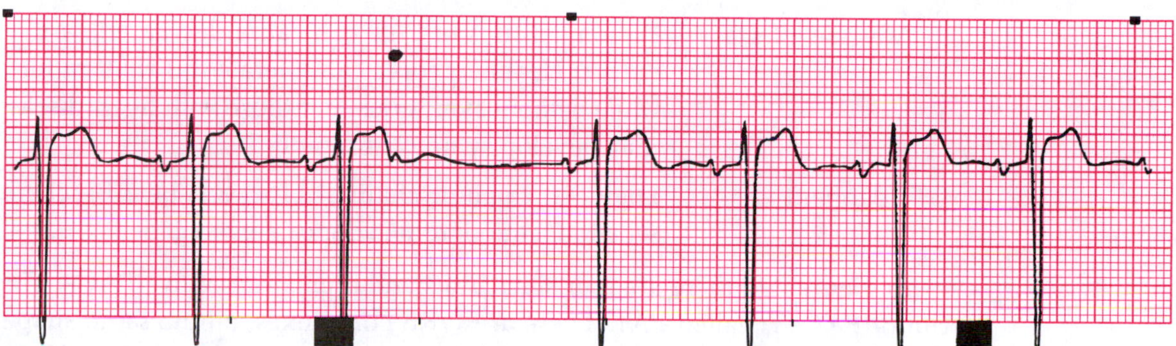

Figure 8-5 Nonconducted PAC.

In Figure 8-5, there are QRS complexes, all the same shape. Regularity is regular but interrupted (by a pause). Heart rate is 43 to 75, with a mean rate of 70. P waves are biphasic (half up, half down) and matching, except for the P wave that's at the end of the third beat's T wave. See the little hump there under the dot? That's a P wave. That P wave is shaped differently from the sinus P waves, and it is premature. How do we know it's premature? Look at the P-P intervals, the distance between consecutive P waves. All the sinus P waves are about four big blocks apart. This abnormal P wave is only $2^1/_2$ blocks from the P wave that precedes it. Thus it is premature. A premature P wave that is not followed by a QRS complex is a **nonconducted PAC**. Note the long pause that this nonconducted PAC causes. *Nonconducted PACs are the most common cause of otherwise unexplained pauses.* It is important to note that many nonconducted PACs do not have such easily noticeable P waves. Much of the time the premature P wave is hidden inside the T wave of the preceding beat, deforming that T wave's shape. PR interval here is 0.16; QRS interval is 0.10. Interpretation: sinus rhythm with a nonconducted PAC.

Paroxysmal Atrial Tachycardia (PAT)

What is it? The term *paroxysmal* refers to a rhythm that starts and stops suddenly. PAT is simply a sudden burst of three or more PACs in a row that usurps the underlying rhythm and then becomes its *own* rhythm for a period of time. PAT resembles sinus tach, but with a faster heart rate. *In order to diagnose PAT, the PAC that initiates it must be seen.*

Rate	160 to 250 on the atrial tachycardia itself. The rhythm it interrupts will have a different rate.
Regularity	The atrial tachycardia itself is regular, but since it interrupts another rhythm, the rhythm strip as a whole will be regular but interrupted.
P waves	The atrial tachycardia Ps will be shaped differently from sinus P waves, but all are the same as each other.
PR	0.12 to 0.20 second, constant.
QRS	<0.12 second (>0.12 s if BBB present).
Cause	Same as PACs or sinus tach.
Adverse effects	Prolonged runs of PAT can cause decreased cardiac output. Healthy people can tolerate this rhythm for a while without symptoms, but those with heart disease may develop symptoms rapidly.
Treatment	Digitalis, calcium channel blockers, beta-blockers, sedation, amiodarone, adenosine, oxygen.

In Figure 8-6, there are four sinus beats and then a run of five PACs. This run of PACs is called PAT. There are QRS complexes, all the same shape. Regularity is regular but interrupted (by a run of premature beats). Heart rate is 75 for the sinus rhythm, and 187 for the atrial tachycardia. P waves precede each QRS complex but are not all the same shape. The sinus beats have one shape of P wave, and the atrial tachycardia has a different shape P that is deforming the T waves. Note the dots over the premature P waves. Wait a minute, you say! What P waves? We can't see them! Here's a rule to help you: If the QRS complexes on the strip look alike, the T waves that follow them should also look alike. A T wave that changes shape when the QRSs don't is hiding a P wave inside it. Look at the T waves of the first four beats. They have rather broad sloping T waves. The PAT's T waves are pointy–totally different in shape. They're hiding a P wave. Now to continue with our interpretation: P-P interval is regular during the sinus rhythm, and regular, though different, during the atrial tachycardia. PR interval of the sinus beats is 0.16. Cannot measure the PR interval of the PAT beats, since the P wave is hidden. QRS 0.08. Interpretation: sinus rhythm with a five-beat run of PAT.

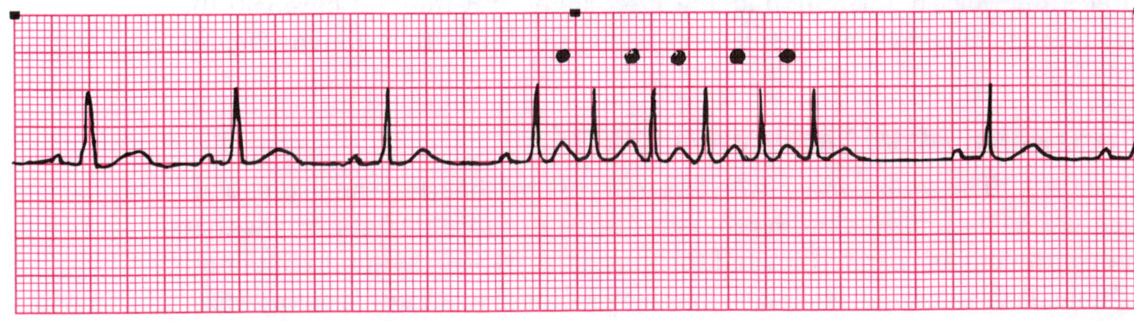

Figure 8-6 Paroxysmal atrial tachycardia.

Atrial Flutter

What is it? Atrial flutter results when one irritable atrial focus fires out regular impulses at a rate so rapid that a fluttery pattern is produced instead of P waves. The atrium is firing out its impulses so fast that the AV node, bombarded with all these impulses, lets some through but blocks others. Imagine a tennis ball machine firing out tennis balls so fast that there's no way you can hit them all. You end up ducking to protect yourself. The AV node is the gatekeeper–the protector–of the ventricles. Impulses must pass through it to reach the ventricles. Impulses that are too fast would provide a dangerously fast heart rate, so the AV node selectively blocks out some of the impulses, only letting some through.

Rate	Atrial rate 250 to 350. Ventricular rate depends on the conduction ratio.
Regularity	Regular if the conduction ratio is constant; irregular if the conduction ratio varies; can look regular but interrupted at times.
P waves	No P waves present. Flutter waves are present instead. These are sawtooth-shaped waves between the QRS complexes. Flutter waves are also described as picket-fence-shaped, V-shaped, or upside-down-V shaped. There will be two or more flutter waves to each QRS. All flutter waves march out–they're all the same distance apart. Flutter waves are always regular. They do not interrupt themselves to allow a QRS complex to pop in. Some flutter waves will therefore be hidden inside QRS complexes or T waves. The easiest way to find all the flutter waves is to find two flutter waves back-to-back and note the distance between the two (measure from either the top or bottom of the flutter waves; go from top to top of the flutter waves or bottom to bottom). Then march out where the rest of the flutter waves should be using this interval. Though most flutter waves will be easily visible using this method, some flutter waves will not be as obvious, as they are hidden inside the QRS or the T wave. Even though you can't see these flutter waves, they are there and they still count.
PR	Not measured, since there are no real P waves.
QRS	<0.12 second (≥0.12 s if BBB present).
Cause	Almost always implies heart disease. Other causes include pulmonary embolus, valvular heart disease, thyrotoxicosis, or lung disease.
Adverse effects	Can be very well tolerated at normal ventricular rates. At higher rates, signs of decreased cardiac output can occur. Cardiac output is influenced not by the atrial rate, but by the heart rate.

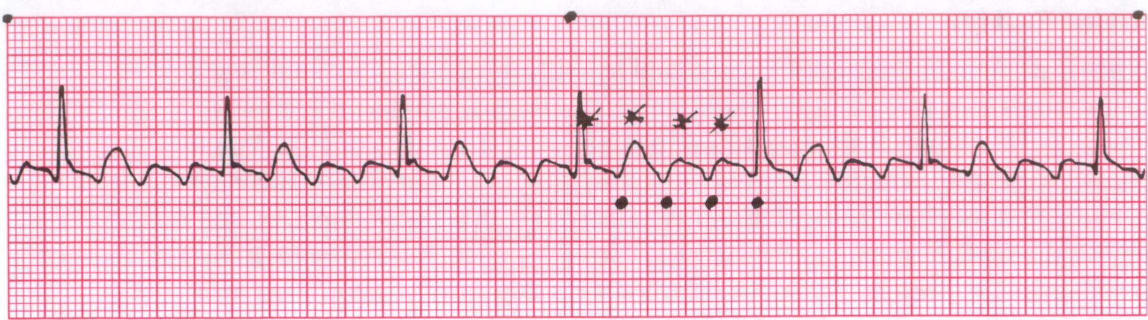

Figure 8-7 Atrial flutter.

Treatment — Digitalis, calcium channel blockers, beta-blockers, adenosine, carotid sinus massage to slow the ventricular rate. Electrical cardioversion can be done if medications are ineffective or the patient's condition deteriorates.

In Figure 8-7, there are QRS complexes, all shaped the same. Regularity is regular. Atrial rate is 250; heart rate is 65. P waves are not present; flutter waves are present instead, as evidenced by the V-shaped waves between the QRS complexes. Flutter waves are all regular. PR interval is not measured in atrial flutter. QRS interval is approximately 0.08, though it's difficult to measure as the flutter waves distort the QRS complex. Interpretation: atrial flutter with 4:1 conduction (four flutter waves to each QRS). See the dots under the flutter waves? There are four dots for each QRS. What if we measured from the top of the flutter waves instead of the bottom? Same thing. See the asterisks above the flutter waves? There are four of them (the fourth flutter wave is *inside* the QRS, but it still counts) to each QRS complex.

Atrial Fibrillation

What is it? In atrial fibrillation there are hundreds of atrial impulses from different locations all firing off at the same time. As a result, the atria depolarize not as a unit as they usually do, but rather in small sections. This causes the atria to wiggle instead of contract. The AV node is bombarded with all these impulses and simply cannot depolarize fast enough to let them all through. Every now and then one of these impulses does get through to the ventricle and provides a QRS.

Rate — Atrial rate is 350 to 700; ventricular rate varies. Atrial fibrillation with a ventricular rate >150 is called uncontrolled atrial fib; a ventricular rate of >100 is called rapid atrial fib; a ventricular rate of <60 is slow atrial fib. Remember ventricular rate is the same as heart rate.

Regularity — Irregularly irregular, completely unpredictable.

P waves — No P waves are present. Fibrillatory waves are present instead. These are undulations or waviness of the baseline between QRSs. If there are P waves, the rhythm is not atrial fibrillation.

PR	Since there are no P waves, there is no PR interval.
QRS	<0.12 second (>0.12 s if BBB present).
Cause	MI, lung disease, valvular heart disease, hyperthyroidism.
Adverse effects	Atrial fibrillation can cause a drop in cardiac output because of the loss of the atrial kick, which accounts for 15% to 30% of the cardiac output. One possible complication of atrial fibrillation is blood clots, which can collect in the sluggish atria. This can result in MI, strokes, or blood clots in the lung.
Treatment	Depends on the duration of atrial fib. If *less than* 48 hours, digitalis, calcium channel blockers, beta-blockers, amiodarone, or electrical cardioversion (small electrical shock to the heart to convert the rhythm back to sinus) can be utilized. In stable patients who have been in atrial fibrillation for *greater than* 48 hours, an anticoagulant (blood-thinner) called Coumadin is given to prevent blood clots from forming and cardioversion is delayed two to three weeks. In emergencies, patients in atrial fib greater than 48 hours will be started on heparin (an anticoagulant) intravenously, given a transesophageal echocardiogram (a sonarlike test using a probe inserted into the esophagus) to rule out blood clots in the atria, then electrically cardioverted. Consider starting oxygen.

In Figure 8-8, there are QRS complexes, all the same shape. Regularity is irregular. Heart rate is 65 to 100, with a mean rate of 90. P waves are absent; fibrillatory waves are present instead. PR interval is not applicable; QRS interval is 0.10. Interpretation: atrial fibrillation.

Supraventricular Tachycardia (SVT)

What is it? SVT is a term given to tachycardias that originate above the ventricles (the prefix supra- means above) in either the sinus node, the atrium, or the AV junction, but whose exact origin cannot be identified because P waves are not discernible.

Rate	About 130 or higher.
Regularity	Regular.

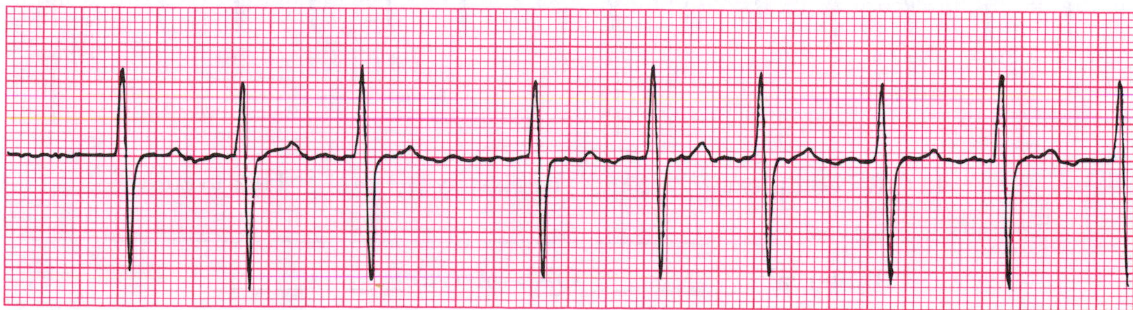

Figure 8-8 Atrial fibrillation.

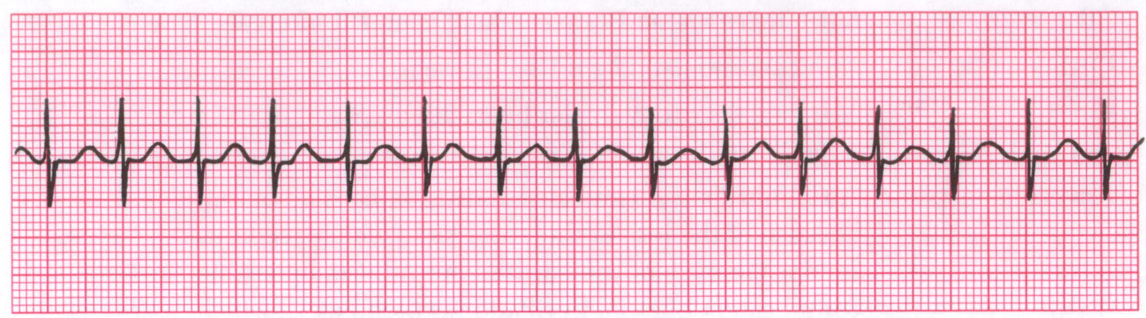

Figure 8-9 Supraventricular tachycardia.

P waves	Not discernible.
PR	Cannot be measured since P waves cannot be positively identified.
QRS	<0.12 second (≥0.12 s if BBB present).
Cause	Same as PAT.
Adverse effects	Decreased cardiac output secondary to the rapid heart rate.
Treatment	Digitalis, ibutilide, calcium channel blockers, beta-blockers. Consider starting oxygen.

In Figure 8-9, there are QRS complexes, all shaped the same. Rhythm is regular. Heart rate is 150. P waves are not identifiable. PR interval is not measurable. QRS interval is 0.08. Interpretation: SVT. Could it be atrial flutter? Sure. Could it be sinus tachycardia with the P inside the T wave? Possibly. The point is the origin of this rhythm is not clear, but we know that it originated in a pacemaker above the ventricle, since the QRS complex is narrow, less than 0.12 second. (Rhythms that originate in the ventricle have a wide QRS complex, greater than 0.12 second.) Bottom line: If the QRS is <0.12 second, the heart rate is around 130 or higher, the rhythm is regular, and you can't pick out the P waves, call the rhythm SVT.

Practice Strips: Atrial Rhythms

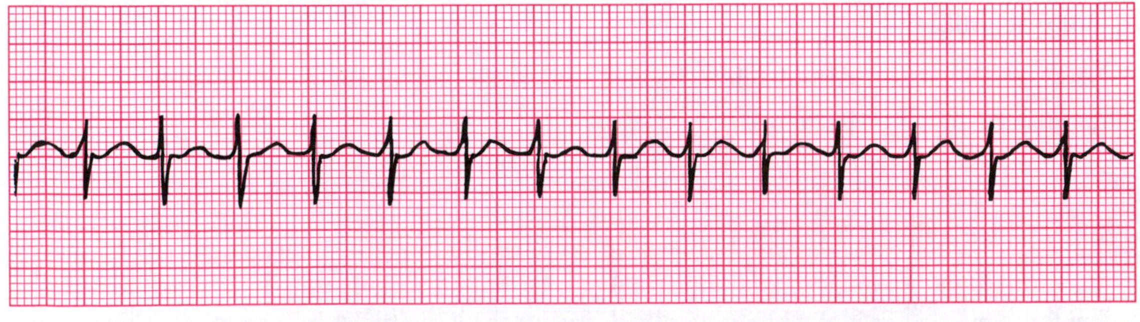

1. QRS complexes ________ Regularity ________ Heart rate ________
   P waves ____
   PR interval __________ QRS interval __________
   Interpretation (name of rhythm) ______________________________

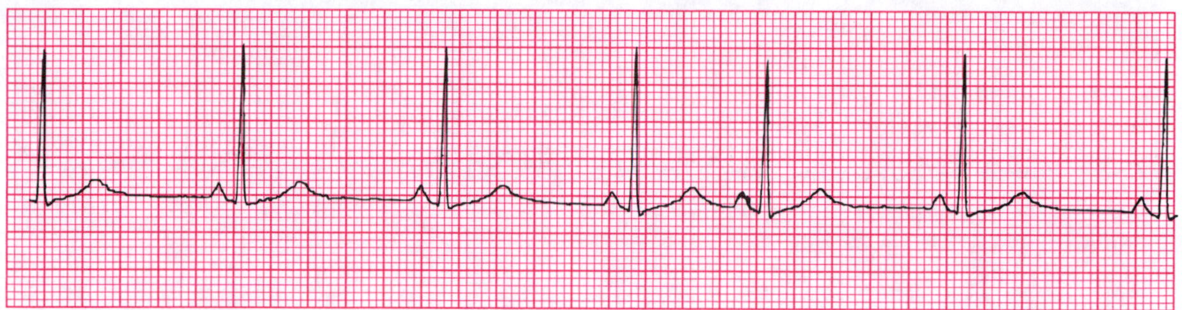

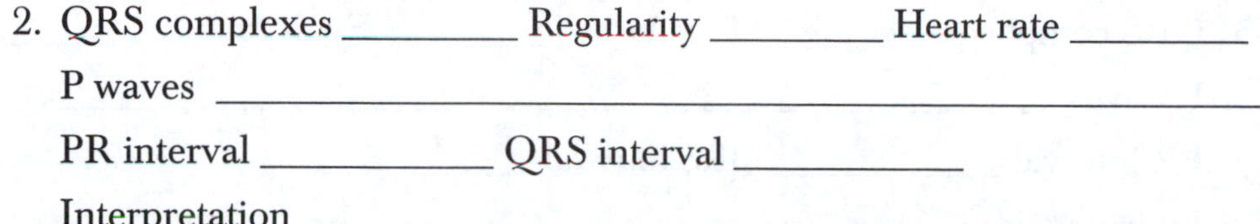

2. QRS complexes ________ Regularity ________ Heart rate ________
   P waves ____
   PR interval __________ QRS interval __________
   Interpretation ____

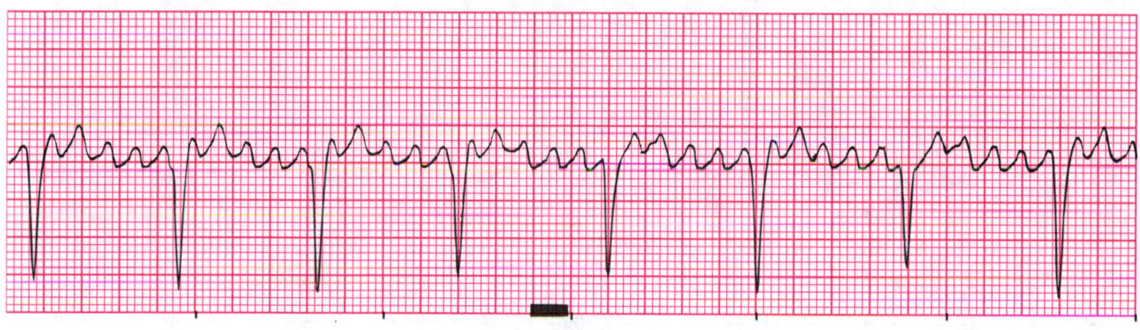

3. QRS complexes ________ Regularity ________ Heart rate ________
   P waves ____
   PR interval __________ QRS interval __________
   Interpretation ____

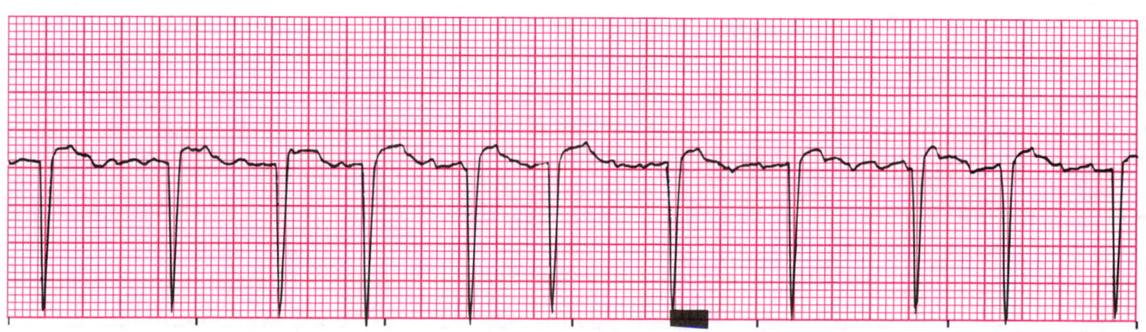

4. QRS complexes ________ Regularity ________ Heart rate ________
   P waves ____
   PR interval __________ QRS interval __________
   Interpretation ____

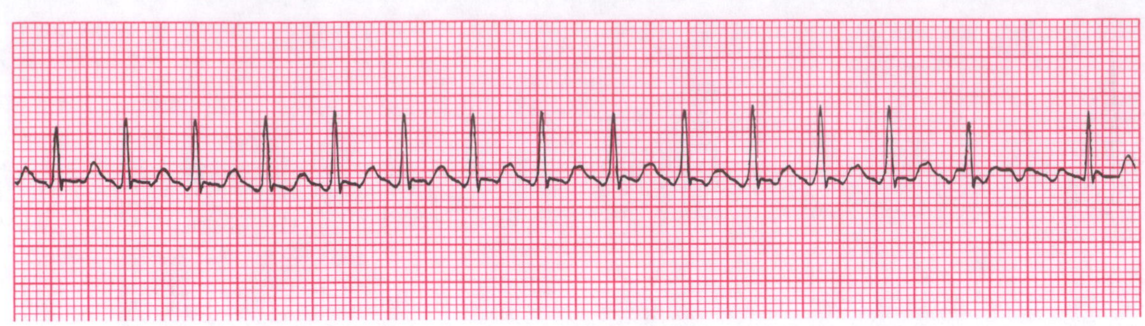

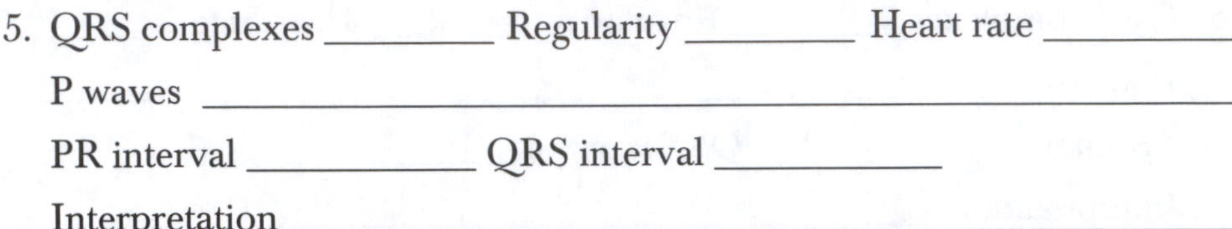

5. QRS complexes ________ Regularity ________ Heart rate ________
   P waves ____
   PR interval ____________ QRS interval ____________
   Interpretation ____

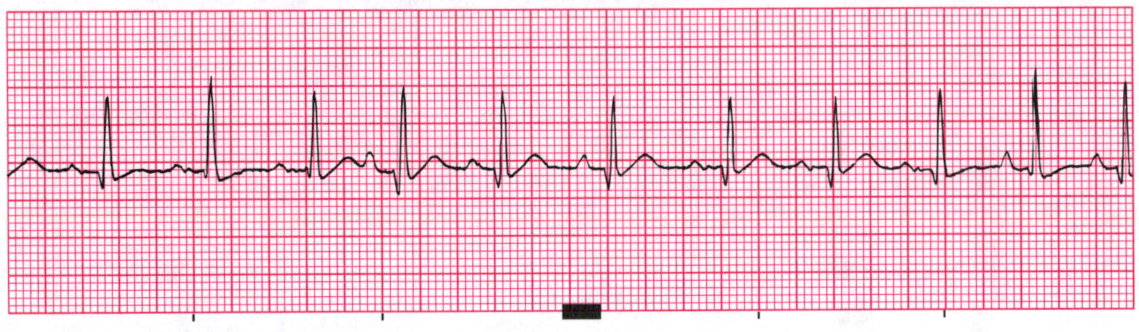

6. QRS complexes ________ Regularity ________ Heart rate ________
   P waves ____
   PR interval ____________ QRS interval ____________
   Interpretation ____

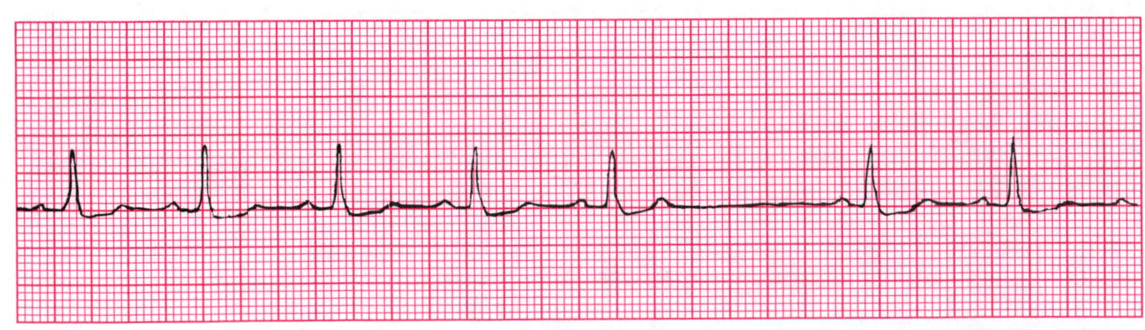

7. QRS complexes ________ Regularity ________ Heart rate ________
   P waves ____
   PR interval ____________ QRS interval ____________
   Interpretation ____

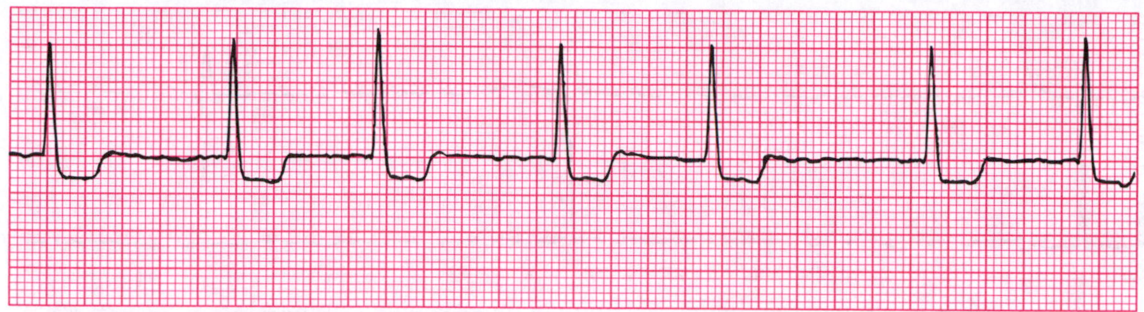

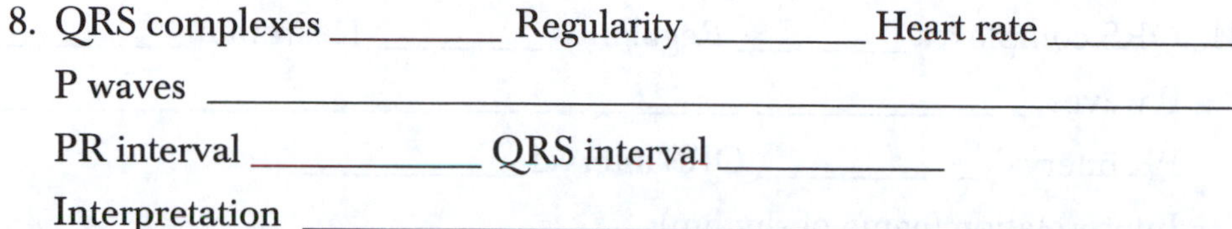

8. QRS complexes ________ Regularity ________ Heart rate ________
   P waves ____
   PR interval __________ QRS interval __________
   Interpretation ____

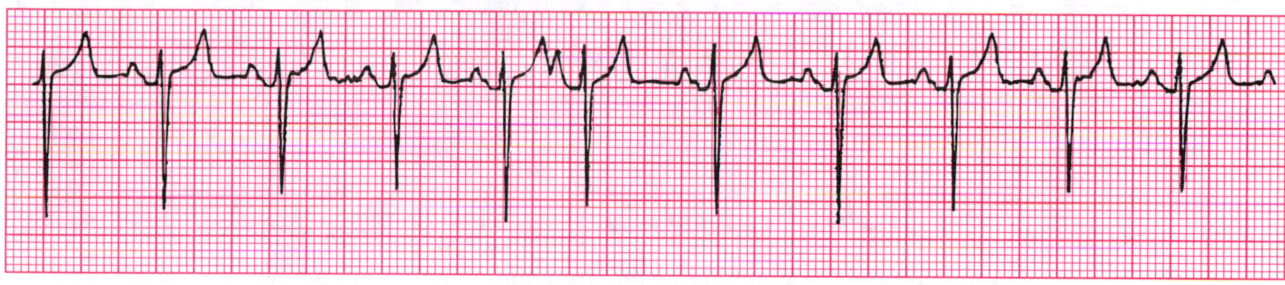

9. QRS complexes ________ Regularity ________ Heart rate ________
   P waves ____
   PR interval __________ QRS interval __________
   Interpretation ____

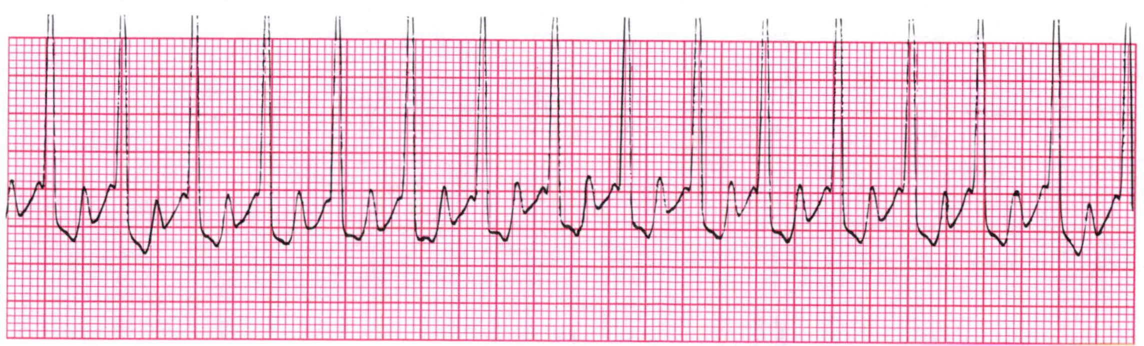

10. QRS complexes ________ Regularity ________ Heart rate ________
    P waves ____
    PR interval __________ QRS interval __________
    Interpretation ____

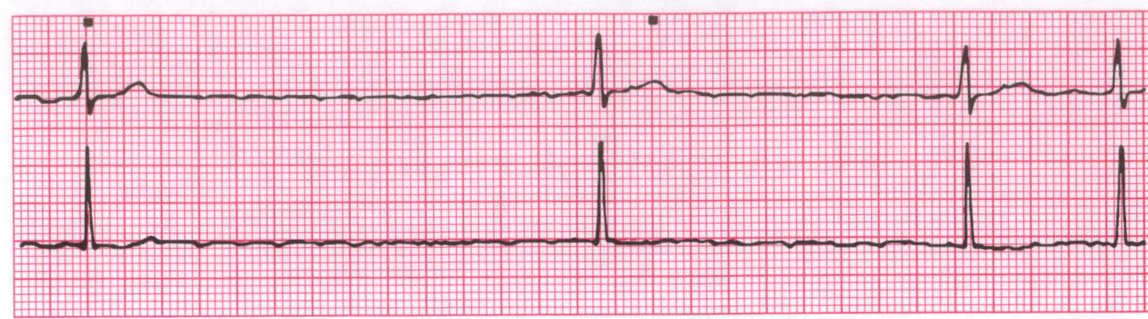

11. QRS complexes ________ Regularity ________ Heart rate ________
P waves ____
PR interval ____________ QRS interval ____________
Interpretation (name of rhythm) ________________________

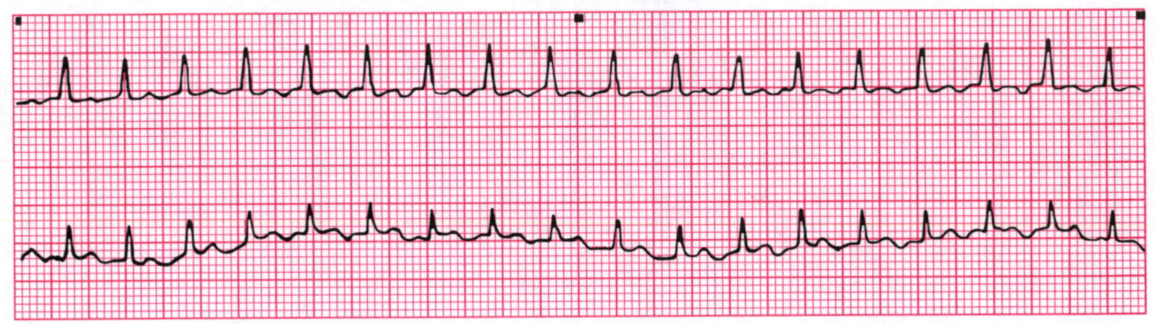

12. QRS complexes ________ Regularity ________ Heart rate ________
P waves ____
PR interval ____________ QRS interval ____________
Interpretation ________________________________

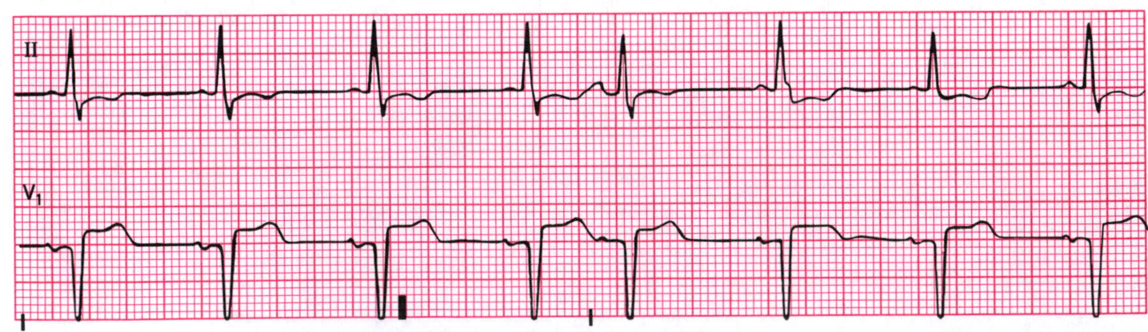

13. QRS complexes ________ Regularity ________ Heart rate ________
P waves ____
PR interval ____________ QRS interval ____________
Interpretation ________________________________

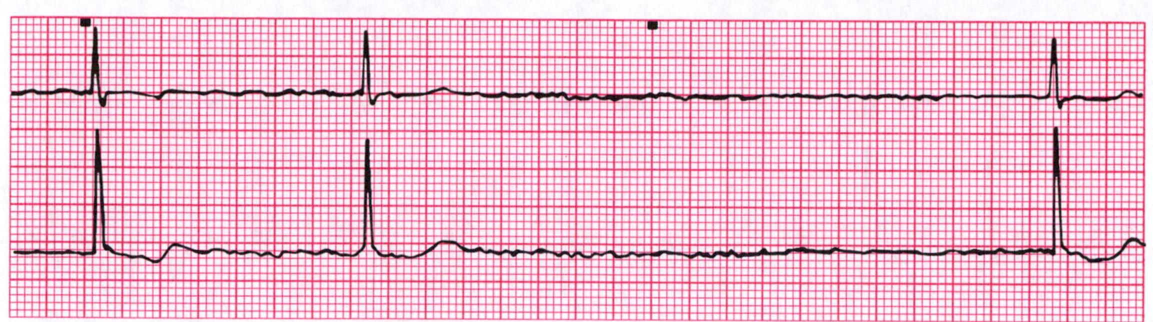

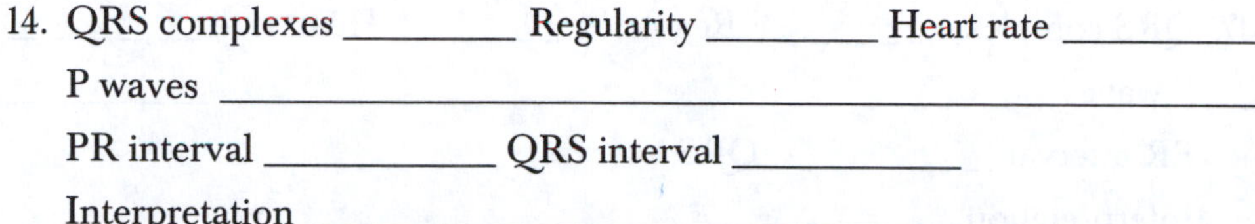

14. QRS complexes ________ Regularity ________ Heart rate ________

P waves ____

PR interval ____________ QRS interval ____________

Interpretation ____

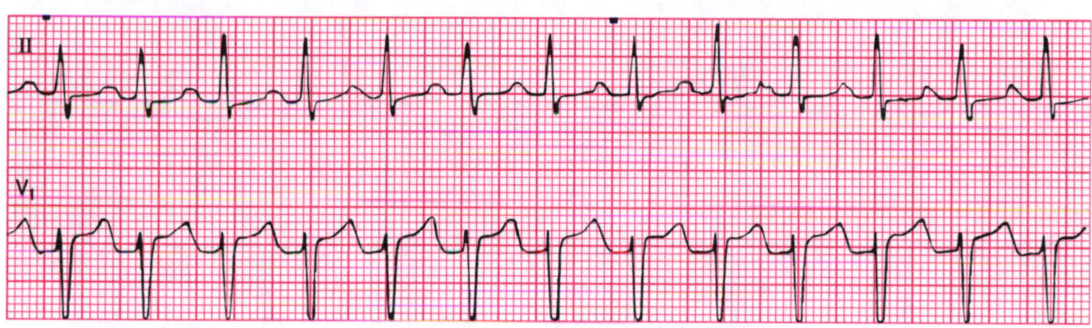

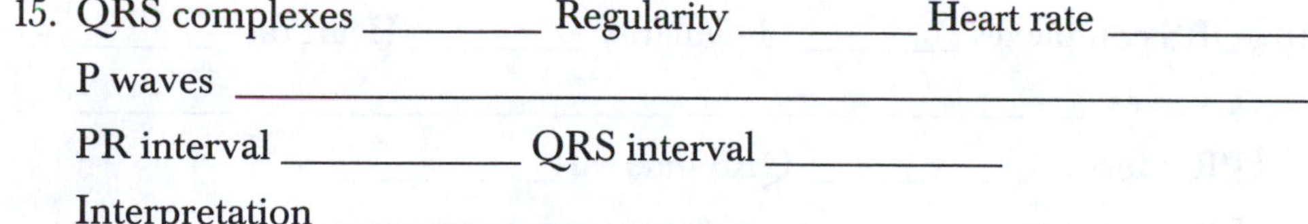

15. QRS complexes ________ Regularity ________ Heart rate ________

P waves ____

PR interval ____________ QRS interval ____________

Interpretation ____

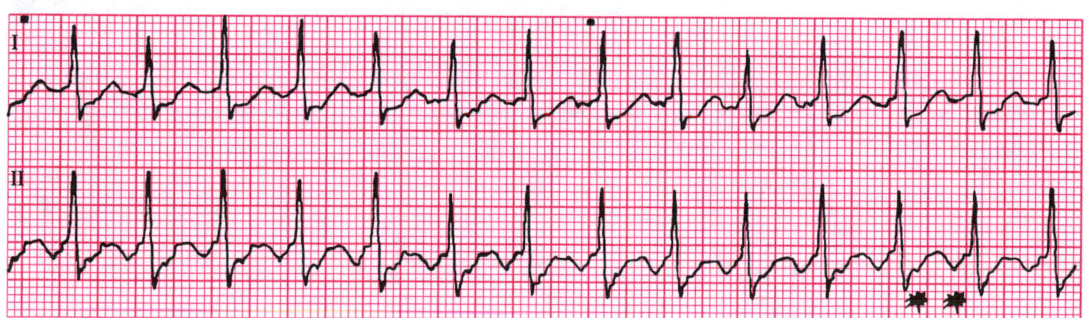

16. QRS complexes ________ Regularity ________ Heart rate ________

P waves ____

PR interval ____________ QRS interval ____________

Interpretation ____

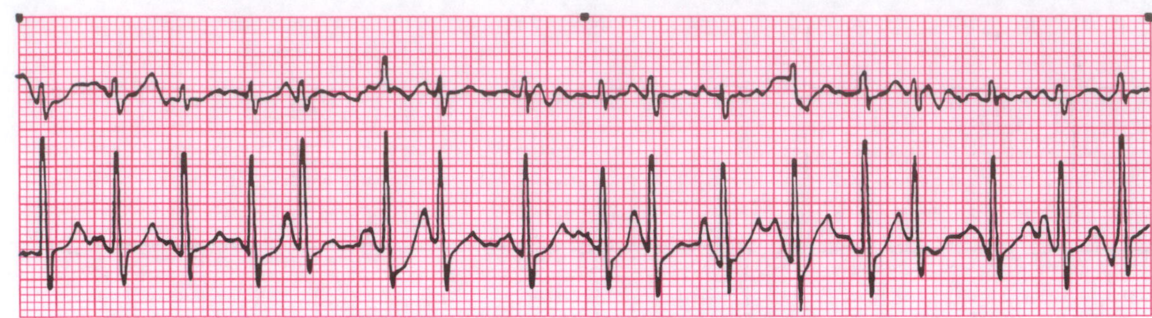

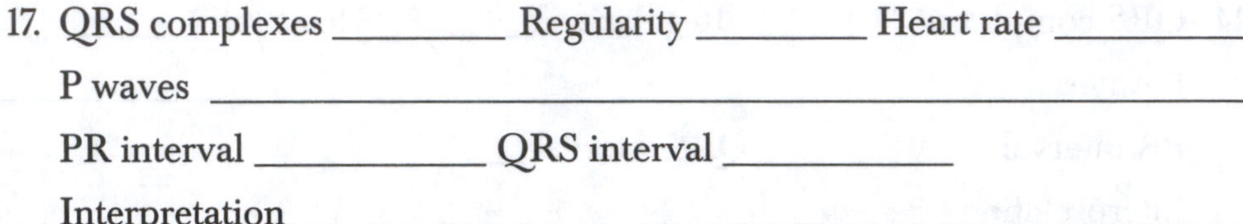

17. QRS complexes ________ Regularity ________ Heart rate ________
P waves ____
PR interval ____________ QRS interval ____________
Interpretation ____

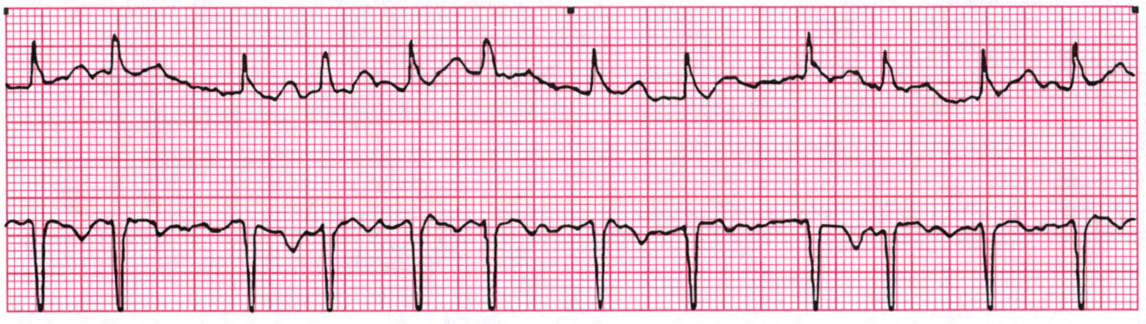

18. QRS complexes ________ Regularity ________ Heart rate ________
P waves ____
PR interval ____________ QRS interval ____________
Interpretation ____

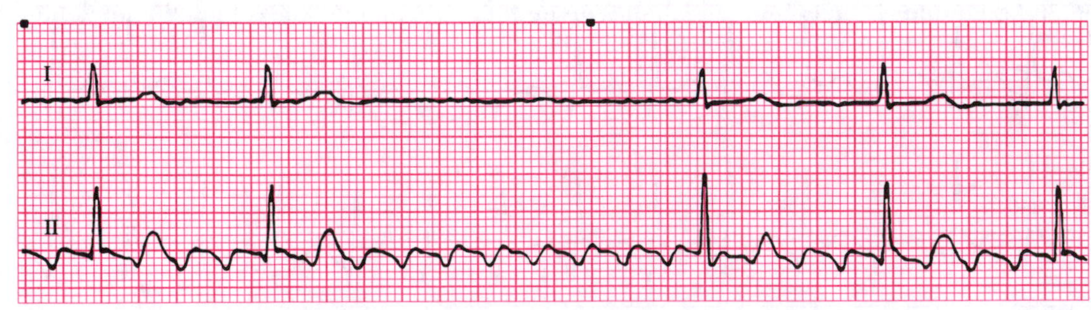

19. QRS complexes ________ Regularity ________ Heart rate ________
P waves ____
PR interval ____________ QRS interval ____________
Interpretation ____

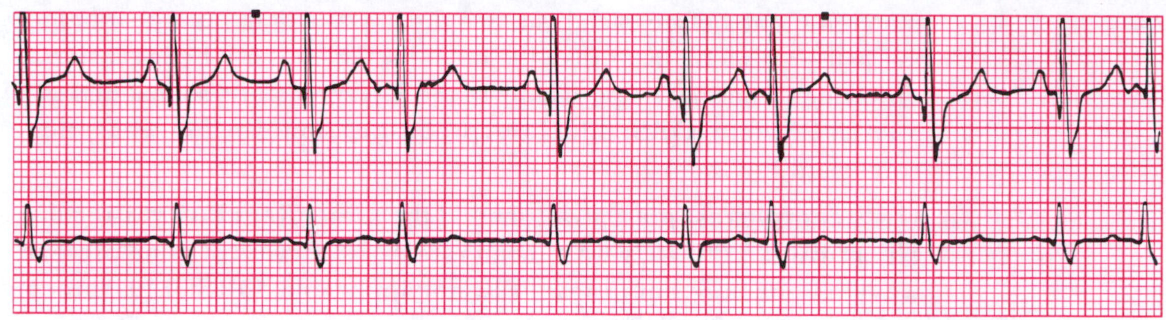

20. QRS complexes ________ Regularity ________ Heart rate ________
P waves ____
PR interval ____________ QRS interval ____________
Interpretation ____

Answers to Atrial Rhythms Practice Strips

1. **QRS complexes:** present, all shaped the same. **Regularity:** regular. **Heart rate:** 150. **P waves:** none visible. **PR:** not applicable. **QRS:** 0.08. **Interpretation:** SVT.
2. **QRS complexes:** present, all shaped the same. **Regularity:** regular but interrupted (by a premature beat). Remember it's normal to have a short pause after a premature beat. **Heart rate:** 56. **P waves:** upright and matching, except for the fourth P wave, which is premature and shaped differently. (There is a tiny notch on the downstroke of the premature P wave.) P-P interval irregular because of the premature beat. **PR:** 0.12. **QRS:** 0.08. **Interpretation:** sinus bradycardia with a PAC.
3. **QRS complexes:** present, all shaped the same. **Regularity:** regular. **Heart rate:** atrial rate 375; ventricular rate 79. **P waves:** none present; flutter waves present instead. **PR:** not applicable. **QRS:** 0.10. **Interpretation:** atrial flutter with 5:1 and 6:1 conduction.
4. **QRS complexes:** present, all shaped the same. **Regularity:** irregular. **Heart rate:** 88 to 137, with a mean rate of 110. **P waves:** none present; wavy baseline present instead. **PR:** not applicable. **QRS:** 0.08. **Interpretation:** atrial fibrillation.
5. **QRS complexes:** present, all shaped the same. **Regularity:** regular but interrupted (by a pause). **Heart rate:** atrial rate 300; ventricular rate 98 to 158, with a mean rate of 150. **P waves:** none present; flutter waves present instead. **PR:** not applicable. **QRS:** 0.08. **Interpretation:** atrial flutter with 2:1 and 4:1 conduction.
6. **QRS complexes:** present, all shaped the same. **Regularity:** irregular. **Heart rate:** 100 to 125, with a mean rate of 110. **P waves:** at least three different shapes. P-P interval irregular. **PR:** varies. **QRS:** 0.08. **Interpretation:** multifocal atrial tachycardia (wandering atrial pacemaker with a heart rate greater than 100).
7. **QRS complexes:** present, all shaped the same. **Regularity:** regular but interrupted (by a pause). **Heart rate:** 43 to 83. **P waves:** upright and

matching, one before each beat. See the T wave of the last beat before the pause? It's a bit taller than the other Ts. There is a P hiding inside it, distorting its normal shape. That P in the T is premature, so that makes it a PAC. **PR:** 0.16. **QRS:** 0.10. **Interpretation:** sinus rhythm with a non-conducted PAC.

8. **QRS complexes:** present, all shaped the same. **Regularity:** irregular. **Heart rate:** 52 to 75, with a mean rate of 70. **P waves:** none present; wavy baseline present instead. **PR:** not applicable. **QRS:** 0.10. **Interpretation:** atrial fibrillation.
9. **QRS complexes:** present, all shaped the same. **Regularity:** regular but interrupted (by a premature beat). **Heart rate:** 100. **P waves:** upright, all matching except for the premature P wave preceding the sixth QRS complex. There is one P wave preceding each QRS complex. P-P interval irregular. **PR:** 0.16. **QRS:** 0.08. **Interpretation:** sinus rhythm with a PAC.
10. **QRS complexes:** present, all shaped the same. **Regularity:** regular. **Heart rate:** about 150. **P waves:** Is that a tall pointy P wave distorting the T waves? Maybe. But it's also a possibility that those are flutter waves between the QRS complexes. We just can't be sure. **PR:** not applicable. **QRS:** 0.08. **Interpretation:** SVT.
11. **QRS complexes:** present, all shaped the same. **Regularity:** irregular. **Heart rate:** 22 to 75, mean rate 40. **P waves:** none noted; wavy baseline present instead. **PR:** not applicable. **QRS:** 0.08. **Interpretation:** atrial fibrillation.
12. **QRS complexes:** present, all shaped the same. **Regularity:** regular. **Heart rate:** 187. **P waves:** not seen. The wave between the QRS complexes may just be a T wave without a P wave. **PR:** not applicable. **QRS:** 0.06. **Interpretation:** SVT.
13. **QRS complexes:** present, all shaped the same. **Regularity:** regular but interrupted (by a premature beat). **Heart rate:** 75. **P waves:** biphasic, all matching except for the premature P wave preceding the fifth QRS. There is one P wave preceding each QRS. P-P interval irregular. **PR:** 0.14. **QRS:** 0.08. **Interpretation:** sinus rhythm with a PAC.
14. **QRS complexes:** present, all shaped the same. **Regularity:** irregular. **Heart rate:** 16 to 44, mean rate 30. **P waves:** none noted; wavy baseline present instead. **PR:** not applicable. **QRS:** 0.08. **Interpretation:** atrial fibrillation.
15. **QRS complexes:** present, all shaped the same. **Regularity:** regular. **Heart rate:** about 136. **P waves:** Is that a pointy P wave distorting the T waves in the top strip? Maybe–can't be sure. There are no hints of a P wave in the bottom strip. **PR:** not applicable. **QRS:** 0.10. **Interpretation:** SVT. This may indeed be a sinus tachycardia with the P wave hidden in the T wave of the preceding beat, but can't be sure.
16. **QRS complexes:** present, all shaped the same. **Regularity:** regular. **Heart rate:** 150. **P waves:** No P waves–those are flutter waves between the QRS complexes. See the asterisks under the flutter waves toward the

end of the strip on the bottom lead. **PR:** not applicable. **QRS:** 0.08. **Interpretation:** atrial flutter with 2:1 conduction. There are two flutter waves to each QRS.

17. **QRS complexes:** present, all shaped the same. **Regularity:** irregular. **Heart rate:** 136 to 231, mean rate 170. **P waves:** at least three different shapes. P-P interval irregular. **PR:** varies. **QRS:** 0.06. **Interpretation:** multifocal atrial tachycardia (rapid wandering atrial pacemaker).
18. **QRS complexes:** present, all shaped the same. **Regularity:** iregular. **Heart rate:** 88 to 150, mean rate 120. **P waves:** none noted; wavy baseline present instead. **PR:** not applicable. **QRS:** 0.08. **Interpretation:** atrial fibrillation.
19. **QRS complexes:** present, all shaped the same. **Regularity:** regular but interrupted by a pause. **Heart rate:** 26 to 65, mean rate 50. **P waves:** none seen. On the top strip is a very fine wavy baseline. The bottom strip has flutter waves. **PR:** not applicable. **QRS:** 0.08. **Interpretation:** This one is up for grabs. Could be either atrial fibrillation or atrial flutter. (Top strip looks like fib, bottom strip like fluttter.) It would help to have more leads to examine. Statistically, it's more likely that this is flutter rather than fib because atrial fib tends to be much more irregular. On this rhythm the QRS complexes are regular except for the pause.
20. **QRS complexes:** present, all shaped the same. **Regularity:** regular but interrupted by premature beats. Remember that premature beats are followed by a short pause that does not make the rhythm irregular. The fourth, seventh, and tenth beats are premature. **Heart rate:** 83. **P waves:** upright, matching except for the P waves on the premature beats. P-P interval irregular. **PR:** 0.14 on the sinus beats, 0.06 on the premature beats. **QRS:** 0.14. **Interpretation:** sinus rhythm with PACs.

Practice Quiz

1. What common complication of atrial fibrillation can be prevented by the use of anticoagulant medications? ______________________________

   ____
2. The rhythm that is the same as wandering atrial pacemaker except for the heart rate is ______________________________________

   ____
3. The rhythm that produces V-shaped waves between QRS complexes is

   ____
4. Atrial rhythms take what path to the ventricles? ________________
5. All rhythms that originate in a pacemaker other than the sinus node are called ____

   ____
6. Treatment for atrial fibrillation is dependent on what factor? __________

   ____

7. True or false: All PACs conduct through to the ventricles.
8. The classic cause of multifocal atrial tachycardia is ________
9. What test can be used in emergencies to determine if atrial blood clots are present? ________
10. If the rhythm is regular, heart rate is 130 or greater, and P waves cannot be identified, the rhythm is called ________
11. If the rhythm is regular, heart rate is 130 or greater, and P waves cannot be identified, the rhythm is called. ________

Putting It All Together—Critical Thinking Exercises

These exercises may consist of diagrams to label, scenarios to analyze, brain-stumping questions to ponder, or other challenging exercises to boost your knowledge of the chapter material.

Let's play with atrial rhythms a bit. The following scenario will provide you with information about a fictional patient and ask you to analyze the situation, answer questions, and decide on appropriate actions.

Mr. Baldo, a 20-year old college student, awoke feeling palpitations in his chest. He arrives at your emergency department an hour later with the following vital signs: BP normal at 130/78, respirations 22, temp 98.0 degrees. Skin is warm and dry. No pain, shortness of breath, or other distress aside from feeling the palpitations off and on. He denies ever having felt anything like this before. His rhythm strip is below, Figure 8-10.

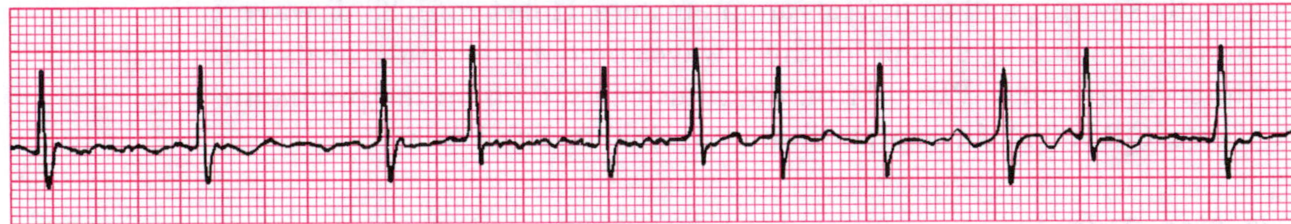

Figure 8-10 Mr. Baldo's initial strip.

1. What is Mr. Baldo's rhythm and heart rate? ________.
2. Is his situation an emergency? Why or why not? ________ ________.
3. Since Mr. Baldo's rhythm started tonight, what medication do we NOT need to consider as a part of his treatment? ________ ________.
4. What treatment would be appropriate for Mr. Baldo's rhythm? ________ ________.

   Mr. Baldo is given medication and, within the hour, the nurse records the following rhythm strip. See Figure 8-11.

5. What's happening on this strip? ________ ________.

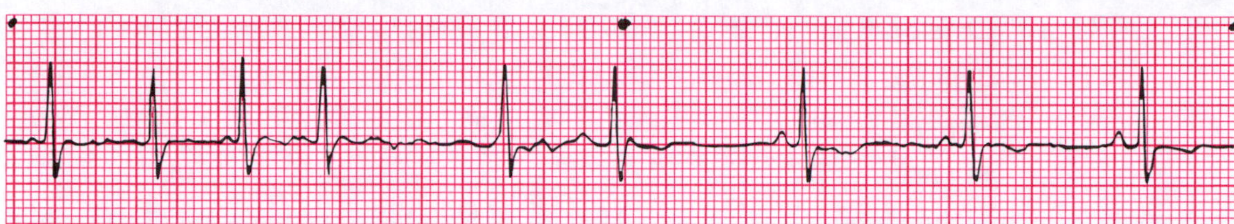

Figure 8-11 Rhythm after medication.

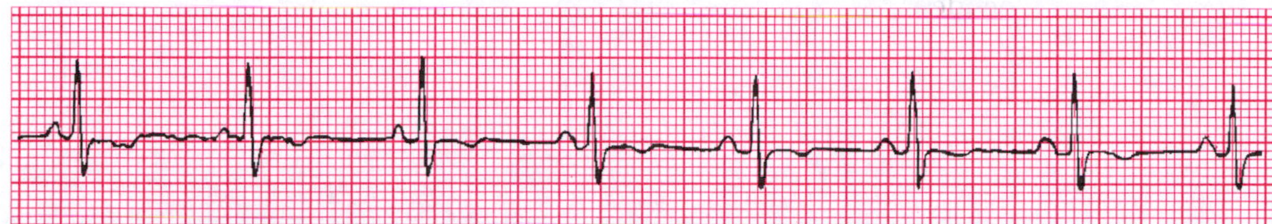

Figure 8-12 Discharge rhythm.

Mr. Baldo is watched in your emergency department for two more hours and then discharged with the following rhythm. See Figure 8-12. He is sent home with medication and told to follow up with a cardiologist for more studies.

6. What is Mr. Baldo's rhythm on discharge?

____

____

____

CHAPTER **9**

Rhythms Originating in the AV Junction

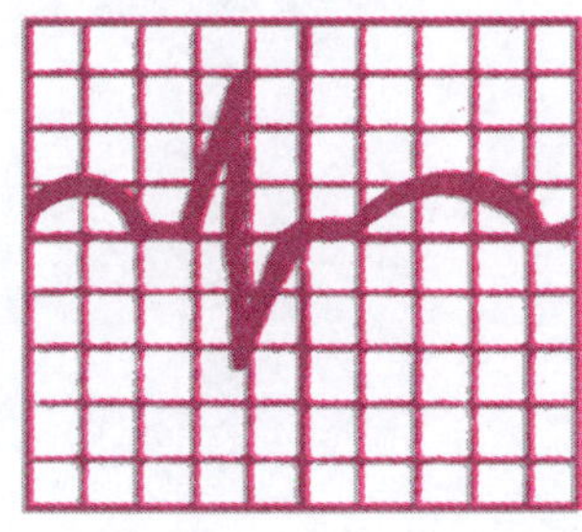

Chapter 9 Objectives

Upon completion of this chapter, the student will be able to:

- State the criteria for each junctional rhythm.
- Differentiate between *high, low,* and *midjunctional.*
- Correctly identify the junctional rhythms using the criteria and the rhythm strip analysis tools.
- State the adverse effects of each junctional rhythm.
- State the possible treatment for the junctional rhythms.
- State which junctional rhythms occur mostly because of escape and which imply usurpation.

Introduction

Though it was once thought that these rhythms originated in the AV node itself, it is now recognized that they arise from the **AV junction,** the tissue located between the right atrium and ventricle and surrounding the AV node. All these rhythms are blanketed under the term **junctional rhythms.**

With junctional rhythms, the impulse originates around the AV node and travels **antegrade,** or forward, toward the ventricle, and **retrograde,** or backward, toward the atria. Thus the impulse travels in two directions. The AV junctional area can be divided into regions–high, mid, and low–and whichever of these regions initiates the impulse will determine the location of the P wave. If the impulse originates high in the AV junction, close to the atria, it will arrive at the atria first and write an **inverted** (upside down) P wave. The P wave is inverted because the impulse is going in a backward direction to reach the atria. Then the forward impulses reach the ventricle and write the QRS complex. The PR interval is short, less than 0.12 second. Because the impulse starts out in the AV junction, halfway to the ventricle, it simply doesn't have as far to go as sinus impulses would. Bottom line: If the impulse originates high in the AV junction, the resultant rhythm or beat will have an inverted P wave preceding the QRS, and the PR interval should be less than 0.12 second.

If the impulse originates midway in the AV junction, the impulses will reach the atria and ventricles simultaneously because both are the same distance from the AV junction. Therefore, the P wave will be swallowed up by the QRS complex. Bottom line: Midjunctional impulses have no visible P waves.

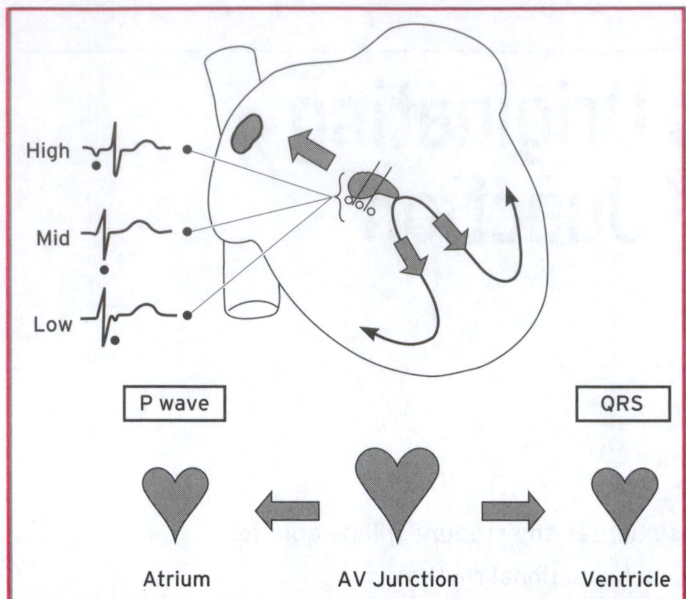

Figure 9-1 Conduction and P wave location in junctional rhythms.

If the impulse originates low in the AV junction, the impulses will reach the ventricle first, writing a QRS complex, and then reaching the atria and writing the P wave. Thus the P wave will follow the QRS and, since the impulses must travel backward to reach the atria, the P wave will be inverted. Bottom line: Impulses originating from low in the AV junction have inverted P waves following the QRS complex. See Figure 9-1.

Junctional rhythms can have inverted P waves preceding or following the QRS, or no visible P wave at all. The high-mid-low terminology is merely to explain why the P waves can be in different locations. It is purely an anatomical distinction and has no bearing on the interpretation of the rhythm.

The Word on Junctional Rhythms

Junctional rhythms are seen less often than sinus or atrial rhythms. Though the inherent rate of the AV junction is 40 to 60, the heart rate may actually be much faster or slower, which can result in symptoms. More normal heart rates are less likely to cause symptoms.

Treatment is aimed at alleviating the cause of the junctional rhythm. More active treatment is not usually necessary unless symptoms develop, at which time the goal is to return the sinus node to control or to return the heart rate to more normal levels.

Junctional rhythms are very easy to identify. Let's look at the criteria, which is a regular rhythm or premature beat with narrow QRS and one of the following:

- Absent P waves
- Inverted P waves following the QRS
- Inverted P waves with short PR interval preceding the QRS

The following junctional rhythms will be covered in this section:

- Premature junctional complexes (PJCs)
- Junctional bradycardia
- Junctional rhythm

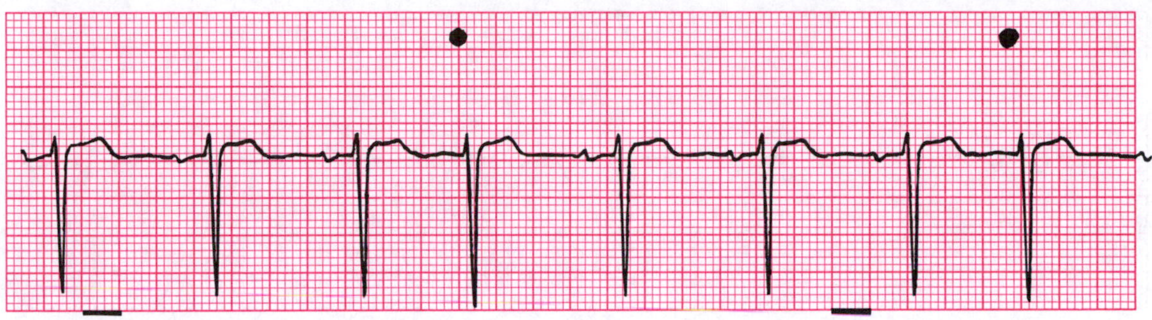

Figure 9-2 PJC.

- Accelerated junctional rhythm
- Junctional tachycardia

Let's look at each of these rhythms in detail.

Premature Junctional Complexes (PJCs)

What are they? PJCs are premature beats that originate in the AV junction before the next sinus beat is due. This is caused by irritable tissue in the AV junction firing off and usurping the sinus node for that beat.

Rate	Can occur at any rate.
Regularity	Regular but interrupted.
P waves	Inverted before or after the QRS, or hidden inside the QRS.
PR	<0.12 second if the P wave precedes the QRS.
QRS	<0.12 second (≥0.12 s if BBB present).
Cause	Stimulants (such as caffeine or drugs), nicotine, hypoxia, heart disease.
Adverse effects	Usually no ill effects.
Treatment	Usually none required aside from removal of the cause.

In Figure 9-2, there are QRS complexes, all shaped the same. Regularity is regular but interrupted (by two premature beats). Heart rate is 71. P waves are matching and biphasic except for the fourth and eighth beats, which are premature and have no P waves. PR interval is 0.16; QRS is 0.10. Interpretation: sinus rhythm with two PJCs.

Junctional Bradycardia

What is it? Junctional bradycardia is a junctional rhythm with a heart rate slower than usual. A higher pacemaker has failed, and the AV junction has to escape to save the patient's life.

Rate	<40.
Regularity	Regular.
P waves	Inverted before or after the QRS, or hidden inside the QRS.

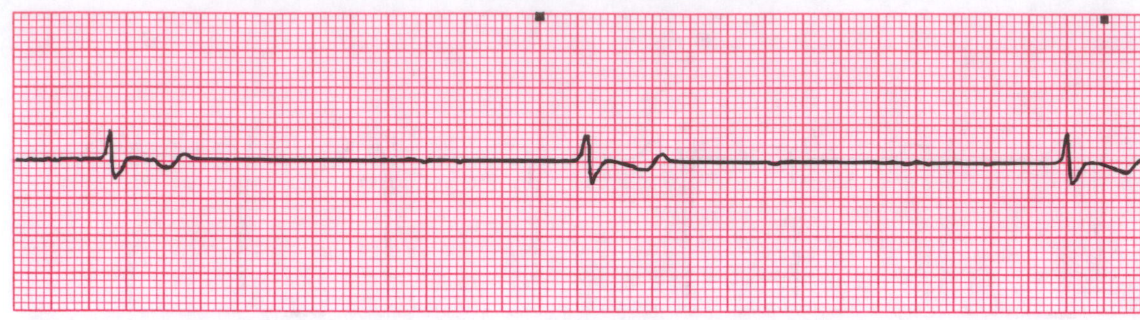

Figure 9-3 Junctional bradycardia.

PR	<0.12 second if the P precedes the QRS.
QRS	<0.12 second (≥0.12 s if BBB present).
Cause	Vagal stimulation, hypoxia, ischemia of the sinus node, heart disease.
Adverse effects	The slow heart rate can cause decreased cardiac output.
Treatment	Atropine if the patient is symptomatic. Hold or withdraw any medications that can slow the heart rate. A pacemaker can be utilized if atropine is unsuccessful and the patient is symptomatic. Start oxygen.

In Figure 9-3, there are QRS complexes, all shaped the same. Regularity is regular. Heart rate is 23. P waves are absent, or at least not visible. There is some somatic tremor artifact causing the baseline to look a bit jittery. PR interval is not applicable. QRS interval is 0.12. Interpretation: junctional bradycardia.

Junctional Rhythm

What is it? Junctional rhythm is a rhythm that originates in the AV junction at its inherent rate of 40 to 60. It is usually an escape rhythm.

Rate	40 to 60.
Regularity	Regular.
P waves	Inverted before or after the QRS, or hidden inside the QRS.
PR	<0.12 second if the P precedes the QRS.
QRS	<0.12 second (≥0.12 s if BBB present).
Cause	Vagal stimulation, hypoxia, sinus node ischemia, heart disease.
Adverse effects	Very often there are no ill effects if the heart rate is closer to the 50s to 60s range. Signs of decreased cardiac output are possible at slower heart rates.
Treatment	Atropine if symptomatic from the slow heart rate. Withdraw or decrease any medications that can slow the heart rate. Consider starting oxygen.

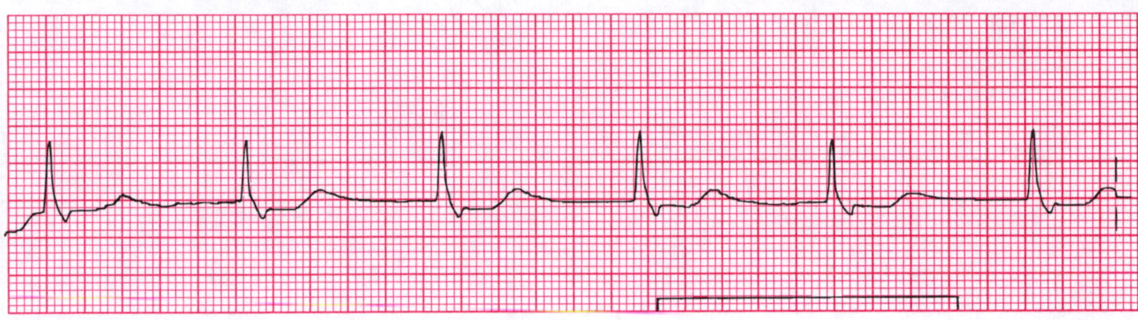

Figure 9-4 Junctional rhythm.

In Figure 9-4, there are QRS complexes, all the same shape. Regularity is regular. Heart rate is 58. P waves are absent. (Those are not P waves after the QRS; those are S waves, a part of the QRS.) PR interval is not applicable. QRS interval is 0.12. Interpretation: junctional rhythm. Though this example of junctional rhythm has no visible P waves, it could just as easily have had an inverted P wave with a short PR interval preceding the QRS, or an inverted P wave following the QRS. Remember, the location of the P wave is dependent on the region of the AV junction in which the impulse originates.

Accelerated Junctional Rhythm

What is it? Accelerated junctional rhythm can occur because of escape or usurpation. If the sinus node slows down, the AV junction can become stimulated to escape and take over as the pacemaker. Or an irritable spot in the AV junction can usurp control from the slower sinus node and become the heart's pacemaker at a heart rate faster than the AV junction normally fires.

Rate	60 to 100.
Regularity	Regular.
P waves	Inverted before or after the QRS, or hidden inside the QRS.
PR	<0.12 second if the P precedes the QRS.
QRS	<0.12 second (≥0.12 s if BBB present).
Cause	Heart disease, stimulant drugs, and caffeine.
Adverse effects	Usually no ill effects because the heart rate is within normal limits.
Treatment	Usually none required aside from removal of the cause.

In Figure 9-5, there are QRS complexes, all the same shape. Regularity is regular. Heart rate is 75. P waves are absent. PR interval is not applicable. QRS interval is 0.08. Interpretation: accelerated junctional rhythm.

Junctional Tachycardia

What is it? An irritable spot in the AV junction has taken over as the pacemaker, and the heart rate is very rapid. This is usually a result of usurpation.

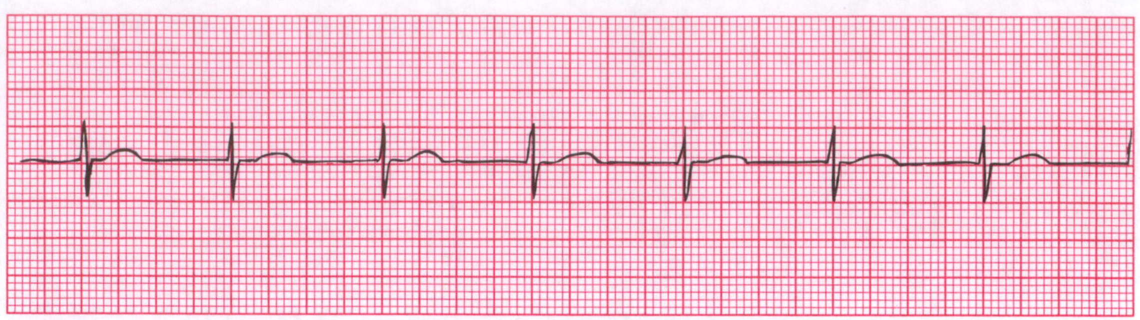

Figure 9-5 Accelerated junctional rhythm.

Junctional tachycardia is best called SVT if there are no visible P waves, as the origin of the rhythm is not identifiable.

Rate	>100.
Regularity	Regular.
P waves	Inverted before or after the QRS, or hidden inside the QRS.
PR	<0.12 second if the P precedes the QRS.
QRS	<0.12 second (≥0.12 s if BBB present).
Cause	Most often caused by digitalis toxicity, but can be caused by heart disease, stimulants, or anything else that stimulates the sympathetic nervous system to speed up the heart rate.
Adverse effects	Decreased cardiac output possible if the heart rate is fast enough.
Treatment	Beta-blockers, calcium channel blockers, adenosine. Consider starting oxygen.

In Figure 9-6, there are QRS complexes, all the same shape. Regularity is regular. Heart rate is 125. P waves are present, inverted, following the QRS complex. PR interval is not applicable. QRS interval is 0.08. Interpretation: junctional tachycardia.

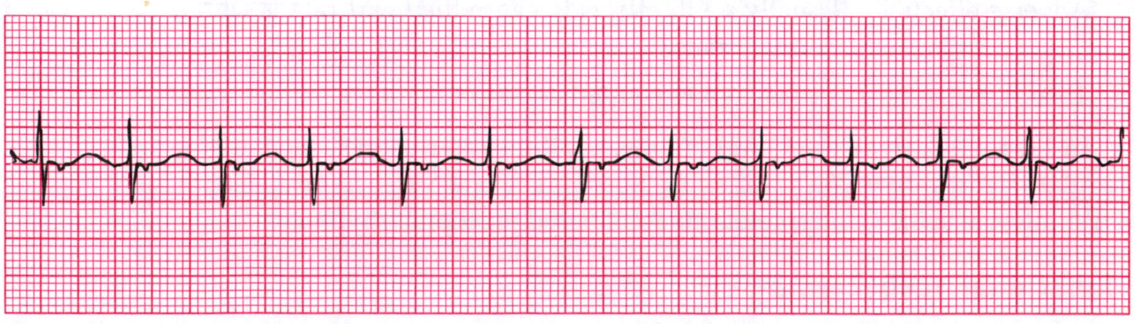

Figure 9-6 Junctional tachycardia.

Practice Strips: Junctional Rhythms

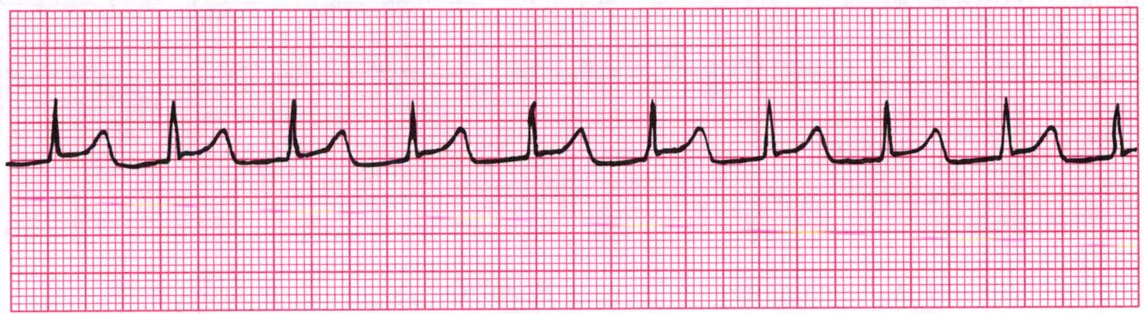

1. QRS complexes ________ Regularity ________ Heart rate ________
   P waves ________________________________
   PR interval __________ QRS interval __________
   Interpretation (name of rhythm) ____________________

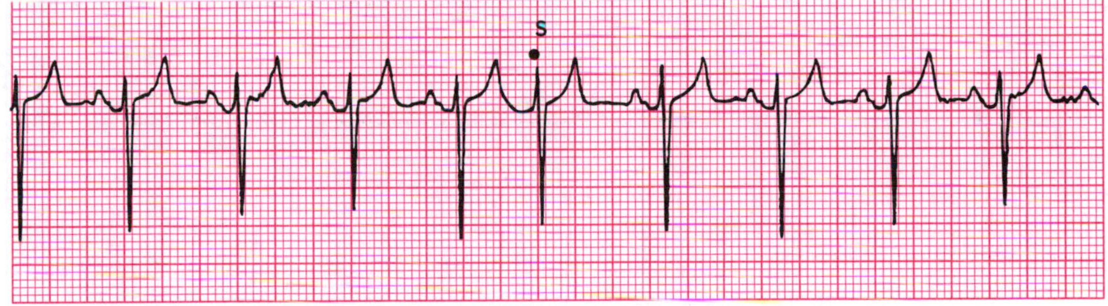

2. QRS complexes ________ Regularity ________ Heart rate ________
   P waves ________________________________
   PR interval __________ QRS interval __________
   Interpretation ____________________

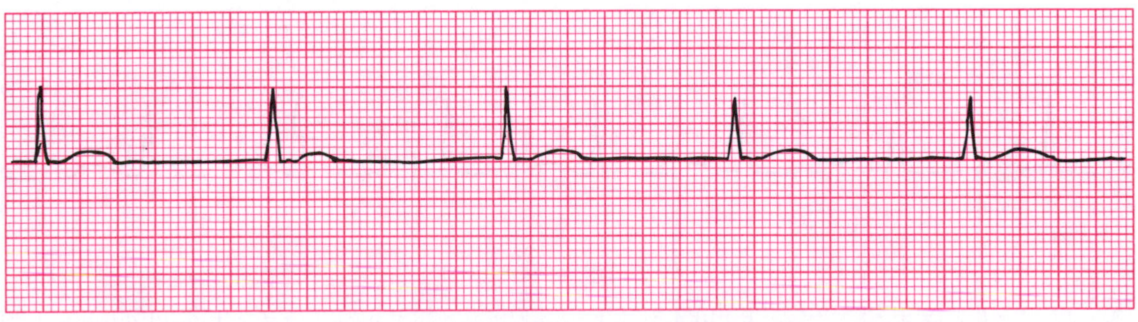

3. QRS complexes ________ Regularity ________ Heart rate ________
   P waves ________________________________
   PR interval __________ QRS interval __________
   Interpretation ____________________

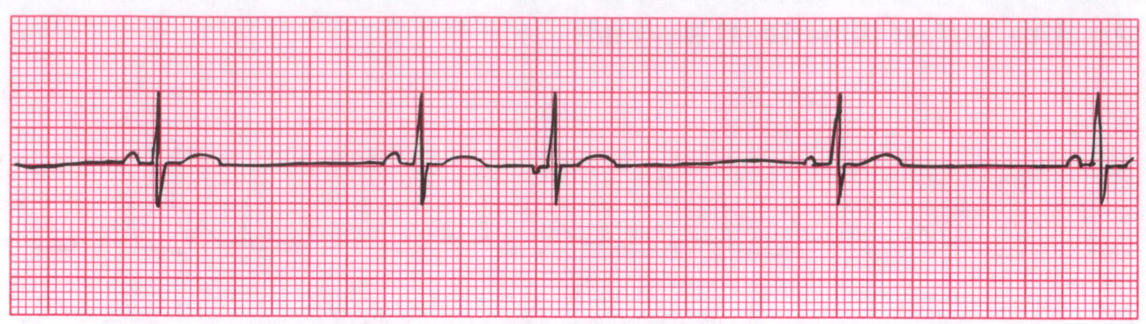

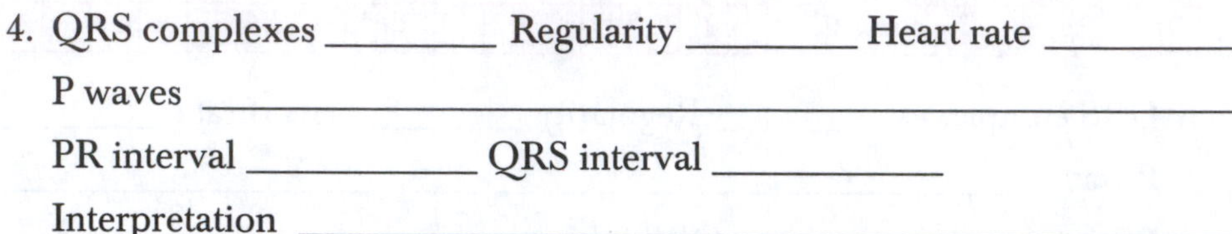

4. QRS complexes ________ Regularity ________ Heart rate ________
   P waves ____
   PR interval ____________ QRS interval ____________
   Interpretation ____

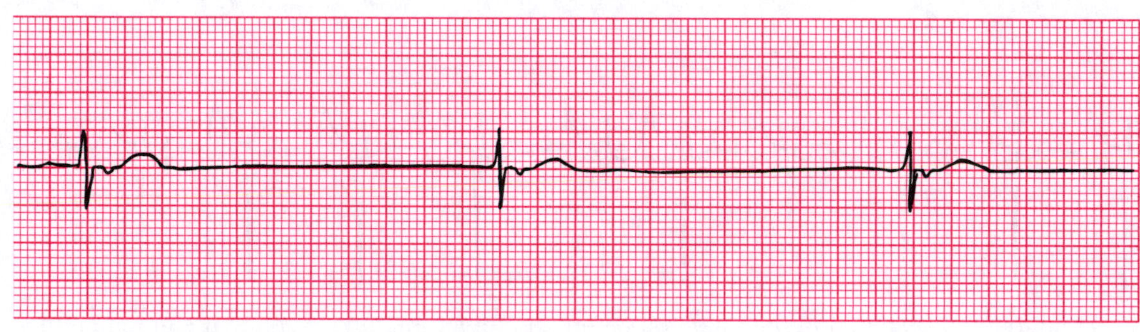

5. QRS complexes ________ Regularity ________ Heart rate ________
   P waves ____
   PR interval ____________ QRS interval ____________
   Interpretation ____

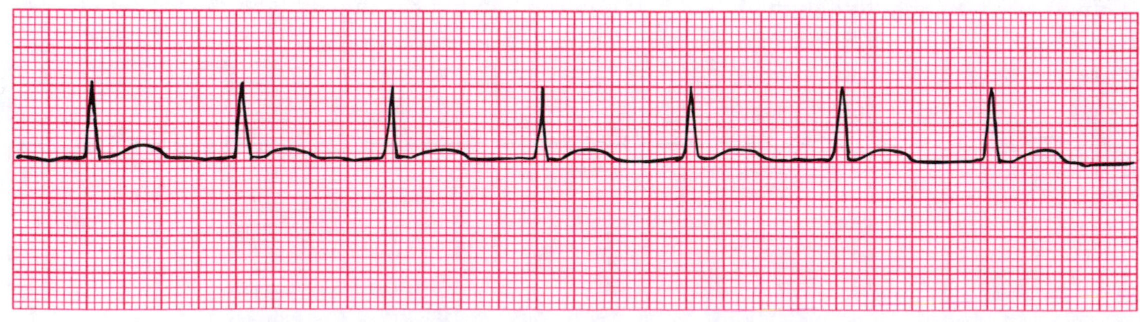

6. QRS complexes ________ Regularity ________ Heart rate ________
   P waves ____
   PR interval ____________ QRS interval ____________
   Interpretation ____

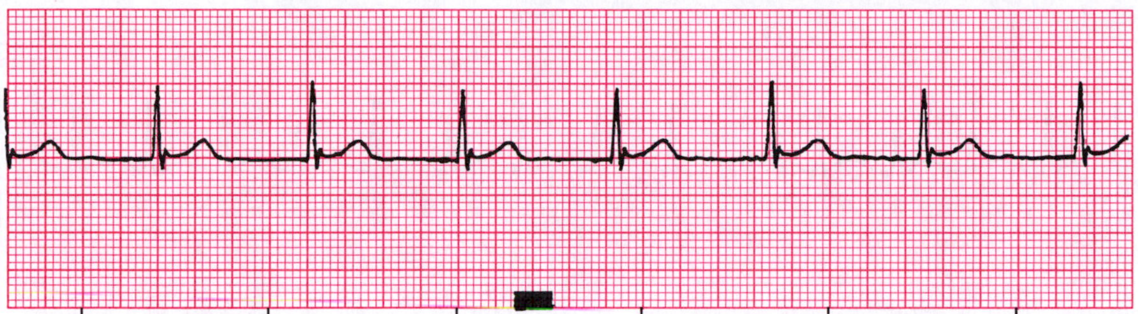

7. QRS complexes ________ Regularity ________ Heart rate __________
P waves ____
PR interval ___________ QRS interval ___________
Interpretation ____

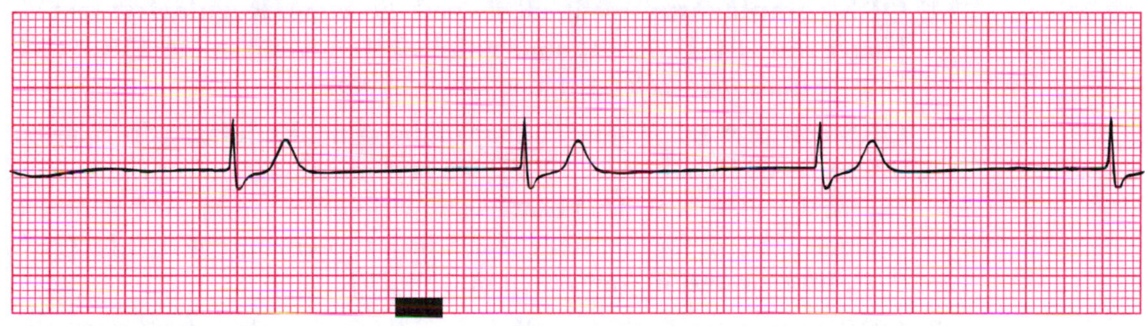

8. QRS complexes ________ Regularity ________ Heart rate __________
P waves ____
PR interval ___________ QRS interval ___________
Interpretation ____

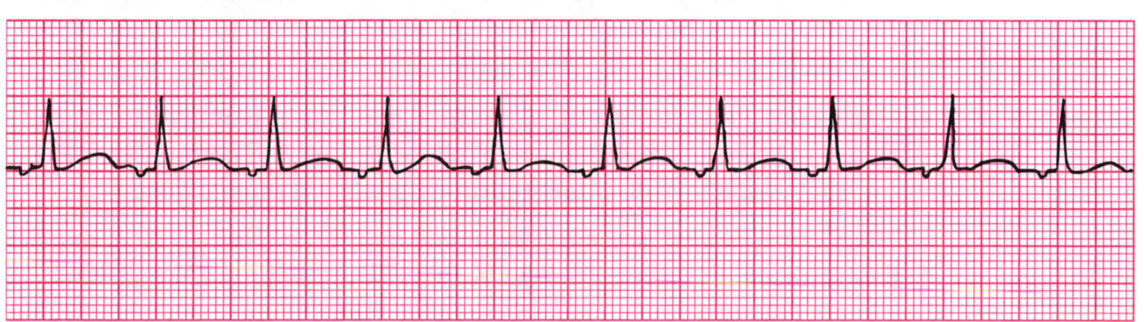

9. QRS complexes ________ Regularity ________ Heart rate __________
P waves ____
PR interval ___________ QRS interval ___________
Interpretation ____

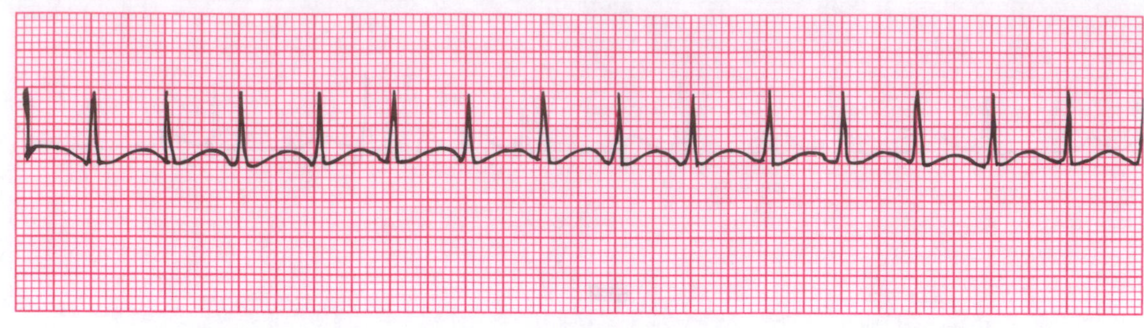

10. QRS complexes ________ Regularity ________ Heart rate ________

    P waves ____

    PR interval ____________ QRS interval ____________

    Interpretation ____

Answers to Junctional Rhythms Practice Strips

1. **QRS complexes:** present, all shaped the same. **Regularity:** regular. **Heart rate:** 94. **P waves:** none visible. **PR:** not applicable. **QRS:** 0.08. **Interpretation:** accelerated junctional rhythm.
2. **QRS complexes:** present, all shaped the same. **Regularity:** regular but interrupted. **Heart rate:** 100. **P waves:** matching and upright on all except the sixth beat. That beat has no visible P wave at all. P-P interval is regular except for that sixth beat, which is premature. **PR:** 0.14. **QRS:** 0.08. **Interpretation:** sinus rhythm with a PJC.
3. **QRS complexes:** present, all shaped the same. **Regularity:** regular. **Heart rate:** 48. **P waves:** none visible. **PR:** not applicable. **QRS:** 0.08. **Interpretation:** junctional rhythm.
4. **QRS complexes:** present, all shaped the same. **Regularity:** regular but interrupted. **Heart rate:** 47. **P waves:** matching upright Ps present except on the third beat, which has an inverted P wave preceding the QRS. **PR:** 0.16 on the beats with upright Ps; 0.06 on the third beat. **QRS:** 0.08. **Interpretation:** sinus bradycardia with a PJC. Remember it is normal for the R-R cycle immediately following a premature beat to be a little longer than usual. Consider this when determining the regularity.
5. **QRS complexes:** present, all shaped the same. **Regularity:** regular. **Heart rate:** 28. **P waves:** inverted following the QRS complexes. **PR:** not applicable. **QRS:** 0.08. **Interpretation:** junctional bradycardia.
6. **QRS complexes:** present, all shaped the same. **Regularity:** regular. **Heart rate:** 75. **P waves:** none visible. **PR:** not applicable. **QRS:** 0.08. **Interpretation:** accelerated junctional rhythm.
7. **QRS complexes:** present, all shaped the same. **Regularity:** regular. **Heart rate:** 72. **P waves:** none visible. **PR:** not applicable. **QRS:** 0.10. **Interpretation:** accelerated junctional rhythm.
8. **QRS complexes:** present, all shaped the same. **Regularity:** regular. **Heart rate:** 38. **P waves:** none visible. **PR:** not applicable. **QRS:** 0.10. **Interpretation:** junctional bradycardia.

9. **QRS complexes:** present, all shaped the same. **Regularity:** regular. **Heart rate:** 100. **P waves:** inverted preceding each QRS. **PR:** 0.10 to 0.12. **QRS:** 0.08. **Interpretation:** accelerated junctional rhythm.
10. **QRS complexes:** present, all shaped the same. **Regularity:** regular. **Heart rate:** 150. **P waves:** none visible. **PR:** not applicable. **QRS:** 0.08. **Interpretation:** SVT. Though this could indeed be a junctional tachycardia, it is best to call this SVT since P waves cannot be seen. Had there been an inverted P wave present, we'd have known for sure the rhythm was junctional in origin. Without those P waves, we can't be sure the rhythm is junctional. It could be atrial or even sinus in origin (with the P waves hidden inside the T waves).

Practice Quiz

1. What are the three possible locations for the P waves in junctional rhythms? ______________________________
____
____
2. Why is the P wave inverted in junctional rhythms? ______________
____
3. A junctional rhythm with a heart rate greater than 100 is __________
4. True or false: PJCs are a sign that the heart is going to develop a lethal arrhythmia.
5. A junctional rhythm with a heart rate less than 40 is ______________
6. Treatment for junctional bradycardia would consist of ____________
____
____
7. PJCs cause the regularity to be ______________________________
8. Is junctional bradycardia usually a result of escape or usurpation? _____
____
9. Junctional tachycardia is best called SVT if the P waves are located where? ______________________________
____
10. Is junctional tachycardia a result of escape or usurpation? __________
____
____

Putting It All Together—Critical Thinking Exercises

These exercises may consist of diagrams to label, scenarios to analyze, brain-stumping questions to ponder, or other challenging exercise to boost your understanding of the chapter material.

Let's play with junctional rhythms a bit. The following scenario will provide you with information about a fictional patient and ask you to analyze the situation, answer questions, and decide on appropriate actions.

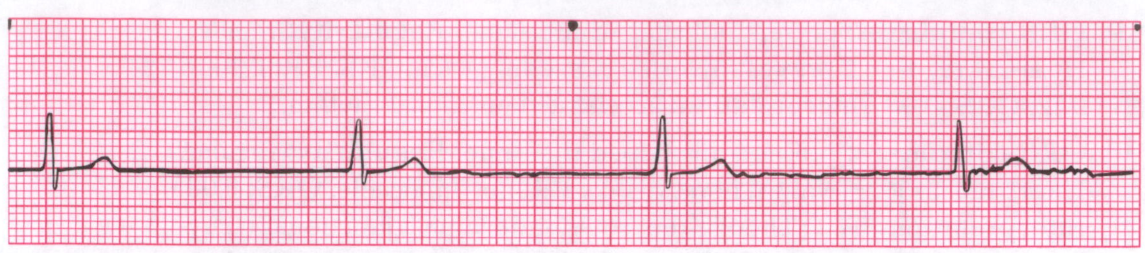

Figure 9-7 Mrs. Dubos's ER rhythm strip.

Mrs. Dubos, age 86, is to be admitted to your intensive care unit. The ER nurse reports to you the following: She'd come to the ER complaining of shortness of breath and chest pain. Examination in the ER found her to be in sinus bradycardia with a heart rate of 47. BP at that time was 76/43 (very low), respirations 34 (fast), and temperature was normal. She was cool and clammy and appeared a bit dazed and confused. After appropriate medication, the heart rate came up to 86, her BP came up to 132/74 (normal) and her respirations slowed to a normal 20. Chest pain and shortness of breath subsided.

1. What medication do you believe was given in the ER to speed up Mrs. Dubos' heart rate? ______________________________.

   When Mrs. Dubos arrives on your floor, you look at the ER rhythm strip. See Figure 9-7.

2. What is the rhythm and rate? ______________________________

   ____

   ______________________________.

3. Was the ER nurse correct in her interpretation of this rhythm and rate? If no, explain why. ______________________________

   ____

   ____

   ______________________________.

4. Do you agree that the treatment rendered in the ER was appropriate for this patient? Why or why not?______________________________

   ____

   ____

   ______________________________.

5. Did Mrs. Dubos have signs of decreased cardiac output in the ER? If yes, what were they? ______________________________

   ____

   ____

   ______________________________.

CHAPTER **10**

Rhythms Originating in the Ventricles

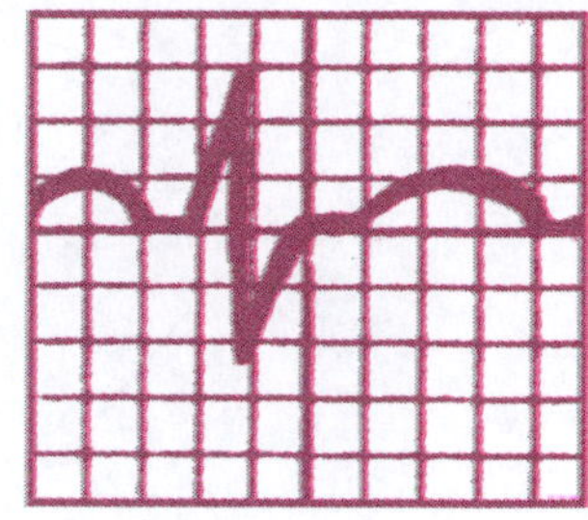

Chapter 10 Objectives

Upon completion of this chapter, the student will be able to:

- State the criteria for each of the ventricular rhythms.
- Using the criteria and the other rhythm analysis tools, correctly identify ventricular rhythms on a variety of strips.
- State the adverse effects for each ventricular rhythm.
- State the possible treatment for the ventricular rhythms.

Introduction

Ventricular rhythms originate in one or more irritable foci in the ventricular tissue and do not have the benefit of the conduction system to speed the depolarization there. The result is that the impulses trudge very slowly, cell by cell, through the ventricle, producing a very wide QRS complex that measures >0.12 seconds. The impulse does sometimes travel backward to depolarize the atria, but the resultant P wave is usually lost in the mammoth QRS complex. Slow ventricular rhythms are the heart's last gasp as a pacemaker, kicking in when the higher pacemakers can't. Rapid ventricular arrhythmias can result in drastically decreased cardiac output, cardiovascular collapse, and death. See Figures 10-1 and 10-2.

The Word on Ventricular Rhythms

Ventricular rhythms are by far the most potentially lethal of all the rhythms. They therefore command great respect from healthcare personnel. Ventricular rhythms can result from escape (you'll recall the inherent rate of the ventricle is 20 to 40) or usurpation, and can have a heart rate varying from 0 to over 250 beats per minute. Though some ventricular rhythms can be well tolerated, most will cause symptoms of decreased cardiac output, if not frank cardiac standstill.

Most ventricular rhythms respond well to medications. Oddly enough, however, some of the very medications used to treat ventricular rhythms can *cause* them in some circumstances. Some ventricular rhythms can only be treated by electric shock to the heart. And others, despite aggressive treatment, are usually lethal.

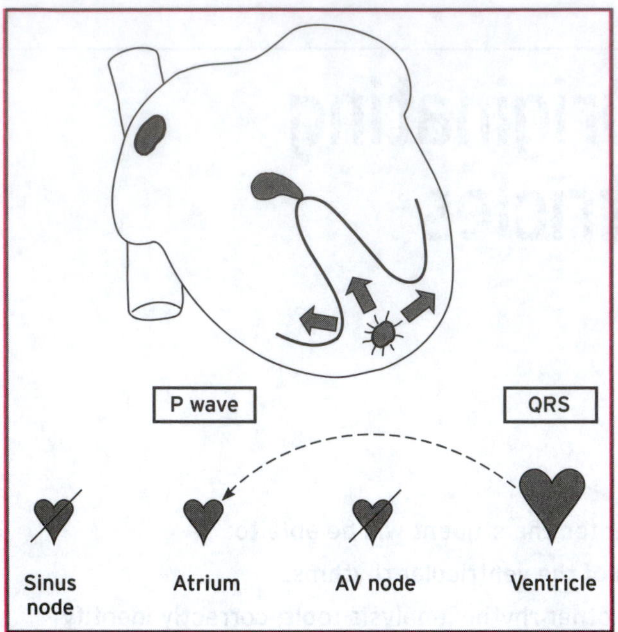

Figure 10-1 Conduction of a single ventricular focus.

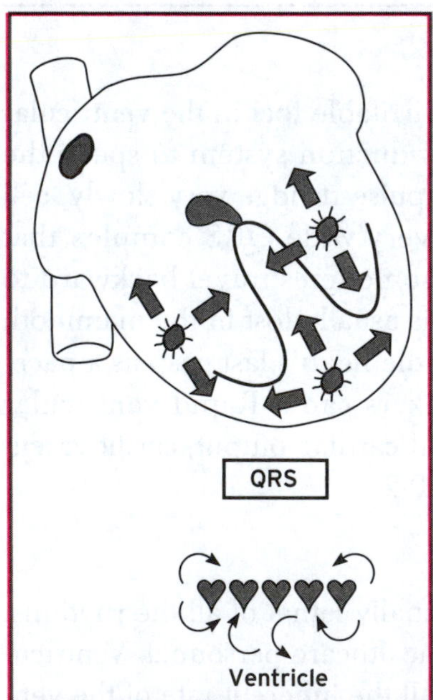

Figure 10-2 Conduction of multiple ventricular foci.

Ventricular beats have wide, bizarre QRS complexes. Some ventricular rhythms, however, have no QRS complexes at all. If the rhythm or beat in question meets *any* of the criteria below, it is ventricular in origin. Let's look at the criteria.

- Wide QRS (>0.12 second) without preceding P wave *or*
- No QRS at all (*or* can't be sure if there are QRS complexes), *or*

- Premature, wide QRS beat without preceding P wave, interrupting another rhythm

The ventricular rhythms that will be covered in this section are the following:

- Premature ventricular complexes (PVCs)
- Agonal rhythm
- Idioventricular rhythm
- Accelerated idioventricular rhythm
- Ventricular tachycardia
- Torsades de pointes
- Ventricular fibrillation
- Asystole
- Pacemaker rhythms

Let's look at each of these rhythms in detail.

Premature Ventricular Complexes (PVCs)

What are they? PVCs are premature beats that originate in irritable ventricular tissue before the next sinus beat is due.

Rate	Can occur at any rate.
Regularity	Regular but interrupted.
P waves	Usually not seen on PVCs.
PR	Not applicable.
QRS	Wide and bizarre in shape. QRS interval >0.12 second. Left-ventricular PVCs have an upward deflection in V_1. Right-ventricular PVCs have a downward deflection in V_1.
T wave	Slopes off in the opposite direction to the QRS. If the QRS points upward, for example, the T wave will point downward.
Cause	The big three causes are heart disease, **hypokalemia** (low blood potassium level), and hypoxia. Other causes include low blood magnesium level, stimulants, caffeine, stress, or anxiety. All these things can cause the ventricle to become irritable and fire off early beats.
Adverse effects	Occasional PVCs are of no concern. Frequent PVCs (six or more per minute) or PVCs that are very close to the preceding T wave can progress to lethal arrhythmias like ventricular tachycardia or ventricular fibrillation. Multifocal PVCs are also cause for concern, since it means that there are multiple irritable areas.

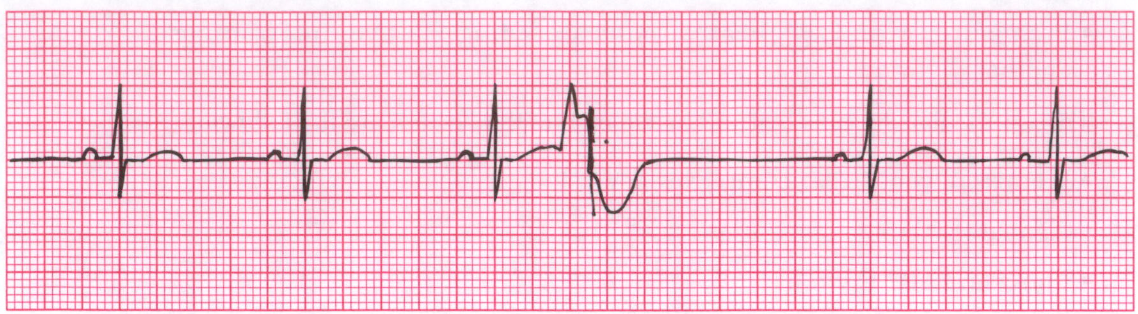

Figure 10-3 PVC.

Treatment

Occasional PVCs don't require treatment. They can occur in normal healthy individuals. If PVCs are more frequent, treat the cause. If the potassium level is low, give supplemental potassium. Start oxygen. Amiodarone is most commonly used to treat PVCs that are frequent or close to the T wave. Procainamide can also be used to decrease ventricular irritability and prevent lethal arrhythmias. Frequent PVCs in the presence of a slow bradycardia are not treated with antiarrhythmics, however. They are treated with atropine. Bradycardic rhythm PVCs are the heart's attempt to increase the heart rate by providing another beat from *somewhere* . . . anywhere. Giving antiarrhythmics would knock out the PVCs, leaving a slower heart rate. Atropine would speed up the underlying rhythm and the PVCs would go away on their own. See Figure 10-3.

In Figure 10-3, there are QRS complexes, all except the fourth beat having the same shape. The fourth beat has a very wide QRS complex. Regularity is regular but interrupted. Heart rate is 60. There are matching upright P waves on all beats except the fourth beat, which has no P wave at all. PR interval is 0.16 on the sinus beats, no PR on the PVC. QRS interval is 0.08 on the sinus beats, 0.14 on the PVC. Interpretation: sinus rhythm with one PVC.

PVCs that come from a single focus all look alike. They're called **unifocal** PVCs. PVCs from different foci look different. They're called **multifocal** PVCs. See Figure 10-4.

Note in Figure 10-4 that A's PVCs are shaped the same–they're unifocal. B's PVCs are shaped differently–they're multifocal.

Two consecutive PVCs are called a **couplet**. Couplets can be either unifocal or multifocal. See Figure 10-5.

PVCs can be very regular at times. If every other beat is a PVC, it's called ventricular **bigeminy**. If every third beat is a PVC, it's called ventricular **trigeminy**. If every fourth beat is a PVC, it's ventricular **quadrigeminy**. See Figure 10-6.

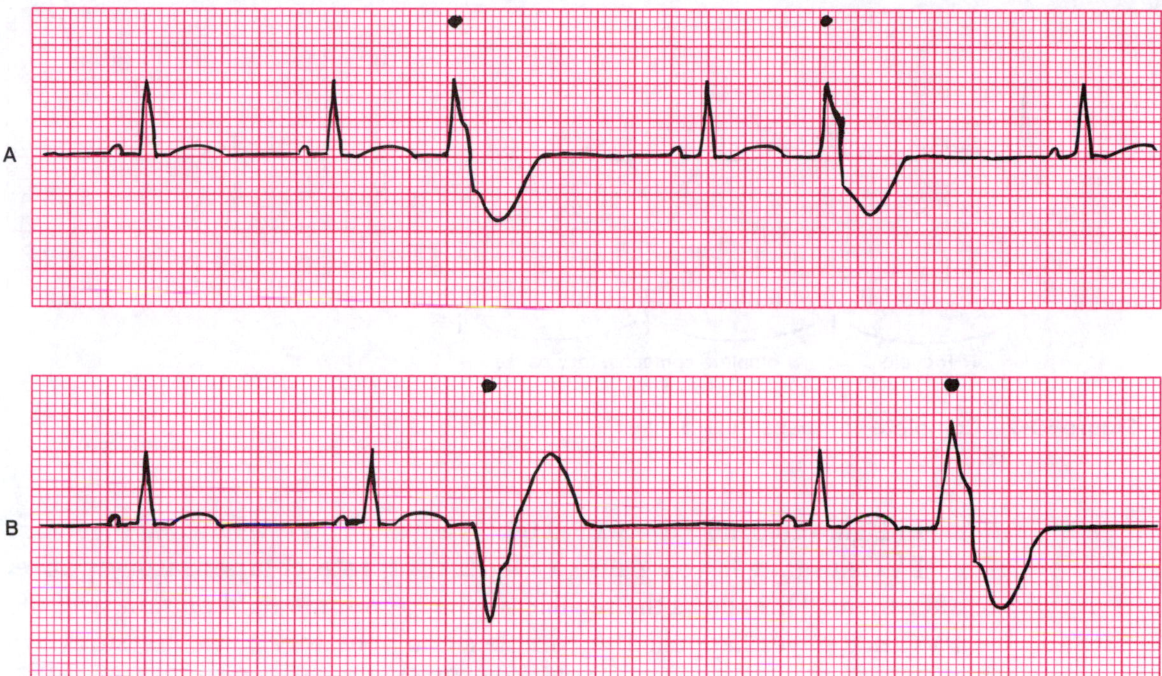

Figure 10-4 (A) Unifocal PVCs; (B) multifocal PVCs.

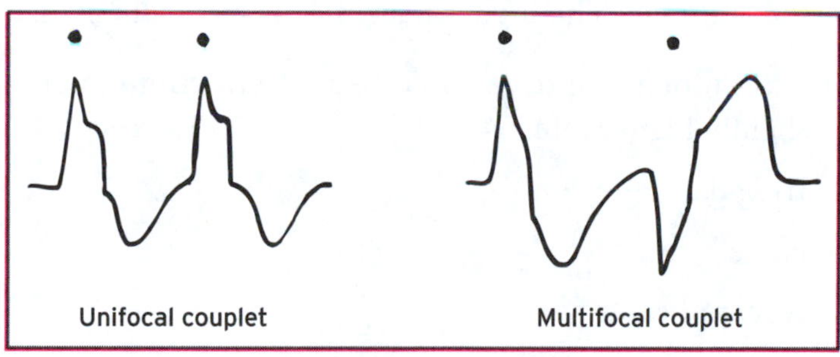

Figure 10-5 Unifocal and multifocal couplets.

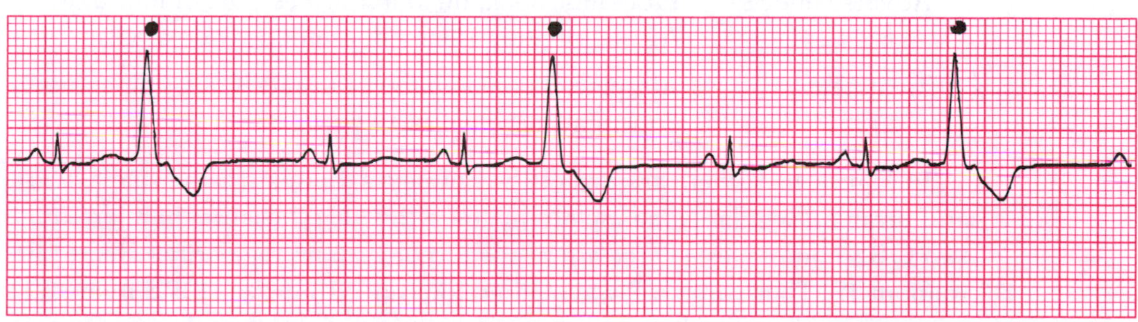

Figure 10-6 Ventricular trigeminy.

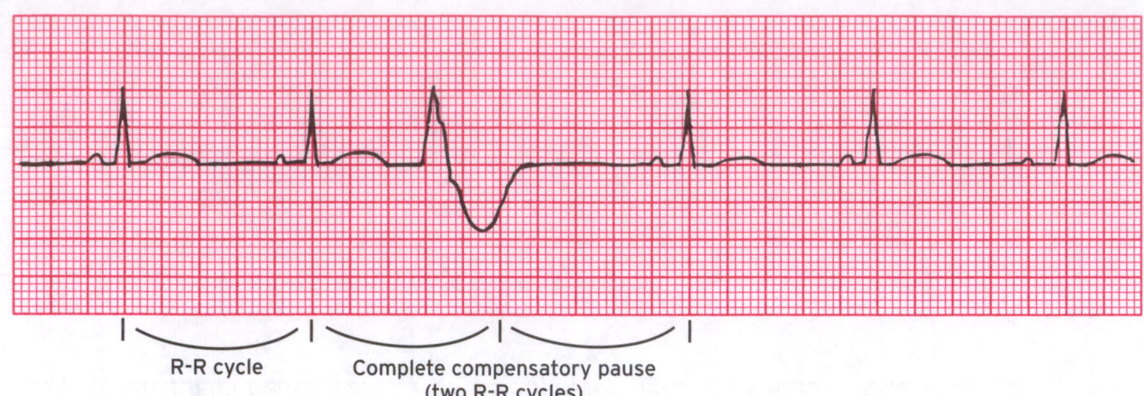

Figure 10-7 Complete compensatory pause.

In Figure 10-6, note every third beat is a PVC. This is ventricular trigeminy.

PVCs usually have a pause, called a **complete compensatory pause,** after them. This allows the regular rhythm to resume right on time as if the PVC had never happened. A complete compensatory pause measures two R-R cycles from the beat preceding the PVC to the beat following the PVC. See Figure 10-7.

Agonal Rhythm (Dying Heart)

What is it? Agonal rhythm is a very irregular rhythm in which the severely impaired heart is only able to "cough out" an occasional beat from its only remaining pacemaker, the ventricle. The higher pacemakers have all failed.

Rate	<20, though an occasional beat might come in at a slightly higher rate.
Regularity	Irregular.
P waves	None.
PR	Not applicable.
QRS	Wide and bizarre, QRS interval >0.12 second.
T wave	Slopes off in the opposite direction to the QRS.
Cause	The patient is dying, usually from profound cardiac or other damage, or from hypoxia.
Adverse effects	Profound shock, unconsciousness; death if untreated. Agonal rhythm usually does not provide a pulse.
Treatment	Atropine to speed up the heart rate, CPR, epinephrine, dopamine, pacemaker, oxygen.

In Figure 10-8, there are two QRS complexes, both the same shape, wide and bizarre. Regularity is indeterminate on this strip because there are only two QRS complexes. (Three are needed to determine regularity.) Heart rate is about 12. There are no P waves, therefore no PR interval. QRS interval is 0.28, extremely wide. Interpretation: agonal rhythm.

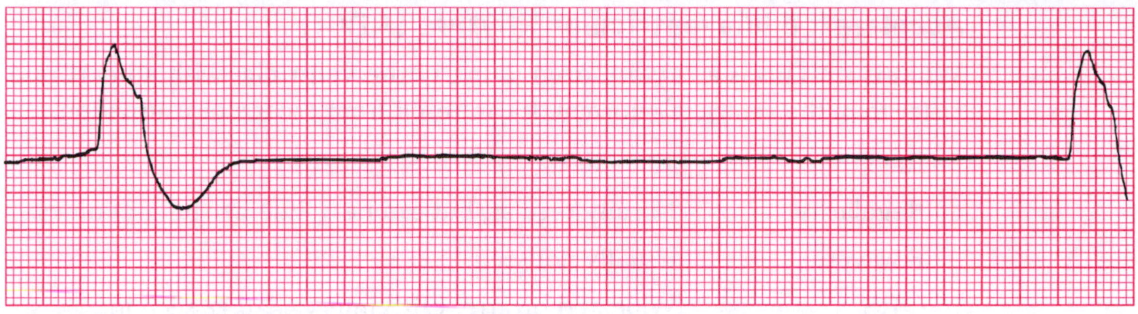

Figure 10-8 Agonal rhythm.

Idioventricular Rhythm (IVR)

What is it? IVR is a rhythm originating in the ventricle at its inherent rate. Higher pacemakers have failed, so the ventricle escapes to save the patient's life.

Rate	20 to 40.
Regularity	Regular.
P waves	None.
PR	Not applicable.
QRS	Wide and bizarre, QRS interval >0.12 second.
T wave	Slopes off in the opposite direction to the QRS.
Cause	Usually implies massive cardiac or other damage, hypoxia.
Adverse effects	Decreased cardiac output, cardiovascular collapse. IVR may or may not result in a pulse.
Treatment	Atropine, epinephrine, pacemaker, oxygen, dopamine. If the patient is pulseless, do CPR.

In Figure 10-9, there are QRS complexes, all wide and bizarre. Regularity is regular. Heart rate is 37. There are no P waves, therefore no PR interval. QRS interval is 0.20, extremely wide. Interpretation: idioventricular rhythm.

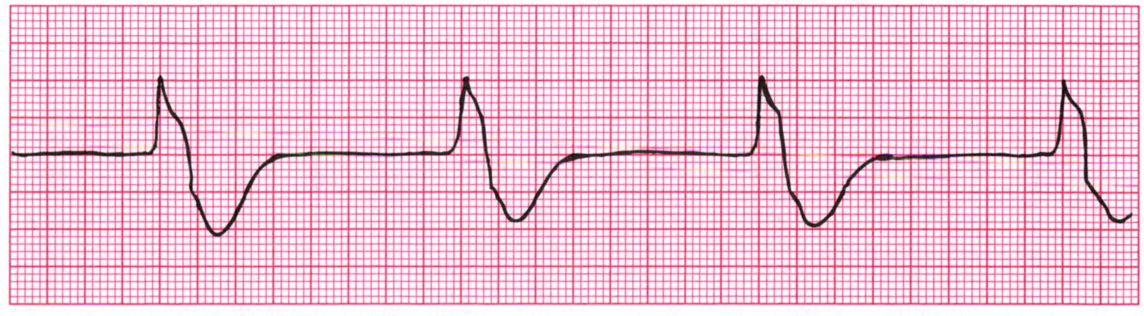

Figure 10-9 Idioventricular rhythm.

Accelerated Idioventricular Rhythm (AIVR)

What is it? This is a rhythm originating in the ventricle, with a heart rate faster than the ventricle's normal. It can result from escape or usurpation.

Rate	40 to 100.
Regularity	Usually regular, but can be a little irregular at times.
P waves	Usually not seen.
QRS	Wide and bizarre, QRS interval >0.12 second.
T wave	Slopes off in the opposite direction to the QRS.
Cause	Very common after an MI. Can be caused by the same things that cause PVCs. AIVR is also very common after administration of thrombolytic (clot-dissolving) medications, and in that context it is considered a **reperfusion dysrhythmia,** meaning it implies the heart muscle is once again getting blood flow. Imagine it this way: Suppose you hadn't eaten anything in several days, and then when you did eat, it was a huge meal. You'd probably feel pretty sick. It's the same with the heart. It's been without blood flow for a period of time because of the blood clot in the coronary artery. Then here comes a tidal wave of blood and oxygen after the thrombolytic medication dissolves the clot. The ventricular tissue becomes a little irritable and goes into AIVR. But just like your stomach, it'll get back to normal soon.
Adverse effects	Usually no ill effects because the heart rate is close to normal.
Treatment	Could be treated with atropine if the heart rate is around 40 and the patient is symptomatic. Consider starting oxygen. Usually no treatment is necessary as AIVR tends to be a self-limiting rhythm.

In Figure 10-10, there are QRS complexes, all wide and bizarre. Regularity is regular. Heart rate is 60. There are no P waves and thus no PR interval. QRS interval is about 0.18, very wide. Interpretation: accelerated idioventricular rhythm.

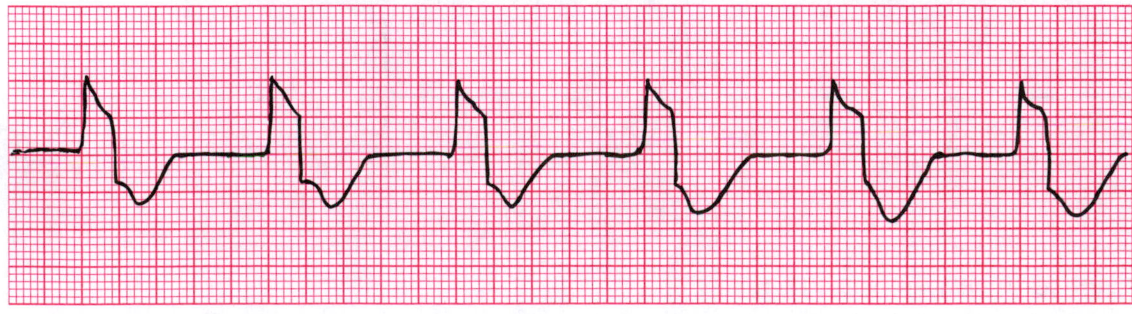

Figure 10-10 AIVR.

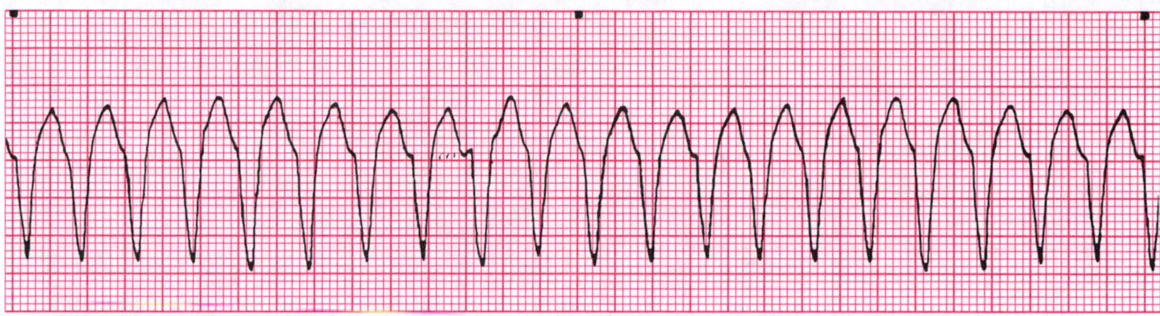

Figure 10-11 Ventricular tachycardia.

Ventricular Tachycardia (V-Tach)

What is it? An irritable focus in the ventricle has usurped the sinus node to become the pacemaker and is firing very rapidly.

Rate	>100.
Regularity	Usually regular, but can be a little irregular at times.
P waves	Usually none, but dissociated from the QRS if present.
PR	Will vary if even present.
QRS	Wide and bizarre, QRS >0.12 second.
T wave	Slopes off in the opposite direction to the QRS.
Cause	Same as PVCs.
Adverse effects	This rhythm may be tolerated for short bursts, but prolonged runs of v-tach can cause profound shock, unconsciousness, and death if untreated.
Treatment	Amiodarone, procainamide, lidocaine. Electric shock to the heart (cardioversion or defibrillation) may be necessary. Also treat the cause (low potassium, magnesium, or oxygen levels, etc.). CPR is indicated if the patient is pulseless.

In Figure 10-11, there are QRS complexes, all wide and bizarre. Regularity is regular. Heart rate is 214. P waves are absent. PR interval is not applicable. QRS interval is 0.13. Interpretation: ventricular tachycardia.

Torsades de Pointes

What is it? *Torsades de pointes* (pronounced *tor-sahd de point*) is a French term meaning "twisting of the points." It's a form of ventricular tachycardia that is recognized primarily by its classic shape–it oscillates around an axis, with the QRS complexes pointing up, then becoming smaller, then rotating around until they point down. Torsades is not usually well tolerated in longer bursts, and often deteriorates into ventricular fibrillation.

Rate	>200.
Regularity	May be regular or irregular.
P waves	None seen.

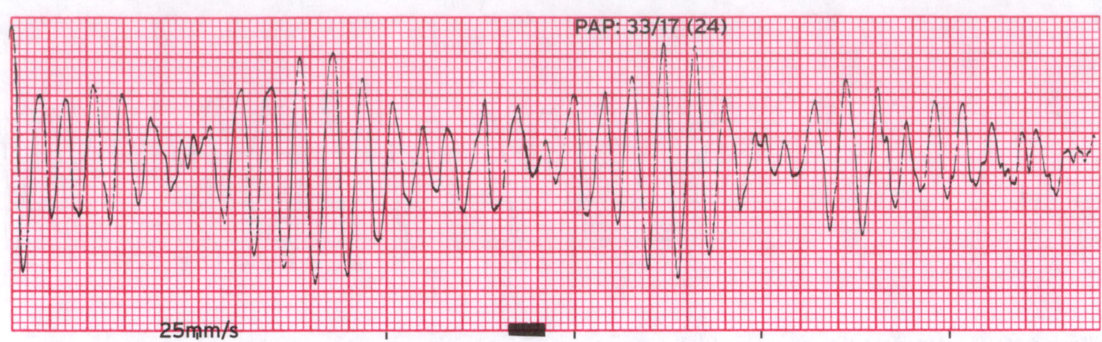

Figure 10-12 Torsades de pointes.

PR	Not applicable.
QRS	Wide and bizarre, >0.12 second; often hard to measure the QRS interval.
T wave	Opposite the QRS, but may not be seen due to the rapidity of the rhythm.
Cause	Can be caused by antiarrhythmic medications such as quinidine or procainamide, which cause an increased QT interval. Otherwise it is caused by the same things that cause v-tach and v-fib.
Adverse effects	May be tolerated for short runs, but usually results in cardiac arrest if sustained.
Treatment	Intravenous magnesium is the usual treatment. Electrical cardioversion may be needed. Isoproterenol is an option if other measures fail. Start oxygen.

In Figure 10-12, there are QRS complexes, not all the same shape. Some point downward, some point upward, and others are very small. Regularity is regular. Heart rate is about 375. P waves are absent, therefore there is no PR interval. QRS interval is 0.16. Interpretation: torsades de pointes. The big clue here is the oscillating character of the QRS complexes–bigger, then smaller, then bigger again, and so on. That's classic for torsades.

Ventricular Fibrillation (V-Fib)

What is it? Hundreds of impulses in the ventricle are firing off, each depolarizing its own little piece of territory. As a result, the ventricles wiggle instead of contract. The heart's electrical system is in chaos, and the resultant rhythm looks like static.

Rate	Cannot be counted
Regularity	None detectable
P waves	None
QRS	None detectable; just a wavy or spiked baseline
T wave	None
Cause	Same as v-tach; also can be caused by drowning, drug overdoses, accidental electric shock

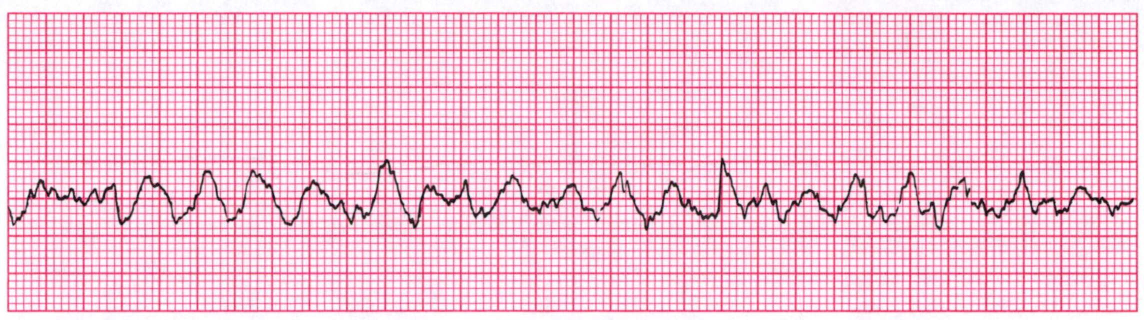

Figure 10-13 Ventricular fibrillation.

Adverse effects	Profound cardiovascular collapse. There is no cardiac output whatsoever. There is no pulse, no breathing, nothing. The patient is functionally dead. New onset v-fib has coarse fibrillatory waves. These waves get progressively finer the longer it lasts.
Treatment	Immediate defibrillation (electric shock to the heart), epinephrine, lidocaine, CPR, procainamide, amiodarone, oxygen. The rhythm will not be converted with just medications. Defibrillation must be done. The medications make the defibrillation more successful and can prevent recurrences of v-fib.

In Figure 10-13, there are no identifiable QRS complexes–just a wavy, spiked baseline resembling static. Regularity is not determinable. Heart rate is not measurable since there are no QRS complexes. P waves are not present. PR and QRS intervals cannot be measured. Interpretation: ventricular fibrillation.

Asystole

What is it? Asystole is flat-line EKG. Every one of the heart's pacemakers has failed.

Rate	Zero.
Regularity	None.
P waves	None.
PR	None.
QRS	None.
T wave	None.
Cause	Profound cardiac or other body system damage; profound hypoxia. Even with vigorous resuscitative efforts, this is usually a terminal rhythm.
Adverse effects	Death if untreated.
Treatment	Atropine to reverse any vagal influence, epinephrine, CPR, pacemaker, dopamine, oxygen.

In Figure 10-14, there are no QRS complexes, only a flat line. There is no regularity. Heart rate is zero. There are no P waves, no PR interval, and no QRS interval. Interpretation: asystole.

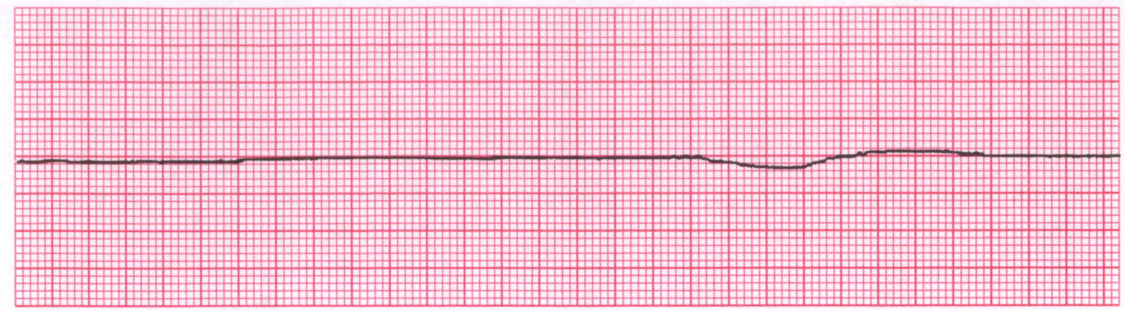

Figure 10-14 Asystole.

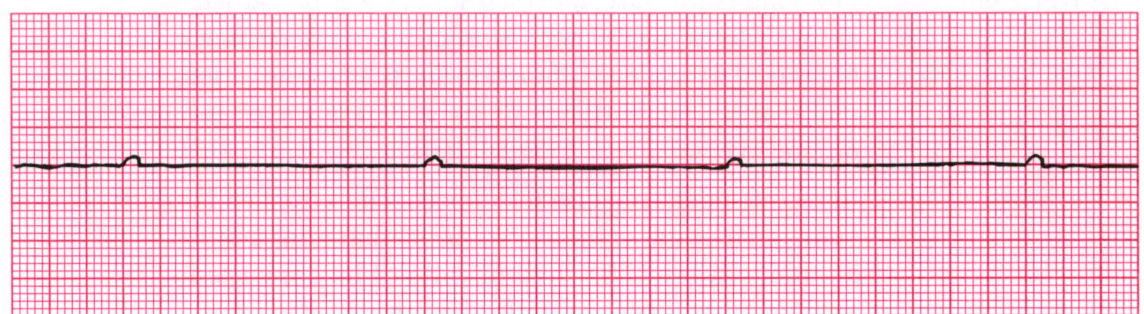

Figure 10-15 P wave asystole.

QuickTip

Do not use electrical shock to treat asystole–it will only result in more asystole. Shocking is used to re-coordinate the heart's electrical activity. In asystole, there is **no electrical activity** to recoordinate.

There is another kind of asystole in which there are no QRS complexes but there are still P waves. This is called **P wave asystole.** The still-functioning sinus node fires out its impulses, but they do not cause ventricular depolarization as the ventricle is too damaged to respond to the stimulus. Since the atria depolarize but the ventricles don't, there is no QRS after the Ps. Eventually the sinus impulses will slow and stop, since there is no cardiac output to feed blood to the sinus node. Remember–if there is no QRS complex, there is no cardiac output. Treatment is the same as for asystole.

In Figure 10-15, there are no QRS complexes. Regularity is not applicable. Heart rate is zero. P waves are present, regular, with an atrial rate of 37. There is no PR interval or QRS interval. Interpretation: P wave asystole.

Pacemakers

Pacemakers are electronic devices that can be implanted into or attached to the patient to send out an electrical impulse to cause the heart to depolarize. Pacemakers are used when the heart is temporarily or permanently unable to generate or transmit its own impulses, or when it does so too slowly to provide a reasonable cardiac output. They can be used to pace the atria, the ventricles, or both.

When the pacemaker sends out its signal, a vertical spike is recorded on the EKG paper. Ventricular pacing provides a spike followed by a wide QRS. Atrial pacing has a spike followed by a P wave. Dual-chamber pacing (both atrium and ventricle) has a spike before both the P and the QRS. See Figure 10-16.

In Figure 10-16(a), there are QRS complexes, all wide, all shaped the same. Each QRS is preceded by a pacemaker spike. Regularity is regular.

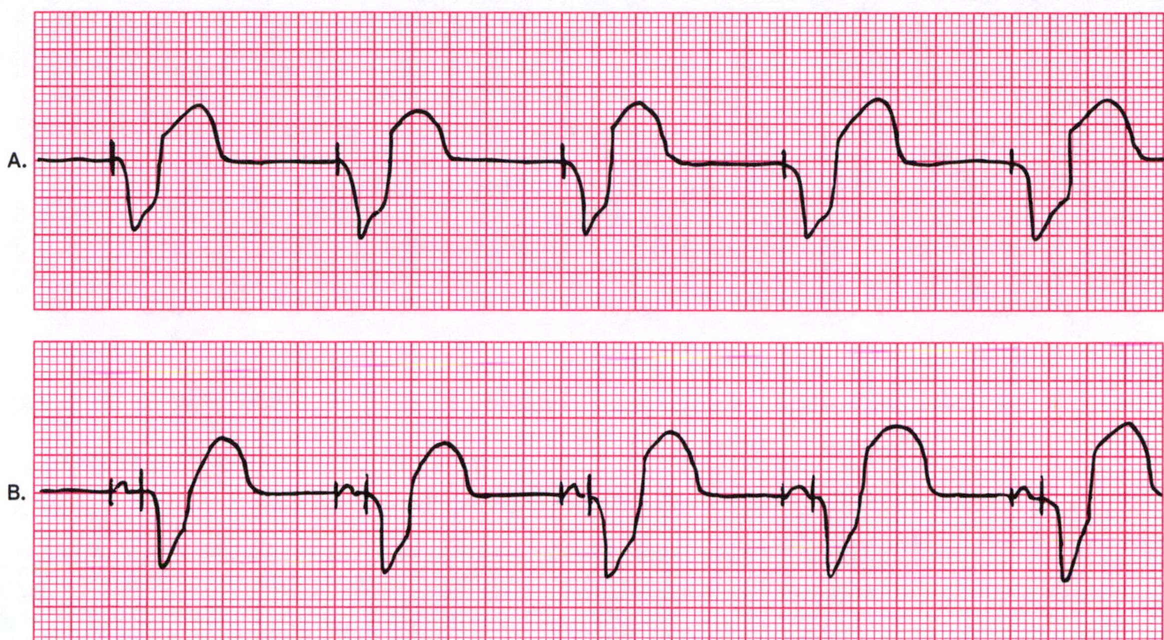

Figure 10-16 Pacemakers: (a) Ventricular pacing; (b) Dual-chamber pacing.

Heart rate is 50. There are no P waves, therefore no PR interval. QRS interval is 0.24 second. Interpretation: ventricular pacing.

In Figure 10-16(b), there are QRS complexes, all wide, all shaped the same. Regularity is regular. Heart rate is 50. There are matching P waves, each preceded by a pacemaker spike. PR interval is not measured in paced rhythms. The **AV interval** (the interval between atrial and ventricular pacing spikes) is 0.16 second and should be constant as this interval is preset when the pacemaker is implanted. QRS interval is 0.24 second. Interpretation: dual-chamber pacing (also called AV pacing).

For in-depth information on pacemakers, see chapter 15.

Practice Strips: Ventricular Rhythms

The first ten strips are single-lead strips; the last ten are double-lead strips.

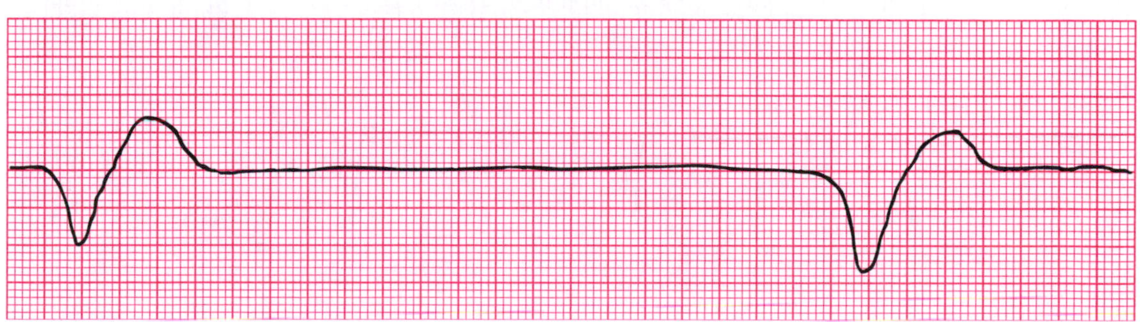

1. QRS complexes ________ Regularity ________ Heart rate ________
   P waves ____
   PR interval ____________ QRS interval ____________
   Interpretation (name of rhythm) ________________________

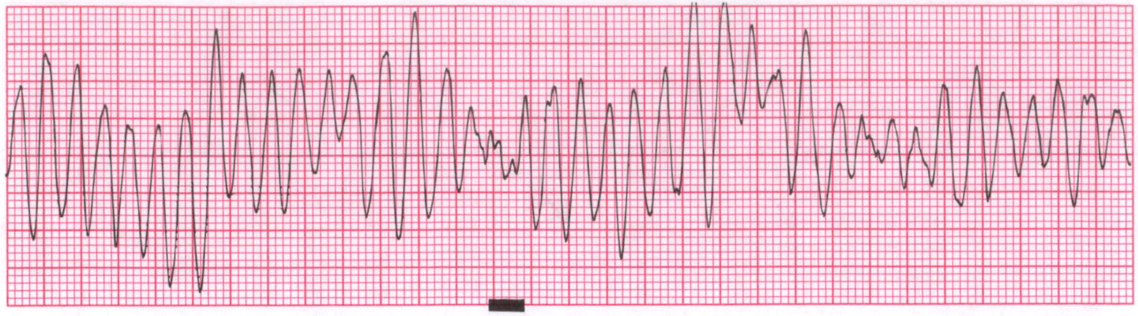

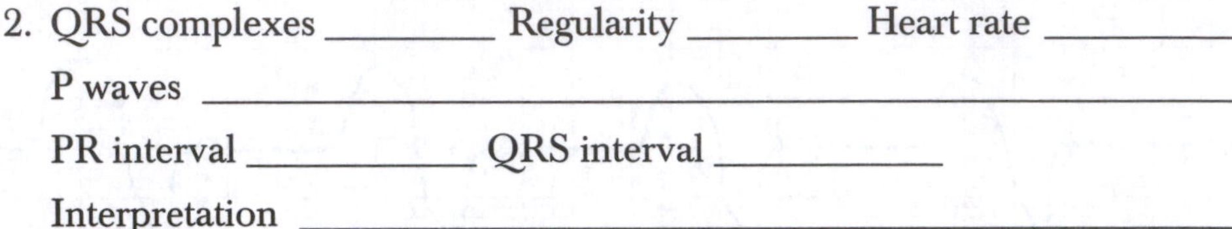

2. QRS complexes ________ Regularity ________ Heart rate ________
   P waves ____
   PR interval ___________ QRS interval ___________
   Interpretation ____

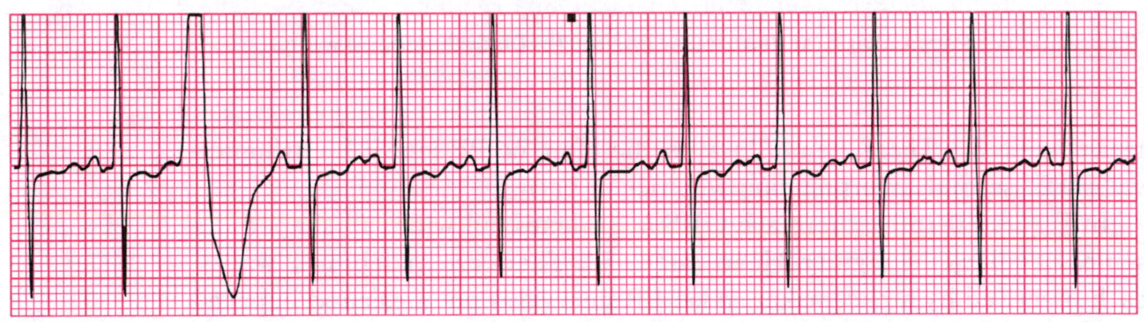

3. QRS complexes ________ Regularity ________ Heart rate ________
   P waves ____
   PR interval ___________ QRS interval ___________
   Interpretation ____

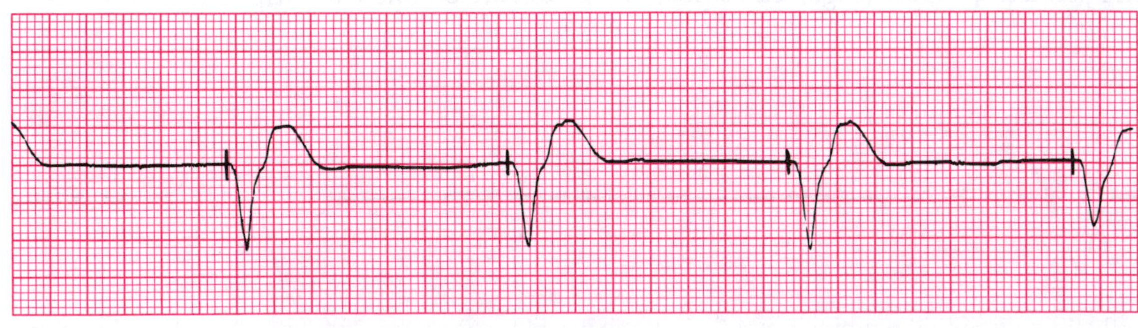

4. QRS complexes ________ Regularity ________ Heart rate ________
   P waves ____
   PR interval ___________ QRS interval ___________
   Interpretation ____

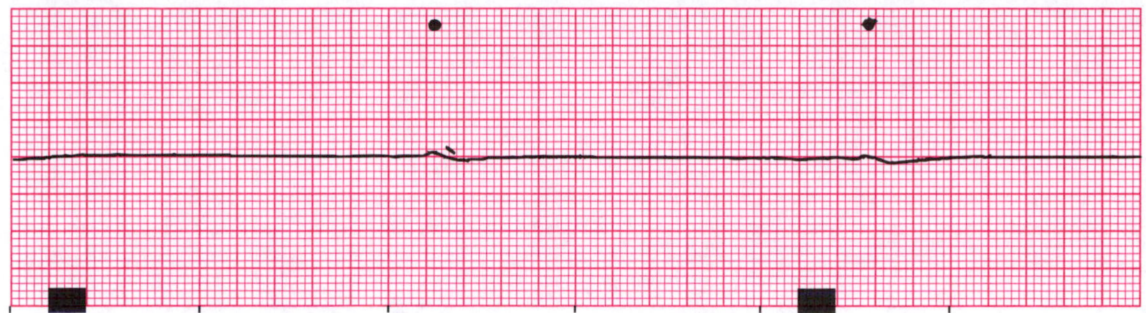

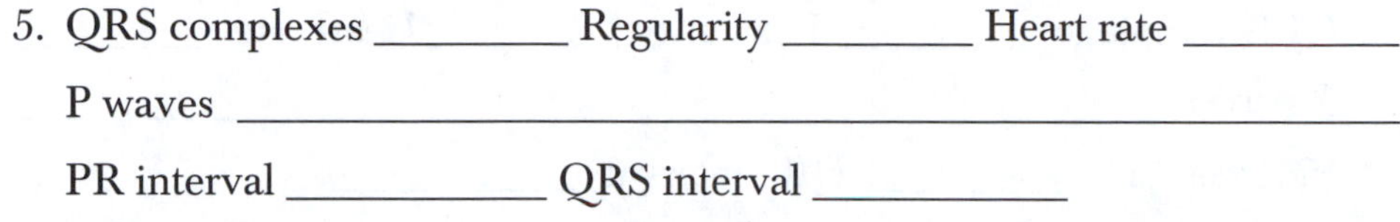

5. QRS complexes ________ Regularity ________ Heart rate __________

   P waves ____

   PR interval ____________ QRS interval ___________

   Interpretation ____

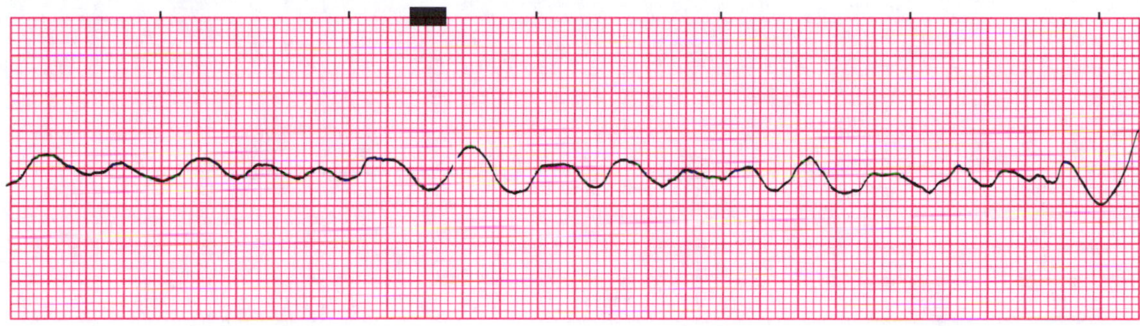

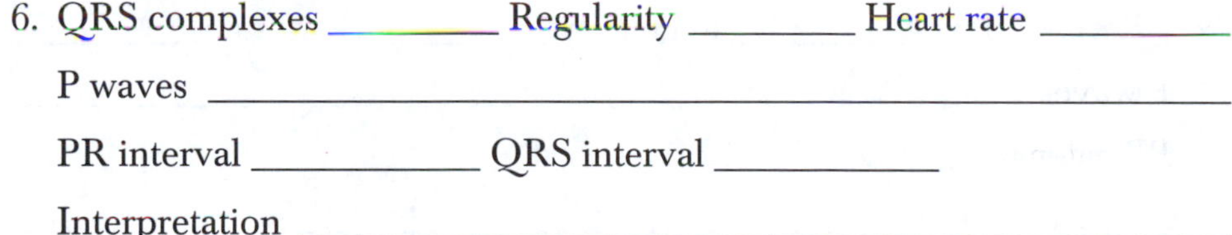

6. QRS complexes ________ Regularity ________ Heart rate __________

   P waves ____

   PR interval ____________ QRS interval ___________

   Interpretation ____

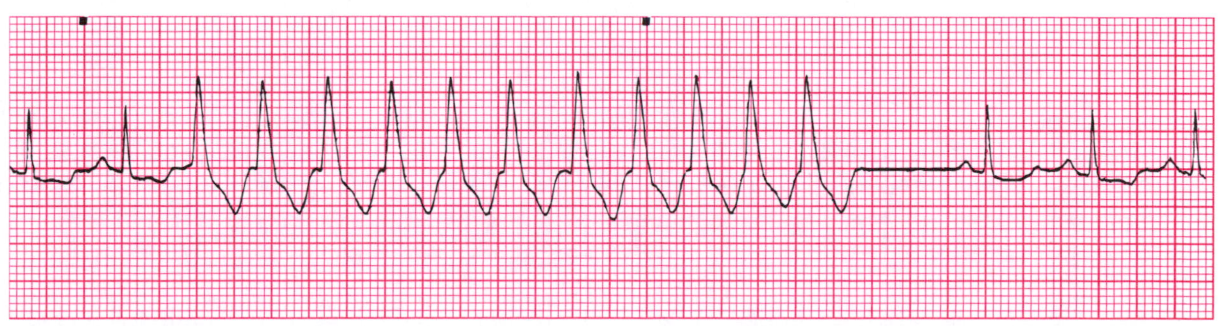

7. QRS complexes ________ Regularity ________ Heart rate __________

   P waves ____

   PR interval ____________ QRS interval ___________

   Interpretation ____

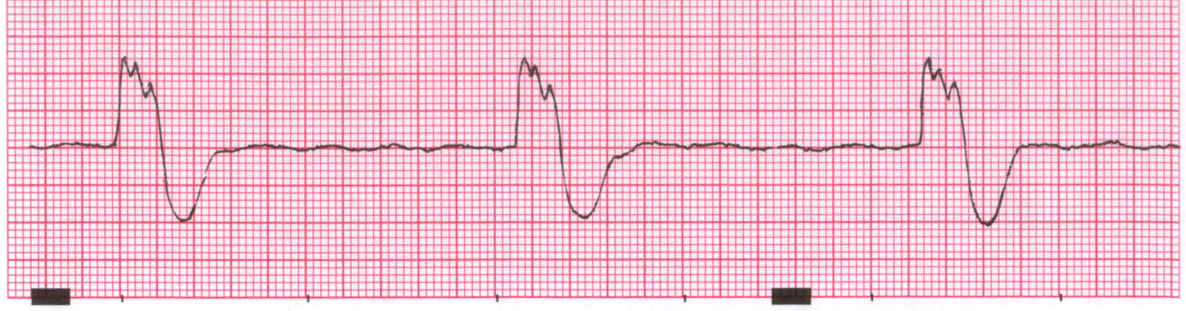

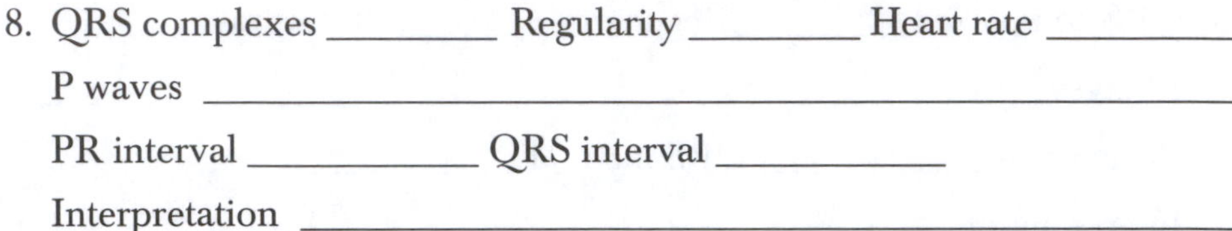

8. QRS complexes ________ Regularity ________ Heart rate ________
   P waves ____
   PR interval __________ QRS interval __________
   Interpretation ____

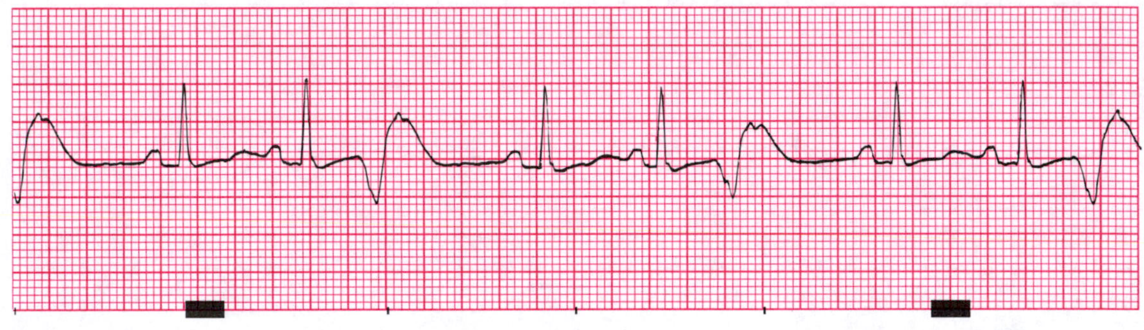

9. QRS complexes ________ Regularity ________ Heart rate ________
   P waves ____
   PR interval __________ QRS interval __________
   Interpretation ____

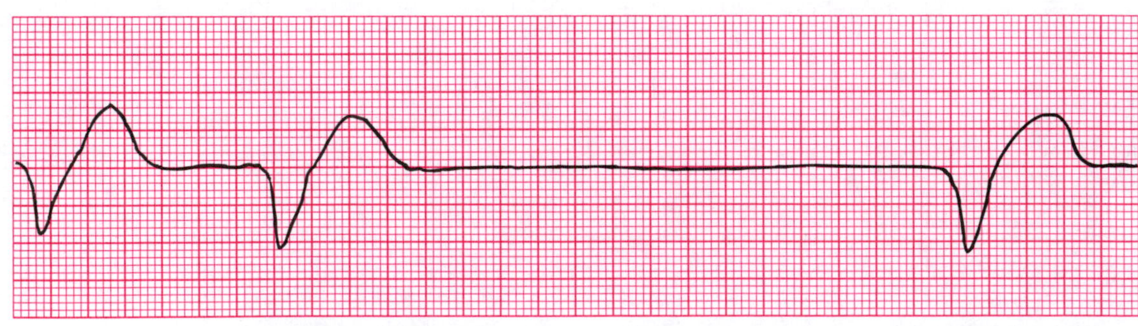

10. QRS complexes ________ Regularity ________ Heart rate ________
    P waves ____
    PR interval __________ QRS interval __________
    Interpretation ____

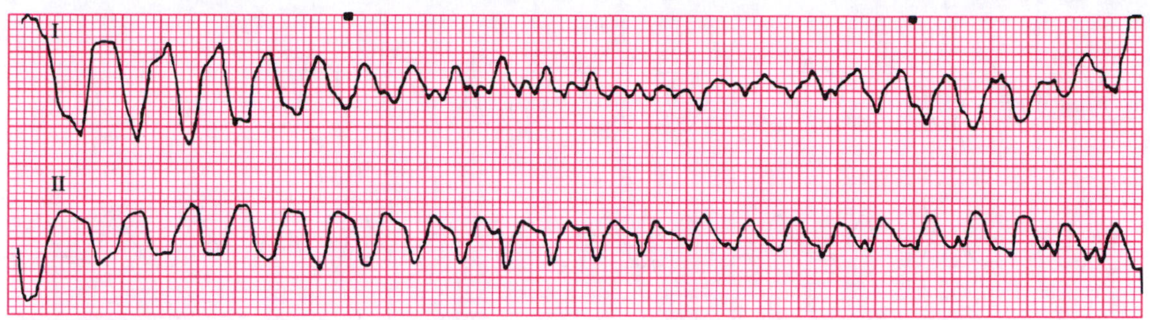

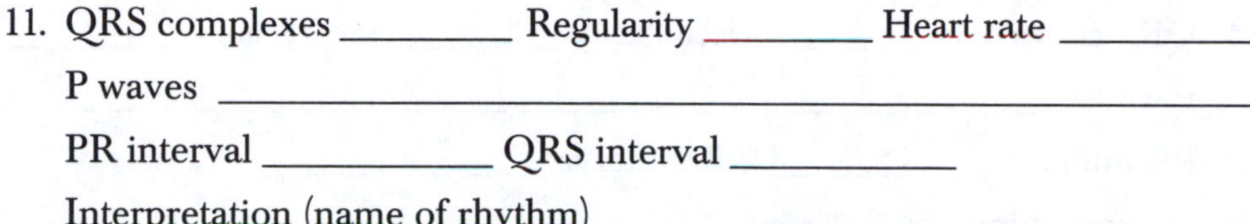

11. QRS complexes ________ Regularity ________ Heart rate _________

P waves ____

PR interval ___________ QRS interval ___________

Interpretation (name of rhythm) ________________________

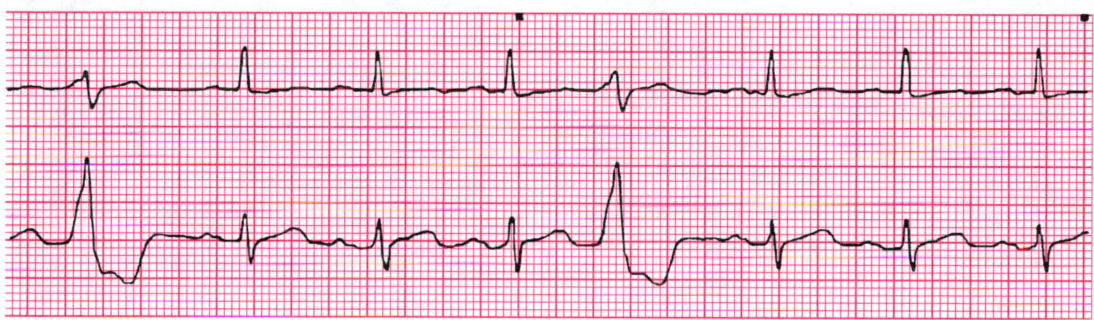

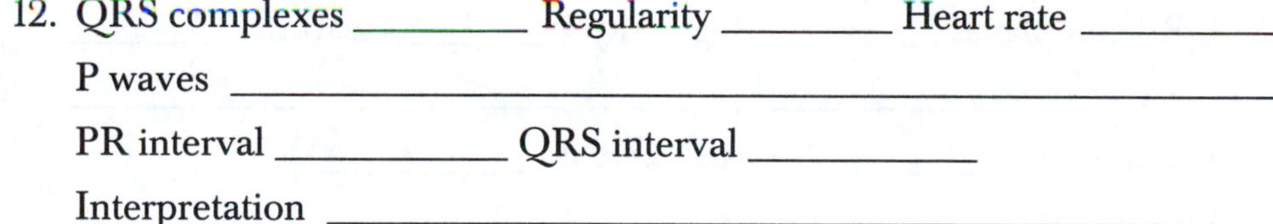

12. QRS complexes ________ Regularity ________ Heart rate _________

P waves ____

PR interval ___________ QRS interval ___________

Interpretation _____________________________________

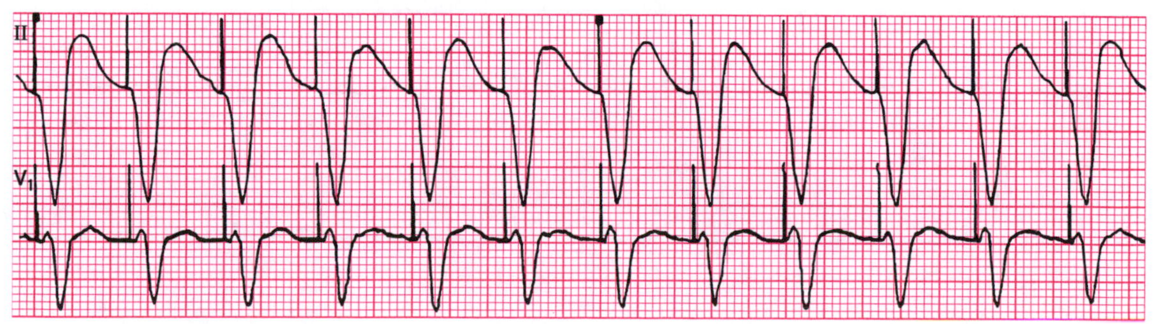

13. QRS complexes ________ Regularity ________ Heart rate _________

P waves ____

PR interval ___________ QRS interval ___________

Interpretation _____________________________________

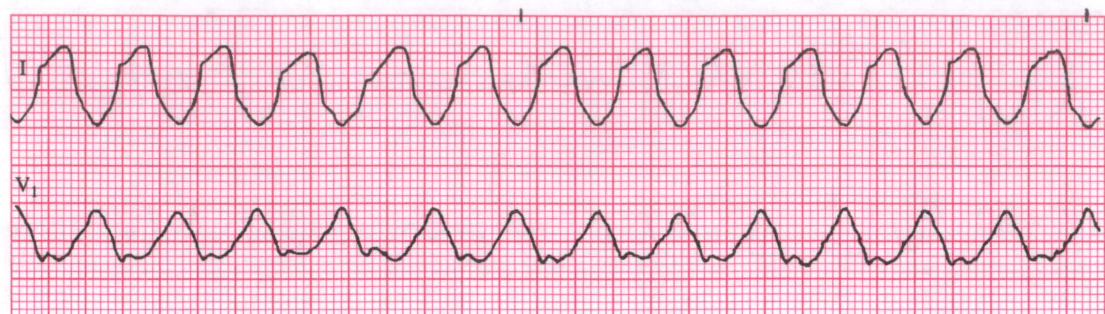

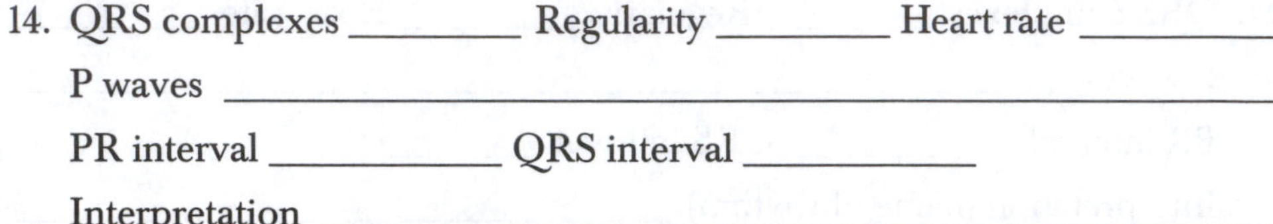

14. QRS complexes ________ Regularity ________ Heart rate ________
P waves ____________________
PR interval ____________ QRS interval ____________
Interpretation ____________________

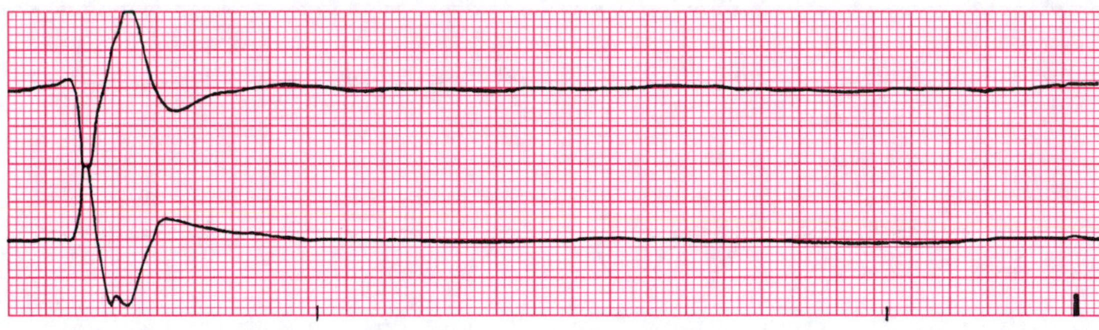

15. QRS complexes ________ Regularity ________ Heart rate ________
P waves ____________________
PR interval ____________ QRS interval ____________
Interpretation ____________________

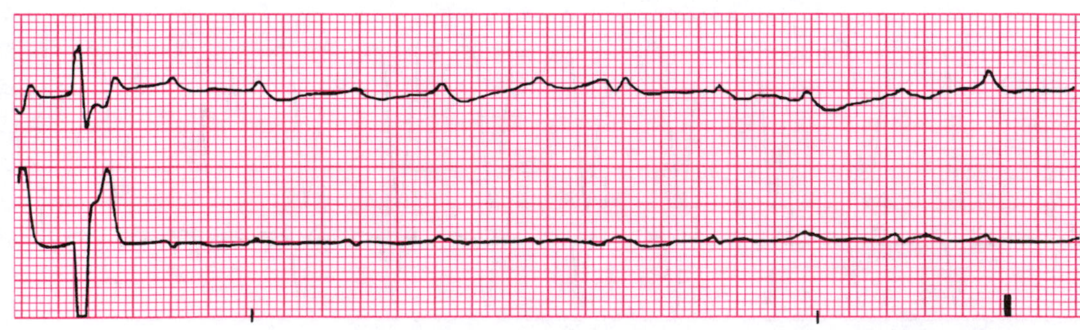

16. QRS complexes ________ Regularity ________ Heart rate ________
P waves ____________________
PR interval ____________ QRS interval ____________
Interpretation ____________________

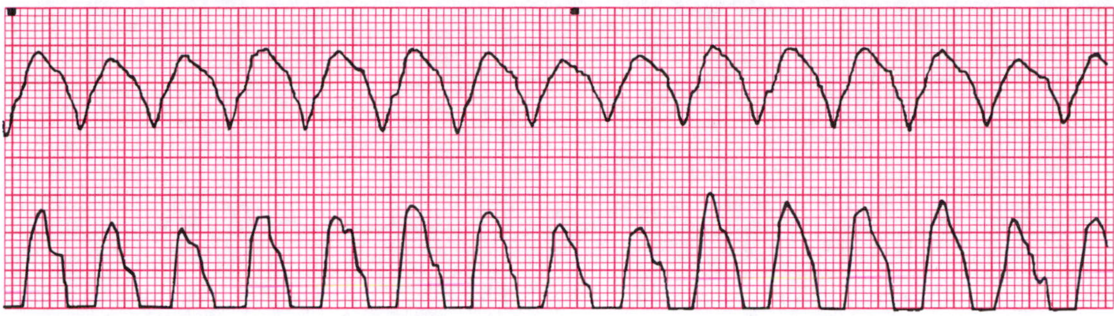

17. QRS complexes ________ Regularity ________ Heart rate ________
    P waves ____
    PR interval __________ QRS interval __________
    Interpretation ____

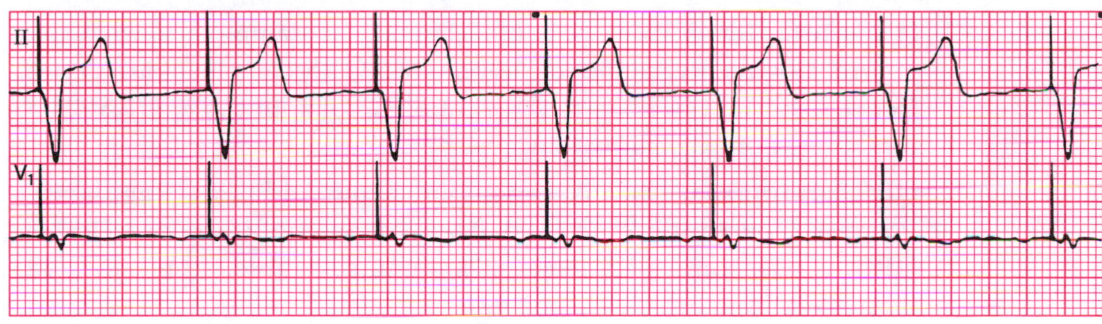

18. QRS complexes ________ Regularity ________ Heart rate ________
    P waves ____
    PR interval __________ QRS interval __________
    Interpretation ____

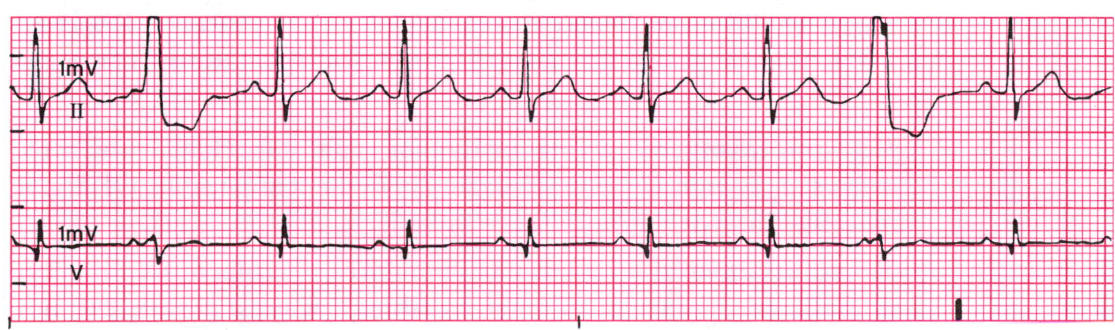

19. QRS complexes ________ Regularity ________ Heart rate ________
    P waves ____
    PR interval __________ QRS interval __________
    Interpretation ____

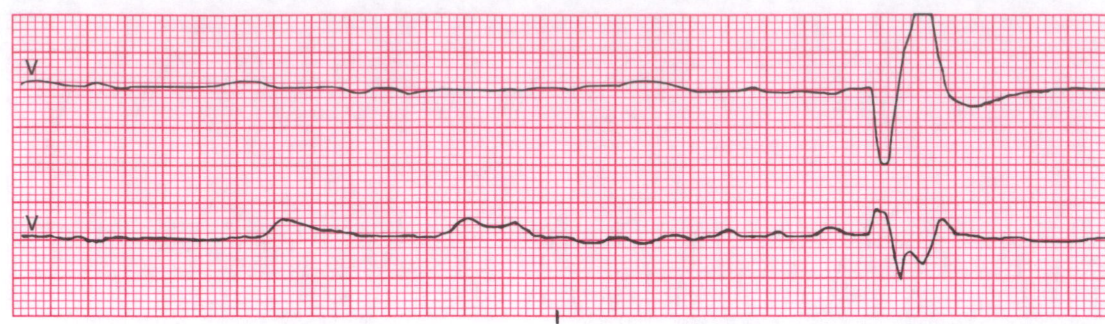

20. QRS complexes ________ Regularity ________ Heart rate ________

P waves ____

PR interval ___________ QRS interval ___________

Interpretation ____

Answers to Ventricular Rhythms Practice Strips

1. **QRS complexes:** present, both shaped the same–very wide and bizarre. **Regularity:** cannot tell as only two QRS complexes are shown. **Heart rate:** 14. **P waves:** not present. **PR:** not applicable. **QRS:** 0.38. **Interpretation:** agonal rhythm.
2. **QRS complexes:** present, varying in shapes and sizes. **Regularity:** irregular. **Heart rate:** 375 to 500. **P waves:** absent. **PR:** not applicable. **QRS:** varies–some QRS intervals are unmeasurable, others are 0.12. **Interpretation:** torsades de pointes.
3. **QRS complexes:** present, all but the third QRS shaped the same. The third QRS is wider. **Regularity:** regular but interrupted (by a premature beat). **Heart rate:** 115. **P waves:** matching and upright on all beats except the third, which has no P wave. **PR:** 0.12 on the sinus beats. **QRS:** 0.10 on the sinus beats; 0.16 on the premature beat. **Interpretation:** sinus tachycardia with one PVC.
4. **QRS complexes:** present, wide, all shaped the same; spike noted preceding each QRS complex. **Regularity:** regular. **Heart rate:** 40. **P waves:** none noted. **PR:** not applicable. **QRS:** 0.16. **Interpretation:** ventricular pacing.
5. **QRS complexes:** absent. **Regularity:** not applicable. **Heart rate:** zero. **P waves:** upright, matching, atrial rate 26. **PR:** not applicable. **QRS:** not applicable. **Interpretation:** P wave asystole.
6. **QRS complexes:** absent; wavy baseline present instead. **Regularity:** not applicable. **Heart rate:** unmeasurable. **P waves:** absent. **PR:** not applicable. **QRS:** not applicable. **Interpretation:** ventricular fibrillation.
7. **QRS complexes:** present, two different shapes–some narrow, others wide and bizarre. **Regularity:** regular but interrupted (by a run of premature beats). **Heart rate:** 107 while in the narrow-QRS rhythm; 187 when in the wide-QRS rhythm. **P waves:** upright and matching on the narrow beats; none noted on the wide beats. **PR:** 0.12 on the narrow

beats; not applicable on the wide beats. **QRS:** 0.06 on the narrow beats; 0.12 on the wide beats. **Interpretation:** sinus tachycardia with an 11-beat run of ventricular tachycardia.

8. **QRS complexes:** present, all shaped the same–extremely wide and bizarre. **Regularity:** regular. **Heart rate:** 28. **P waves:** absent. **PR:** not applicable. **QRS:** 0.28. **Interpretation:** idioventricular rhythm.
9. **QRS complexes:** present, every third beat wider than the rest. **Regularity:** regular but interrupted (by premature beats). **Heart rate:** 94. **P waves:** matching and upright on all narrow beats. P waves are noted in the T waves of the wide beats. **PR:** 0.16. **QRS:** 0.06 on the narrow beats; 0.14 on the wide beats. **Interpretation:** sinus rhythm with PVCs in trigeminy.
10. **QRS complexes:** present, all shaped the same–wide QRS complexes. **Regularity:** irregular. **Heart rate:** 16 to 47, with a mean rate of 30. **P waves:** none noted. **PR:** not applicable. **QRS:** 0.28. **Interpretation:** agonal rhythm. Though in places this rate exceeds 20, the very irregular nature of it points to agonal rhythm rather than idioventricular rhythm.
11. **QRS complexes:** none seen–just a coarse zigzag baseline. **Regularity:** not applicable. **Heart rate:** unmeasurable. **P waves:** absent. **PR:** not applicable. **QRS:** not applicable. **Interpretation:** ventricular fibrillation. (But there could be an argument for torsades de pointes. The rhythm does appear to oscillate toward the middle. It would be helpful to have a longer strip for a better look at the rhythm.)
12. **QRS complexes:** present, all but two shaped the same. Two are wider than the others. **Regularity:** regular but interripted by premature beats. **Heart rate:** 88. **P waves:** upright and matching on the narrow-QRS beats, no P wave preceding the wide-QRS beats. **PR:** 0.20. **QRS:** 0.06 on the narrow-QRS beats, 0.16 on the wide-QRS beats. **Interpretation:** sinus rhythm with two PVCs.
13. **QRS complexes:** present, all shaped the same–very wide with a preceding spike. **Regularity:** regular. **Heart rate:** 115. **P waves:** one present–noted on the downstroke of the second T wave on the strip. **PR:** not applicable. **QRS:** 0.16. **Interpretation:** ventricular pacing.
14. **QRS complexes:** present, all shaped the same–very wide and bizarre. **Regularity:** regular. **Heart rate:** 136. **P waves:** not present. **PR:** not applicable. **QRS:** 0.28. **Interpretation:** ventricular tachycardia. Note the unusually wide QRS complexes–this is often a sign that the patient's blood potassium level is extremely high, a condition seen most often in renal failure.
15. **QRS complexes:** only one present–very wide and bizarre. **Regularity:** not applicable as only one QRS complex is shown. **Heart rate:** zero after that one beat. **P waves:** not present. **PR:** not applicable. **QRS:** 0.20. **Interpretation:** agonal rhythm, then asystole.
16. **QRS complexes:** only one present. **Regularity:** not applicable as only one QRS complex is shown. **Heart rate:** zero after that one beat. **P waves:** upright, matching, one preceding the QRS complex and then continuing

on, P-P interval irregular. **PR:** 0.24 on the one beat with a QRS. **QRS:** 0.08. **Interpretation:** one beat, then P wave asystole.

17. **QRS complexes:** present, all shaped the same–very wide and bizarre. **Regularity:** regular. **Heart rate:** 150. **P waves:** not present. **PR:** not applicable. **QRS:** 0.20. If you measured a bit wider than that, rest assured it is often difficult to measure QRS complexes when they merge into the T wave so well–hard to tell where the QRS ends and the T wave begins. **Interpretation:** ventricular tachycardia.
18. **QRS complexes:** present, all shaped the same–wide and preceded by a spike. **Regularity:** regular. **Heart rate:** 68. **P waves:** upright, matching, one preceding each QRS spike. P-P interval regular. **PR:** 0.20. **QRS:** 0.12. **Interpretation:** ventricular pacing.
19. **QRS complexes:** present, all but two shaped the same–two are wide and bizarre. **Regularity:** regular but interrupted by premature beats. **Heart rate:** 94. **P waves:** upright and matching preceding the narrow-QRS beats. None preceding the wide-QRS beats. **PR:** 0.16. **QRS:** 0.06 on the narrow beats, 0.12 on the wide beats. **Interpretation:** sinus rhythm with two PVCs.
20. **QRS complexes:** only one present–very wide and bizarre. **Regularity:** not applicable as only one QRS complex is shown. **Heart rate:** zero after that one beat. **P waves:** not present. **PR:** not applicable. **QRS:** 0.16. **Interpretation:** agonal rhythm.

Practice Quiz

1. The three main causes of PVCs are ______________________________

____

____

2. The rhythm that has no QRS complexes, but instead has a wavy, static-looking baseline is ______________________________

____

3. Appropriate treatment for PVCs interrupting a sinus bradycardia with a heart rate of 32 would be ______________________________
4. Torsades de pointes is a French term that means ______________
5. How does asystole differ from P wave asystole? ______________

____

6. Your patient has a ventricular rhythm with a heart rate of 39, but no pulse. What treatment would be appropriate? ______________

____

7. True or false: Asystole is treated with electric shock to the heart.
8. The treatment of choice for ventricular fibrillation is ______________

____

9. True or false: Pacemakers can pace the atrium, the ventricle, or both.
10. True or false: Lidocaine should be given to treat agonal rhythm.

Putting It All Together–Critical Thinking Exercises

These exercise may consist of diagrams to label, scenarios to analyze, brainstumping questions to ponder, or other challenging exercise to boost your understanding of the chapter material.

Let's play with ventricular rhythms a bit. The following scenario will provide you with information about a fictional patient and ask you to analyze the situation, answer questions, and decide on appropriate actions.

Harvey Winston, age 45, arrives in your ER complaining of intermittent dizziness. He feels he has come close to passing out a few times in the last 24 hours. Other than a past medical history of diet-controlled diabetes, he's been healthy. See his initial rhythm strip in the ER, Figure 10-17. Vital signs are stable. Mr. Winston denies feeling dizzy at this time.

1. What is this rhythm? ______________________________.
2. Does this rhythm require emergency treatment? ______________.
3. Name three things that can cause this rhythm. ________________

   ____.

   Lab tests reveal Mr. Winston's potassium level to be 1.9, extremely low. The physician orders potassium to be given intravenously. Half an hour later, an alarm sounds and the following rhythm strip prints out. See Figure 10-18.

4. What is this rhythm? ______________________________.
5. Does this rhythm require emergency treatment? ______________.
6. Mr. Winston has no breathing and no pulse. What intervention must be employed to terminate this rhythm?

   ____.

   After successful intervention, Mr. Winston returns to sinus rhythm and has no more problems. After an uneventful course in the intensive care unit, Mr. Winston goes home taking Amiodarone.

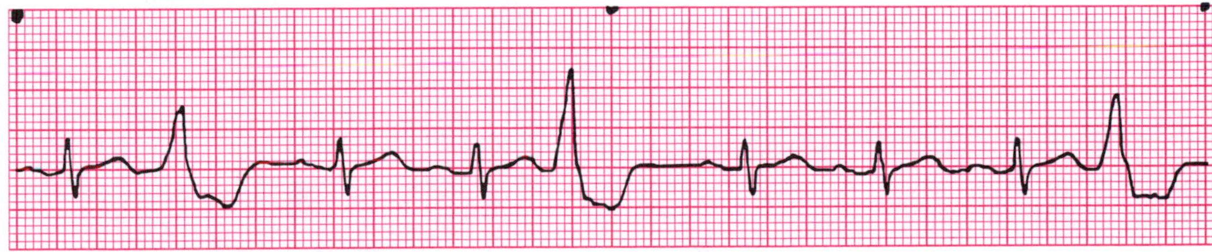

Figure 10-17 Mr. Winston's initial strip.

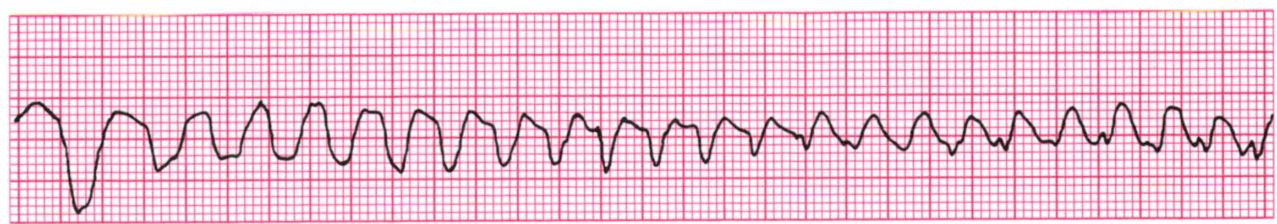

Figure 10-18 Rhythm causing alarm.

AV Blocks

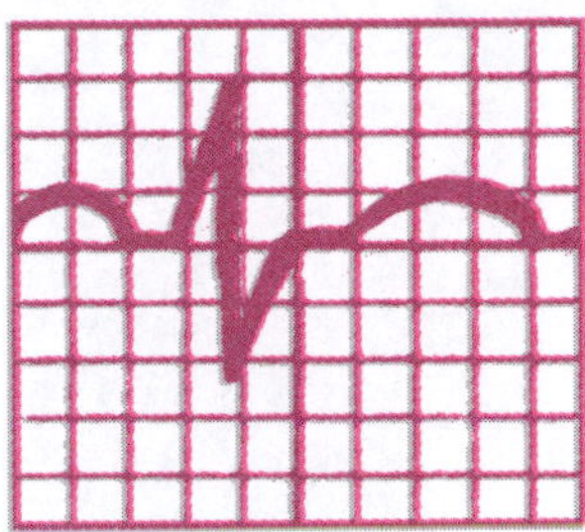

Chapter 11 Objectives

Upon completion of this chapter, the student will be able to:

- State the criteria for each type of AV block.
- State whether the block is at the AV node or the bundle branches.
- Identify each type of AV block using the criteria and the rhythm strip analysis tools.
- State the adverse effects for each type of AV block.
- State the possible treatment for each type of AV block.

Introduction

With AV (atrioventricular) blocks, the sinus node fires out its impulses as usual, but there is a partial or complete interruption in the transmission of these impulses to the ventricles. The site of the block is either at the AV node or at the bundle branches. See Figures 11-1 and 11-2.

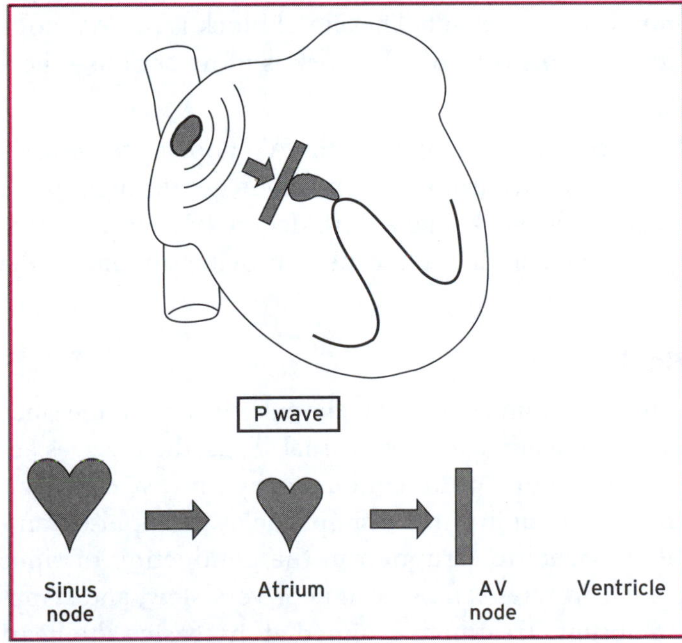

Figure 11-1 Block at the AV node.

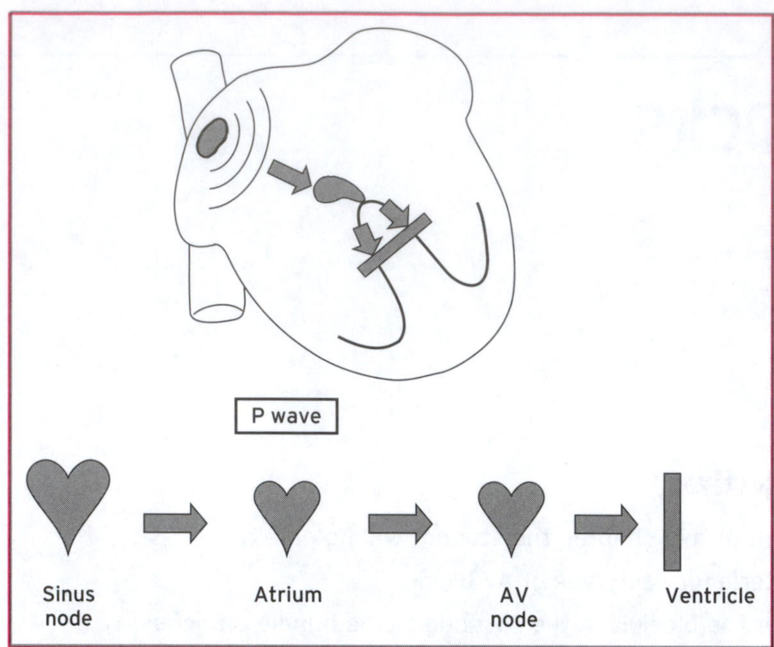

Figure 11-2 Block at the bundle branches.

Degrees of AV Block

There are three degrees of block, varying in severity from benign to life-threatening.

- **First-degree AV block.** Just as a first-degree burn is the least dangerous type of burn, a first-degree AV block is the least dangerous type of AV block. There is a delay in impulse transmission from the sinus node to the ventricles, but every impulse does get there–it just takes a little longer. The site of block is the AV node.
- **Second-degree AV block.** Some impulses from the sinus node get through to the ventricles; some don't. The site of block is the AV node or the bundle branches. This type of AV block is more serious–like a second-degree burn.
- **Third-degree AV block.** Due to a block at the AV node or the bundle branches, **none** of the impulses from the sinus node get through to the ventricles. Third-degree AV block, like a third-degree burn, can be life-threatening. A lower pacemaker has to escape to provide stimulus to the ventricle.

The Word on AV Blocks

In AV blocks, the underlying rhythm is sinus. The impulse is born in the sinus node and heads down the conduction pathway as usual. Thus, the P waves are normal sinus P waves. Further down the conduction pathway, however, there is a roadblock. This can result in either a simple delay in impulse transmission or a complete or partial interruption in the conduction of sinus impulses to the ventricle. Heart rates can be normal or very slow, and symptoms may be present or absent. Treatment is aimed at increasing the heart rate and improving AV conduction.

There are two possible criteria for AV blocks. *If either of these criteria is met, there is an AV block.* Let's look at the criteria:

- PR interval prolonged (>0.20 s) in some kind of sinus rhythm, *or*
- Some Ps not followed by a QRS; P-P interval regular

The following AV blocks will be covered in this section:

- First-degree AV block
- Type I second-degree AV block (Wenckebach)
- Type II second-degree AV block
- 2:1 AV block
- Third-degree AV block

Let's look at each of these rhythms in detail.

First-Degree AV Block

What is it? First-degree AV block is a prolonged PR interval that results from a delay in the AV node's conduction of sinus impulses to the ventricle. All the sinus impulses do get through; they just take longer than normal because the AV node is ischemic or otherwise suppressed.

Rate	Can occur at any rate.
Regularity	Depends on the underlying rhythm.
P waves	Upright, matching; one P to each QRS.
PR interval	Prolonged (>0.20 s), constant.
QRS	<0.12 second (≥0.12 s if BBB present).
Cause	AV node ischemia, digitalis toxicity, or a side effect of other medications such as beta-blockers or calcium channel blockers. This is a benign type of block, but be alert for worsening AV block. First-degree block is usually seen only with rhythms originating in the sinus node.
Adverse effects	The first-degree AV block itself causes no symptoms.
Treatment	Remove any medication causing it. Otherwise, treat the cause.

In Figure 11-3, there are QRS complexes, all shaped the same. Regularity is regular. Heart rate is 62. P waves are upright, matching, one to each QRS.

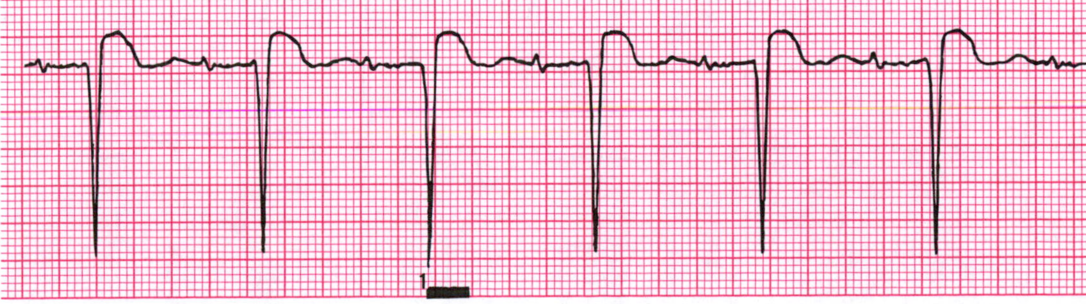

Figure 11-3 First-degree AV block.

PR interval is 0.28. QRS interval is 0.08. Interpretation is sinus rhythm with a first-degree AV block.

Type I Second-Degree AV Block (Wenckebach)

What is it? Usually a transient block, Wenckebach usually lasts only a few days. It occurs when the AV node becomes progressively sicker and less able to conduct the sinus impulses until finally it is unable to send the impulse down to the ventricle at all. As a result, the PR intervals grow progressively longer until there is a P wave that has no QRS behind it.

Rate	Atrial rate usually 60 to 100; ventricular rate less than the atrial rate due to nonconducted beats.
Regularity	Usually irregular, but can look regular but interrupted at times. A hallmark of Wenckebach is groups of beats, then a pause.
P waves	Normal sinus P waves. All Ps except the blocked P are followed by a QRS. P-P interval is regular. There may be P waves that are hidden in the QRS complex or the T wave. Find two consecutive P waves and then march out where the rest of the P waves are, keeping in mind they will all have the same P-P interval, so they'll all be the same distance apart.
PR interval	The PR gradually prolongs until a QRS is dropped.
QRS	<0.12 second (≥ 0.12 s if BBB present).
Cause	Myocardial infarction (MI), digitalis toxicity, medication side effects.
Adverse effects	Usually no ill effects. Watch for worsening block.
Treatment	Atropine if the heart rate is slow and the patient is symptomatic. A pacemaker can be used if atropine is unsuccessful. Most patients with Wenckebach require nothing more than cautious observation.

In Figure 11-4, there are QRS complexes, all shaped the same. Regularity is irregular. Heart rate is 50 to 83, with a mean rate of 70. P waves are matching, upright, some not followed by a QRS. Some Ps are at the end of the T waves. P-P interval is regular. Atrial rate is 83. PR interval varies from 0.04 to 0.28.

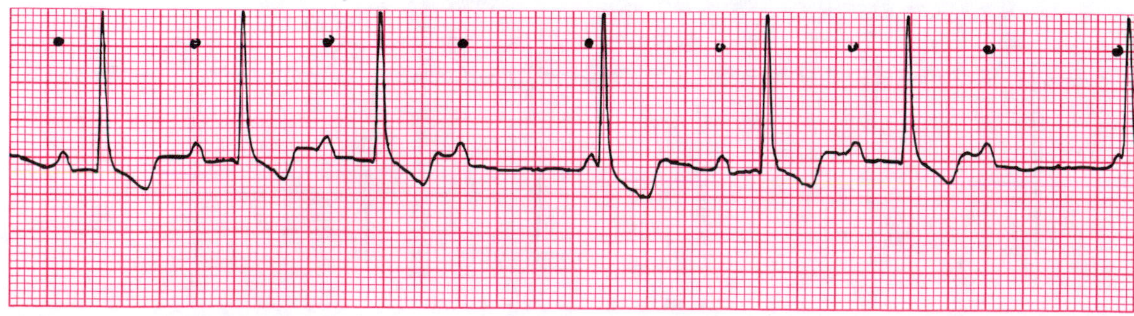

Figure 11-4 Wenckebach.

Note the relatively short PR of the first beat on the strip. Compare this to the third beat. The PR interval prolongs from beat to beat until the fourth P wave does not conduct through to the ventricle at all. We know it doesn't get through to the ventricle because that P wave is not followed by a QRS complex. The cycle then repeats, with prolonging PR intervals, until the eighth P wave is not conducted. QRS interval is 0.10. Interpretation: sinus rhythm with type I second-degree AV block (Wenckebach). Where did the sinus rhythm part of the interpretation come from? Remember, the underlying rhythm in all AV blocks is a sinus rhythm of some sort. The atrial rate will tell you which sinus rhythm it is. An atrial rate of 60 to 100 would be sinus rhythm, an atrial rate of less than 60 would be sinus bradycardia, and an atrial rate greater than 100 would be sinus tachycardia.

Type II Second-Degree AV Block

What is it? Type II results from an intermittent block at the AV node or the bundle branches, preventing some sinus impulses from getting to the ventricles. With AV node block, the resultant QRS complexes will be narrow. With block at the bundle branches, the QRS will be wide. Usually, type II patients already have a bundle branch block, meaning one of their bundle branches does not let impulses through. They are therefore dependent on the other bundle branch to conduct the impulses through to the ventricles. When that other bundle branch becomes suddenly blocked, none of the sinus impulses can get through. Some sinus P waves conduct through normally to the ventricles when the one bundle branch is open, and others never get through at all when both bundle branches are blocked. The impulses that do get through do so with an unchanging PR interval.

Rate	Atrial rate usually 60 to 100; ventricular rate less than atrial rate due to dropped beats.
Regularity	May be regular, irregular, or regular but interrupted.
P waves	Normal sinus P waves. All Ps except the blocked Ps have a QRS behind them. P-P interval is regular. Some P waves may be hidden inside QRS complexes or T waves.
PR interval	Unchanging on the conducted beats.
QRS	<0.12 second if the block is at the AV node, ≥0.12 second if the block is at the bundle branches.
Cause	MI, conduction system lesion, medication side effect, hypoxia.
Adverse effects	Since the heart rate can be very slow, the patient may have signs of decreased cardiac output. Type II can progress to third-degree block if untreated.
Treatment	Atropine first. Depending on where the block is, atropine may or may not work. Atropine speeds up the rate of sinus node firing and improves AV node conduction. If the block is at the AV node, atropine

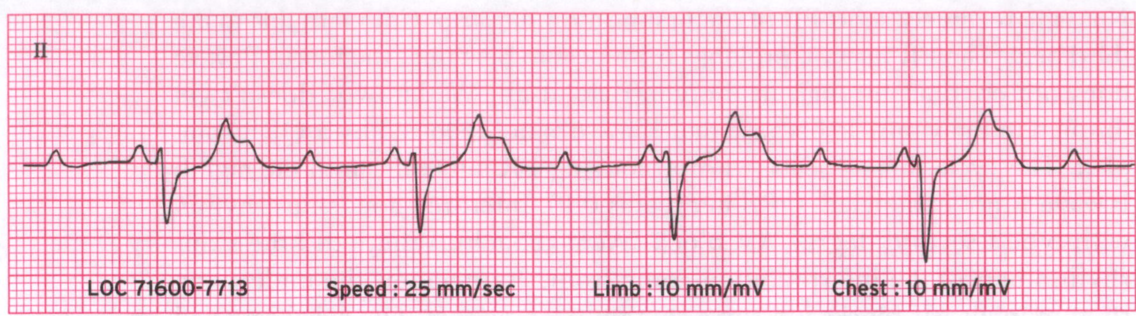

Figure 11-5 Type II second-degree AV block.

will improve the conduction, and the impulse will travel on down the pathway. If the block is at the bundle branches, however, the impulse will blast through the AV node and head down the pathway only to find that both bundle branches are still blocked. Atropine has no effect on the bundle branches. Patients with type II will usually receive epinephrine to increase their heart rate until a temporary pacemaker can be inserted, because the risk is very high that they will soon be in a worse block. Consider starting oxygen.

In Figure 11-5, there are QRS complexes, all the same shape. Regularity is regular. Heart rate is 44. P waves are upright, matching, some not followed by a QRS. P-P interval is regular. Atrial rate is 137. PR interval is constant at 0.12. QRS interval is 0.12. Interpretation is sinus tachycardia with type II second-degree AV block and a BBB.

2:1 AV Block

What is it? 2:1 AV block is a type of second-degree block in which there are two P waves to each QRS complex. The first P wave in each pair of P waves is blocked. 2:1 AV block can be caused by either Wenckebach or type II.

Rate	Atrial rate 60 to 100; ventricular rate half the atrial rate.
Regularity	Regular.
P waves	Normal sinus P waves; two Ps to each QRS; P-P interval is regular.
QRS	<0.12 second (≥0.12 s if BBB present).
Cause	Same as Wenckebach or type II.
Adverse effects	Decreased cardiac output if the heart rate is too slow.
Treatment	Atropine first if the patient is symptomatic; epinephrine, dopamine, pacemaker if the block continues and symptoms are present. Consider starting oxygen.

In Figure 11-6, there are QRS complexes, all the same shape. Regularity is regular. Heart rate is 37. Atrial rate is 75. P waves are upright and matching, two to each QRS. P-P interval is regular. PR interval is 0.16. QRS interval is 0.08. Interpretation: 2:1 AV block.

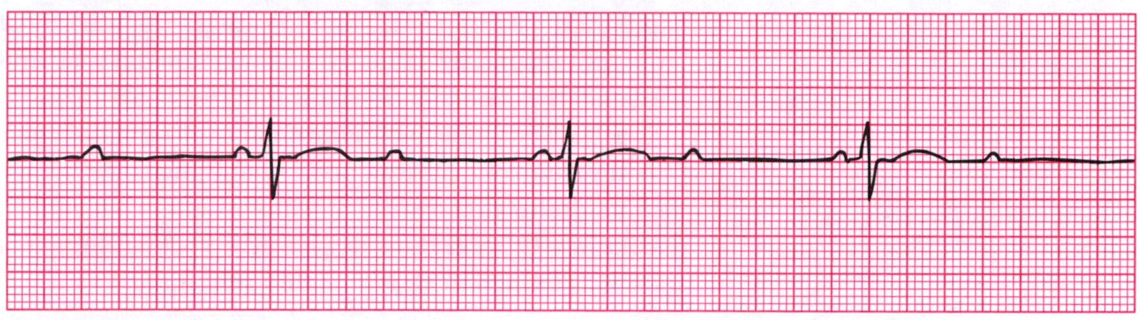

Figure 11-6 2:1 AV block.

Third-Degree AV Block (Complete Heart Block)

What is it? In third-degree block, the sinus node sends out its impulses as usual, *but not a single one of them ever gets to the ventricles,* because there is a complete block at the AV node or the bundle branches. Meanwhile, the AV node and the ventricle wait patiently for the sinus impulses to reach them. When it's obvious that the sinus impulse isn't coming, the lower pacemakers assume the sinus node has failed. One of them then escapes and assumes pacemaking control to provide a QRS complex. If the AV node is the location of the block, a lower spot in the AV junction takes over as pacemaker and provides a heart rate of 40 to 60. If the block is at the bundle branches, the only pacemaker left below that is the ventricle, with a heart rate of 20 to 40. Even though the lower pacemaker has assumed control of providing the QRS complex, the sinus node is unaware of that, so it continues firing out its impulses as usual, providing P waves.

Rate	Atrial rate usually 60 to 100; ventricular rate usually 20 to 60.
Regularity	Regular.
P waves	Normal sinus P waves; P-P interval is regular; P waves may be hidden inside QRS complexes or T waves. P waves are not associated with any of the QRS complexes, even though there may at times appear to be a relationship. This is called **AV dissociation**, and it is a hallmark of third-degree block. AV dissociation means the sinus node is firing at its normal rate, and the lower pacemaker is firing at its slower rate, and the two have nothing to do with each other. AV dissociation results in independent beating of the atria and the ventricles. Here's another way to describe AV dissociation as seen in third-degree AV block: Imagine the lower pacemaker that controls the ventricles as an old man jogging around a circular racetrack at 2 miles per hour. The sinus node is an 18-year-old boy sprinting at 4 miles per hour. Since the boy is going faster than the old man, he will periodically catch up with him

and then pass him. An onlooker might see the boy at the split second he's side by side with the old man and assume they are together and that there is a relationship between the two. There isn't, of course. Their being side by side was just coincidence, just as it's coincidence that a sinus P wave might land right in front of a QRS in third-degree AV block and make it seem as though there is a relationship there.

PR interval	Varies.
QRS	Normal (<0.12 s) or wide (>0.12 s), depending on the location of the block. If the block is at the AV node, the junction will become the pacemaker and the QRS will be narrow. If the block is at the bundle branches, the ventricle will become the pacemaker, with a wide QRS.
Cause	MI, conduction system lesion, medication side effects, hypoxia.
Adverse effects	Signs of low cardiac output may occur. The patient with third-degree block may be very symptomatic or may feel fine, depending on the heart rate.
Treatment	A temporary pacemaker will usually be necessary until the rhythm returns to normal or until a permanent pacemaker can be inserted. Atropine, epinephrine, or dopamine can be given until a pacemaker can be inserted. Start oxygen.

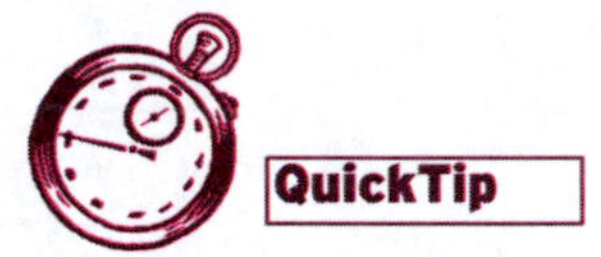

Here's a quick way to differentiate the AV blocks.
1st degree AVB–no dropped QRS, PR interval > 0.20 secs.
Wenckebach (type I 2nd degree AVB)–gradually prolonging PR intervals until a QRS is dropped.
Type II 2nd degree AVB–PR intervals constant, some QRS complexes dropped.
2:1 AVB–two P waves to every QRS.
3rd degree AVB–PR intervals vary, some QRS complexes dropped, R-R interval constant.

In Figure 11-7, there are QRS complexes, all shaped the same. Regularity is regular. Heart rate is 37. P waves are upright and matching. Atrial rate is 60. P-P interval is regular. One P wave is hidden in the ST segment of the third QRS complex. PR interval varies. QRS interval is 0.20. Interpretation: sinus rhythm with third-degree AV block and an idioventricular rhythm. Idioventricular rhythm? We know the sinus node is controlling the atria and providing the P waves. We also know, since the QRS is wide, that the ventricle is the pacemaker controlling the ventricles. Since the ventricular rate is between 20 and 40, the rhythm is idioventricular rhythm. Put the two together and we come up with our interpretation. If the AV junction had been the pacemaker, the QRS would have been narrow.

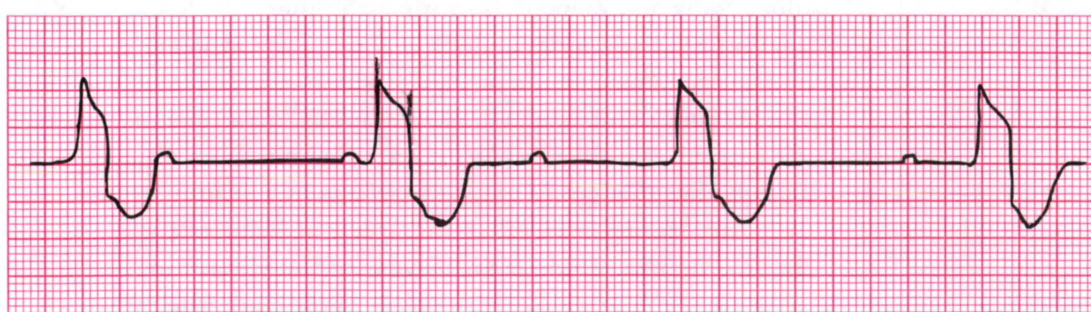

Figure 11-7 Third-degree AV block.

Practice Strips: AV Blocks

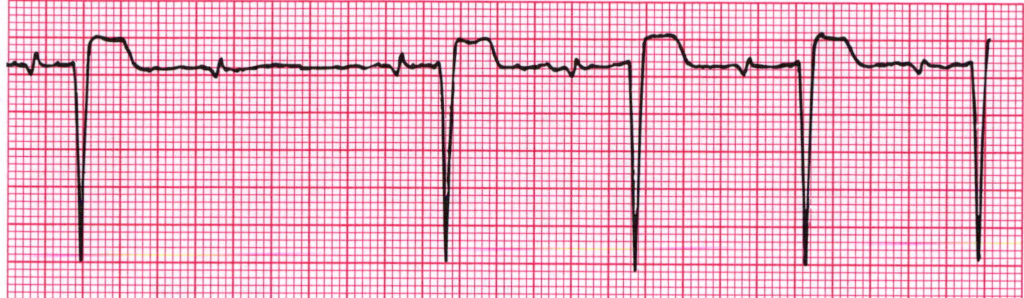

1. QRS complexes ________ Regularity ________ Heart rate ________

   P waves ____

   PR interval ____________ QRS interval ____________

   Interpretation (name of rhythm) ______________________

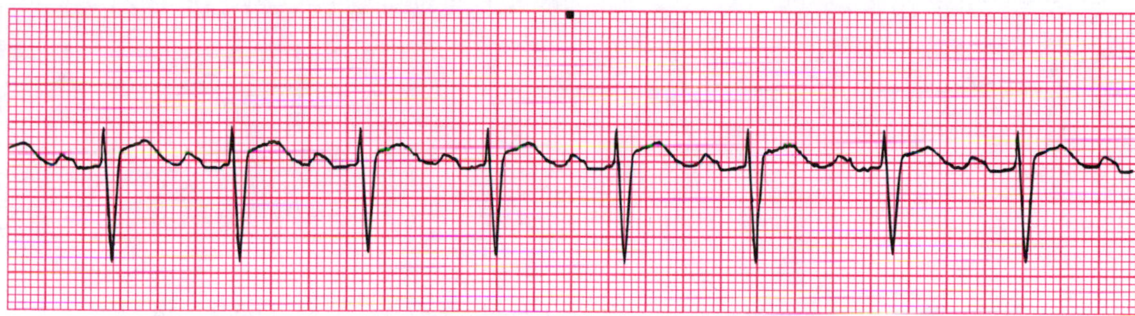

2. QRS complexes ________ Regularity ________ Heart rate ________

   P waves ____

   PR interval ____________ QRS interval ____________

   Interpretation ______________________________

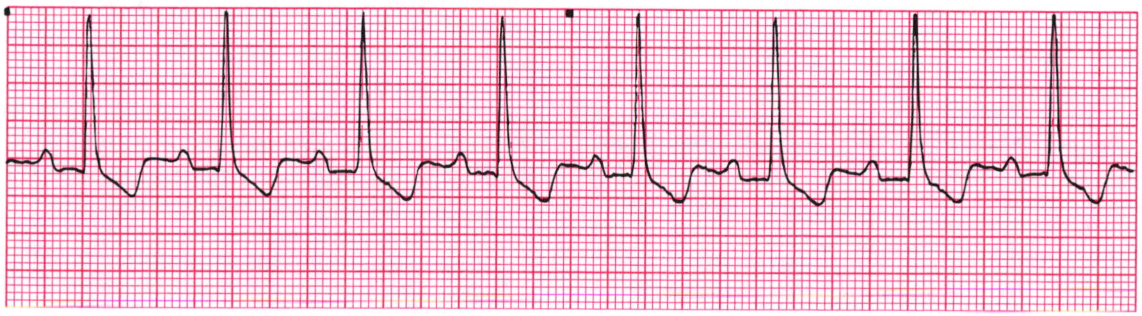

3. QRS complexes ________ Regularity ________ Heart rate ________

   P waves ____

   PR interval ____________ QRS interval ____________

   Interpretation ______________________________

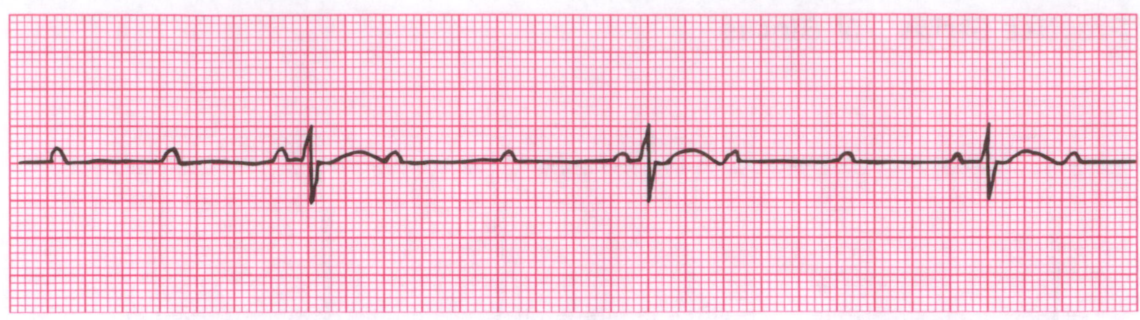

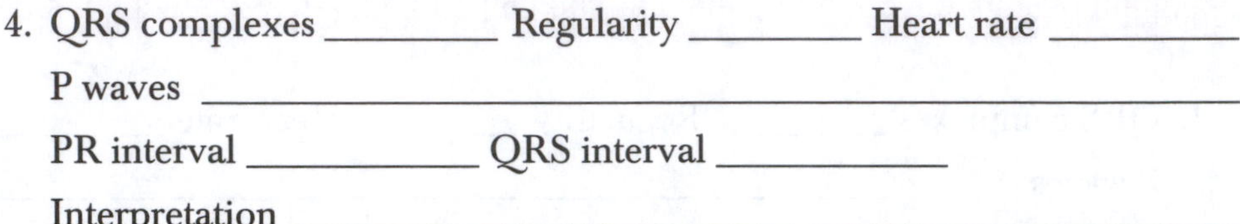

4. QRS complexes ________ Regularity ________ Heart rate ________
   P waves ____
   PR interval ___________ QRS interval ___________
   Interpretation ____

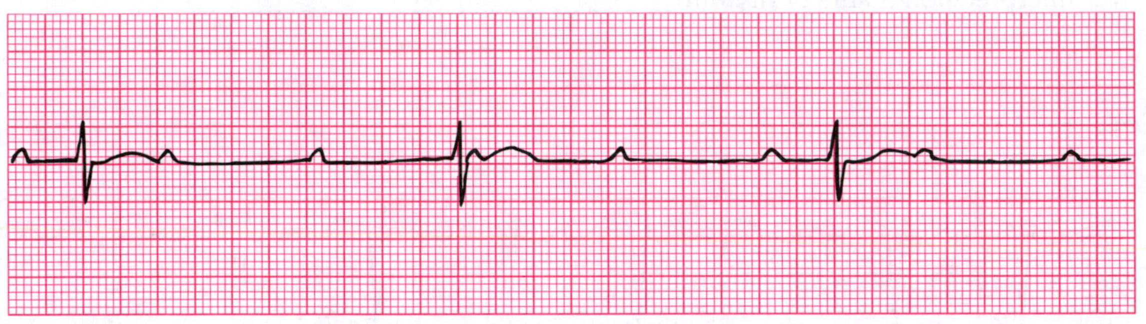

5. QRS complexes ________ Regularity ________ Heart rate ________
   P waves ____
   PR interval ___________ QRS interval ___________
   Interpretation ____

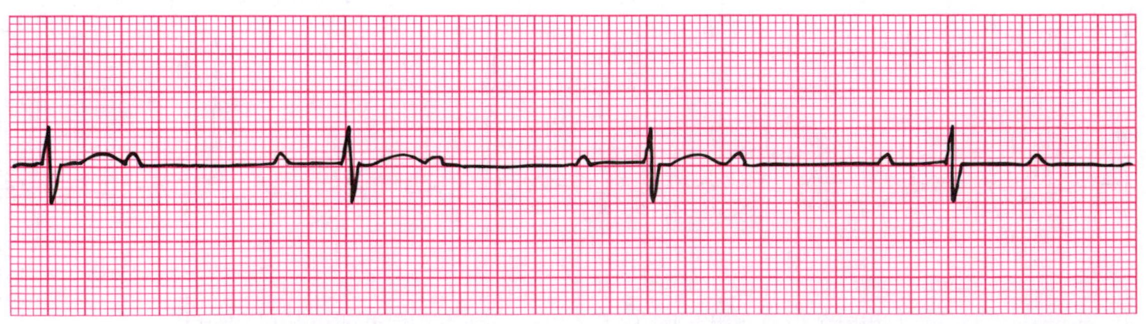

6. QRS complexes ________ Regularity ________ Heart rate ________
   P waves ____
   PR interval ___________ QRS interval ___________
   Interpretation ____

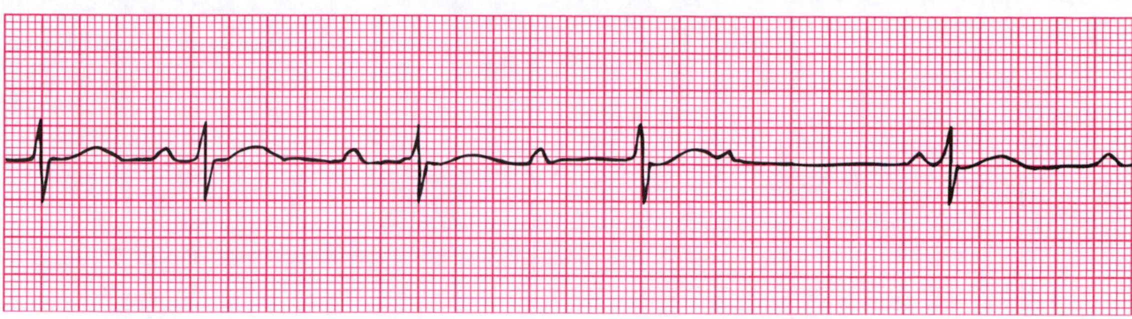

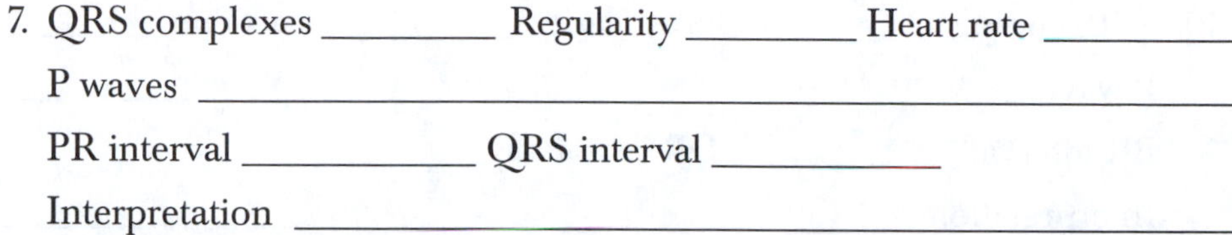

7. QRS complexes ________ Regularity ________ Heart rate ________

   P waves ____

   PR interval ____________ QRS interval ____________

   Interpretation ____

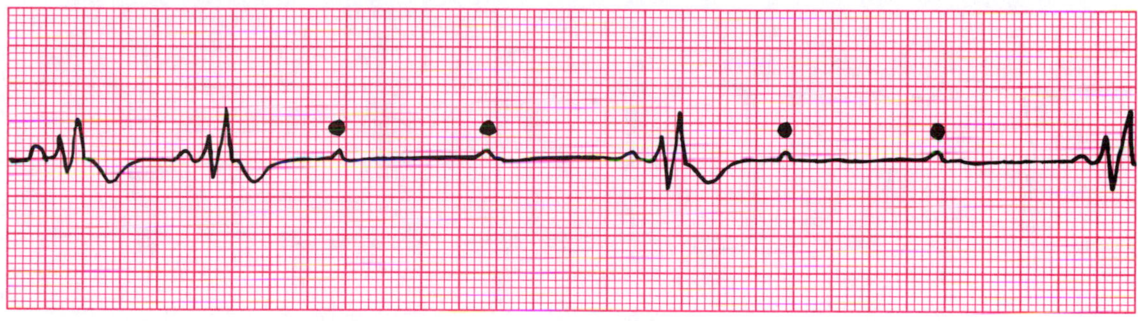

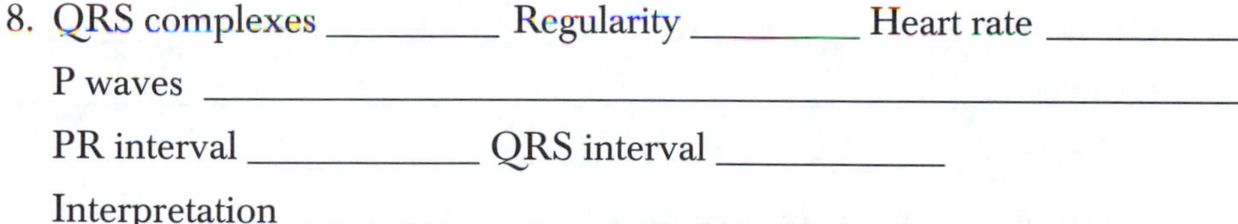

8. QRS complexes ________ Regularity ________ Heart rate ________

   P waves ____

   PR interval ____________ QRS interval ____________

   Interpretation ____

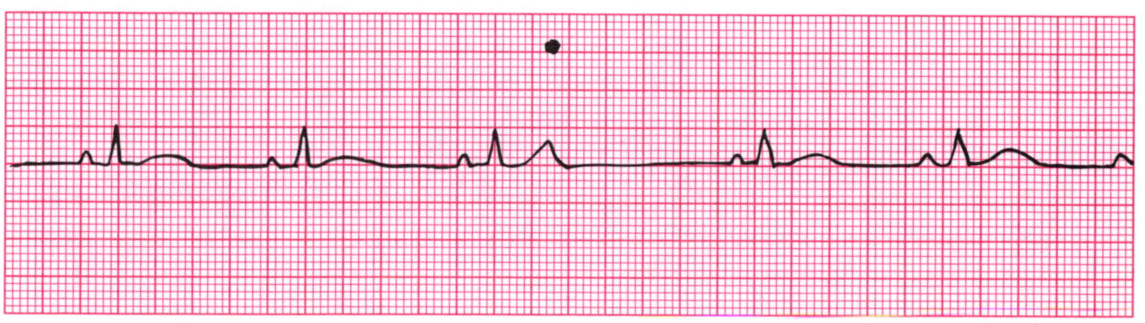

9. QRS complexes ________ Regularity ________ Heart rate ________

   P waves ____

   PR interval ____________ QRS interval ____________

   Interpretation ____

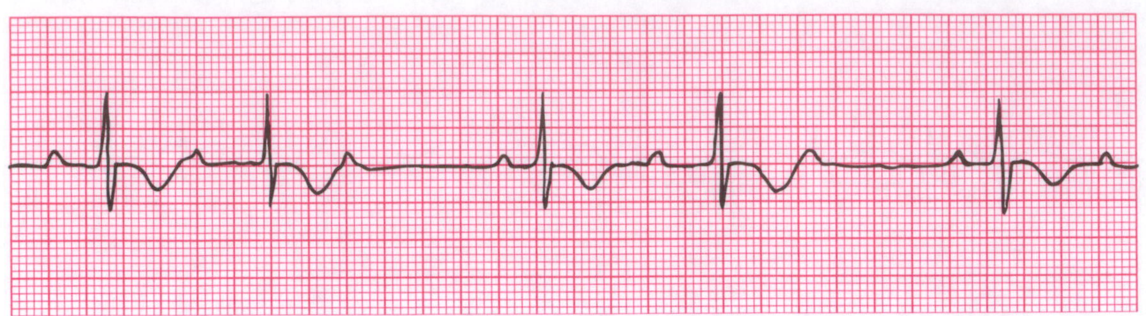

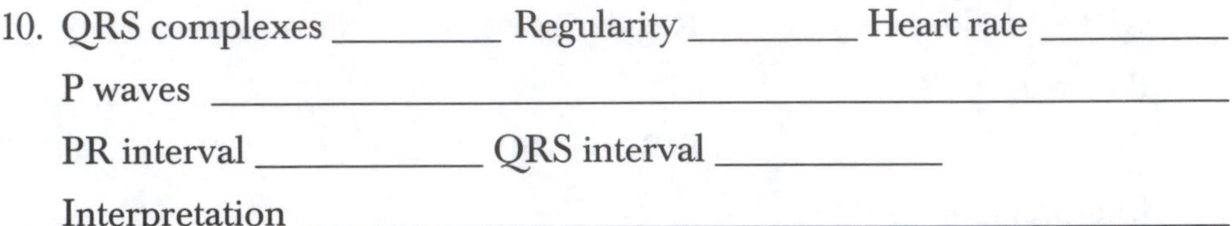

10. QRS complexes ________ Regularity ________ Heart rate ________
P waves ____
PR interval ____________ QRS interval ____________
Interpretation ____

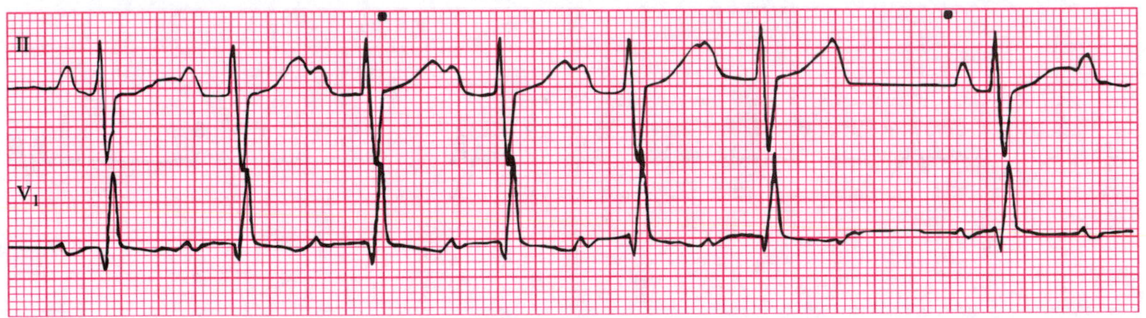

11. QRS complexes ________ Regularity ________ Heart rate ________
P waves ____
PR interval ____________ QRS interval ____________
Interpretation (name of rhythm) ____________________________

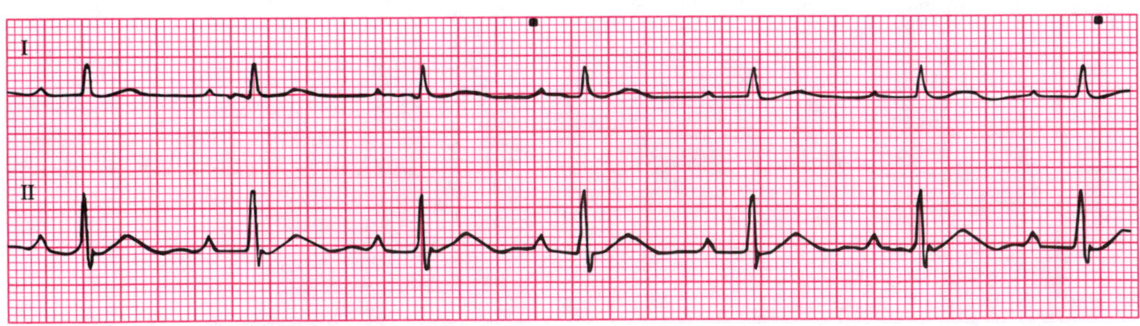

12. QRS complexes ________ Regularity ________ Heart rate ________
P waves ____
PR interval ____________ QRS interval ____________
Interpretation ____

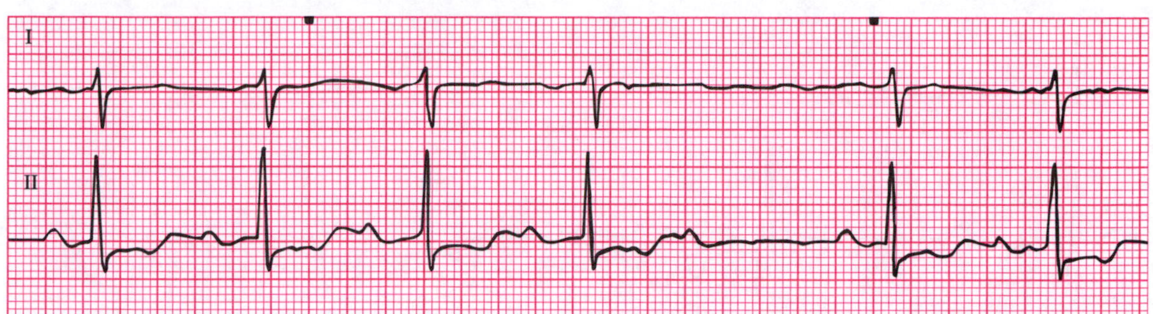

13. QRS complexes ________ Regularity ________ Heart rate ________
    P waves ________
    PR interval ________ QRS interval ________
    Interpretation ________

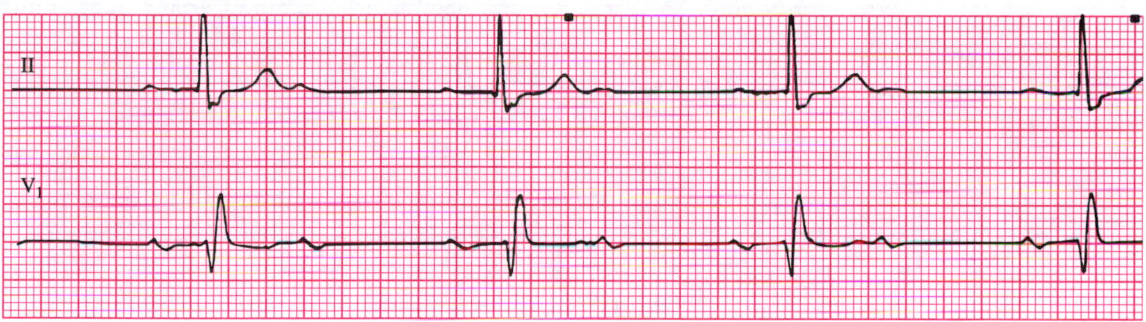

14. QRS complexes ________ Regularity ________ Heart rate ________
    P waves ________
    PR interval ________ QRS interval ________
    Interpretation ________

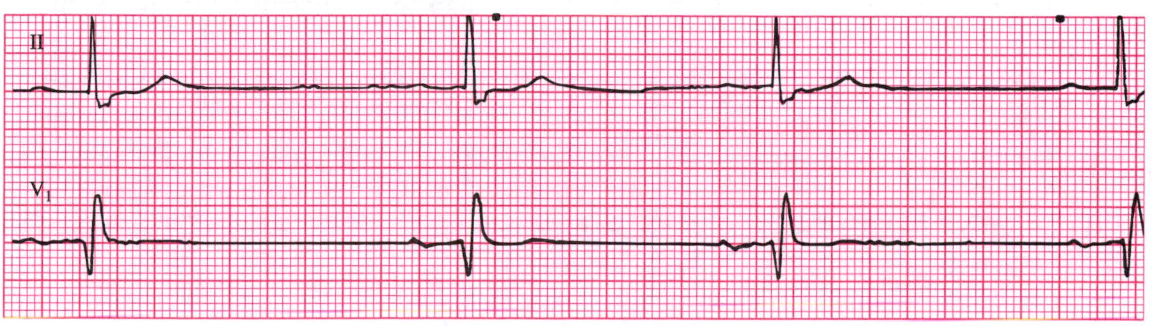

15. QRS complexes ________ Regularity ________ Heart rate ________
    P waves ________
    PR interval ________ QRS interval ________
    Interpretation ________

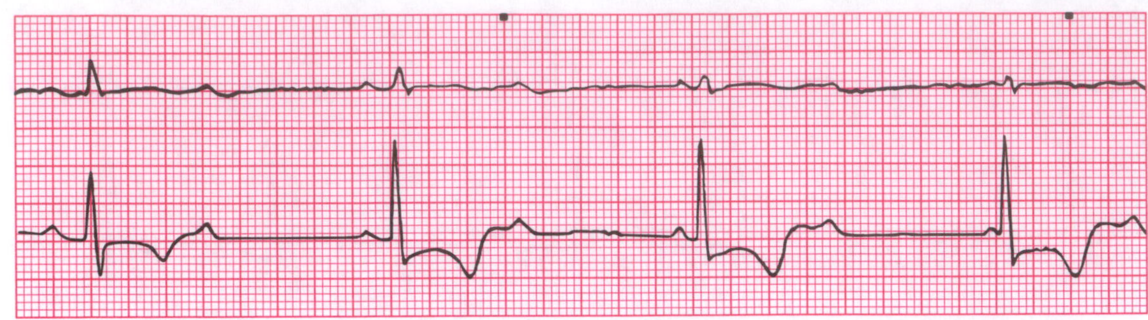

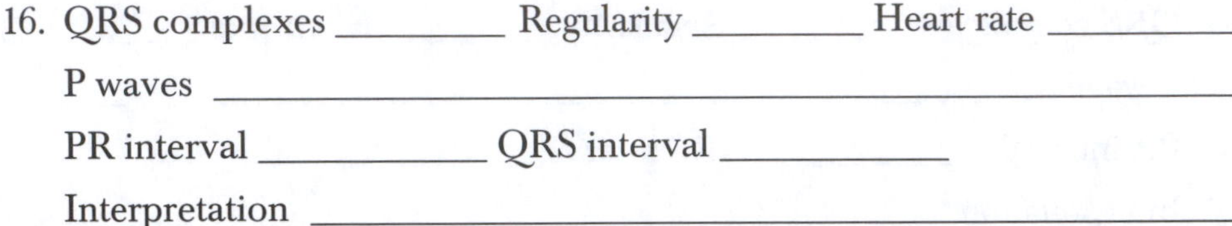

16. QRS complexes ________ Regularity ________ Heart rate ________
    P waves ____
    PR interval ____________ QRS interval ____________
    Interpretation ____

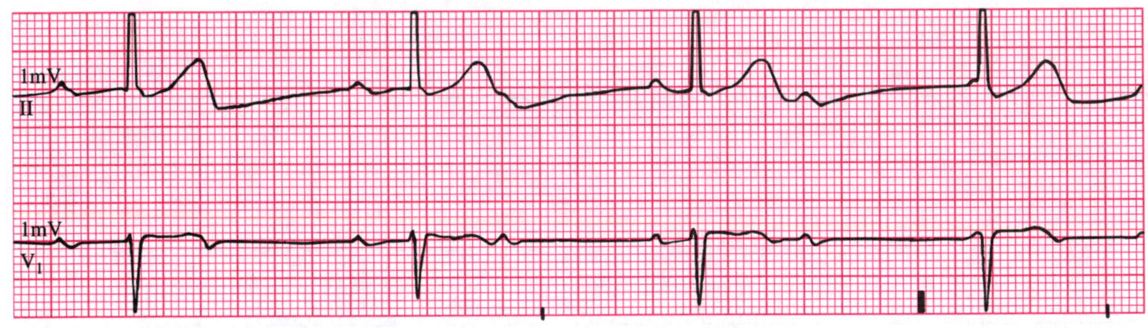

17. QRS complexes ________ Regularity ________ Heart rate ________
    P waves ____
    PR interval ____________ QRS interval ____________
    Interpretation ____

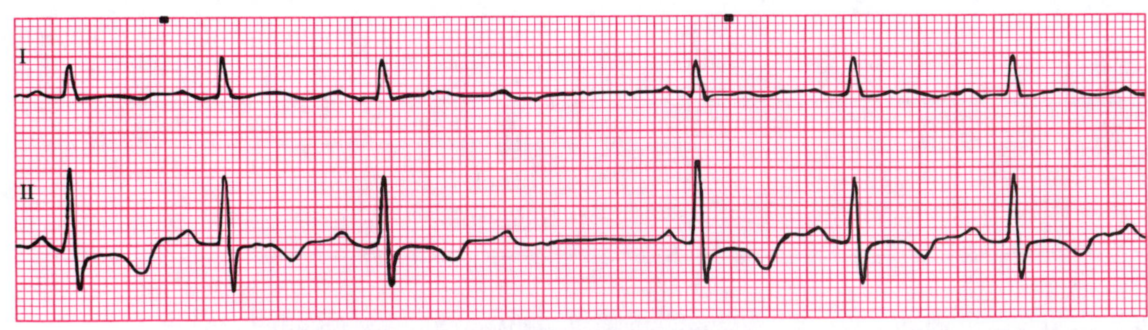

18. QRS complexes ________ Regularity ________ Heart rate ________
    P waves ____
    PR interval ____________ QRS interval ____________
    Interpretation ____

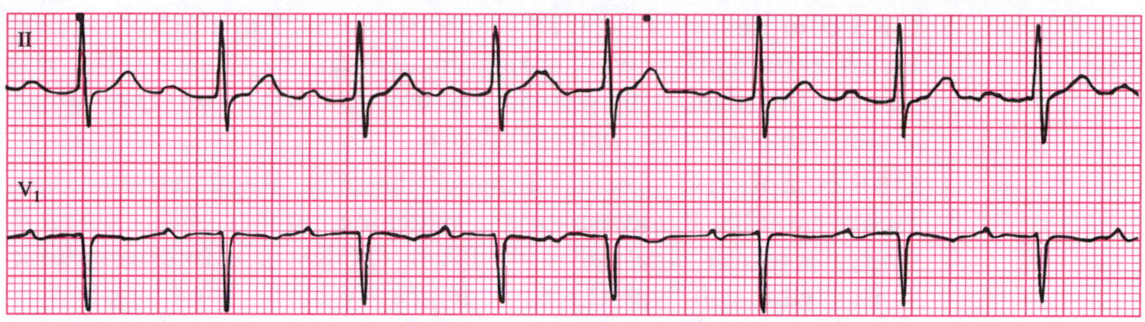

19. QRS complexes ________ Regularity ________ Heart rate ________

P waves ____

PR interval ____________ QRS interval ________

Interpretation ____

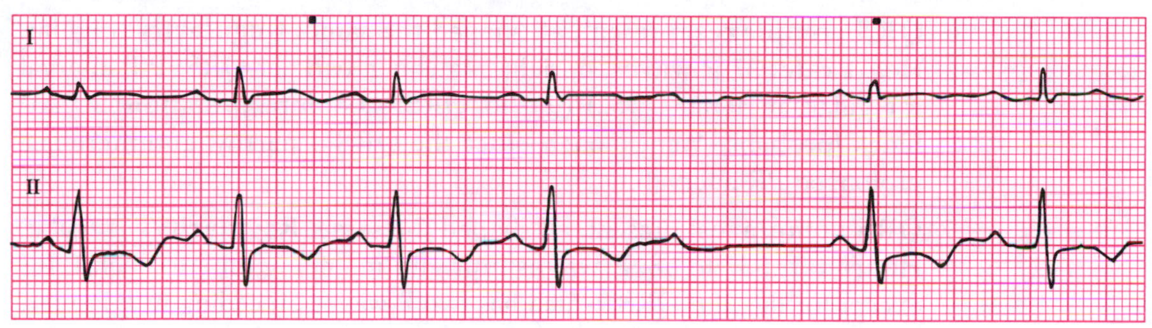

20. QRS complexes ________ Regularity ________ Heart rate ________

P waves ____

PR interval ____________ QRS interval ________

Interpretation ____

Answers to AV Blocks Practice Strips

1. **QRS complexes:** present, all shaped the same. **Regularity:** regular but interrupted (by a pause). **Heart rate:** 31 to 68, with a mean rate of 50. **P waves:** biphasic, matching, more than one per QRS at times. P-P interval is regular. Atrial rate is 62. **PR:** varies. **QRS:** 0.08. **Interpretation:** sinus rhythm with type I second-degree AV block (Wenckebach). Look at the P directly preceding the second QRS complex. The PR interval there is 0.24. The PR preceding the last QRS on the strip is 0.28. The PR interval prolongs and there are blocked P waves. The rhythm starts out as 2:1 AV block, then becomes an obvious Wenckebach. The 2:1 AV block here is therefore also Wenckebach.

2. **QRS complexes:** present, all shaped the same. **Regularity:** regular. **Heart rate:** 88. **P waves:** upright, matching, one to each QRS complex; atrial rate is 88; P-P interval is regular. **PR:** 0.24. **QRS:** 0.10. **Interpretation:** sinus rhythm with first-degree AV block.

3. **QRS complexes:** present, all shaped the same. **Regularity:** regular. **Heart rate:** 83. **P waves:** upright, matching, one to each QRS; P-P interval is regular; atrial rate is 83. **PR:** 0.24. **QRS:** 0.10. **Interpretation:** sinus rhythm with first-degree AV block.
4. **QRS complexes:** present, all shaped the same. **Regularity:** regular. **Heart rate:** 33. **P waves:** upright, matching, three to each QRS; P-P interval is regular; atrial rate is 100. **PR:** 0.16. **QRS:** 0.08. **Interpretation:** sinus rhythm with type II second-degree AV block. The block here is probably at the AV node, as evidenced by the narrow QRS. This can also be called a **high-grade AV block,** as more than half the P waves are not conducted.
5. **QRS complexes:** present, all shaped the same. **Regularity:** regular. **Heart rate:** 30. **P waves:** upright, matching, more than one per QRS; P-P interval is regular; atrial rate is 75. **PR:** varies. **QRS:** 0.08. **Interpretation:** Sinus rhythm with third-degree AV block and a junctional bradycardia.
6. **QRS complexes:** present, all shaped the same. **Regularity:** regular. **Heart rate:** 37. **P waves:** upright, matching, two per QRS; P-P interval is regular; atrial rate is 75. **PR:** 0.36. **QRS:** 0.08. **Interpretation:** 2:1 AV block (probably Wenckebach, since the QRS is narrow and there is a prolonged PR interval).
7. **QRS complexes:** present, all shaped the same. **Regularity:** irregular. **Heart rate:** 37 to 68. **P waves:** upright, matching, one to each QRS except for the fifth QRS, which has two P waves preceding it; P-P interval is regular; atrial rate is 60. **PR:** varies–prolongs progressively. **QRS:** 0.08. **Interpretation:** sinus rhythm with type I second-degree AV block (Wenckebach).
8. **QRS complexes:** present, all the same shape. **Regularity:** irregular. **Heart rate:** 25 to 75, with a mean rate of 40. **P waves:** matching, upright, one for the first two QRS complexes, then three per QRS; P-P interval is regular; atrial rate is 75. **PR:** 0.16. **QRS:** 0.16. **Interpretation:** sinus rhythm with type II second-degree AV block and a bundle branch block. The first two beats are sinus rhythm with BBB, then suddenly the other bundle branch goes down and the sinus impulses can't get through. When they do finally get through, they do so with the same PR interval they started with.
9. **QRS complexes:** present, all shaped the same. **Regularity:** regular but interrupted (by a pause). **Heart rate:** 42 to 60, with a mean rate of 50. **P waves:** matching, upright, one preceding each QRS except the fourth QRS, which has two P waves preceding it (there's a P in the T wave of the third beat); P-P interval is *irregular;* atrial rate is 60 to 125. **PR:** 0.16. **QRS:** 0.108. **Interpretation:** sinus rhythm with a nonconducted PAC. "Wait a minute," you exclaim. "That's not fair! We're doing AV blocks, not atrial rhythms!" *Mea culpa.* But there's a method to this madness. Do you see how easy it is to mistake a nonconducted PAC for an AV block?

How do you tell the difference? Simple. AV blocks have regular P-P intervals. Here the P-P is *not regular,* is it? One P is premature. That makes it a PAC. And since there's no QRS following it, that makes it a nonconducted PAC. Piece of cake. . . .

10. **QRS complexes:** present, all shaped the same. **Regularity:** regular but interrupted (by pauses). **Heart rate:** 42 to 68, with a mean rate of 50. **P waves:** upright, matching, more than one per QRS at times; P-P interval is regular; atrial rate is 75. **PR:** varies. **QRS:** 0.08. **Interpretation:** sinus rhythm with type I second-degree AV block (Wenckebach).

11. **QRS complexes:** present, all shaped the same within each lead. **Regularity:** regular but interrupted (by a pause). **Heart rate:** 48 to 79, with a mean rate of 70. **P waves:** upright, matching, more than one per QRS at times. P-P interval is regular. Atrial rate is 88. **PR:** varies. **QRS:** 0.12. **Interpretation:** sinus rhythm with type I second-degree AV block (Wenckebach). Look at the P wave directly preceding the first QRS complex. The PR interval there is 0.22. The PR preceding the sixth QRS (the last QRS before the pause) is 0.32. The PR interval prolongs until a P wave is blocked. This is typical of Wenckebach.

12. **QRS complexes:** present, all shaped the same within each lead. **Regularity:** regular. **Heart rate:** 68. **P waves:** upright, matching, one per QRS. P-P interval is regular. **PR:** 0.24. **QRS:** 0.08. **Interpretation:** sinus rhythm with first-degree AV block.

13. **QRS complexes:** present, all shaped the same within each lead. **Regularity:** regular but interrupted (by a pause). **Heart rate:** 38 to 68, with a mean rate of 60. **P waves:** upright, matching, more than one per QRS at times. P-P interval is regular. Atrial rate is 75. **PR:** varies. **QRS:** 0.08. **Interpretation:** sinus rhythm with type I second-degree AV block (Wenckebach). Look at the first PR interval on the strip–it's 0.24. The PR preceding the fourth QRS is 0.36. The PR interval prolongs and there is a blocked P wave–classic Wenckebach.

14. **QRS complexes:** present, all shaped the same within each lead. **Regularity:** regular. **Heart rate:** 38. **P waves:** upright in top strip, biphasic in bottom, matching, two P waves per QRS (except first QRS only has one because the start of the strip cut off the other P wave). P-P interval is regular. Atrial rate is 79. **PR:** 0.28. **QRS:** 0.12. **Interpretation:** sinus rhythm with 2:1 AV block.

15. **QRS complexes:** present, all shaped the same within each lead. **Regularity:** irregular. **Heart rate:** 30 to 37, with a mean rate of 40. **P waves:** biphasic, matching, one per QRS. P-P interval is irregular. **PR:** 0.28. **QRS:** 0.13. **Interpretation:** sinus arrhythmia with first degree AV block.

16. **QRS complexes:** present, all shaped the same within each lead. **Regularity:** regular. **Heart rate:** 37. **P waves:** upright, matching, two per QRS. P-P interval is regular. Atrial rate is 75. **PR:** varies. **QRS:** 0.09.

Interpretation: sinus rhythm with third degree AV block. This is not 2:1 AV block because the PR intervals are not constant here, as they should be for 2:1 AV block. Notice the first PR interval on the strip is 0.20 and the last one is 0.06, with the P wave "crawling up onto" the QRS complex.

17. **QRS complexes:** present, all shaped the same within each lead. **Regularity:** regular. **Heart rate P waves:** upright in top strip, biphasic in bottom, matching, more than one per QRS. P-P interval is regular. Atrial rate is 79. **PR:** varies. **QRS:** 0.08. **Interpretation:** sinus rhythm with third degree AV block.
18. **QRS complexes:** present, all shaped the same within each lead. **Regularity:** regular but interrupted (by a pause). **Heart rate:** 37 to 75, with a mean rate of 60. **P waves:** upright, matching, more than one per QRS at times. P-P interval is regular. Atrial rate is 75. **PR:** varies. **QRS:** 0.10. **Interpretation:** sinus rhythm with type I second-degree AV block (Wenckebach). Note the first PR interval on the strip is shorter than the second and third, then there is a blocked P wave. After the pause the PR is short again, but lengthens by the next beat.
19. **QRS complexes:** present, all shaped the same within each lead. **Regularity:** regular but interrupted (by a premature beat). **Heart rate:** 81. **P waves:** upright, all but the fifth matching (the fifth is a premature P wave of a different shape). P-P interval is irregular. **PR:** 0.28. **QRS:** 0.08. **Interpretation:** sinus rhythm with a PAC (the fifth QRS is premature) and first degree AV block.
20. **QRS complexes:** present, all shaped the same within each lead. **Regularity:** regular but interrupted (by a pause). **Heart rate:** 36 to 75, with a mean rate of 60. **P waves:** upright, matching, more than one per QRS at times. P-P interval is regular. Atrial rate is 75. **PR:** varies. **QRS:** 0.10. **Interpretation:** sinus rhythm with type I second-degree AV block (Wenckebach). The PR intervals prolong until a P wave is blocked.

Practice Quiz

1. Name the two typical locations of the block in AV blocks. ____________

   ____
2. True or false: People with a first-degree AV block need a pacemaker inserted.
3. Wenckebach is another name for which kind of block? ____________

   ____
4. AV dissociation is a hallmark of which kind of AV block? ____________

   ____
5. True or false: Atropine is effective in all types of AV blocks, whether the block is at the AV node or the bundle branches.

6. The AV block that merely provides a prolonged PR interval is ________
____
7. What is atropine's mode of action? ________
____
8. The most dangerous type of AV block is ________
9. The least dangerous type of AV block is ________
10. True or false: All AV blocks require atropine or epinephrine to increase the heart rate.

Putting It All Together—Critical Thinking Exercises

These exercises may consist of diagrams to label, scenarios to analyze, brain-stumping questions to ponder, or other challenging exercises to boost your understanding of the chapter material.

Let's play with AV blocks a bit. The following scenario will provide you with information about a fictional patient and will ask you to analyze the situation, answer questions, and decide on appropriate actions.

Ms. Watson, age 89, presents to her physician's office complaining of feeling weak and tired for the past three days. She has a history of atrial fibrillation and has been taking digoxin for years. She also takes insulin for diabetes and beta-blockers for high blood pressure. Vital signs are stable and within normal limits. Suspecting that Ms. Watson's atrial fib has again gotten out of control, the nurse records the rhythm strip below. See Figure 11-8.

1. What is the rhythm and heart rate? ________.
2. Does this rhythm require emergency treatment? ________.

   Suddenly, Ms. Watson says " I feel funny," and the nurse helps her lie back on the examining table. Vital signs are still within normal limits, but her BP has dropped some. Her repeat rhythm strip is seen in Figure 11-9.

3. What has happened? ________.
4. Which of Ms. Watson's medications could be responsible for this rhythm?
   ____
   ________.

   The physician admits Ms. Watson to the telemetry floor and orders a digoxin level, which comes back elevated. Further questioning of Ms. Watson reveals that she'd doubled up on her digoxin the past three days cause she thought it would help her feel better.

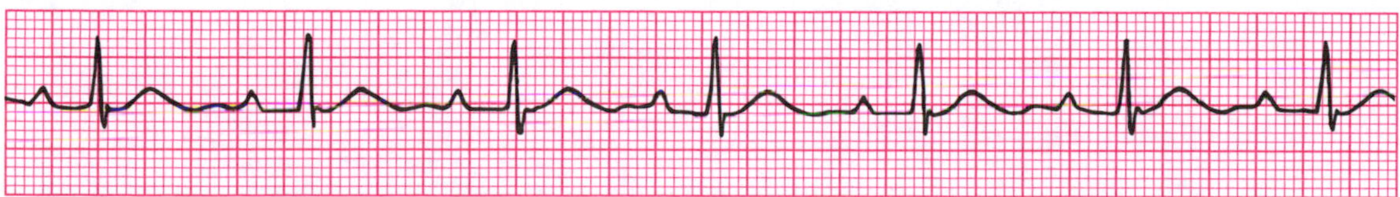

Figure 11-8 Ms. Watson's initial strip.

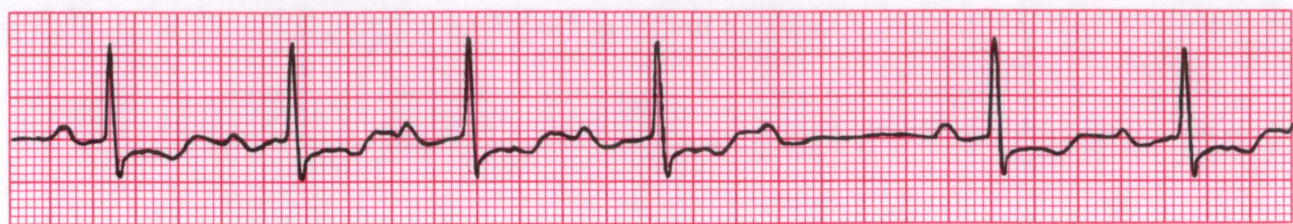

Figure 11-9 Ms. Watson's "funny" strip.

5. Given this latest information, what treatment is appropriate for this rhythm? ____
____.

CHAPTER **12**

Rhythm Practice Strips

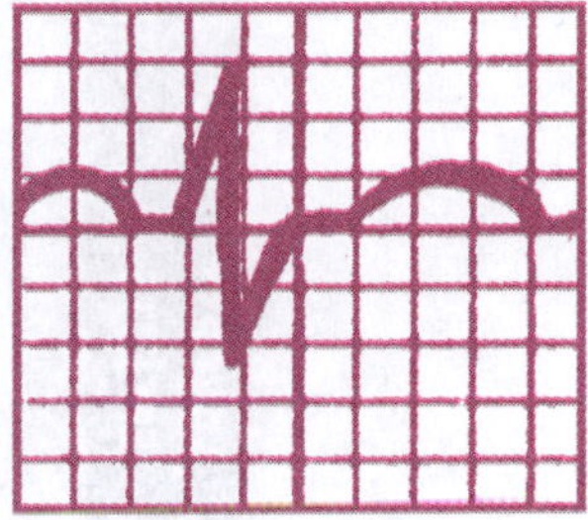

Chapter 12 Objectives

At the conclusion of this chapter the student will be able to:

- Correctly identify the rhythms.
- Identify any weak areas for further study.

Introduction

This chapter focus on the interpretation of rhythm strips utilizing the five steps you learned in chapter 6 and the rhythm descriptions in chapters 7 through 11. Additionally, two other analysis tools are included here to help you analyze rhythms: **Rhythm summary sheets** present a summary of all the rhythm criteria along with a pictorial review, so you can turn to this section for a quick comparison of criteria. And the **rhythm regularity summary** points out the type of regularity of each rhythm. For example, if you know the rhythm is irregular but aren't sure what rhythm it is, you can turn to this summary to determine which rhythms are irregular and which are not.

Rhythm Summary Sheets

Rhythm Summary: Sinus Rhythms

	RATE	REGULARITY	P WAVE	PR INTERVAL	QRS INTERVAL	CAUSE	ADVERSE EFFECTS	TREATMENT
Sinus rhythm	60-100	Regular	Upright, one per QRS, all shaped the same	0.12-0.20 Constant	<0.12 unless BBB	Normal	None	None
Sinus brady	<60	Regular	Upright, one per QRS, all shaped the same	0.12-0.20 Constant	<0.12 unless BBB	MI, vagal stimulation, hypoxia	None necessarily; maybe decreased cardiac output	Atropine if symptoms Consider O_2
Sinus tachy-cardia	101-160	Regular	Upright, one per QRS, all shaped the same	0.12-0.20 Constant	<0.12 unless BBB	SNS stimulation, MI, hypoxia, pulmonary embolus, CHF, thyroid storm, fever, vagal inhibition	Maybe none; maybe decreased cardiac output	Treat the cause Consider O_2 and beta blockers
Sinus arrhyth-mia	Varies-↑ with inspiration, ↓ with expiration	Irregular, R-R varies by ≥0.16 s	Upright, one per QRS, all shaped the same	0.12-0.20 Constant	<0.12 unless BBB	The breathing pattern	Usually none	Atropine if HR slow and symptoms
Sinus arrest	Can occur at any rate	Regular but interrupted	Normal before the pause, may be different or absent after	Normal before pause, may be different or absent after	<0.12 unless BBB or ventricular escape beat present	Sinus node ischemia, hypoxia,digitoxicity, excessive vagal tone, medication side effects	Maybe none; maybe decreased cardiac output; lower pacemaker may take over after pause	Consider O_2; atropine or pacemaker if symptoms
Sinus exit block	Can occur at any rate	Regular but interrupted	Normal before and after the pause, all shaped the same	0.12-0.20	<0.12 unless BBB	Medication side effects, excessive vagal tone, hypoxia	Same as sinus arrest; pause is a multiple of R-R; Sinus resumes after pause	Consider O_2; atropine or pacemaker if symp-toms

Sinus Rhythms Pictorial Review

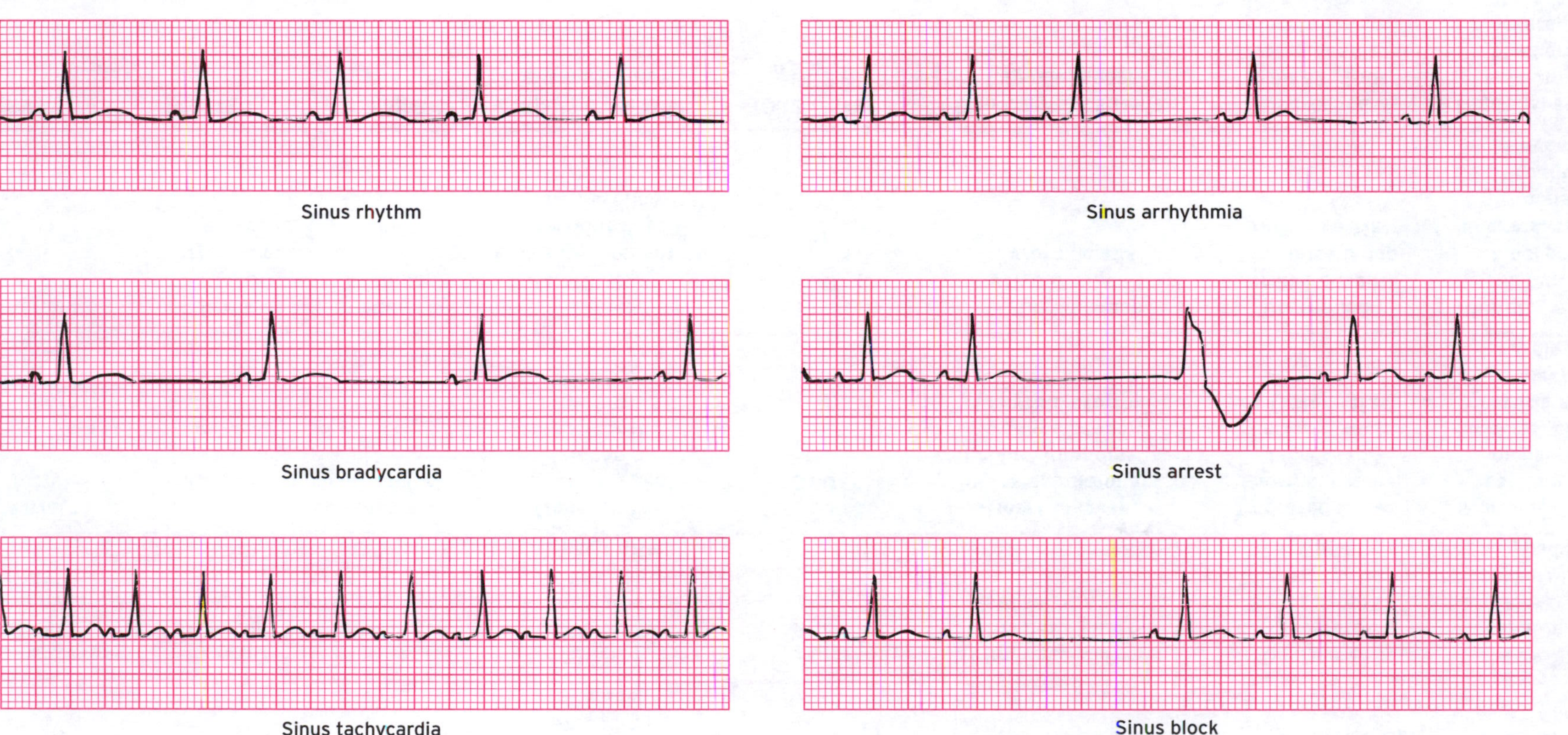

Rhythm Summary: Atrial Rhythms

	RATE	REGULARITY	P WAVE	QRS INTERVAL	CAUSE	ADVERSE EFFECTS	TREATMENT
Wandering atrial pacemaker	< 100	Irregular	At least three different shapes, sometimes no P at all on some beats	<0.12 unless BBB	MI, medication side effects, hypoxia, vagal stimulation	Usually no ill effects	Usually none. Atropine if HR slow and symptoms
PACs	Can occur at any rate	Regular but interrupted	Shaped differently than sinus Ps; often hidden in preceding T wave	<0.12 unless BBB; absent after non-conducted PAC	Stimulants, caffeine, hypoxia, heart disease, or normal	None if occasional; can be a sign of early heart failure	Omit the causes; consider O_2, digitalis, calcium channel blockers
Paroxysmal atrial tachycardia (PAT)	161-250 once in atrial tach	Regular but interrupted	Shaped differently than sinus Ps but same as each other	<0.12 unless BBB	Stimulants, caffeine, hypoxia, heart disease, or normal	Decreased cardiac output; some people tolerate OK for a while	Digitalis, amiodarone, calcium channel blockers, beta-blockers, sedation, O_2, adenosine
Atrial flutter	Atria: 251-350 Ventri-cle: varies	Regular or irregular	None; flutter waves present (zigzag or sawtooth waves)	<0.12 unless BBB	Heart disease, hypoxia, pulmonary embolus, lung disease, valve disease, thyroid storm	Tolerated OK at normal rate; decreased cardiac output at faster rates	Digitalis, amiodarone, calcium channel blockers, beta-blockers, consider O_2, carotid massage, electrical cardioversion
Atrial fib	Atria: 350-700 Ventri-cle: varies	Irregularly irregular	None; fibrillatory waves present (waviness of the baseline)	<0.12 unless BBB	MI, lung disease, valve disease, thyrotoxicosis	Decreased cardiac output; can cause blood clots in atria	Digitalis, amiodarone, calcium channel blockers, beta-blockers, consider O_2; consider anticoagulation to prevent clots
SVT	$\geq$ 130	Regular	May be present but hard to see	<0.12 unless BBB	Stimulants, caffeine, hypoxia, heart disease, or normal	Decreased cardiac output; some people tolerate OK for a while	Digitalis, amiodarone, calcium channel blockers, beta-blockers, sedation, O_2, adenosine

Atrial Rhythms Pictorial Review

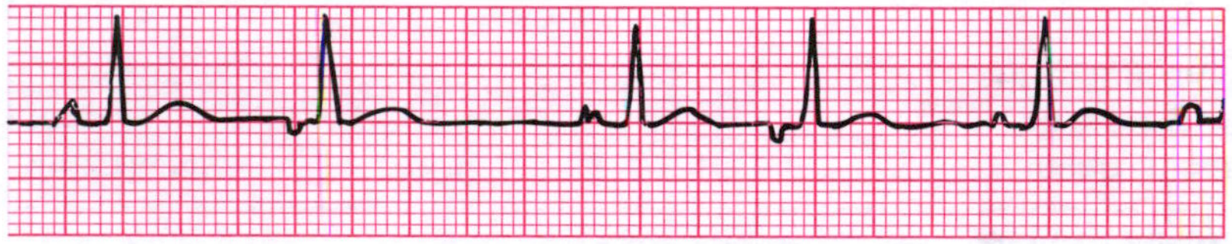

Wandering atrial pacemaker

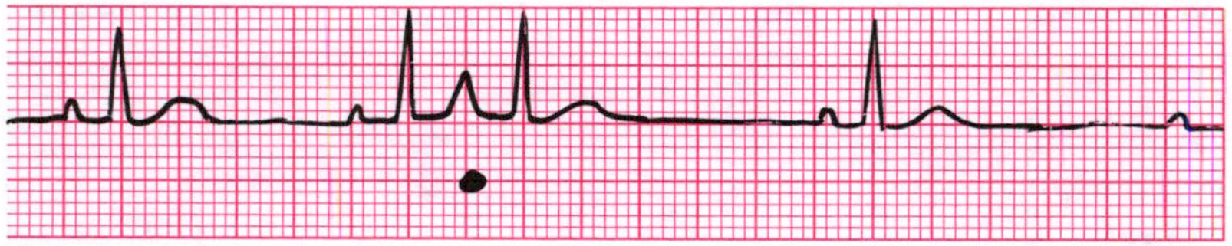

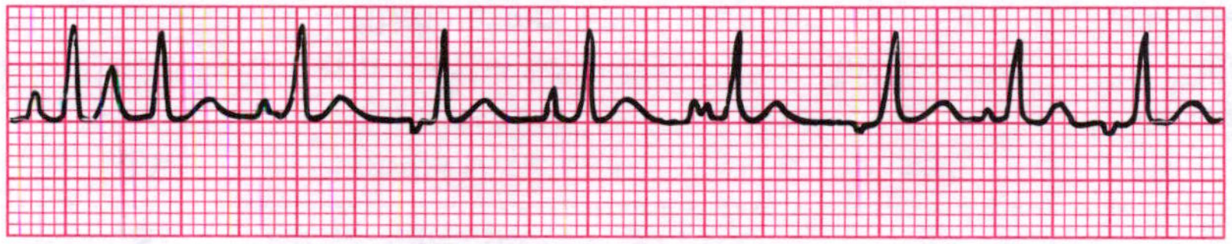

Multifocal atrial tachycardia

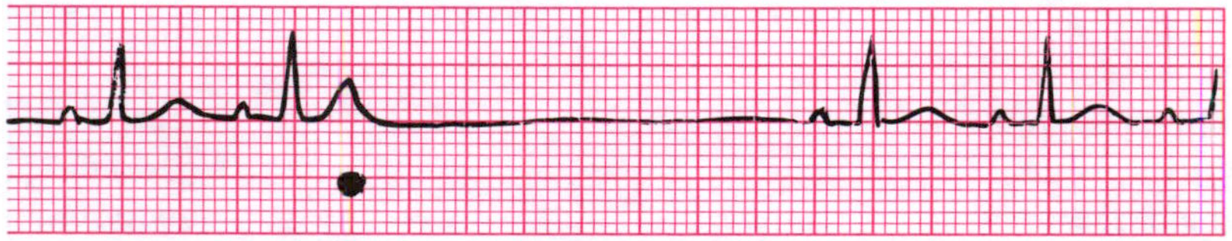

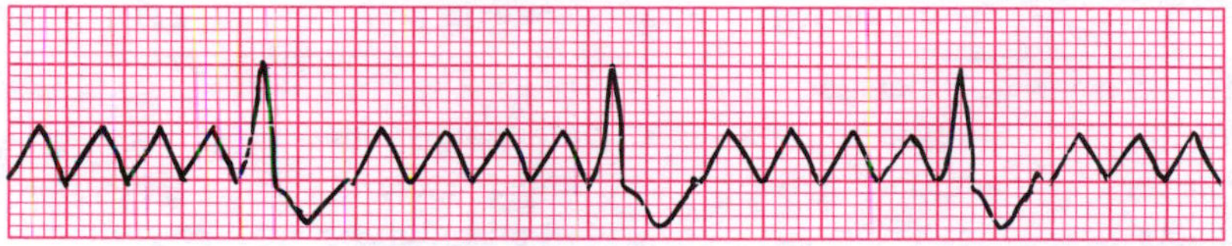

PAC

Atrial flutter

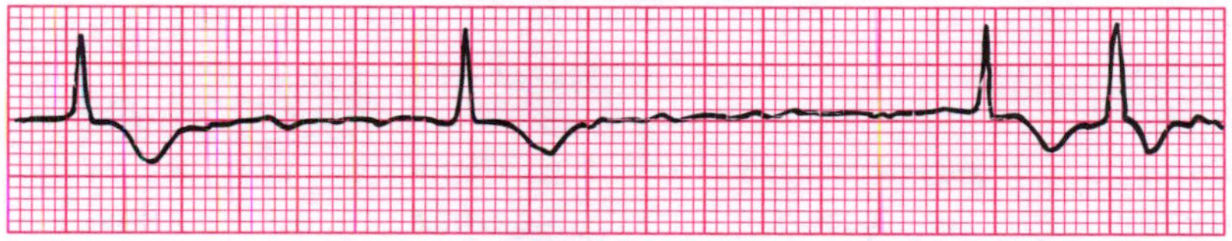

Nonconducted PAC

Atrial fibrillation

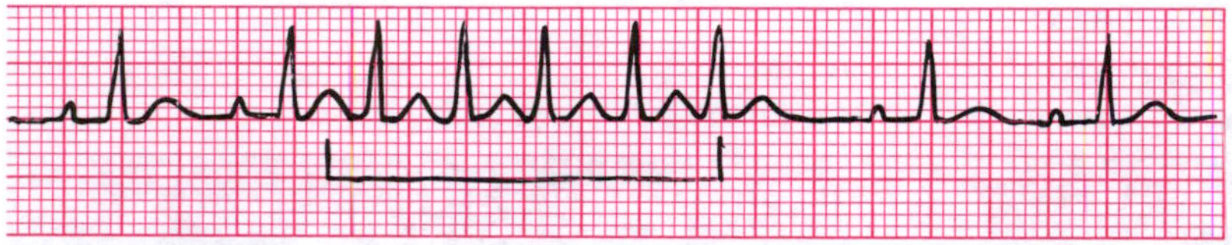

Paroxysmal atrial tachycardia

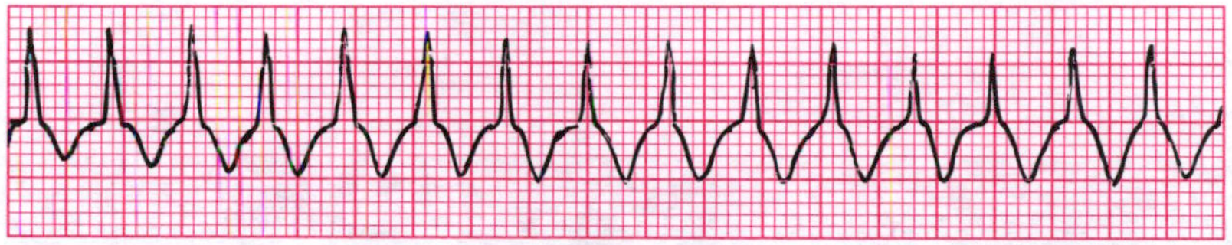

SVT

Rhythm Summary: Junctional Rhythms

	RATE	REGULARITY	P WAVE	QRS	CAUSE	ADVERSE EFFECTS	TREATMENT
PJCs	Can occur at any rate	Regular but interrupted	Inverted before or after QRS or hidden inside QRS	<0.12 unless BBB	Stimulants, caffeine, hypoxia, heart disease, or normal	Usually no ill effects	Usually none required
Junctional bradycardia	<40	Regular	Inverted before or after QRS or hidden inside QRS	<0.12 unless BBB	Vagal stimulation, hypoxia, sinus node ischemia, MI	Decreased cardiac output	Atropine if symptoms; hold medications that can slow the HR; start O_2
Junctional rhythm	40-60	Regular	Inverted before or after QRS or hidden inside QRS	<0.12 unless BBB	Vagal stimulation, hypoxia, sinus node ischemia, MI	Well tolerated if HR closer to 50-60; decreased cardiac output possible	Atropine if symptoms; hold medications that can slow the HR; start O_2
Accelerated junctional	60-100	Regular	Inverted before or after QRS or hidden inside QRS	<0.12 unless BBB	Heart disease, stimulant drugs, caffeine	Usually no ill effects	Usually none needed
Junctional tach	>100	Regular	Inverted before or after QRS or hidden inside QRS	<0.12 unless BBB	Digitalis toxicity, heart disease, stimulants, SNS stimulation	Decreased cardiac HR too fast	Beta-blockers, calcium channel blockers, adenosine; consider O_2

Junctional Rhythms Pictorial Review

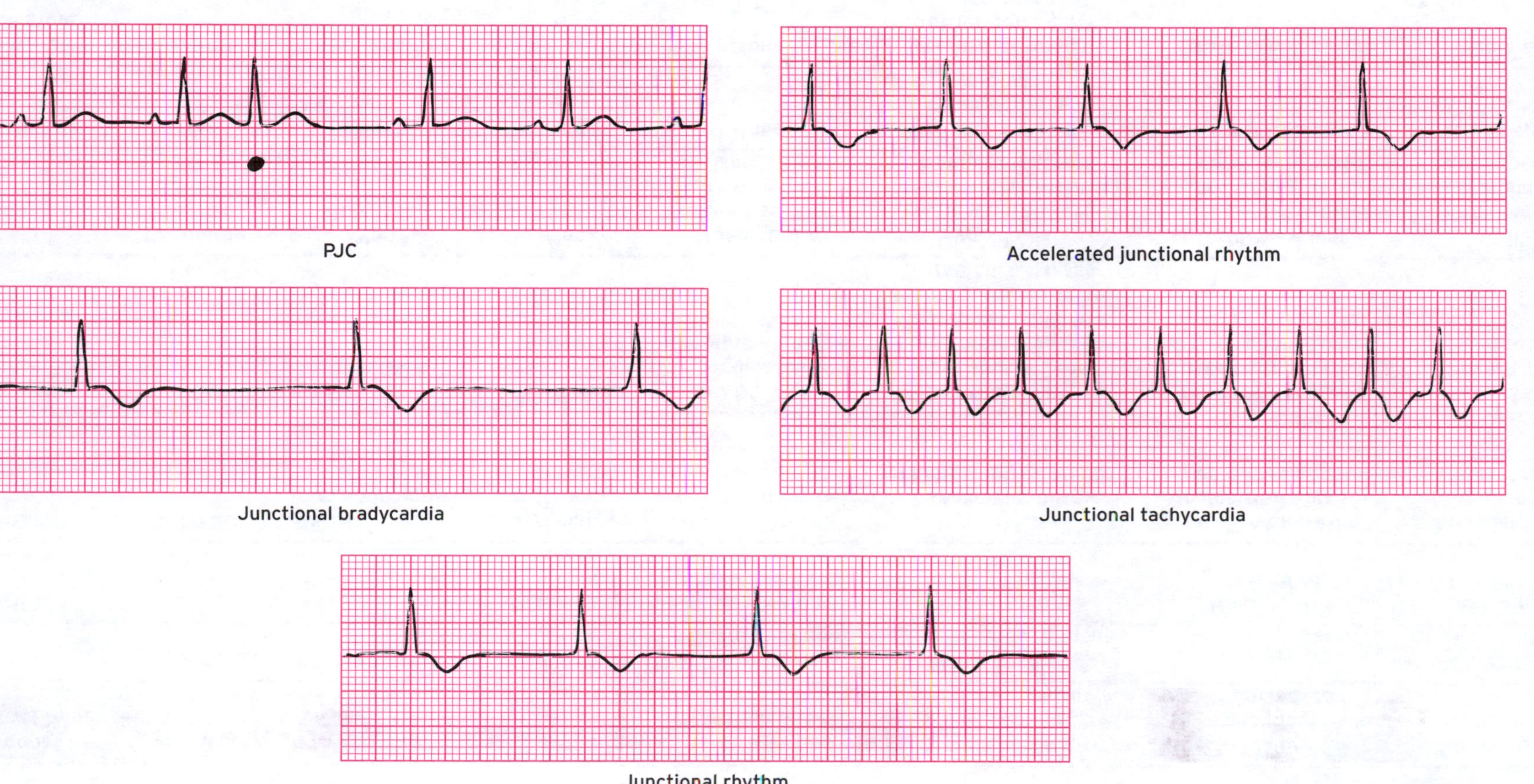

PJC

Accelerated junctional rhythm

Junctional bradycardia

Junctional tachycardia

Junctional rhythm

Rhythm Summary: Ventricular Rhythms

	RATE	REGULARITY	P WAVE	QRS	CAUSE	ADVERS EEFFECTS	TREATMENT
PVCs	Can occur at any rate	Regular but interrupted	Usually none	>0.12, wide and bizarre in shape	Hypoxia, MI, hypokalemia; low magnesium, caffeine, stimulants, stress	Occasional are no problem; can lead to lethal arrhythmias if frequent or after an MI	Amiodarone, O_2, procainamide; atropine for bradycardic PVCs
Agonal rhythm	<20	Irregular	None	>0.12, wide and bizarre in shape	Profound cardiac or other damage, profound hypoxia	Shock, unconsciousness, death if untreated	Atropine, epinephrine, CPR, O_2, pacemaker
IVR	20-40	Regular	None	>0.12, wide and bizarre in shape	Massive cardiac or other damage hypoxia	↓ CO	Atropine, epinephrine, O_2, pacemaker
AIVR	40-100	Usually regular–can be irregular at times	Dissociated if even present	>0.12, wide and bizarre in shape	Reperfusion after TPA, MI	Usually well tolerated	Atropine if HR low and symptoms
V-tach	100-250	Usually regular–can be irregular at times	Dissociated if even present	>0.12, wide and bizarre in shape	Hypoxia, MI, hypokalemia; low magnesium, caffeine, stimulants, stress	May be tolerated OK for short bursts; can cause shock, unconsciousness, and and death if untreated	Amiodarone, lidocaine, O_2, procainamide, cardioversion or defib; CPR if no pulse
Torsades de pointes	>200	Regular or irregular	None seen	>0.12, QRS oscillates around an axis	Medications such as quinidine or procainamide; Hypoxia, MI, hypokalemia; low magnesium, caffeine, stimulants, stress	Circulatory collapse if sustained; tolerated OK for short bursts	IV magnesium, overdrive pacing, Isuprel, O_2
V-fib	Cannot be counted	None detectable	None	None; just a wavy baseline that looks like static	Hypoxia, MI, hypokalemia; low magnesium, caffeine, stimulants, stress	Cardiovascular collapse; no pulse, breathing, zero cardiac output	Defibrillation, lidocaine, amiodarone, procainamide, epinephrine, O_2, CPR
Asystole	Zero	None	None	None	Profound cardiac or other damage, hypoxia	Death if untreated	Atropine, epinephrine, CPR, pacemaker, O_2
P wave asystole	Zero	Ps regular	Sinus Ps	None	Profound cardiac or other damage, hypoxia	Death if untreated	Same as asystole

Ventricular Rhythms Pictorial Review

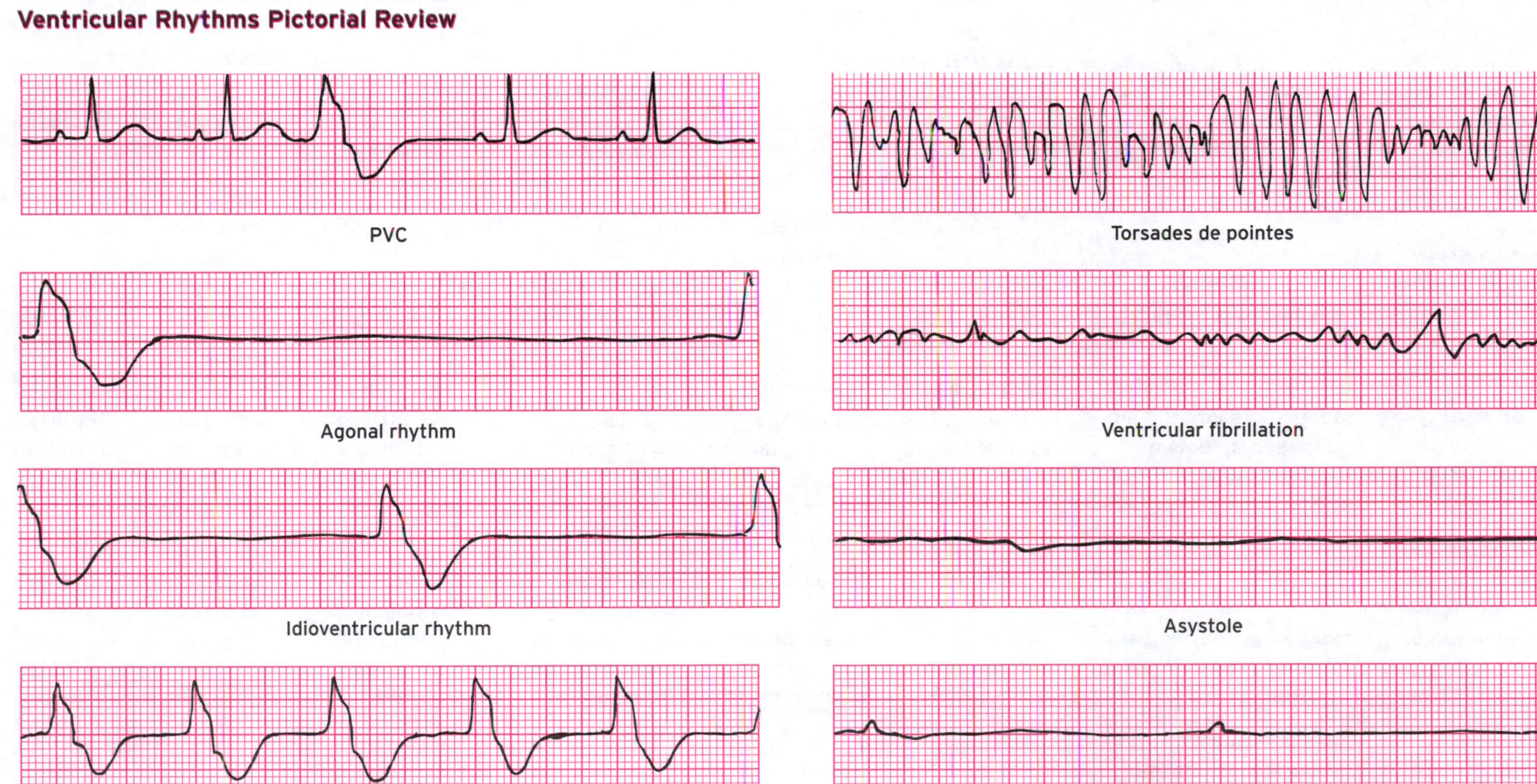

Rhythm Summary: AV Blocks

	RATE	REGULARITY	P WAVE	PR INTERVAL	QRS INTERVAL	CAUSE	ADVERSE EFFECTS	TREATMENT
First-degree AVB	Can occur at any rate	Depends on underlying rhythm	Normal; one per QRS; all shaped the same	>0.20; constant	<0.12 unless BBB	AV node ischemia, prolonged bundle branch depolarization time, digitalis toxicity, other medication side effects	Usually no ill effects	Remove the cause
Type I second-degree AVB	Atria: 60–100 Ventricle: less than atrial rate	Regular but interrupted or irregular; groups of beats, then a pause	Normal; one not followed by a QRS; all shaped the same	Gradually prolongs till a QRS is dropped	<0.12 unless BBB	MI, digitalis toxicity, medication side effects	Usually well tolerated, but watch for worsening AV block	Atropine if symptoms from low HR
Type II second-degree AVB	Atria: 60–100 Ventricle: less than atrial rate	Regular, regular but interrupted, or irregular	Normal; some not followed by a QRS	Constant on the conducted beats	<0.12 if block at AV node, ≥0.12 if block at bundle branches	MI, conduction system lesion, hypoxia, medication side effects	Decreased cardiac output if HR slow	Atropine, pacemaker, O_2
2:1 AVB	Atria: 60–100 Ventricle: half the atrial rate	Regular	Normal; two Ps to each QRS	Constant on the conducted beats	<0.12 unless BBB	Same as Wenckebach and type II	Decreased cardiac output if HR slow	Atropine, pacemaker; consider O_2
Third-degree AVB	Atria: 60–100 Ventricle: 20–60	Regular	Normal; dissociated from QRS	Varies	<0.12 if AV node is the pace-maker, >0.12 if ventricle is the pacemaker	MI, conduction system lesion, hypoxia, medication side effect	Decreased cardiac output if HR slow	Atropine, pacemaker, O_2

AV Blocks Pictorial Review

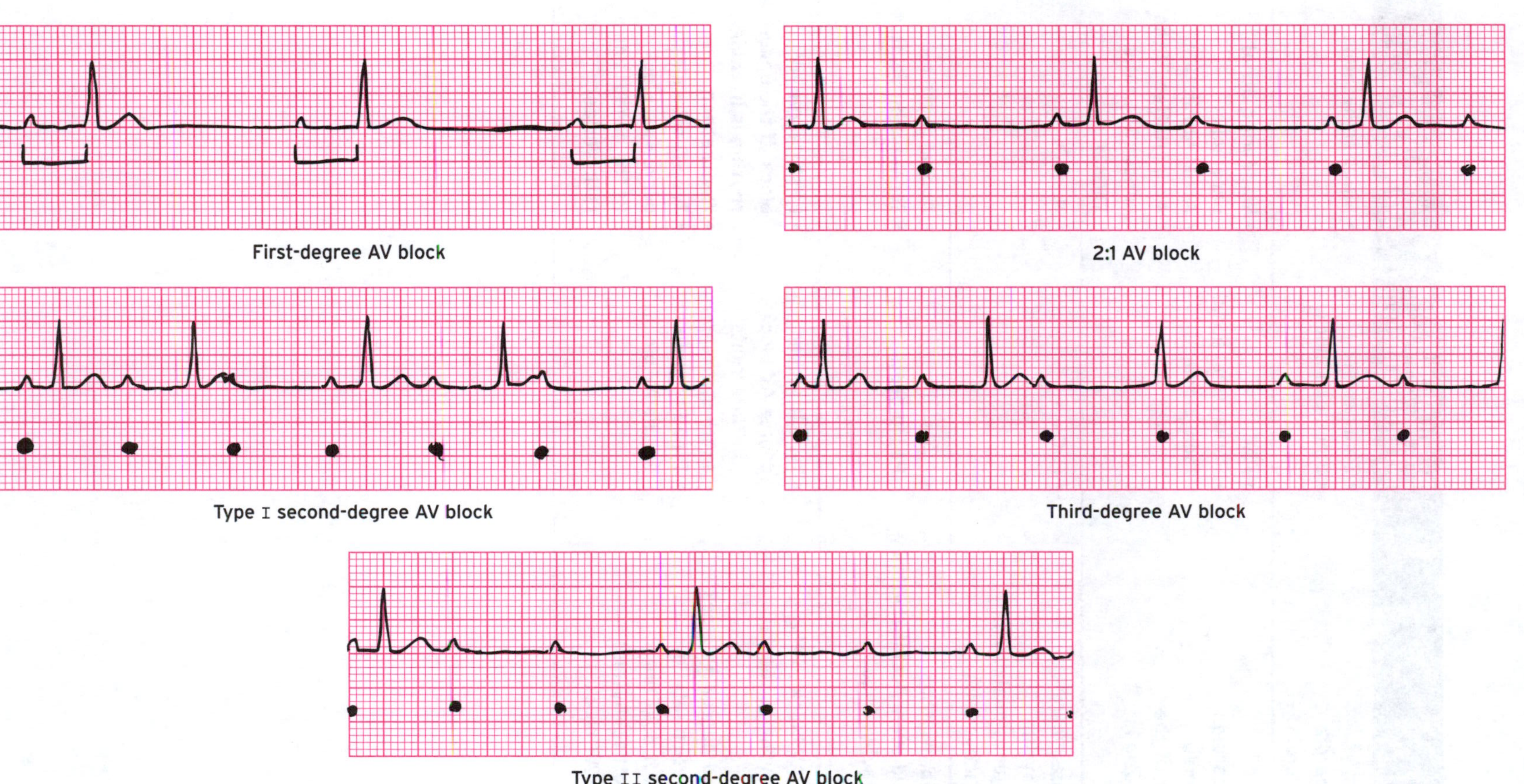

Rhythm Regularity Summary

The following table points out the type of regularity of each rhythm. *Only rhythms with QRS complexes are shown here.*

ORIGIN OF RHYTHM	REGULAR	REGULAR BUT INTERRUPTED	IRREGULAR
Sinus	• Sinus rhythm • Sinus bradycardia • Sinus tachycardia	• Sinus arrest • Sinus exit block	• Sinus arrhythmia
Atrial	• SVT • Atrial tachycardia (nonparoxysmal) • Atrial flutter (if the conduction ratio is constant)	• PACs • Paroxysmal atrial tachycardia	• Wandering atrial pacemaker • Atrial fibrillation • Atrial flutter (if the conduction ratio varies)
Junctional	• Junctional bradycardia • Junctional rhythm • Accelerated junctional rhythm • Junctional tachycardia	• PJCs	• None
Ventricular	• Idioventricular rhythm • Accelerated idioventricular rhythm • Ventricular tachycardia • Paced rhythm	• PVCs • Paced beats	• Agonal rhythm • Torsades de pointes
AV blocks	• First-degree AV block (if the underlying rhythm is regular) • 2:1 AV block • Type II second-degree AV block (if the conduction ratio is constant and it does not interrupt another rhythm) • Third-degree AV block	• Type II second-degree AV block (if it interrupts another rhythm) • Type I second-degree AV block	• First-degree AV block (if the underlying rhythm is irregular) • Wenckebach • Type II second-degree AV block (if the conduction ratio varies)

Rhythms for Practice

Ok, let's get down to work. Some rhythms in this chapter are on single-lead strips, while others are on double-lead strips. Remember that on double-lead strips, both leads represent the same rhythm seen in different leads. Thus the heart rate, interval measurements, and other interpretation will be the same whether you assess the top lead or the bottom lead. Use either lead you prefer to do your interpretation.

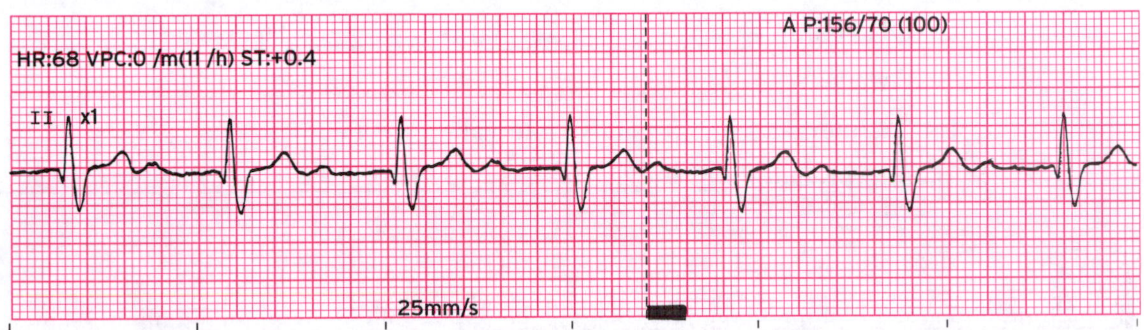

1. QRS complexes ________ Regularity ________ Heart rate ________
   P waves ____
   PR interval ________ QRS interval ________
   Interpretation ____

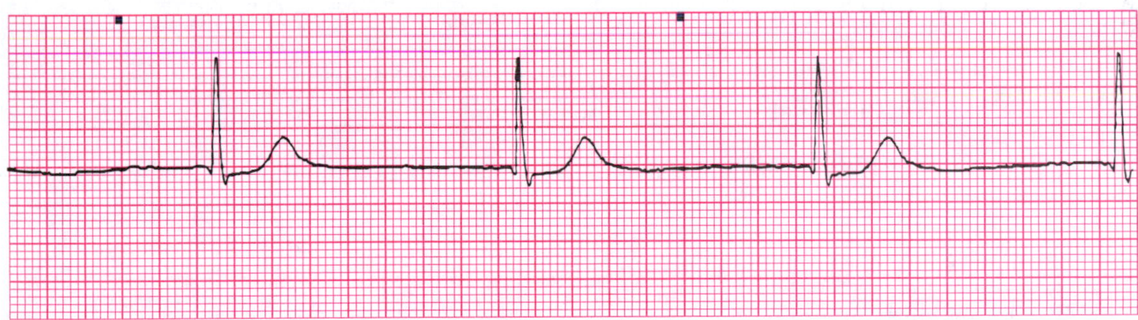

2. QRS complexes ________ Regularity ________ Heart rate ________
   P waves ____
   PR interval ________ QRS interval ________
   Interpretation ____

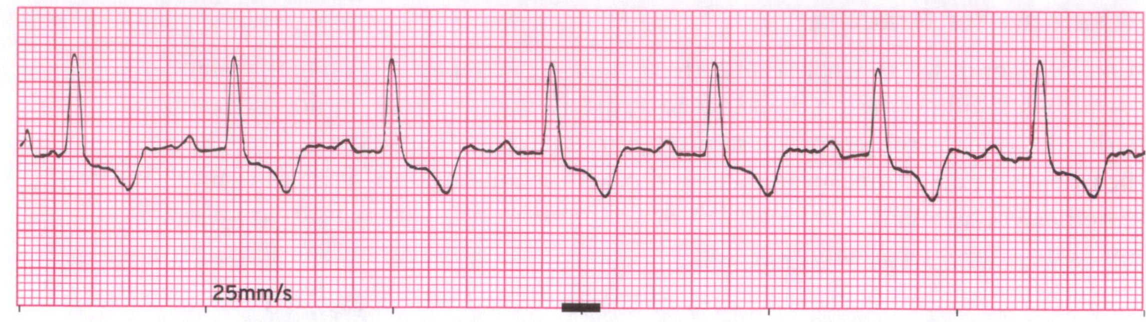

3. QRS complexes ________ Regularity ________ Heart rate ________
   P waves ____
   PR interval ________ QRS interval ________
   Interpretation ____

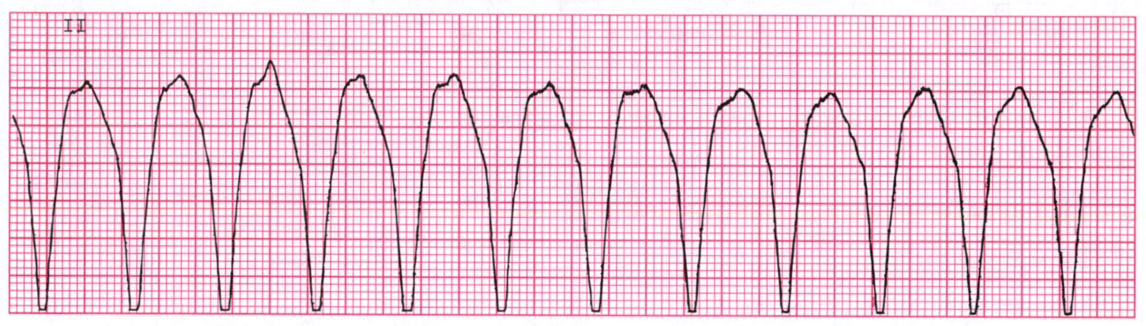

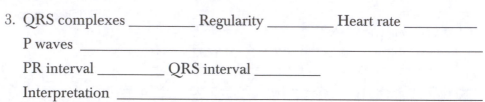

4. QRS complexes ________ Regularity ________ Heart rate ________
   P waves ____
   PR interval ________ QRS interval ________
   Interpretation ____

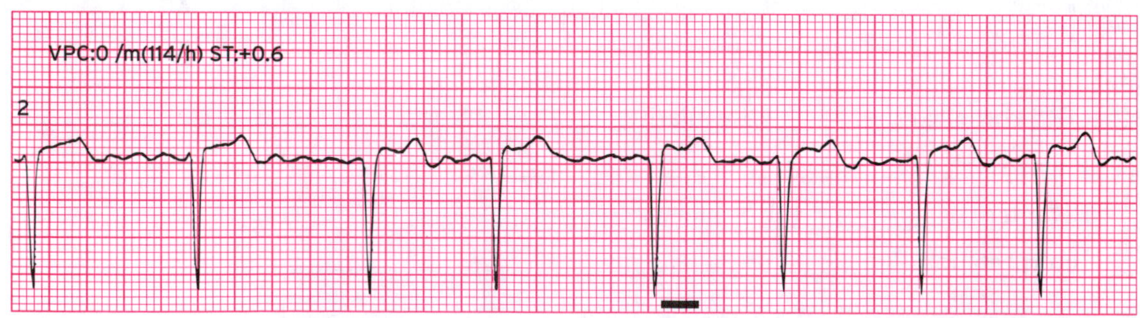

5. QRS complexes ________ Regularity ________ Heart rate ________
   P waves ____
   PR interval ________ QRS interval ________
   Interpretation ____

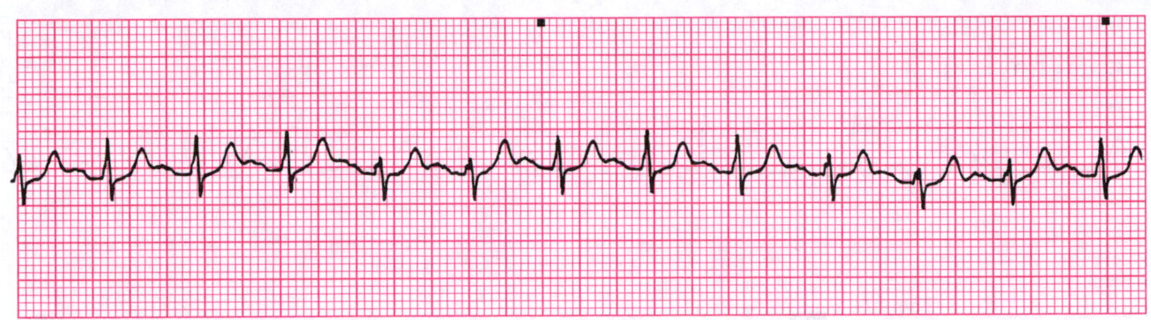

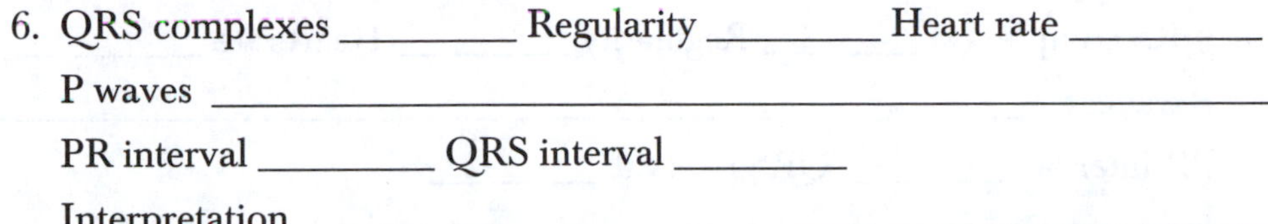

6. QRS complexes ________ Regularity ________ Heart rate ________
   P waves ____
   PR interval ________ QRS interval ________
   Interpretation ____

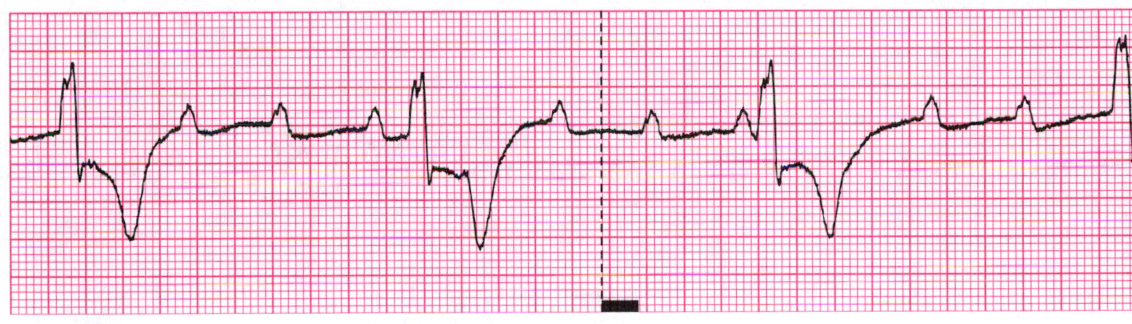

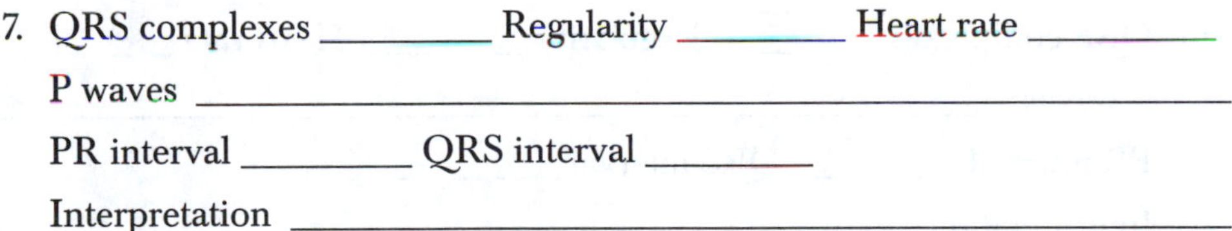

7. QRS complexes ________ Regularity ________ Heart rate ________
   P waves ____
   PR interval ________ QRS interval ________
   Interpretation ____

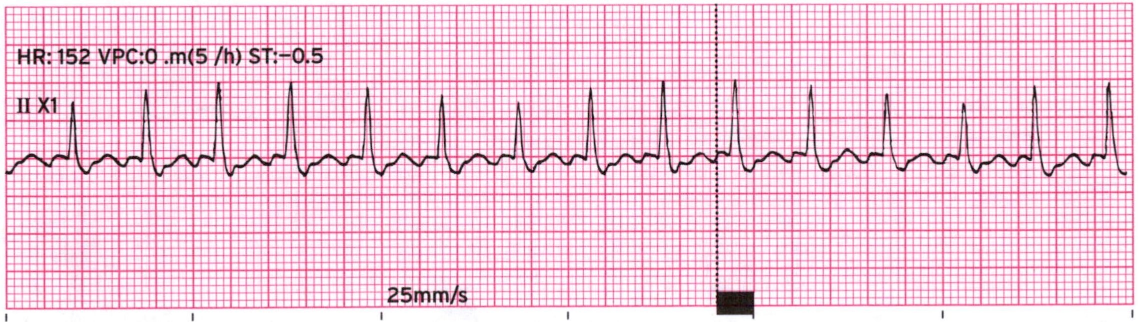

8. QRS complexes ________ Regularity ________ Heart rate ________
   P waves ____
   PR interval ________ QRS interval ________
   Interpretation ____

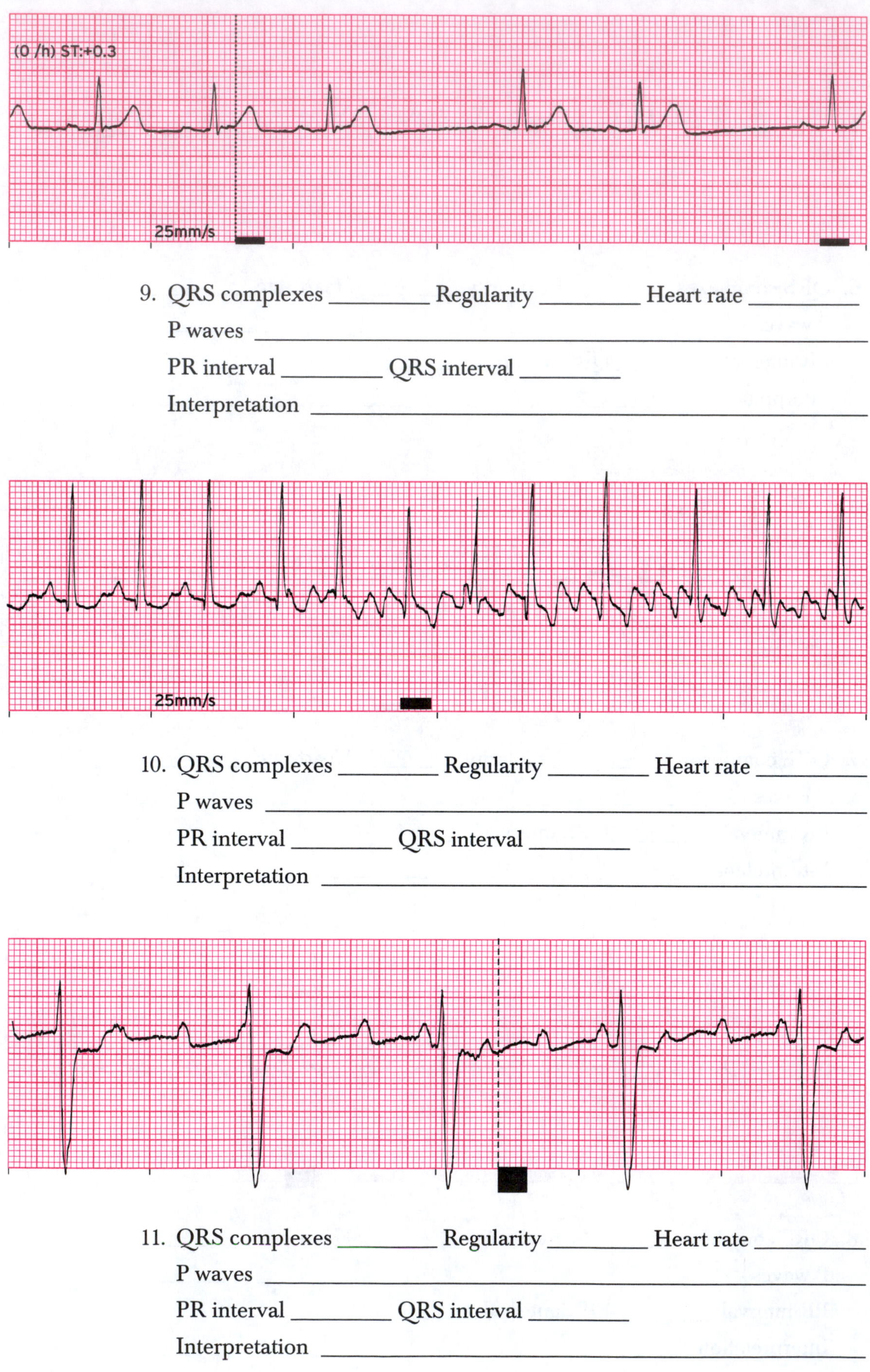

9. QRS complexes ________ Regularity ________ Heart rate ________
P waves ____________________
PR interval ________ QRS interval ________
Interpretation ____________________

10. QRS complexes ________ Regularity ________ Heart rate ________
P waves ____________________
PR interval ________ QRS interval ________
Interpretation ____________________

11. QRS complexes ________ Regularity ________ Heart rate ________
P waves ____________________
PR interval ________ QRS interval ________
Interpretation ____________________

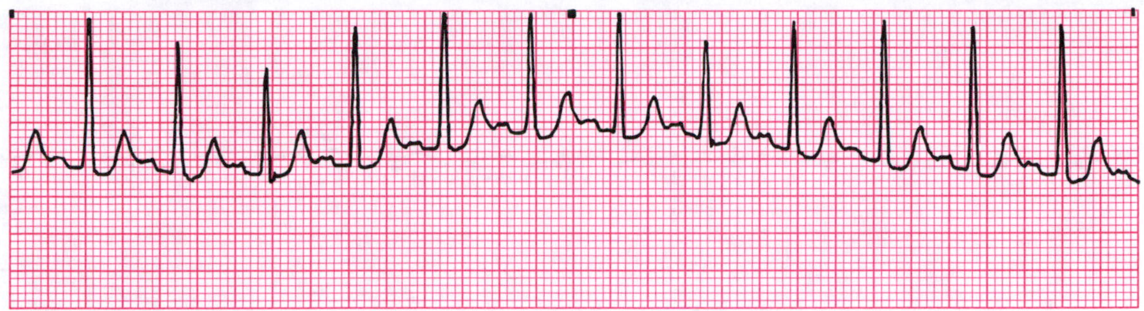

12. QRS complexes ________ Regularity ________ Heart rate __________
    P waves ____
    PR interval ________ QRS interval ________
    Interpretation ____

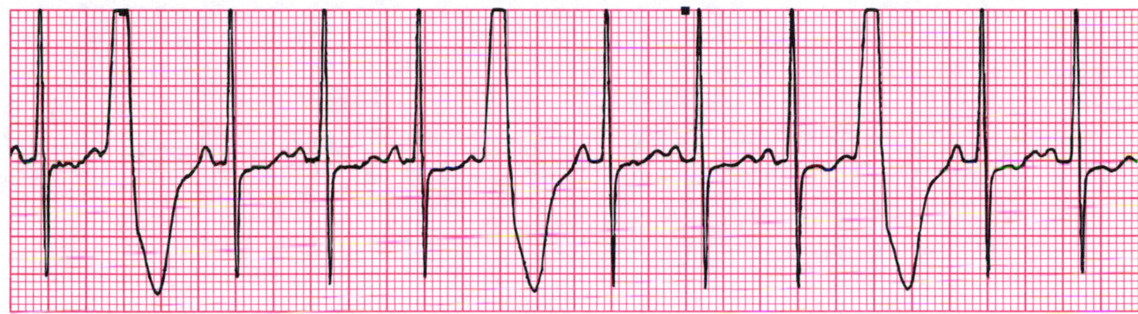

13. QRS complexes ________ Regularity ________ Heart rate __________
    P waves ____
    PR interval ________ QRS interval ________
    Interpretation ____

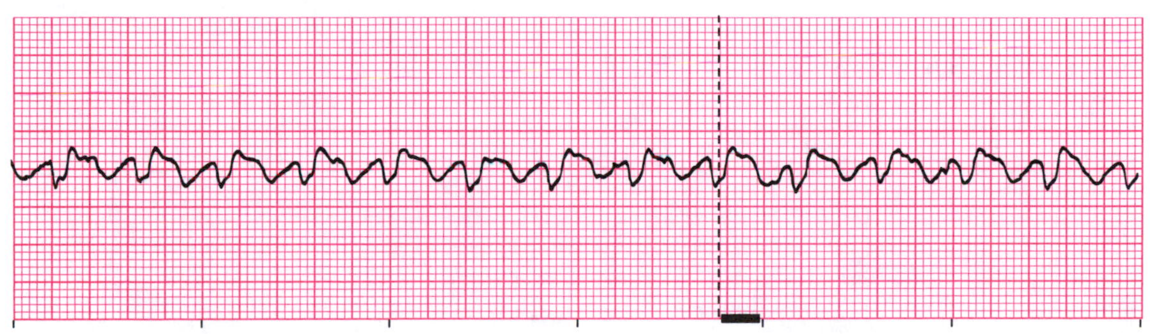

14. QRS complexes ________ Regularity ________ Heart rate __________
    P waves ____
    PR interval ________ QRS interval ________
    Interpretation ____

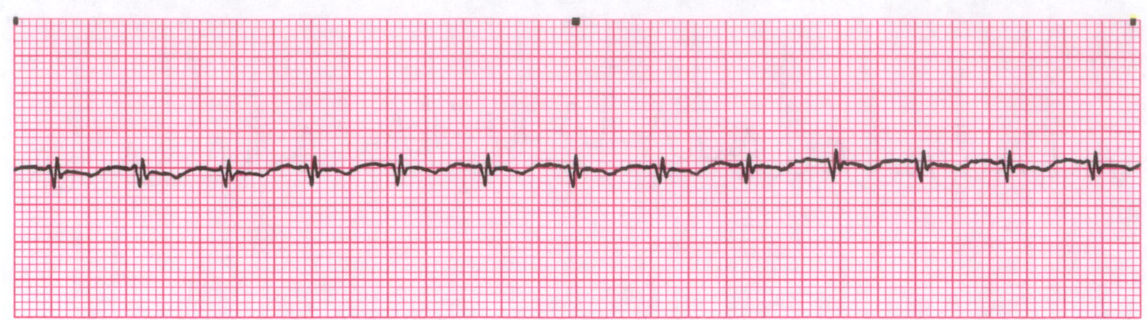

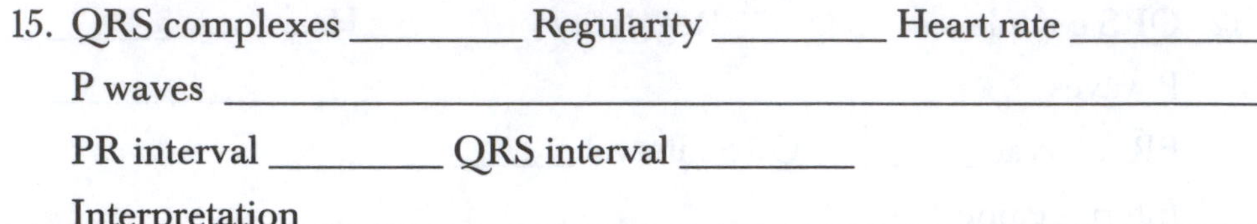

15. QRS complexes ________ Regularity ________ Heart rate ________

    P waves ____

    PR interval ________ QRS interval ________

    Interpretation ____

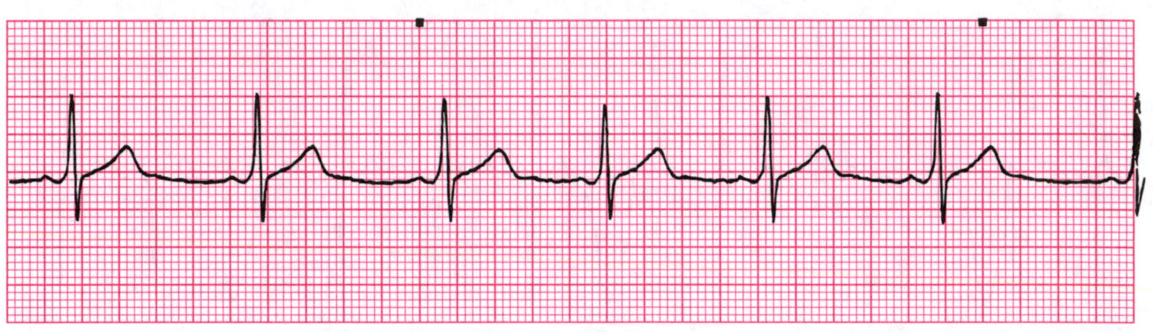

16. QRS complexes ________ Regularity ________ Heart rate ________

    P waves ____

    PR interval ________ QRS interval ________

    Interpretation ____

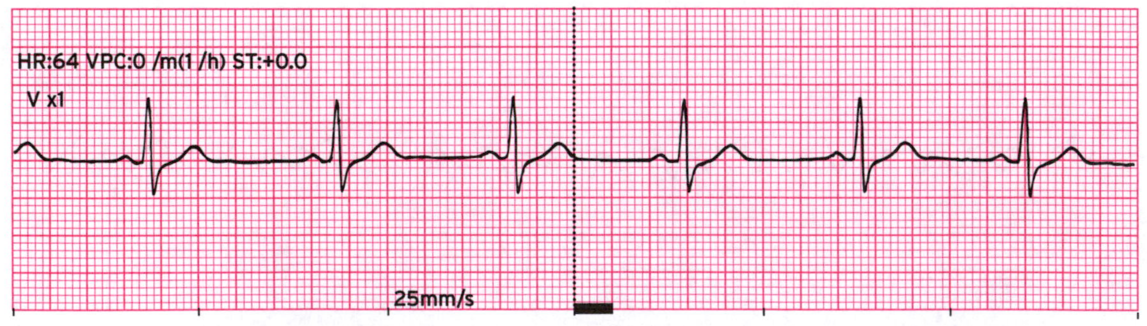

17. QRS complexes ________ Regularity ________ Heart rate ________

    P waves ____

    PR interval ________ QRS interval ________

    Interpretation____

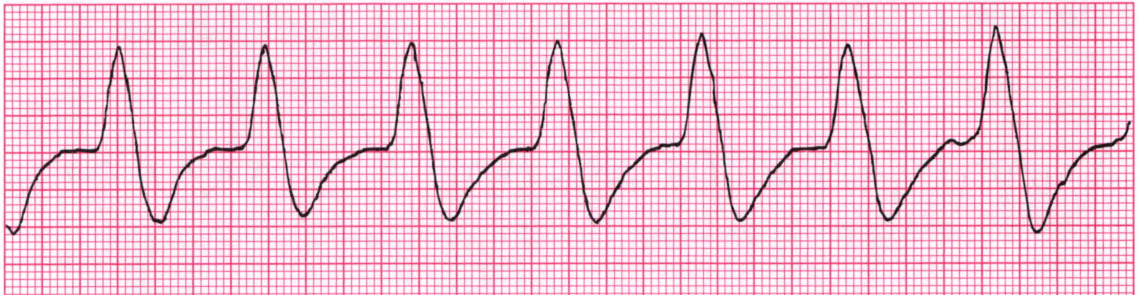

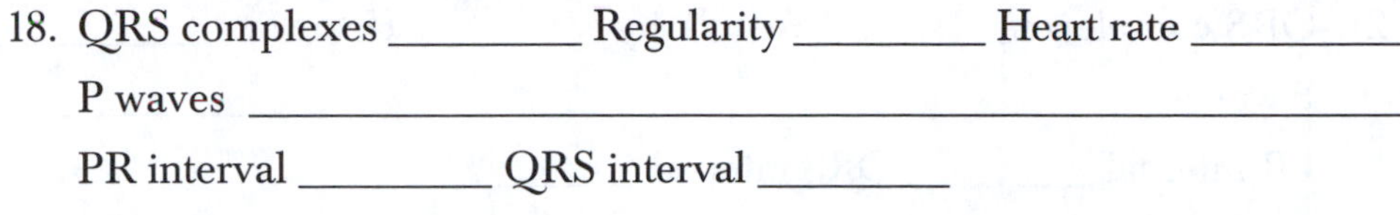

18. QRS complexes ________ Regularity ________ Heart rate ________

    P waves ____

    PR interval ________ QRS interval ________

    Interpretation ______________________________________

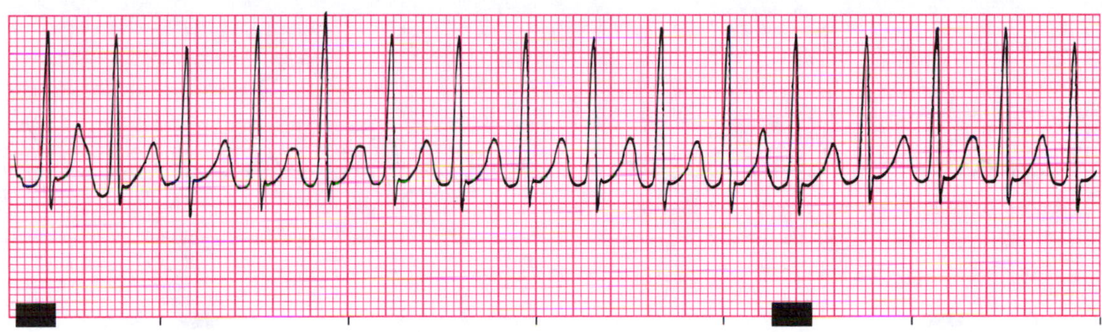

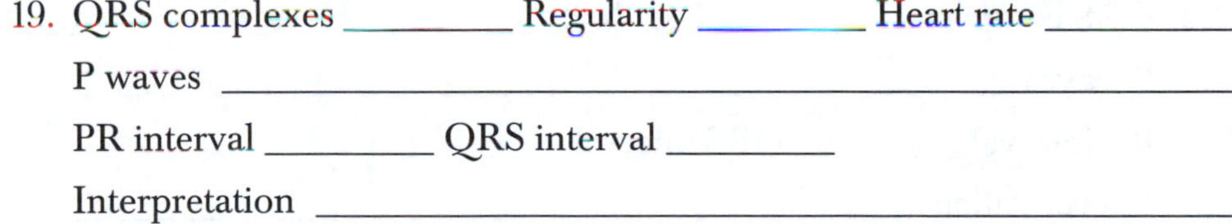

19. QRS complexes ________ Regularity ________ Heart rate ________

    P waves ____

    PR interval ________ QRS interval ________

    Interpretation ______________________________________

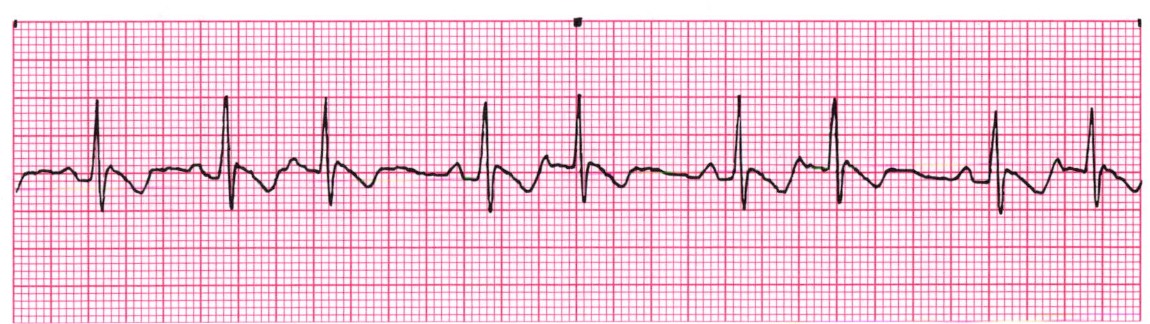

20. QRS complexes ________ Regularity ________ Heart rate ________

    P waves ____

    PR interval ________ QRS interval ________

    Interpretation ______________________________________

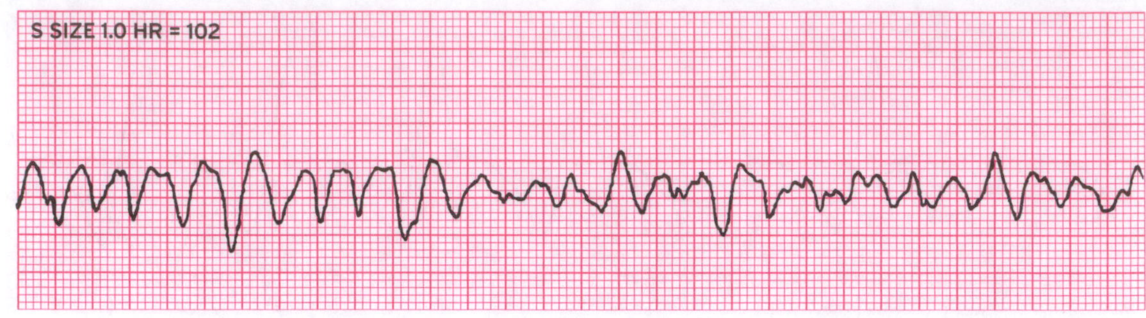

21. QRS complexes ________ Regularity ________ Heart rate ________
    P waves ____
    PR interval ________ QRS interval ________
    Interpretation ____

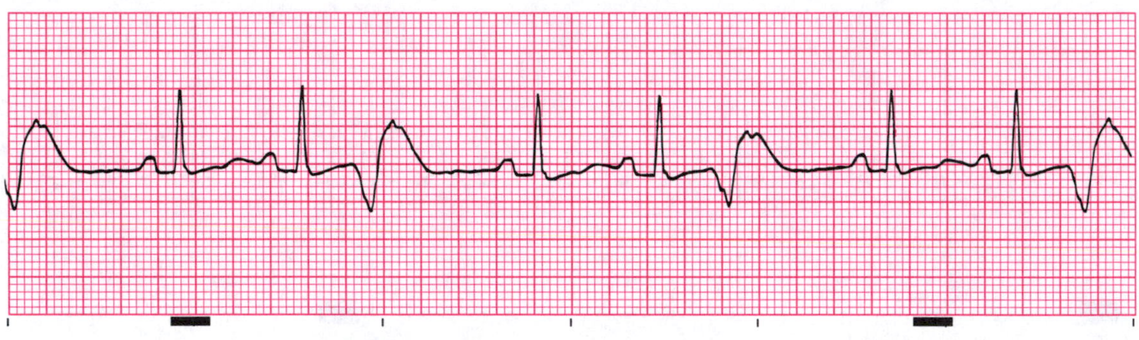

22. QRS complexes ________ Regularity ________ Heart rate ________
    P waves ____
    PR interval ________ QRS interval ________
    Interpretation ____

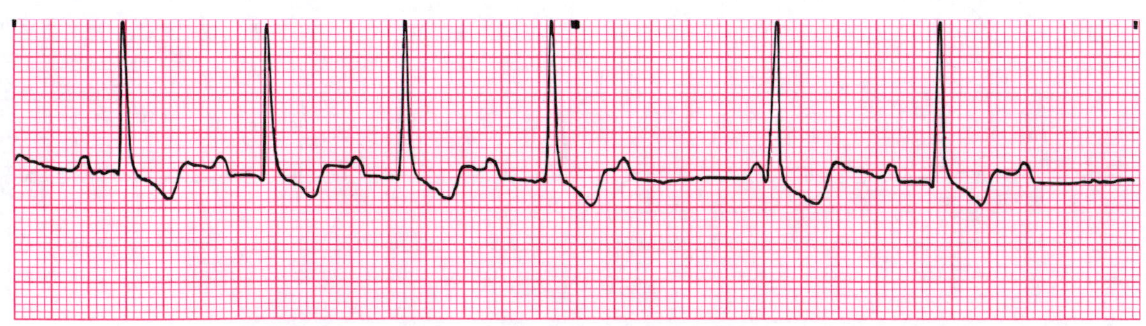

23. QRS complexes ________ Regularity ________ Heart rate ________
    P waves ____
    PR interval ________ QRS interval ________
    Interpretation ____

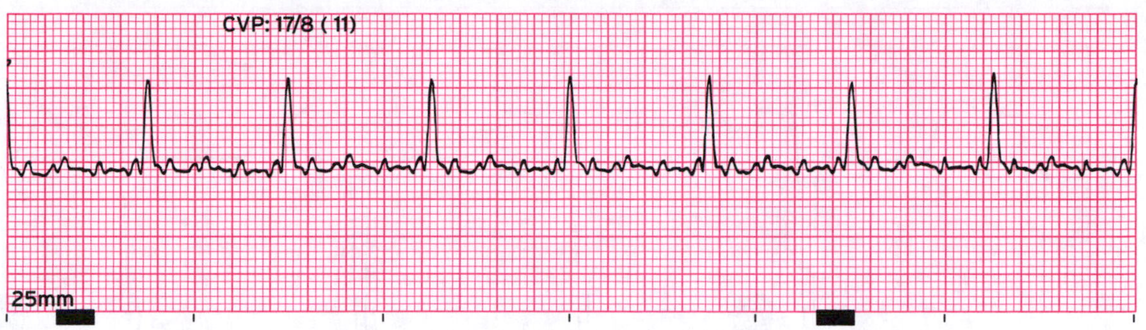

24. QRS complexes ________ Regularity ________ Heart rate ________
    P waves ____
    PR interval ________ QRS interval ________
    Interpretation ____

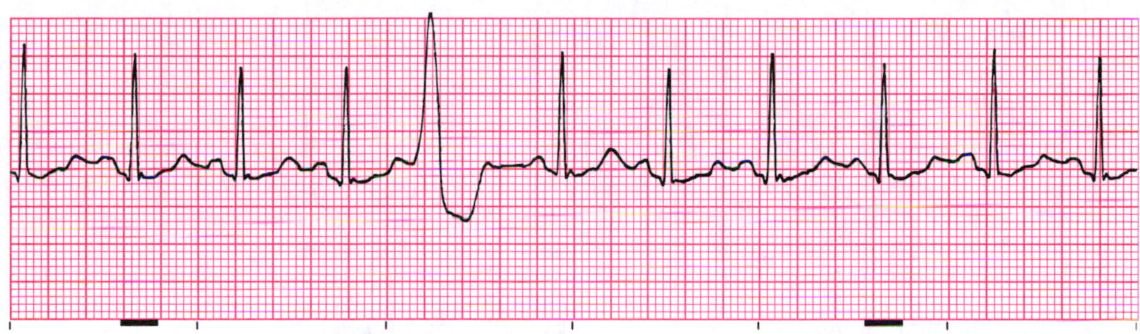

25. QRS complexes ________ Regularity ________ Heart rate ________
    P waves ____
    PR interval ________ QRS interval ________
    Interpretation ____

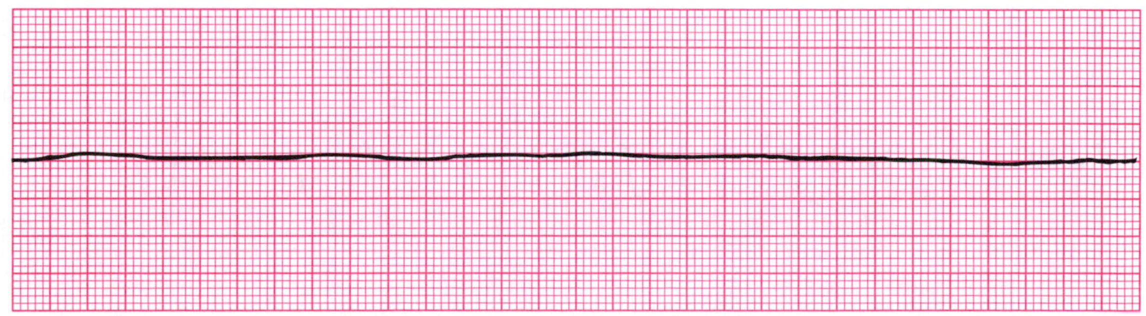

26. QRS complexes ________ Regularity ________ Heart rate ________
    P waves ____
    PR interval ________ QRS interval ________
    Interpretation ____

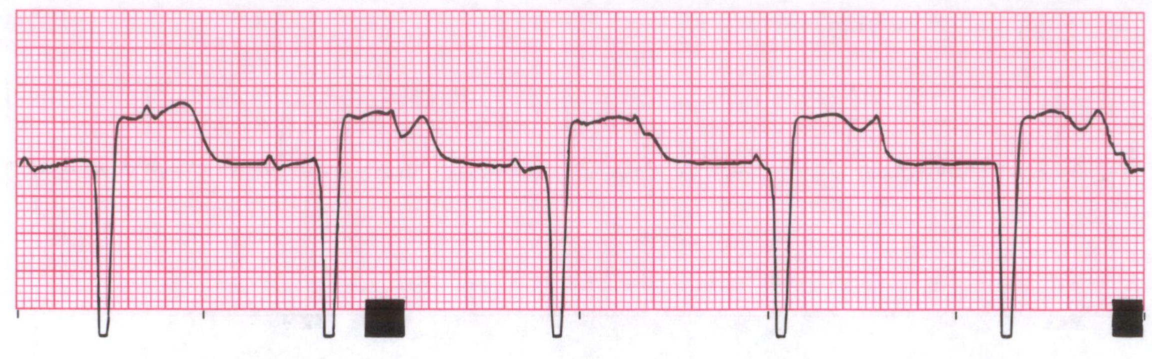

27. QRS complexes ________ Regularity ________ Heart rate ________
    P waves ________________________________
    PR interval ________ QRS interval ________
    Interpretation ________________________________

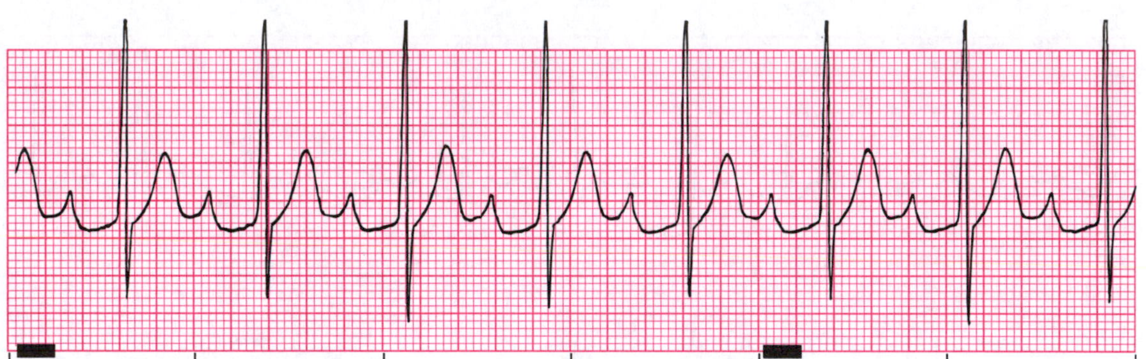

28. QRS complexes ________ Regularity ________ Heart rate ________
    P waves ________________________________
    PR interval ________ QRS interval ________
    Interpretation ________________________________

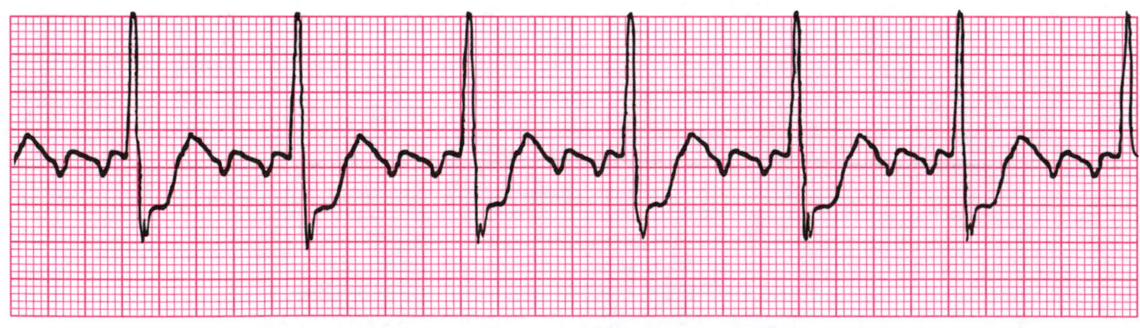

29. QRS complexes ________ Regularity ________ Heart rate ________
    P waves ________________________________
    PR interval ________ QRS interval ________
    Interpretation ________________________________

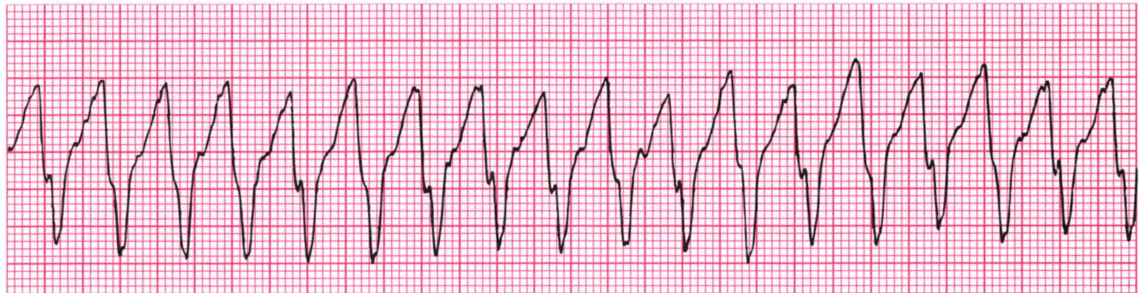

30. QRS complexes ________ Regularity ________ Heart rate ________

P waves ____

PR interval ________ QRS interval ________

Interpretation ____

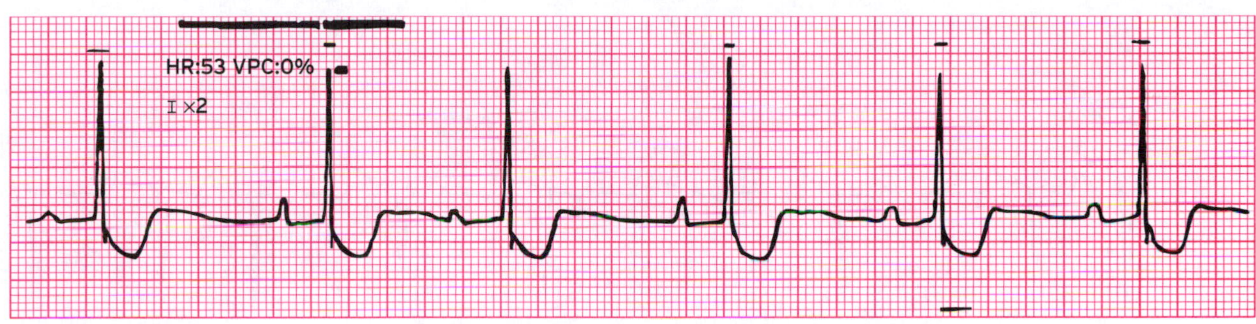

31. QRS complexes ________ Regularity ________ Heart rate ________

P waves ____

PR interval ________ QRS interval ________

Interpretation ____

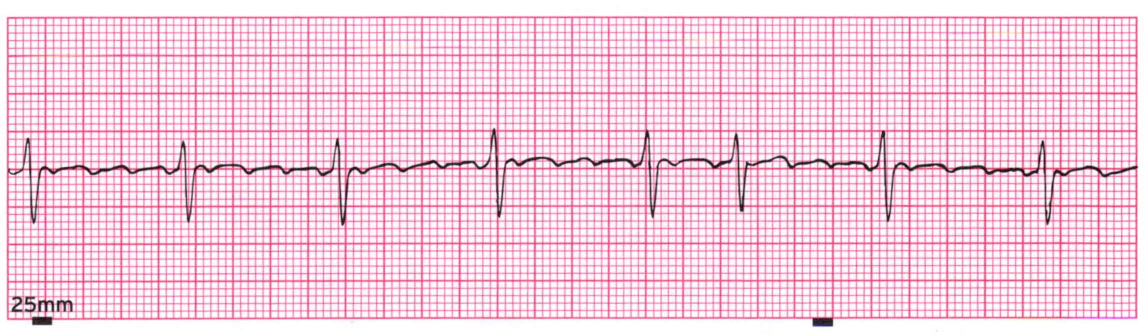

32. QRS complexes ________ Regularity ________ Heart rate ________

P waves ____

PR interval ________ QRS interval ________

Interpretation ____

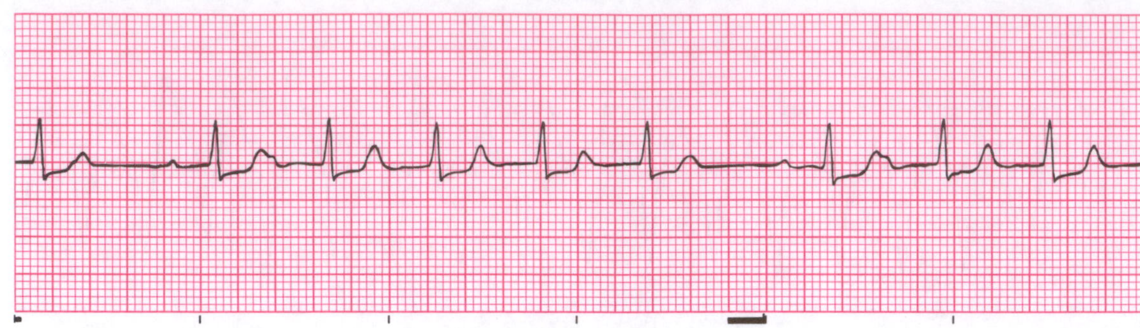

33. QRS complexes ________ Regularity ________ Heart rate ________
    P waves ____
    PR interval ________ QRS interval ________
    Interpretation ____

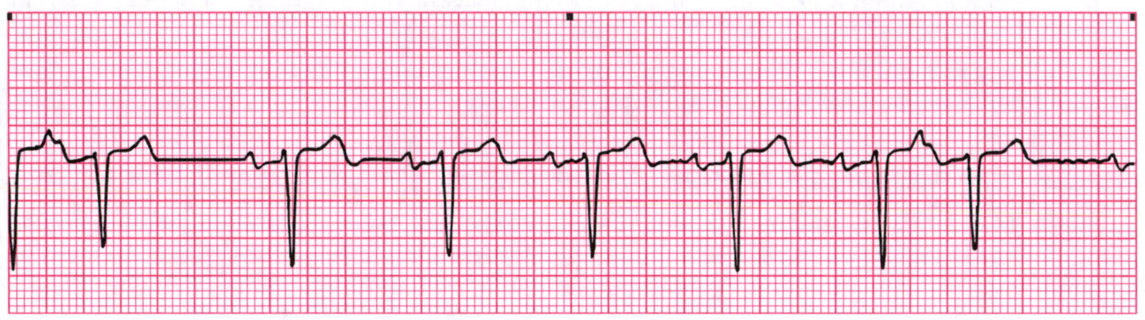

34. QRS complexes ________ Regularity ________ Heart rate ________
    P waves ____
    PR interval ________ QRS interval ________
    Interpretation ____

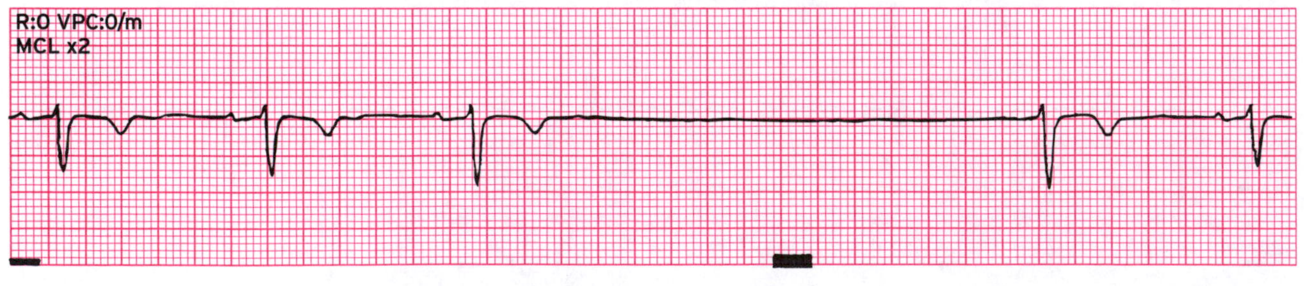

35. QRS complexes ________ Regularity ________ Heart rate ________
    P waves ____
    PR interval ________ QRS interval ________
    Interpretation ____

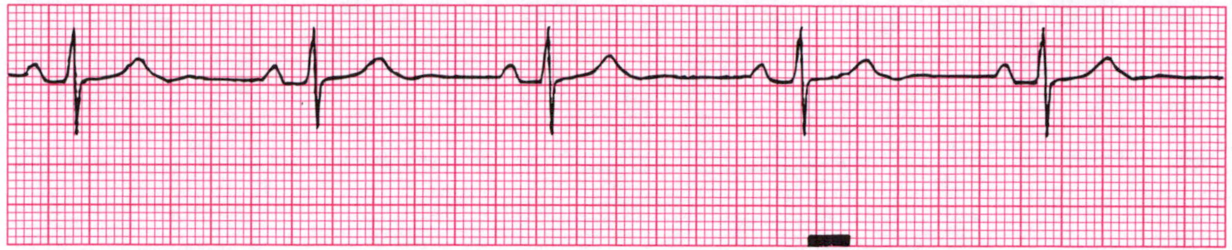

36. QRS complexes ________ Regularity ________ Heart rate ________
    P waves ____
    PR interval ________ QRS interval ________
    Interpretation ______________________________________

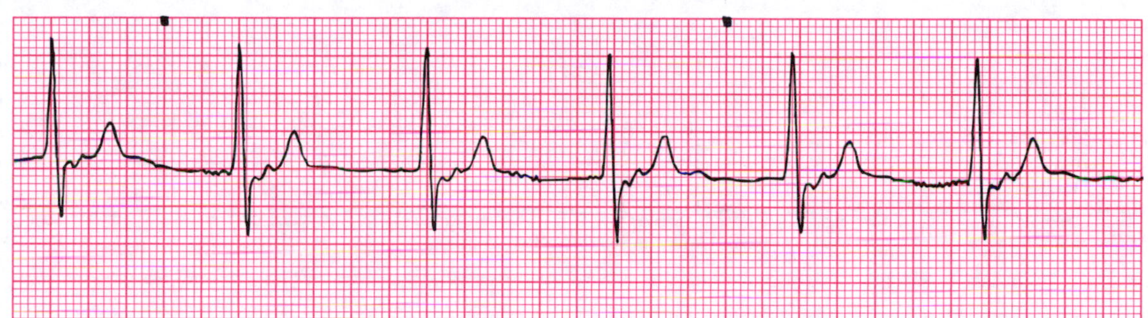

37. QRS complexes ________ Regularity ________ Heart rate ________
    P waves ____
    PR interval ________ QRS interval ________
    Interpretation ______________________________________

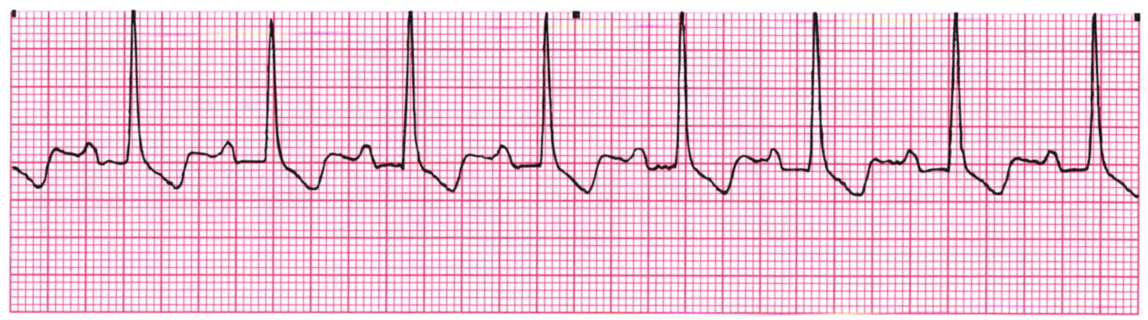

38. QRS complexes ________ Regularity ________ Heart rate ________
    P waves ____
    PR interval ________ QRS interval ________
    Interpretation ______________________________________

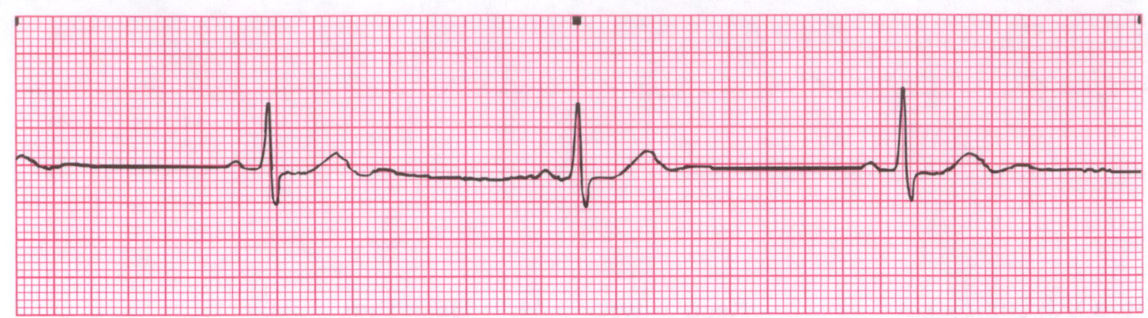

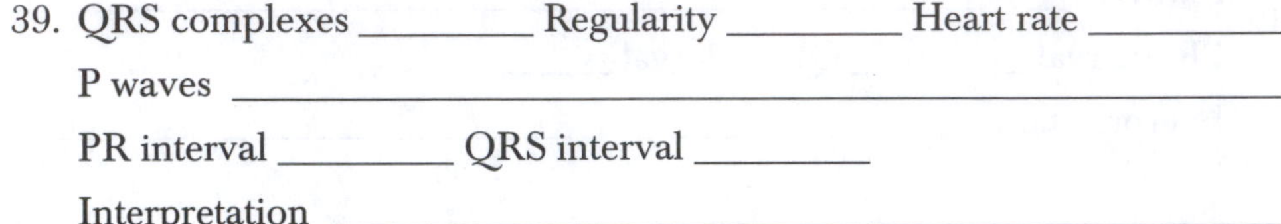

39. QRS complexes ________ Regularity ________ Heart rate ________

    P waves ____

    PR interval ________ QRS interval ________

    Interpretation ____

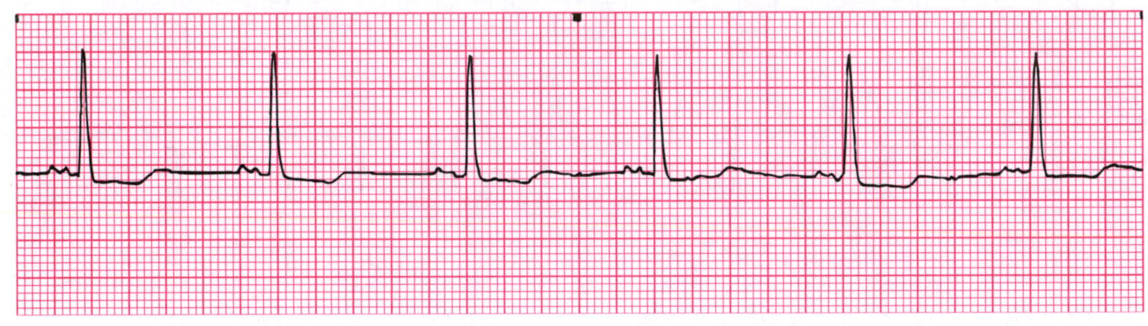

40. QRS complexes ________ Regularity ________ Heart rate ________

    P waves ____

    PR interval ________ QRS interval ________

    Interpretation ____

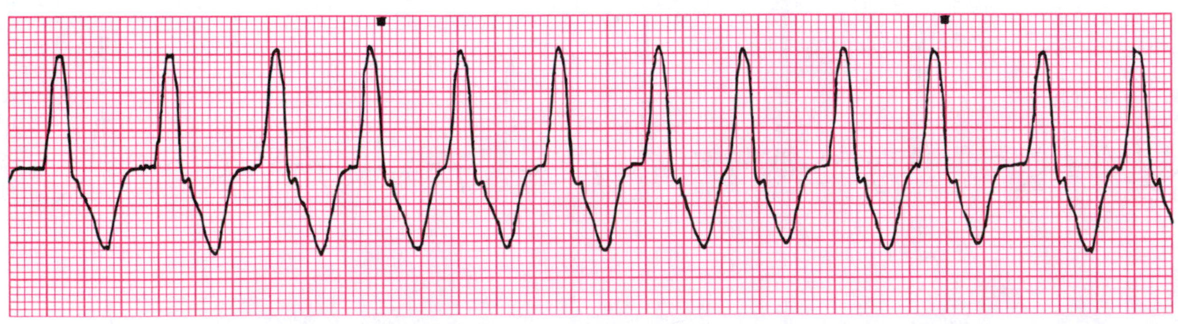

41. QRS complexes ________ Regularity ________ Heart rate ________

    P waves ____

    PR interval ________ QRS interval ________

    Interpretation ____

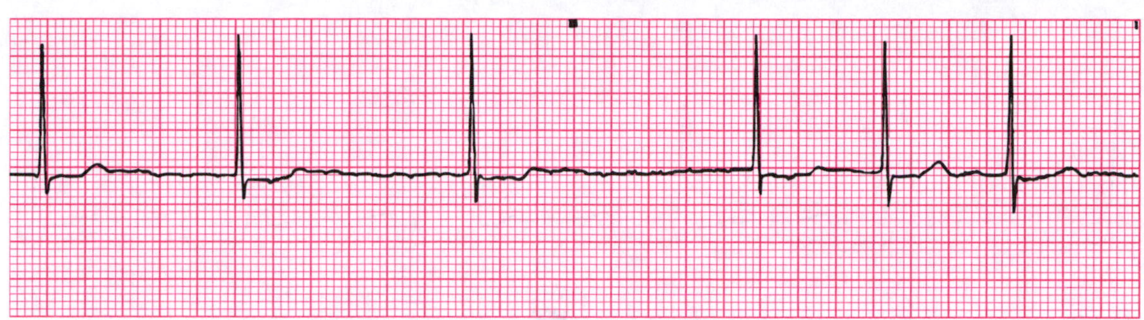

42. QRS complexes ________ Regularity ________ Heart rate ________
    P waves ____
    PR interval ________ QRS interval ________
    Interpretation ____

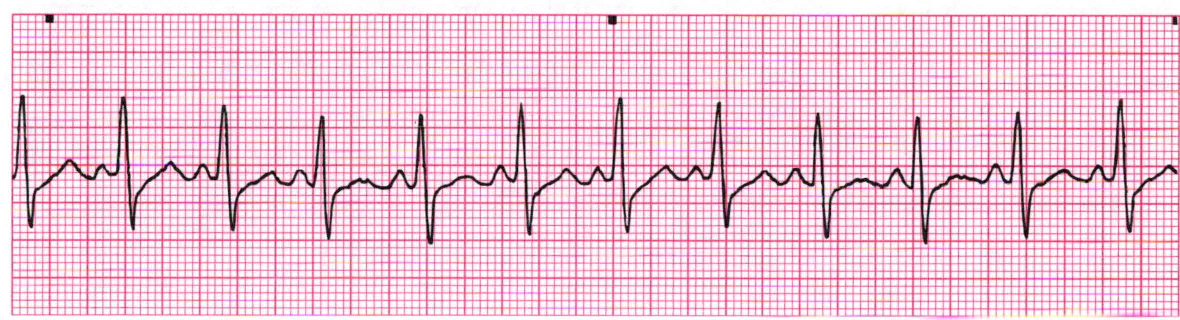

43. QRS complexes ________ Regularity ________ Heart rate ________
    P waves ____
    PR interval ________ QRS interval ________
    Interpretation ____

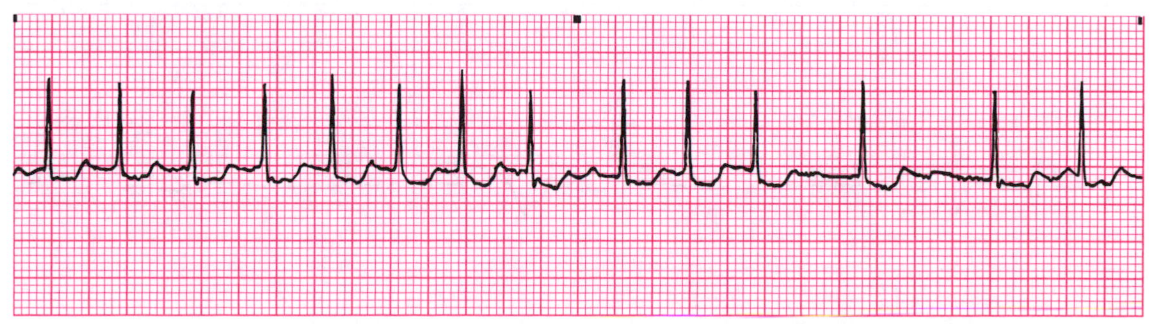

44. QRS complexes ________ Regularity ________ Heart rate ________
    P waves ____
    PR interval ________ QRS interval ________
    Interpretation ____

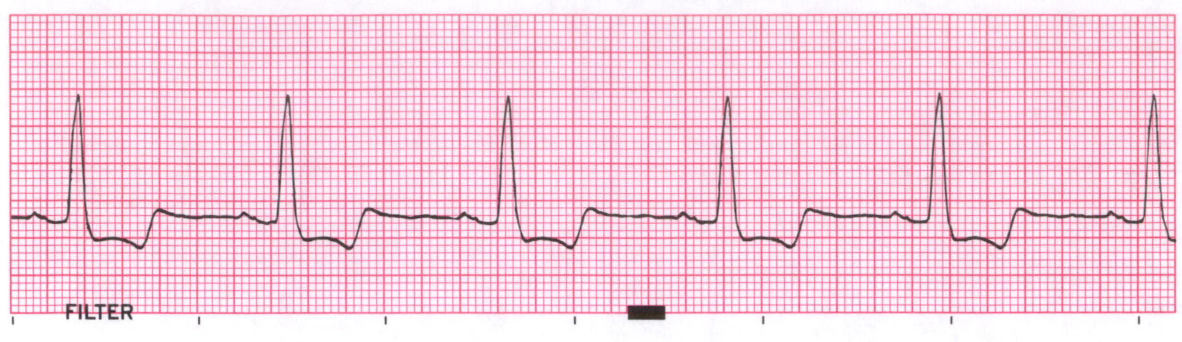

45. QRS complexes ________ Regularity ________ Heart rate ________
P waves ________________________________
PR interval ________ QRS interval ________
Interpretation ________________________________

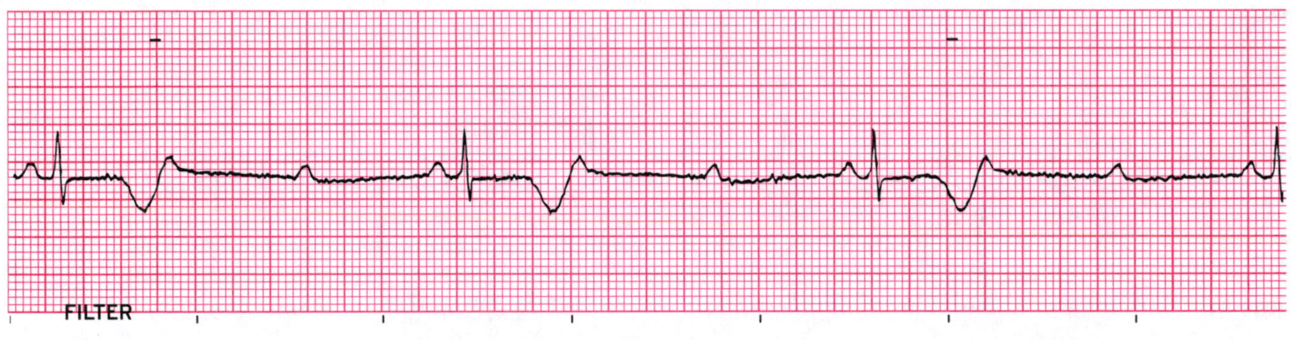

46. QRS complexes ________ Regularity ________ Heart rate ________
P waves ________________________________
PR interval ________ QRS interval ________
Interpretation ________________________________

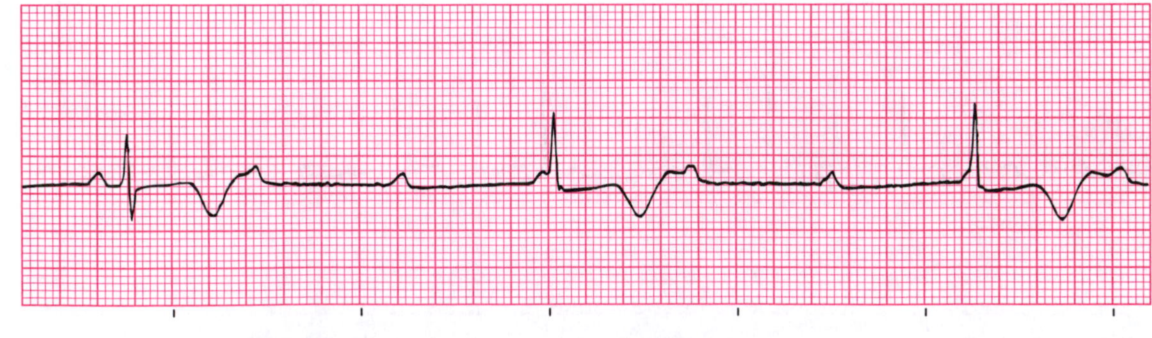

47. QRS complexes ________ Regularity ________ Heart rate ________
P waves ________________________________
PR interval ________ QRS interval ________
Interpretation ________________________________

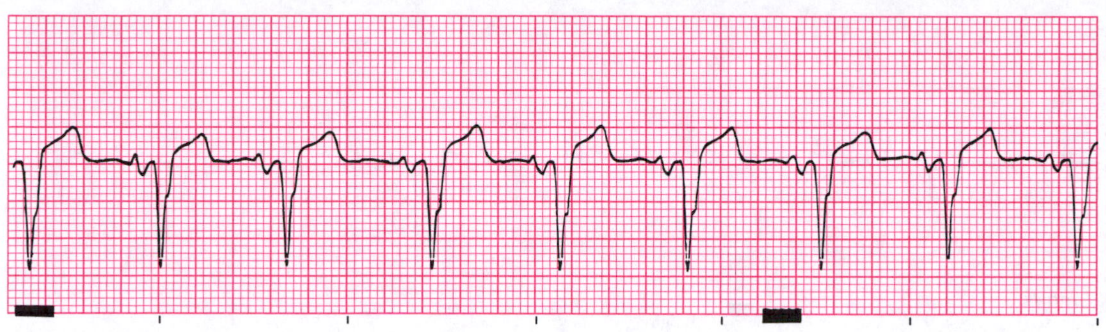

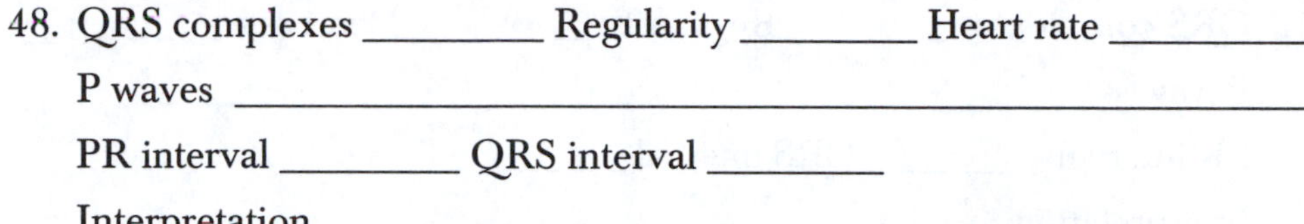

48. QRS complexes ________ Regularity ________ Heart rate ________

P waves ____

PR interval ________ QRS interval ________

Interpretation ____

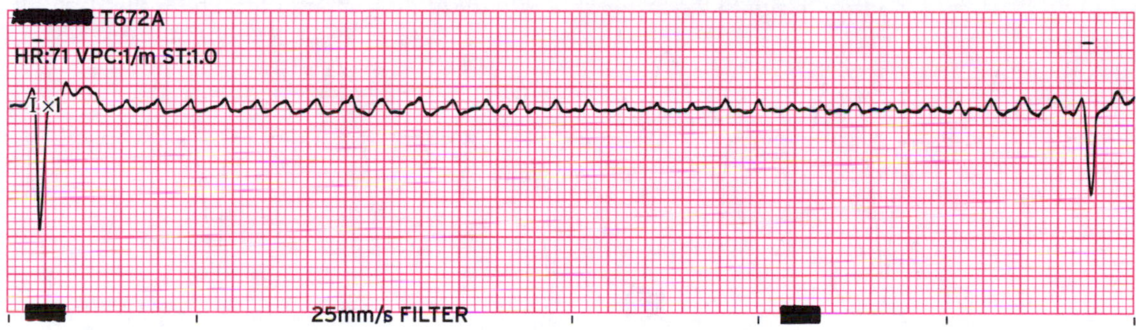

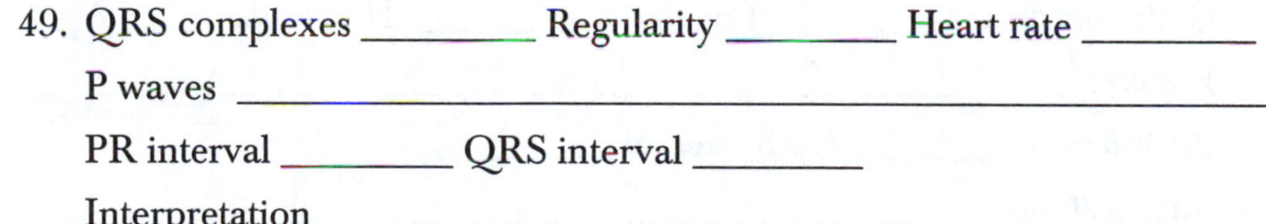

49. QRS complexes ________ Regularity ________ Heart rate ________

P waves ____

PR interval ________ QRS interval ________

Interpretation ____

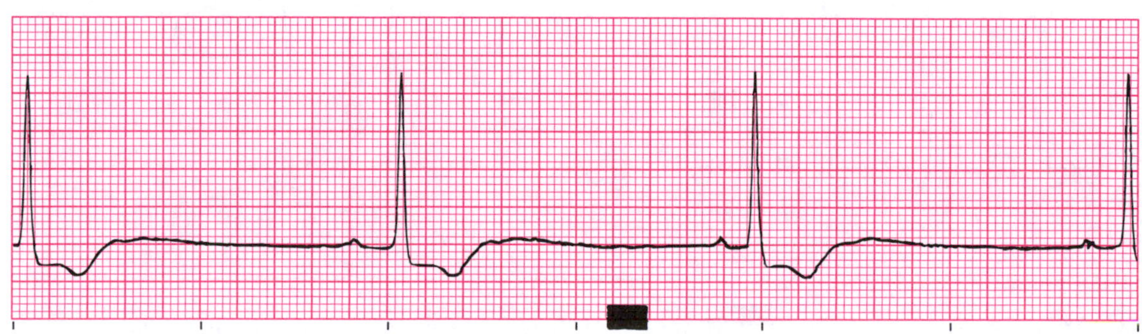

50. QRS complexes ________ Regularity ________ Heart rate ________

P waves ____

PR interval ________ QRS interval ________

Interpretation ____

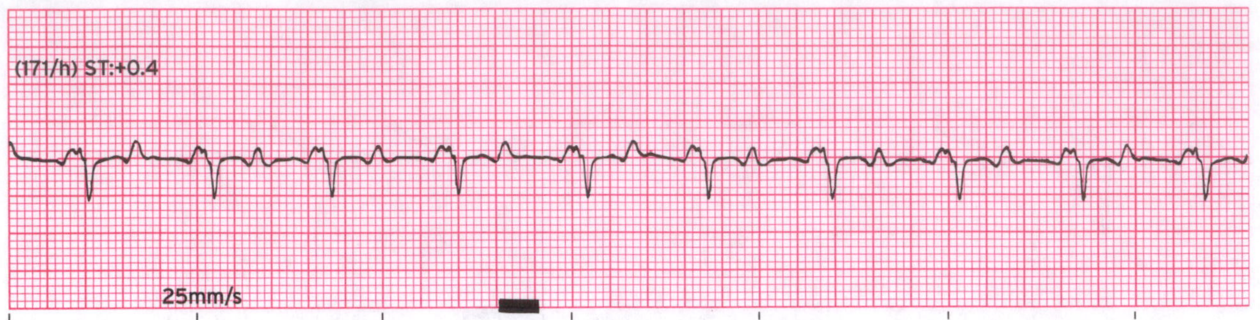

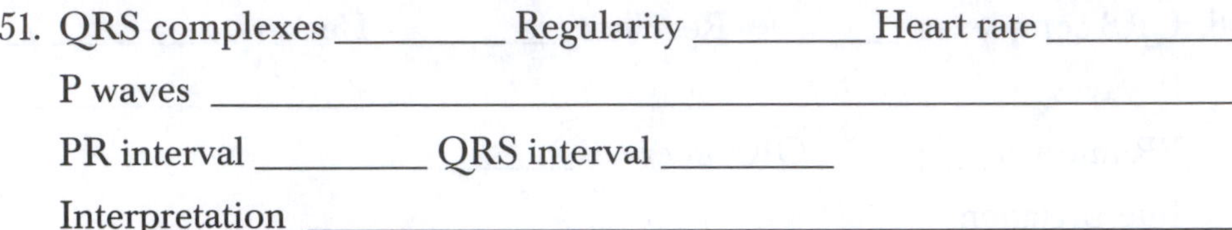

51. QRS complexes ________ Regularity ________ Heart rate ________
P waves ______________________________
PR interval ________ QRS interval ________
Interpretation ______________________________

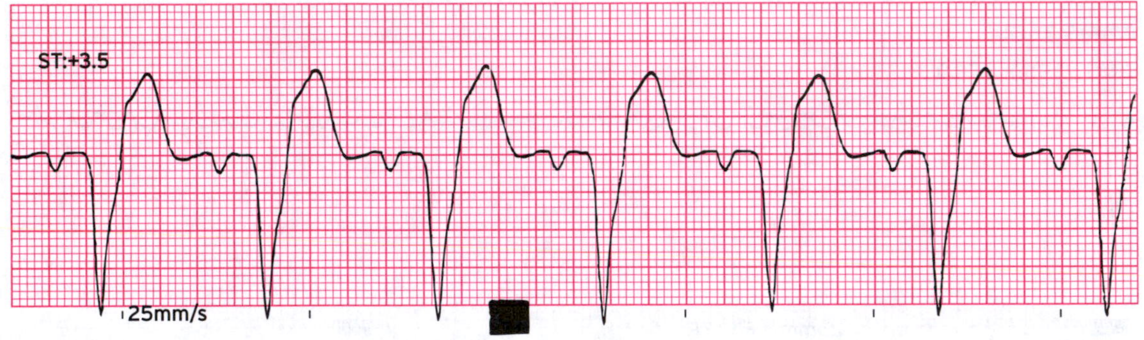

52. QRS complexes ________ Regularity ________ Heart rate ________
P waves ______________________________
PR interval ________ QRS interval ________
Interpretation ______________________________

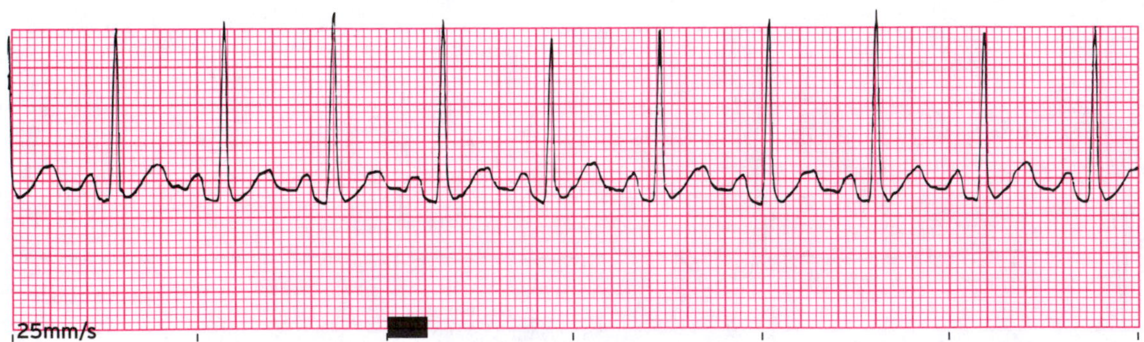

53. QRS complexes ________ Regularity ________ Heart rate ________
P waves ______________________________
PR interval ________ QRS interval ________
Interpretation ______________________________

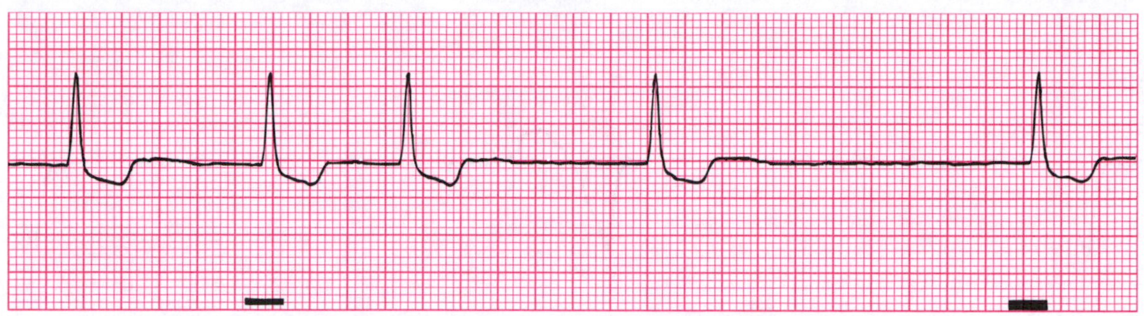

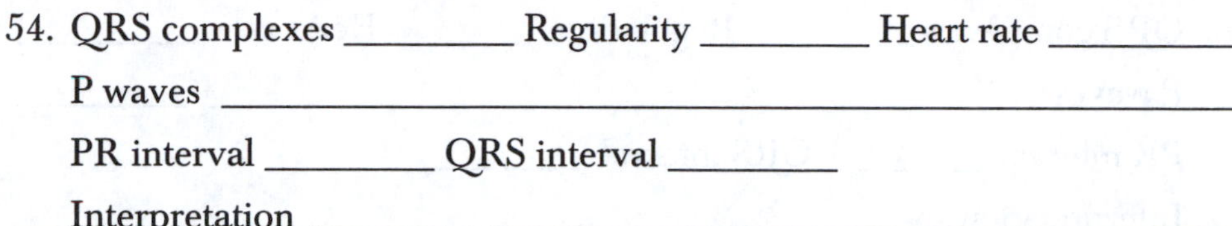

54. QRS complexes ________ Regularity ________ Heart rate ________
P waves ____
PR interval ________ QRS interval ________
Interpretation ____

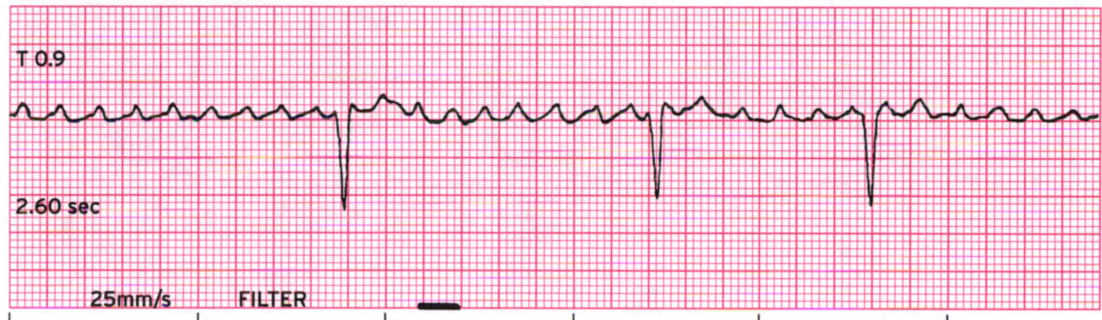

55. QRS complexes ________ Regularity ________ Heart rate ________
P waves ____
PR interval ________ QRS interval ________
Interpretation ____

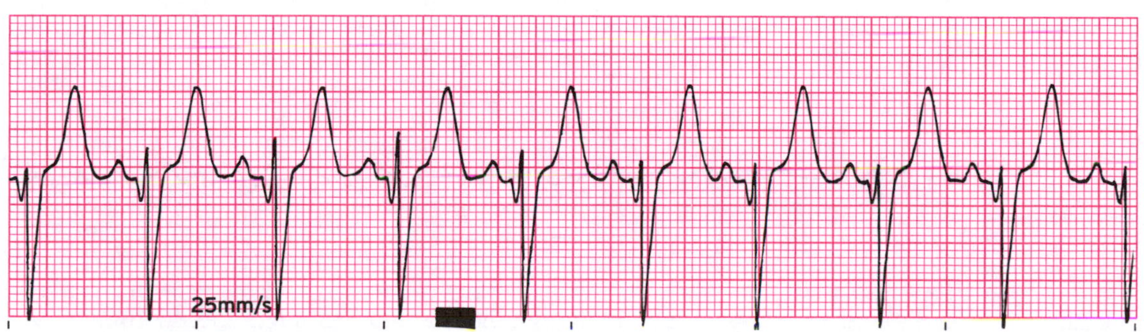

56. QRS complexes ________ Regularity ________ Heart rate ________
P waves ____
PR interval ________ QRS interval ________
Interpretation ____

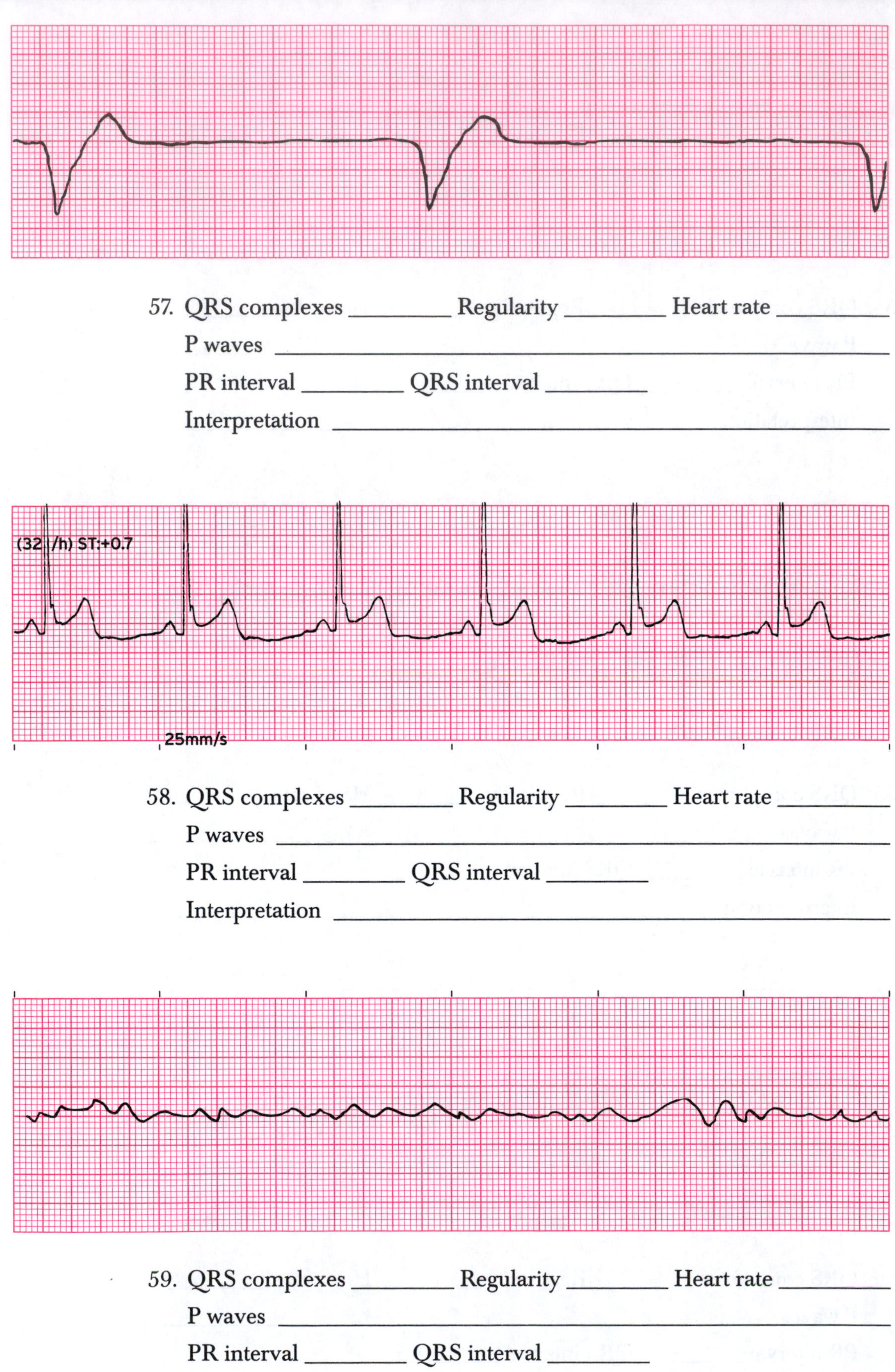

57. QRS complexes ________ Regularity ________ Heart rate ________
P waves ____
PR interval ________ QRS interval ________
Interpretation ____

58. QRS complexes ________ Regularity ________ Heart rate ________
P waves ____
PR interval ________ QRS interval ________
Interpretation ____

59. QRS complexes ________ Regularity ________ Heart rate ________
P waves ____
PR interval ________ QRS interval ________
Interpretation ____

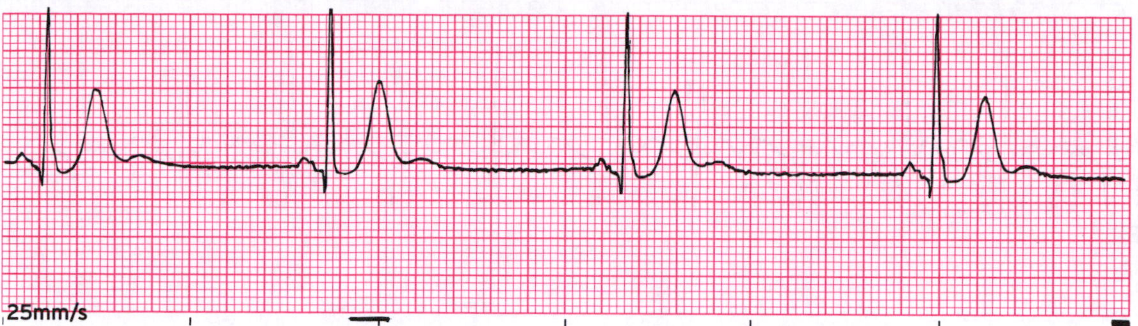

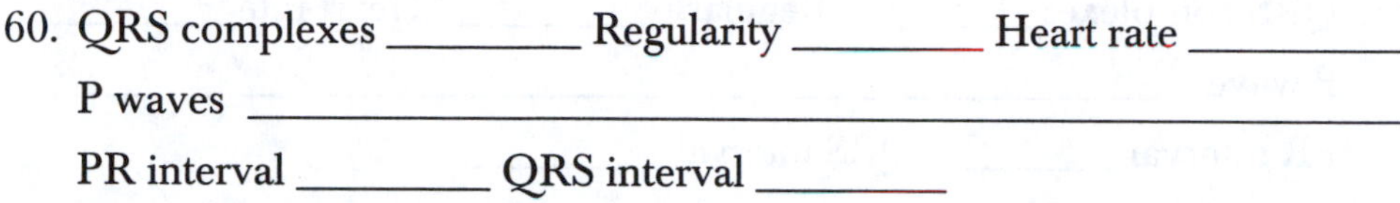

60. QRS complexes ________ Regularity ________ Heart rate ________
    P waves ____
    PR interval ________ QRS interval ________
    Interpretation ____

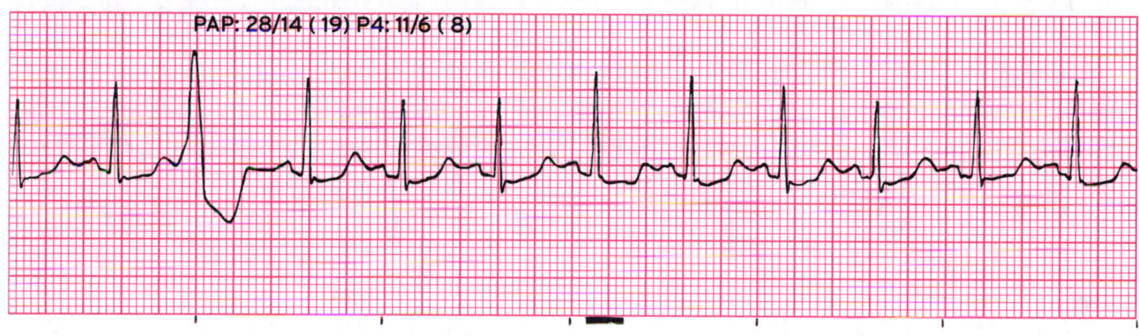

61. QRS complexes ________ Regularity ________ Heart rate ________
    P waves ____
    PR interval ________ QRS interval ________
    Interpretation ____

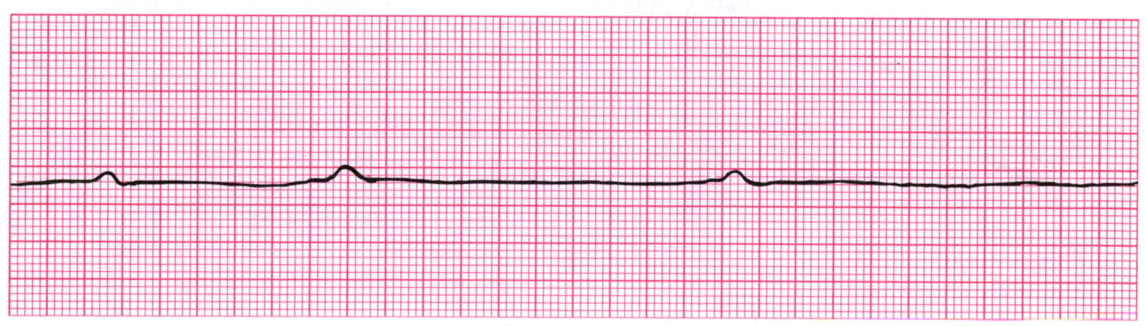

62. QRS complexes ________ Regularity ________ Heart rate ________
    P waves ____
    PR interval ________ QRS interval ________
    Interpretation ____

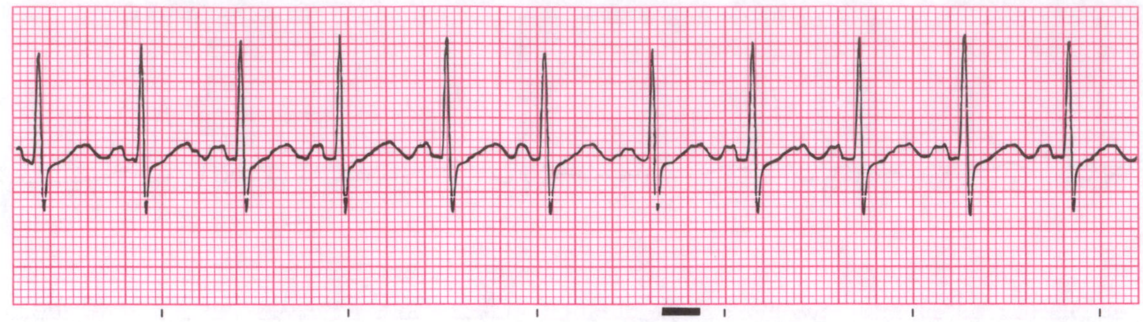

63. QRS complexes ________ Regularity ________ Heart rate ________
P waves ________________________________
PR interval ________ QRS interval ________
Interpretation ________________________________

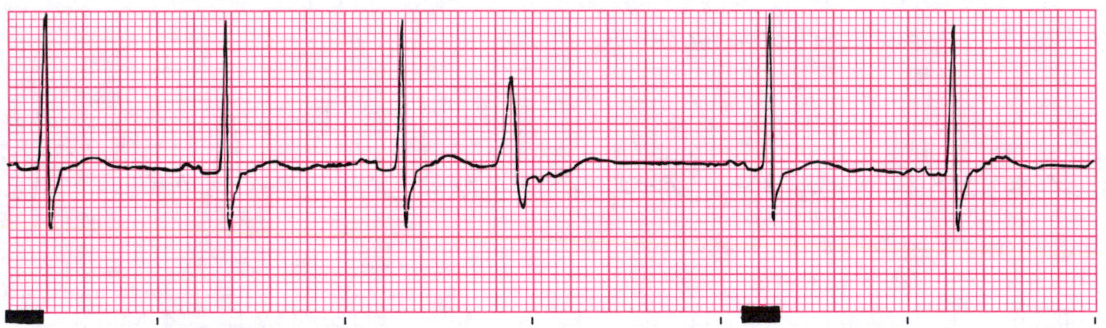

64. QRS complexes ________ Regularity ________ Heart rate ________
P waves ________________________________
PR interval ________ QRS interval ________
Interpretation ________________________________

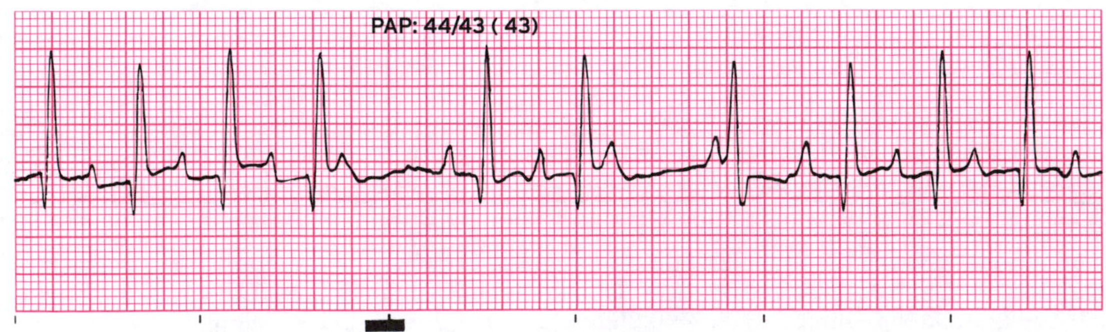

65. QRS complexes ________ Regularity ________ Heart rate ________
P waves ________________________________
PR interval ________ QRS interval ________
Interpretation ________________________________

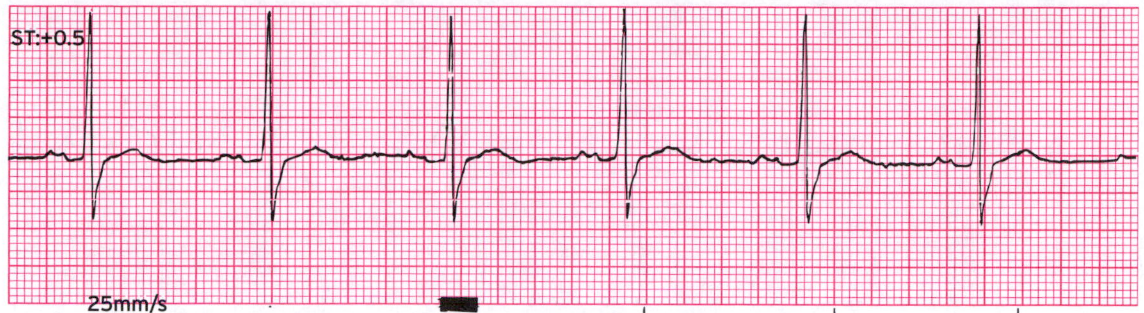

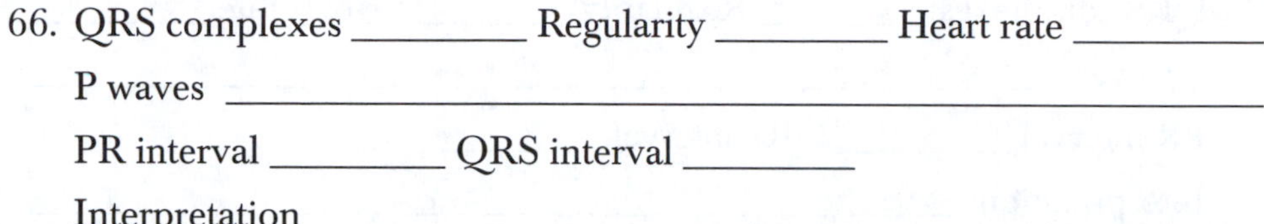
66. QRS complexes ________ Regularity ________ Heart rate ________
P waves ________________________________
PR interval ________ QRS interval ________
Interpretation ________________________________

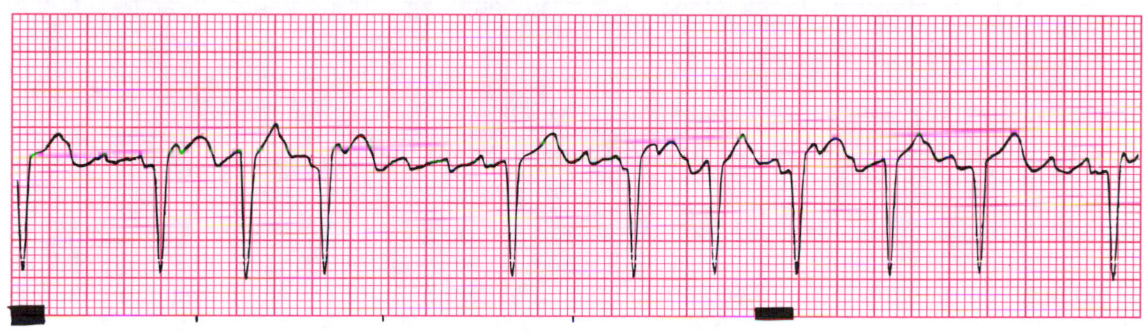

67. QRS complexes ________ Regularity ________ Heart rate ________
P waves ________________________________
PR interval ________ QRS interval ________
Interpretation ________________________________

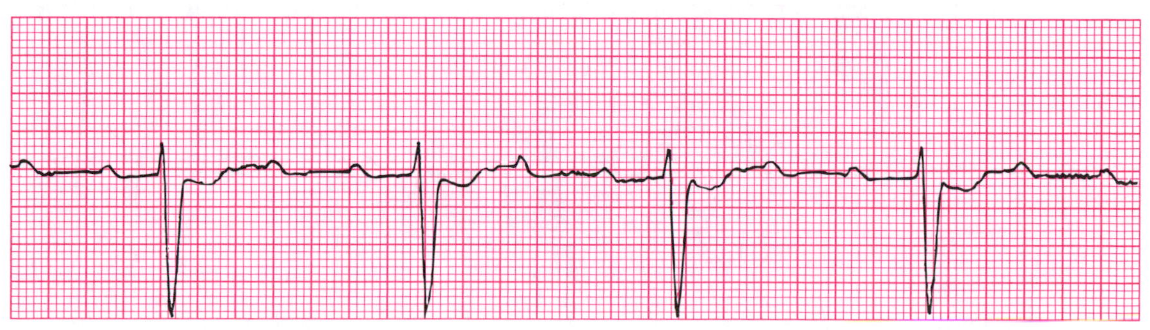

68. QRS complexes ________ Regularity ________ Heart rate ________
P waves ________________________________
PR interval ________ QRS interval ________
Interpretation ________________________________

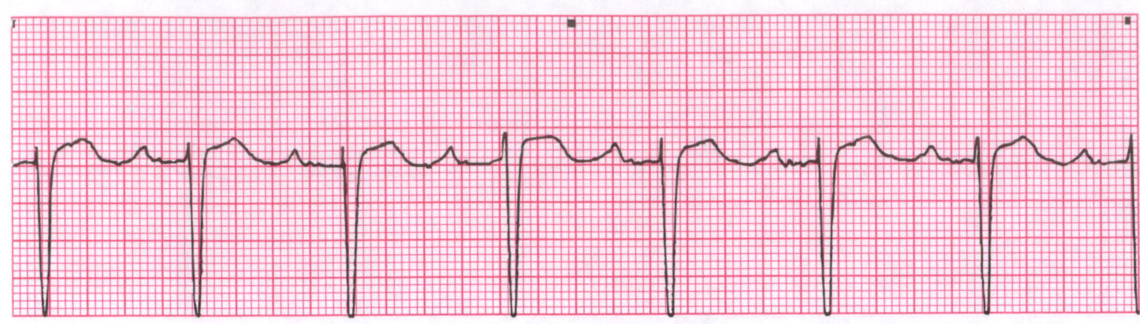

69. QRS complexes ________ Regularity ________ Heart rate ________
P waves ________________________________
PR interval ________ QRS interval ________
Interpretation ________________________________

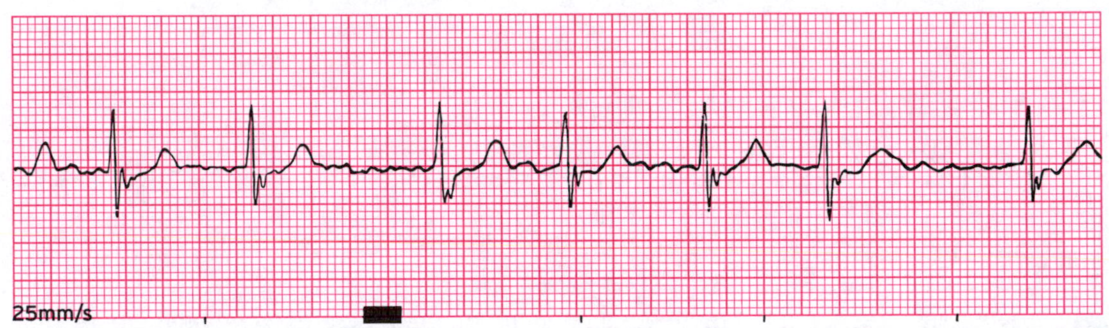

70. QRS complexes ________ Regularity ________ Heart rate ________
P waves ________________________________
PR interval ________ QRS interval ________
Interpretation ________________________________

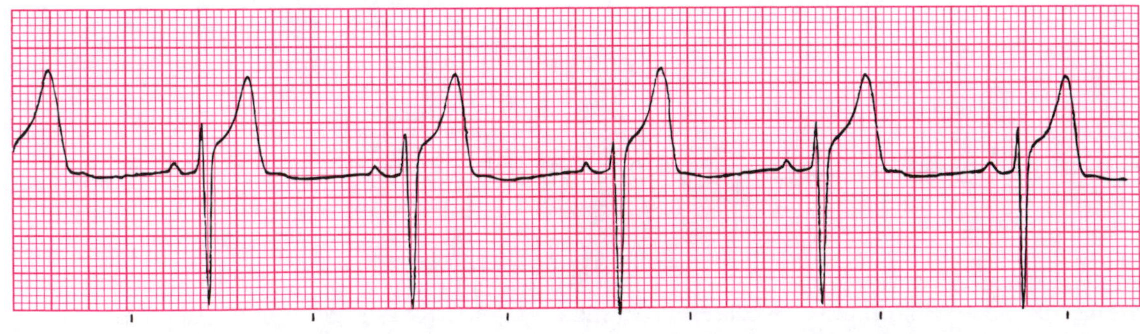

71. QRS complexes ________ Regularity ________ Heart rate ________
P waves ________________________________
PR interval ________ QRS interval ________
Interpretation ________________________________

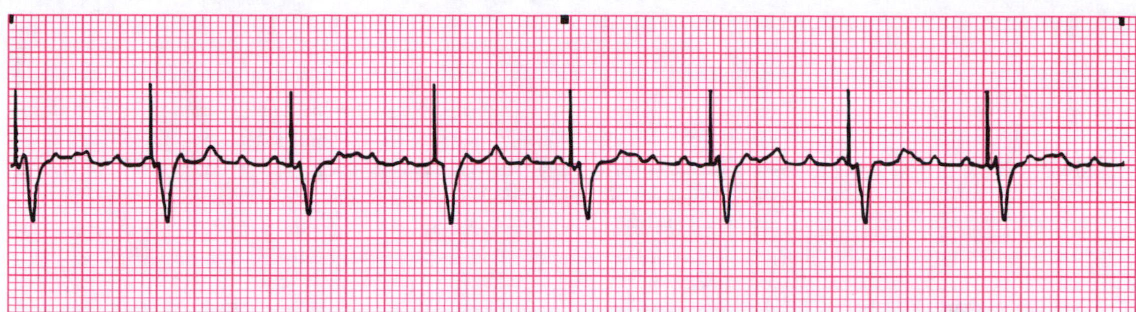

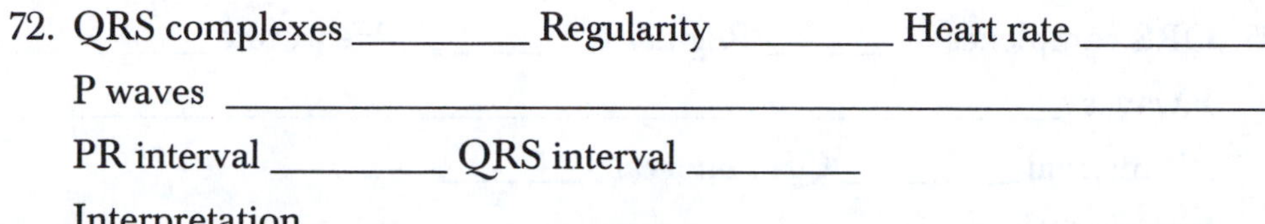

72. QRS complexes ________ Regularity ________ Heart rate ________

P waves ____

PR interval ________ QRS interval ________

Interpretation ____

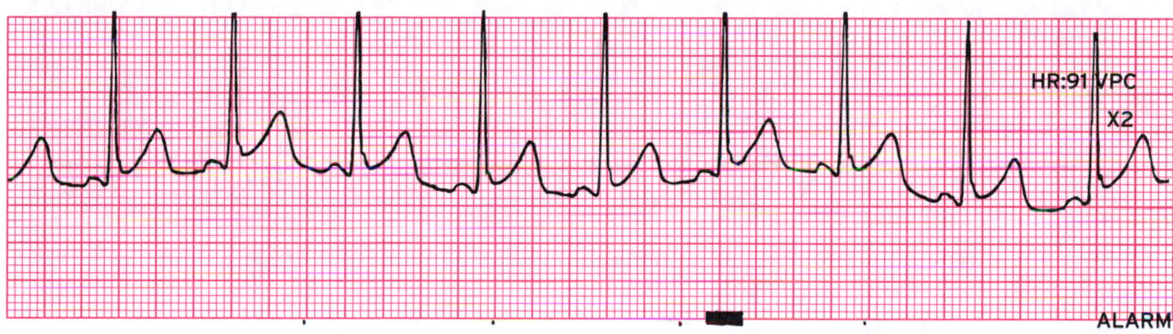

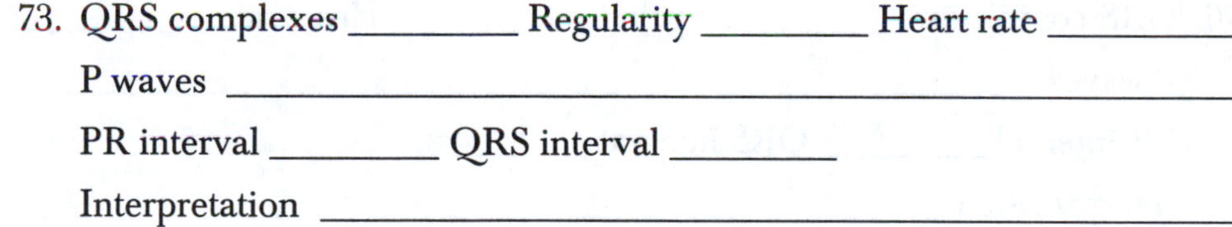

73. QRS complexes ________ Regularity ________ Heart rate ________

P waves ____

PR interval ________ QRS interval ________

Interpretation ____

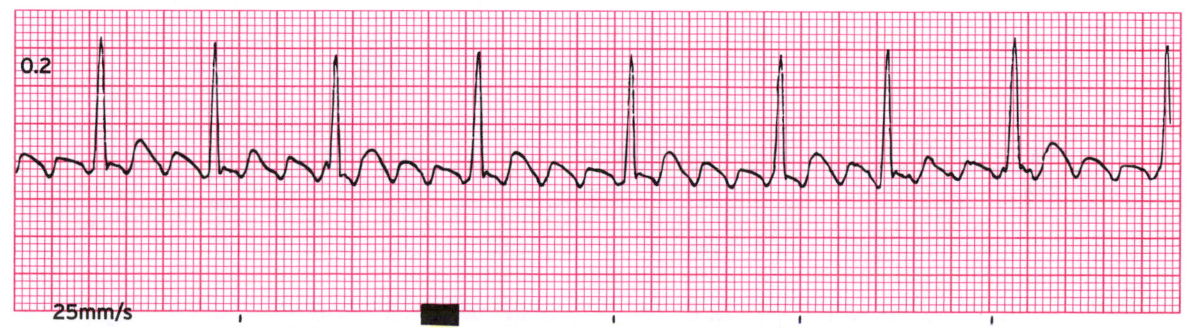

74. QRS complexes ________ Regularity ________ Heart rate ________

P waves ____

PR interval ________ QRS interval ________

Interpretation ____

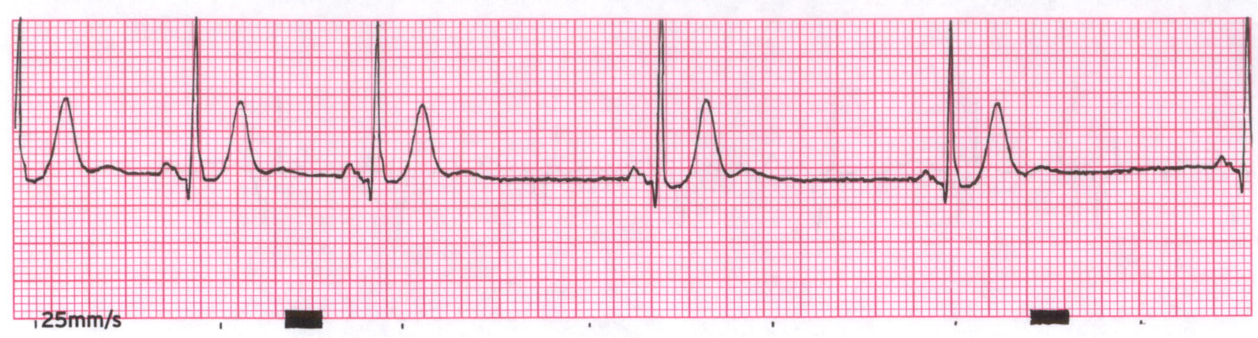

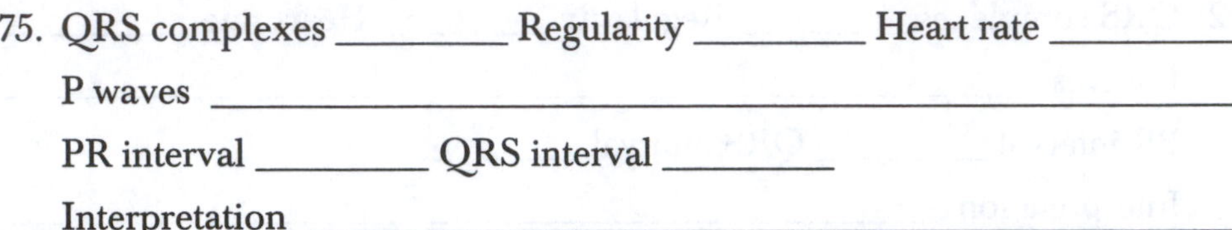

75. QRS complexes ________ Regularity ________ Heart rate ________

P waves ____

PR interval ________ QRS interval ________

Interpretation ____

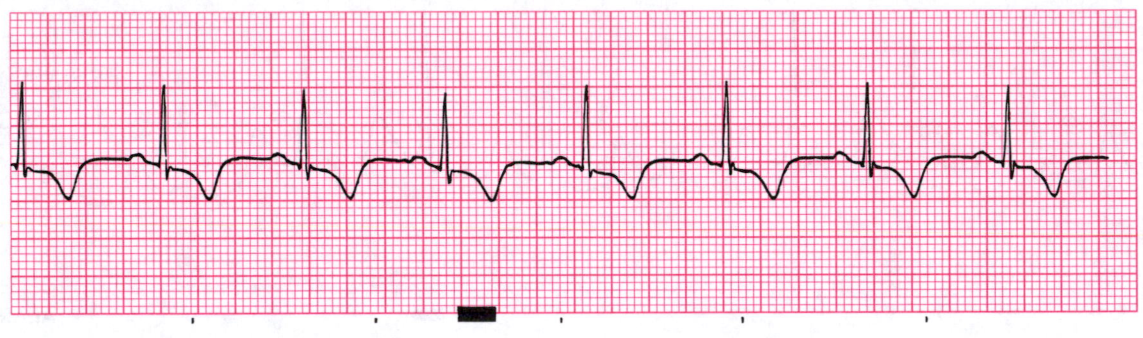

76. QRS complexes ________ Regularity ________ Heart rate ________

P waves ____

PR interval ________ QRS interval ________

Interpretation ____

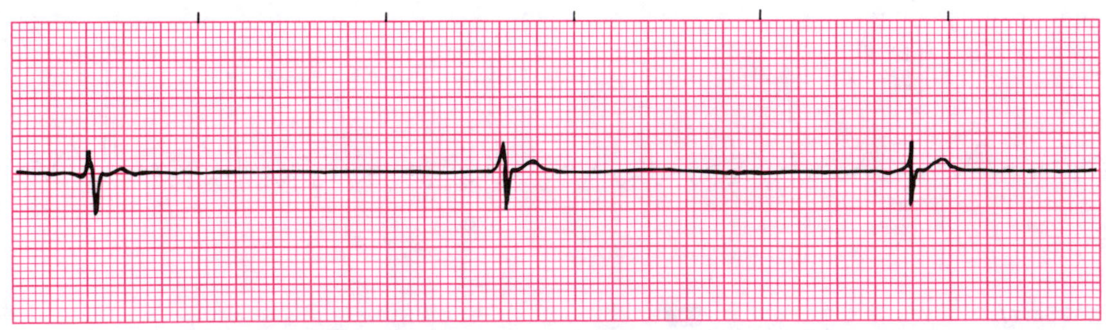

77. QRS complexes ________ Regularity ________ Heart rate ________

P waves ____

PR interval ________ QRS interval ________

Interpretation ____

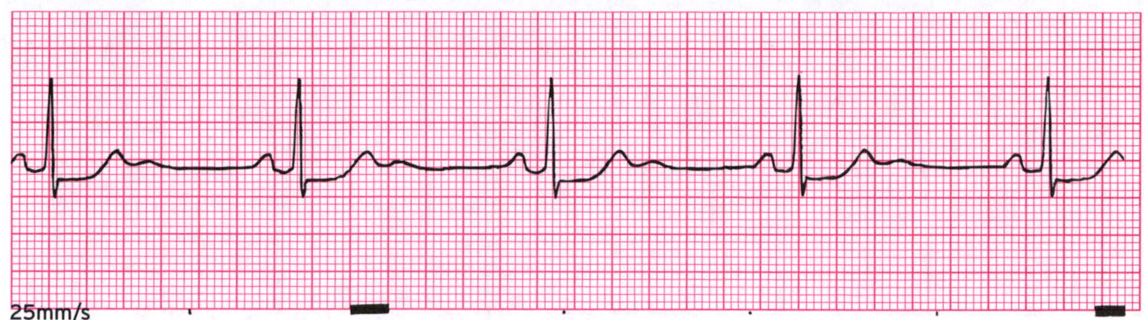

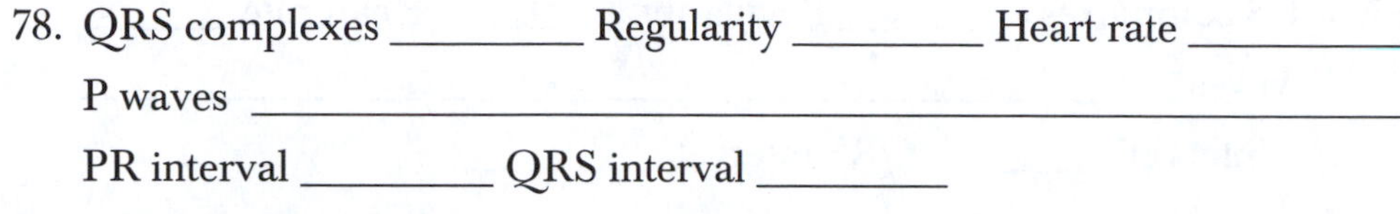
78. QRS complexes ________ Regularity ________ Heart rate ________
P waves ____
PR interval ________ QRS interval ________
Interpretation ____

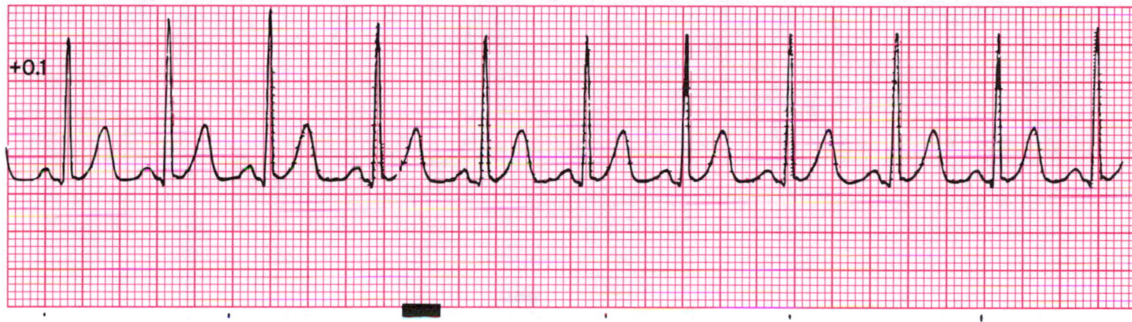

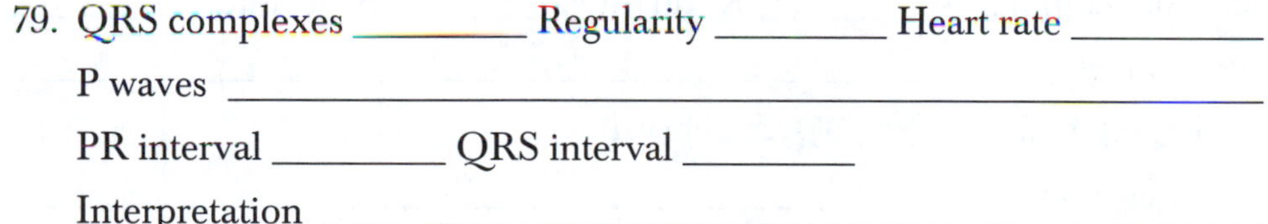
79. QRS complexes ________ Regularity ________ Heart rate ________
P waves ____
PR interval ________ QRS interval ________
Interpretation ____

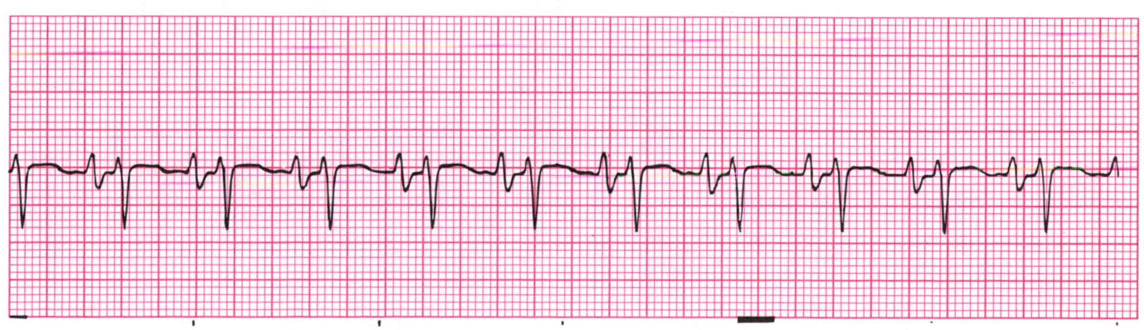

80. QRS complexes ________ Regularity ________ Heart rate ________
P waves ____
PR interval ________ QRS interval ________
Interpretation ____

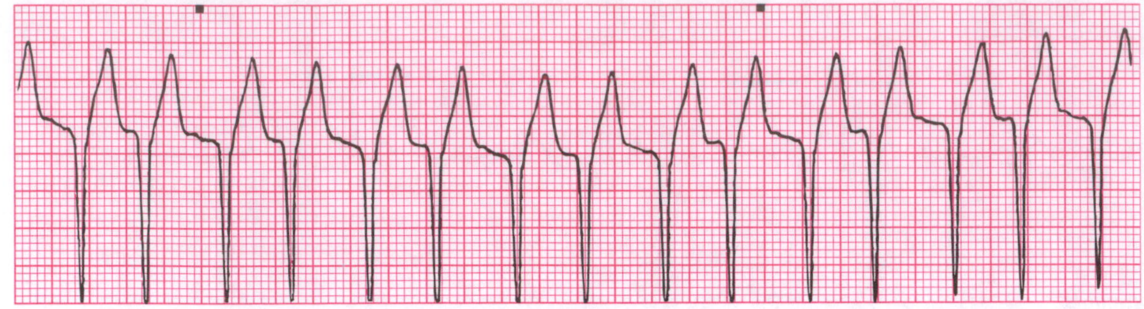

81. QRS complexes ________ Regularity ________ Heart rate ________
P waves ____
PR interval ________ QRS interval ________
Interpretation ____

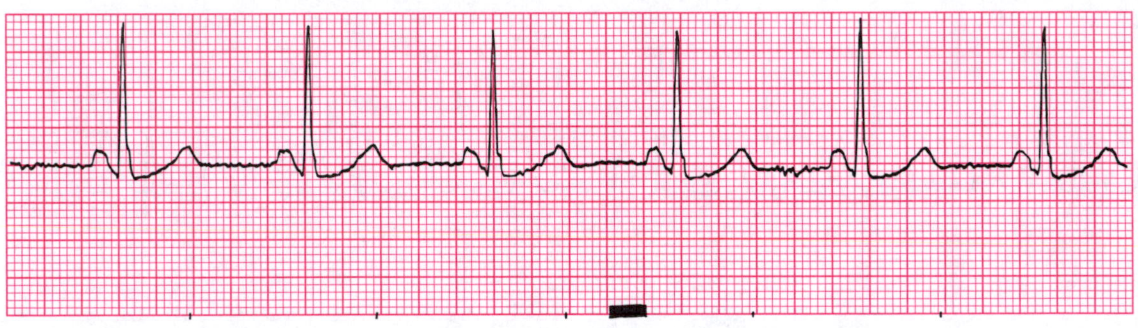

82. QRS complexes ________ Regularity ________ Heart rate ________
P waves ____
PR interval ________ QRS interval ________
Interpretation ____

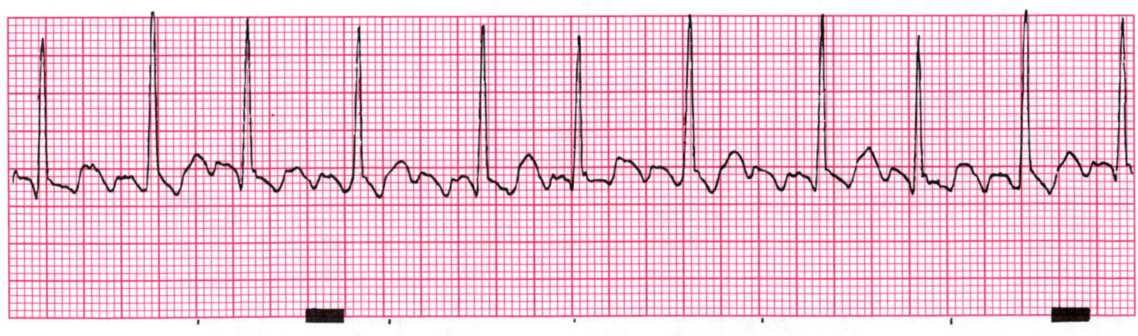

83. QRS complexes ________ Regularity ________ Heart rate ________
P waves ____
PR interval ________ QRS interval ________
Interpretation ____

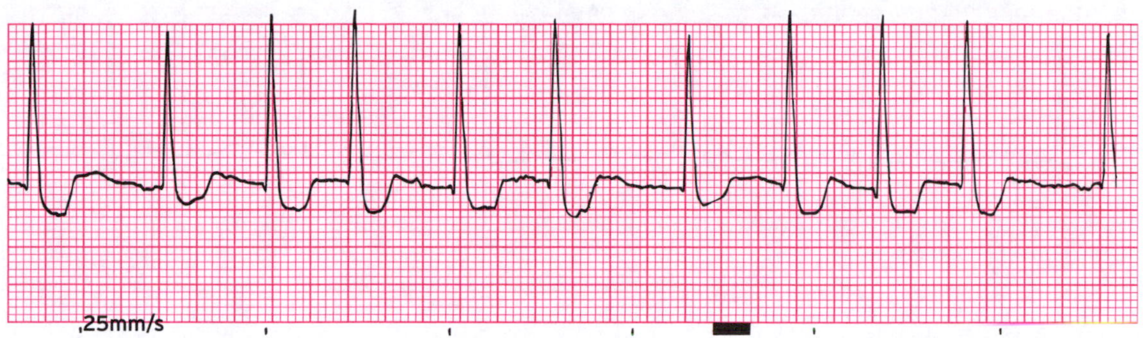

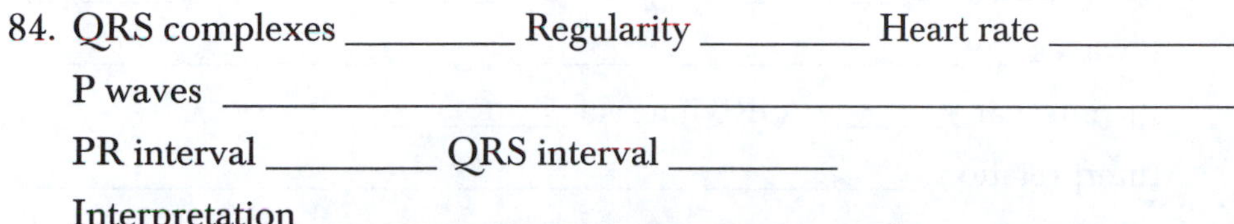

84. QRS complexes ________ Regularity ________ Heart rate ________

P waves ____

PR interval ________ QRS interval ________

Interpretation ____

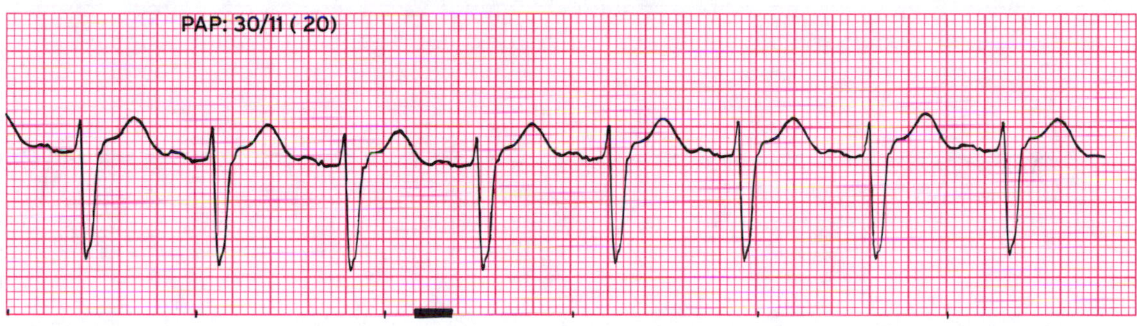

85. QRS complexes ________ Regularity ________ Heart rate ________

P waves ____

PR interval ________ QRS interval ________

Interpretation ____

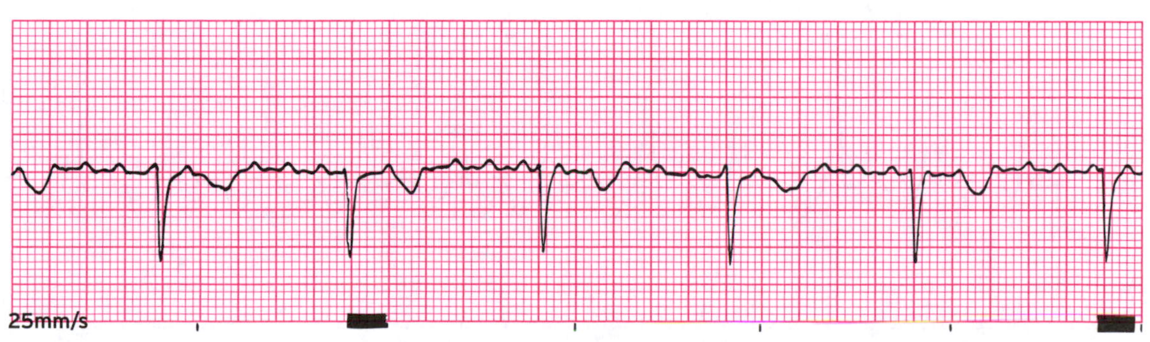

86. QRS complexes ________ Regularity ________ Heart rate ________

P waves ____

PR interval ________ QRS interval ________

Interpretation ____

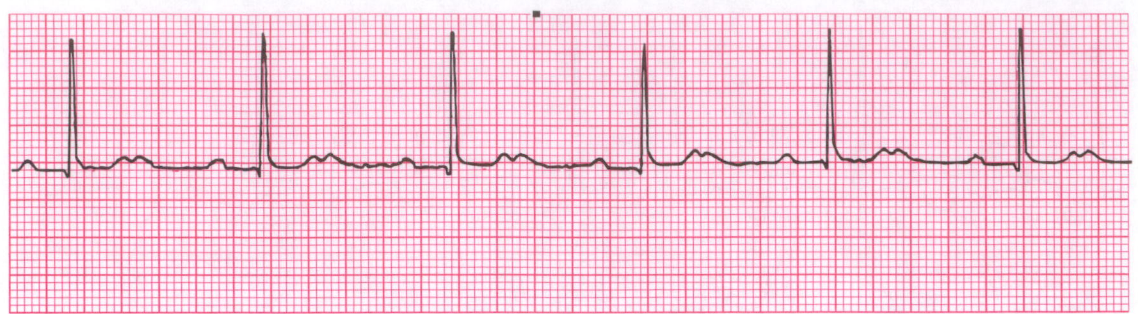

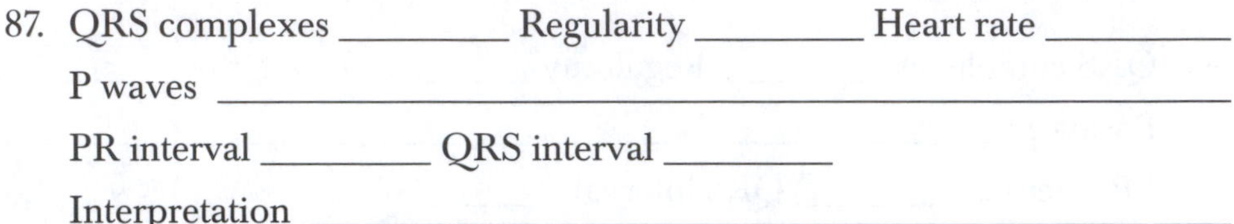

87. QRS complexes ________ Regularity ________ Heart rate ________
P waves ____
PR interval ________ QRS interval ________
Interpretation ____

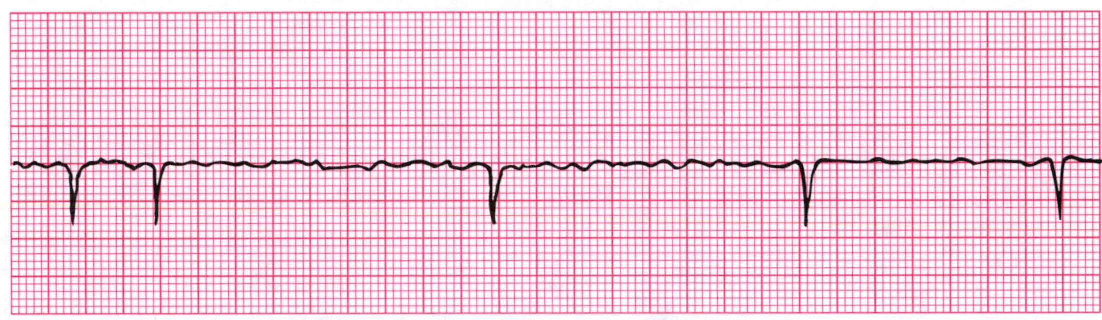

88. QRS complexes ________ Regularity ________ Heart rate ________
P waves ____
PR interval ________ QRS interval ________
Interpretation ____

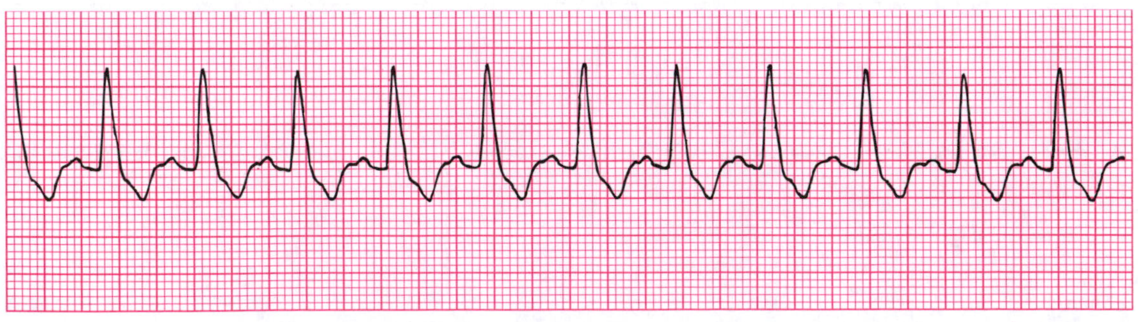

89. QRS complexes ________ Regularity ________ Heart rate ________
P waves ____
PR interval ________ QRS interval ________
Interpretation ____

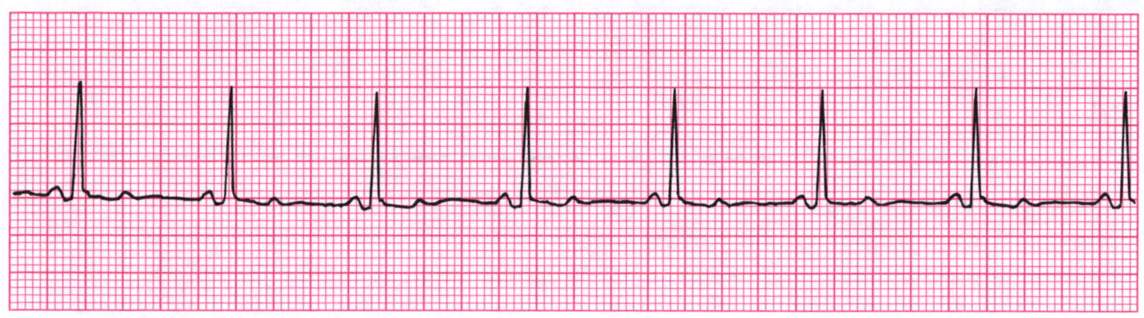

90. QRS complexes ________ Regularity ________ Heart rate ________
P waves ____
PR interval ________ QRS interval ________
Interpretation ____

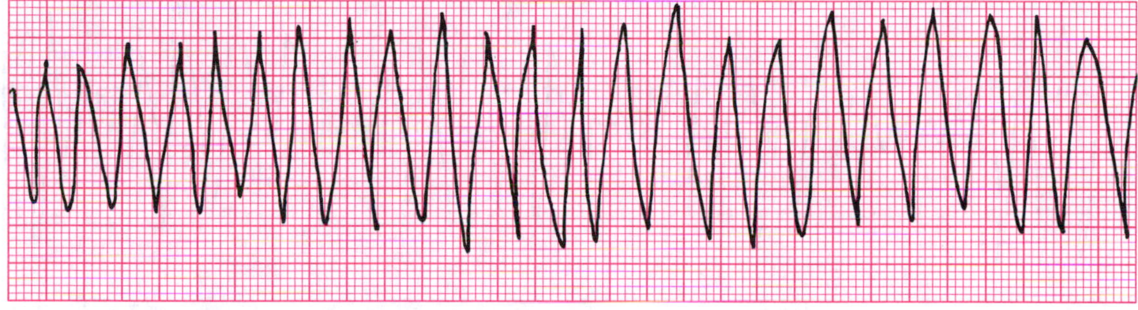

91. QRS complexes ________ Regularity ________ Heart rate ________
P waves ____
PR interval ________ QRS interval ________
Interpretation ____

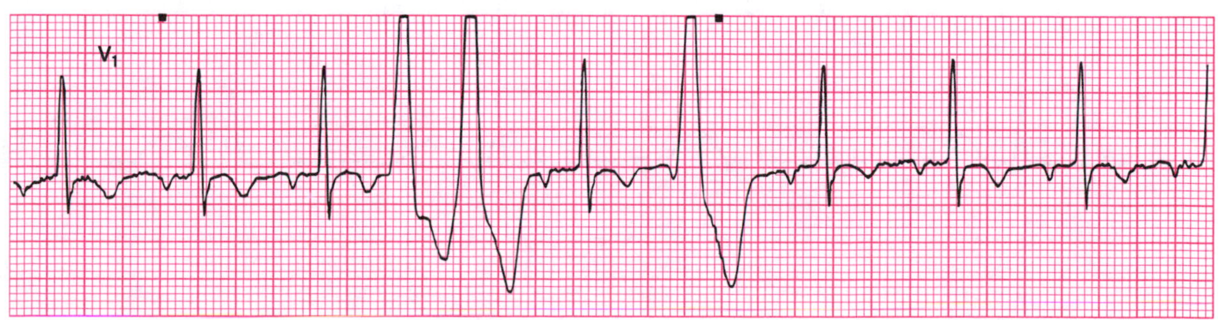

92. QRS complexes ________ Regularity ________ Heart rate ________
P waves ____
PR interval ________ QRS interval ________
Interpretation ____

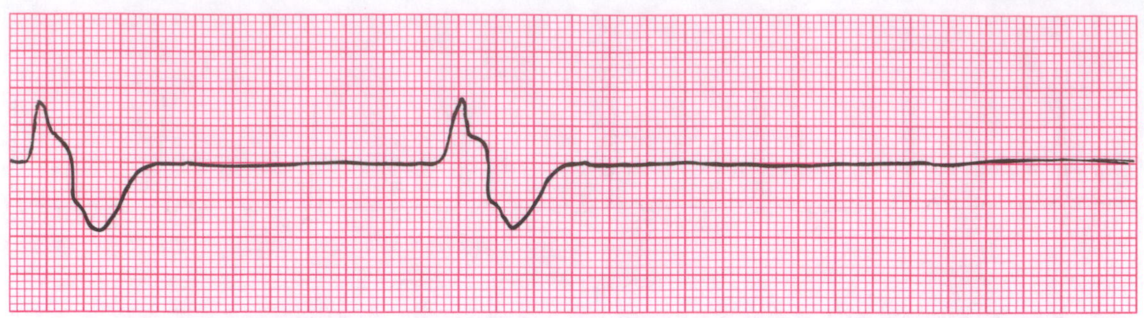

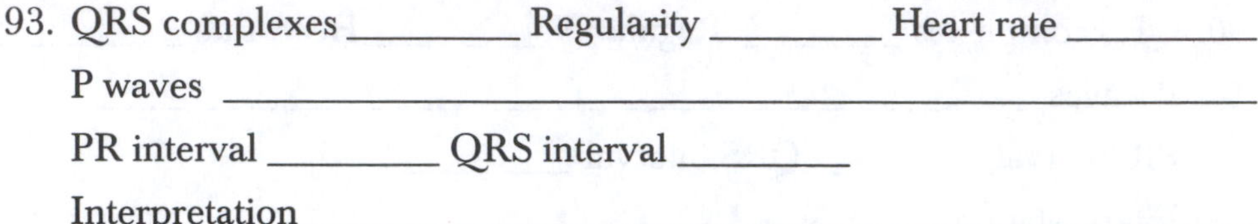

93. QRS complexes ________ Regularity ________ Heart rate ________
    P waves ____
    PR interval ________ QRS interval ________
    Interpretation ____

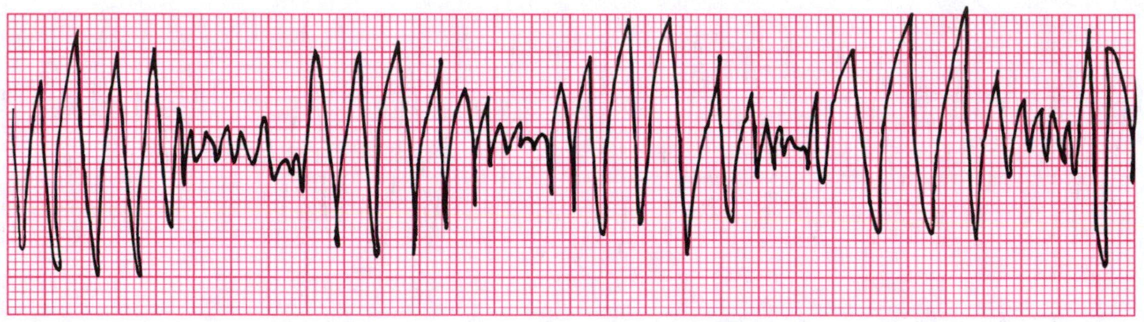

94. QRS complexes ________ Regularity ________ Heart rate ________
    P waves ____
    PR interval ________ QRS interval ________
    Interpretation ____

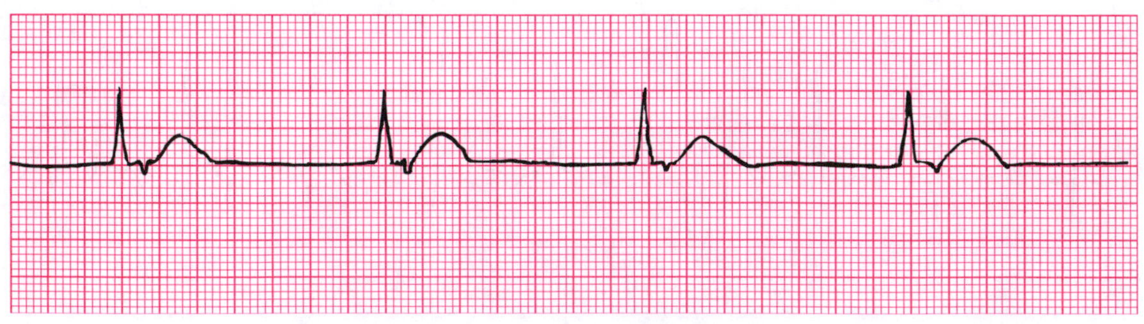

95. QRS complexes ________ Regularity ________ Heart rate ________
    P waves ____
    PR interval ________ QRS interval ________
    Interpretation ____

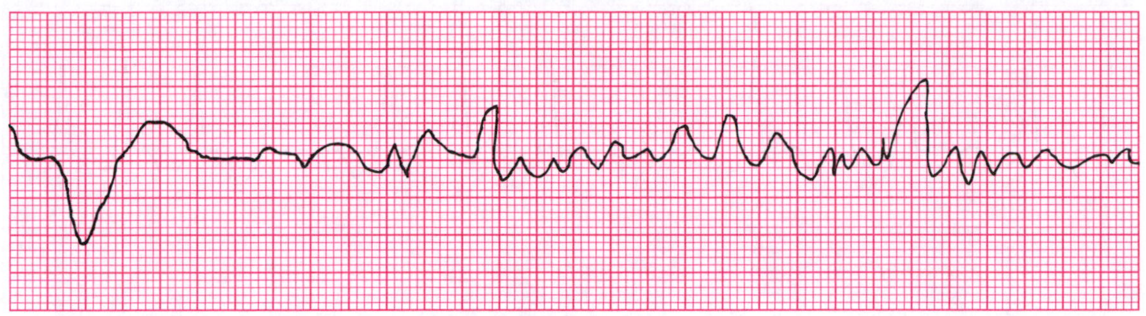

96. QRS complexes ________ Regularity ________ Heart rate ________
    P waves ____
    PR interval ________ QRS interval ________
    Interpretation ____

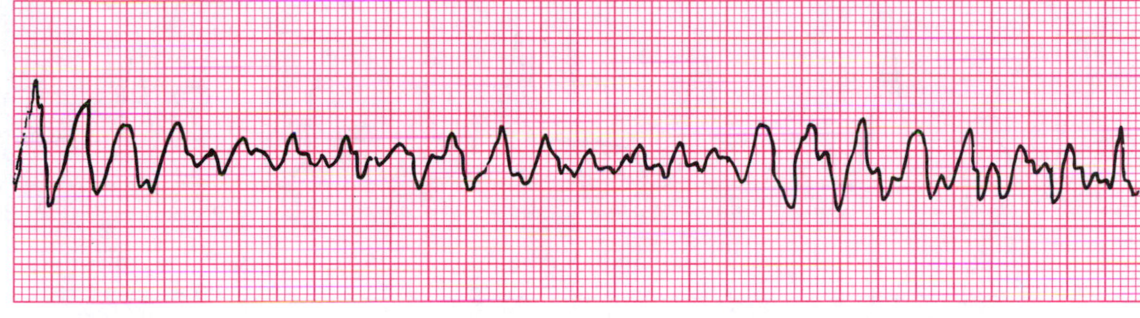

97. QRS complexes ________ Regularity ________ Heart rate ________
    P waves ____
    PR interval ________ QRS interval ________
    Interpretation ____

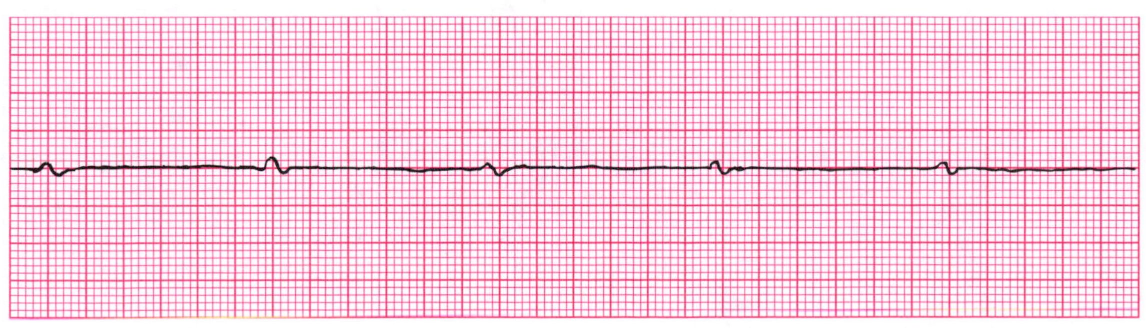

98. QRS complexes ________ Regularity ________ Heart rate ________
    P waves ____
    PR interval ________ QRS interval ________
    Interpretation ____

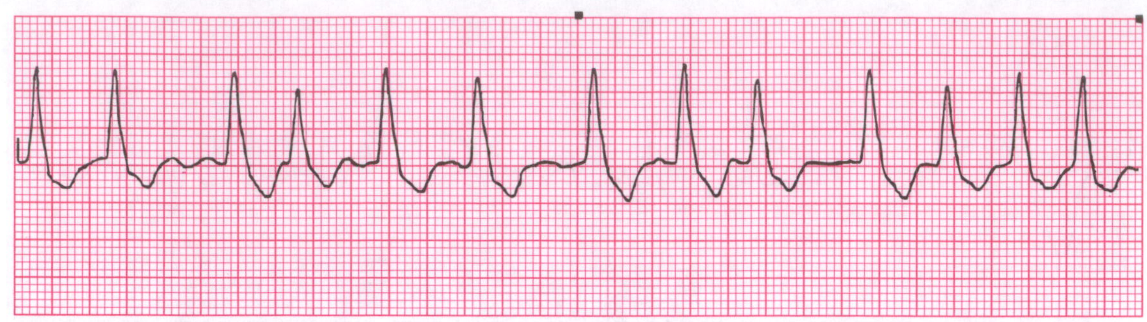

99. QRS complexes ________ Regularity ________ Heart rate ________
P waves ____
PR interval ________ QRS interval ________
Interpretation ____

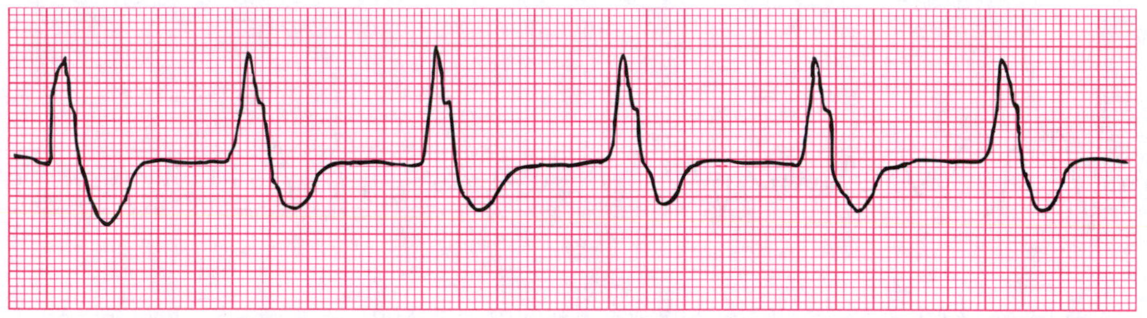

100. QRS complexes ________ Regularity ________ Heart rate ________
P waves ____
PR interval ________ QRS interval ________
Interpretation ____

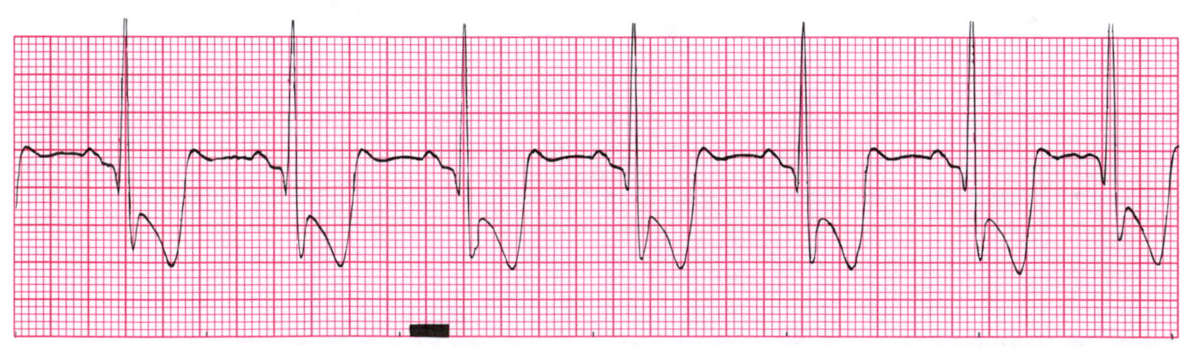

101. QRS complexes ________ Regularity ________ Heart rate ________
P waves ____
PR interval ________ QRS interval ________
Interpretation ____

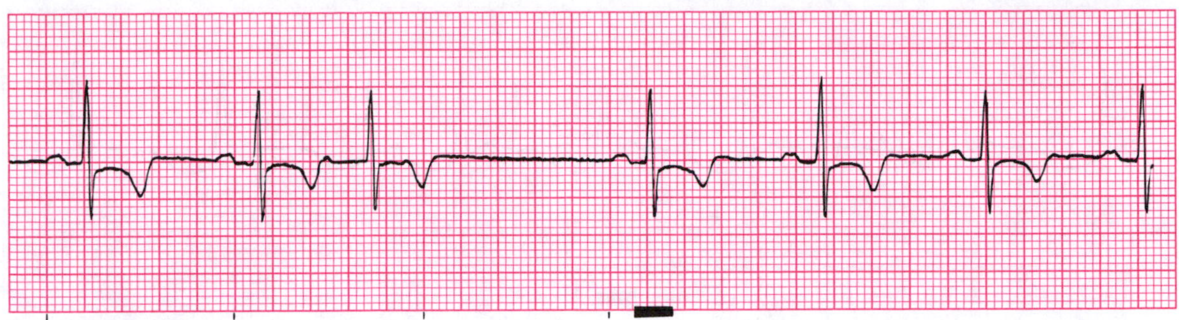

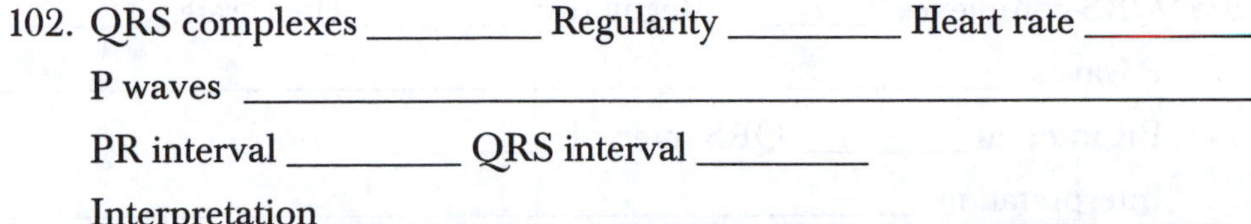

102. QRS complexes ________ Regularity ________ Heart rate ________

P waves ____

PR interval ________ QRS interval ________

Interpretation ____

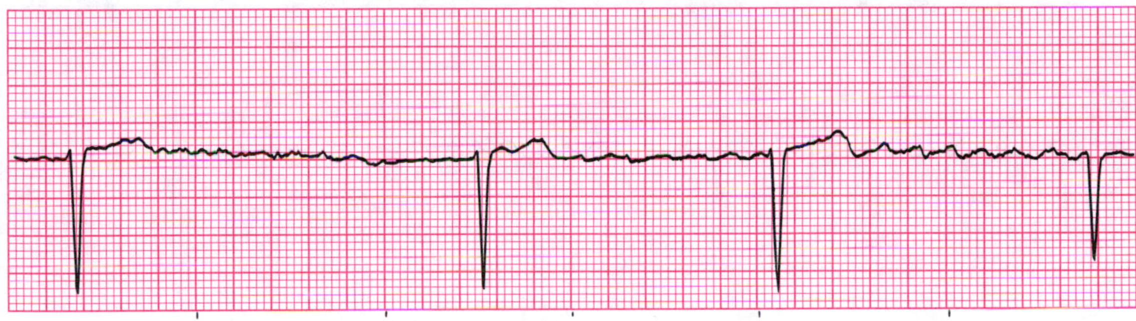

103. QRS complexes ________ Regularity ________ Heart rate ________

P waves ____

PR interval ________ QRS interval ________

Interpretation ____

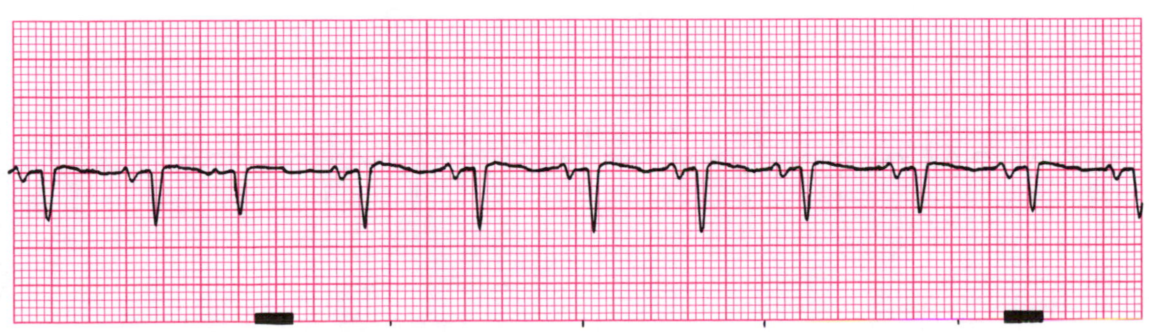

104. QRS complexes ________ Regularity ________ Heart rate ________

P waves ____

PR interval ________ QRS interval ________

Interpretation ____

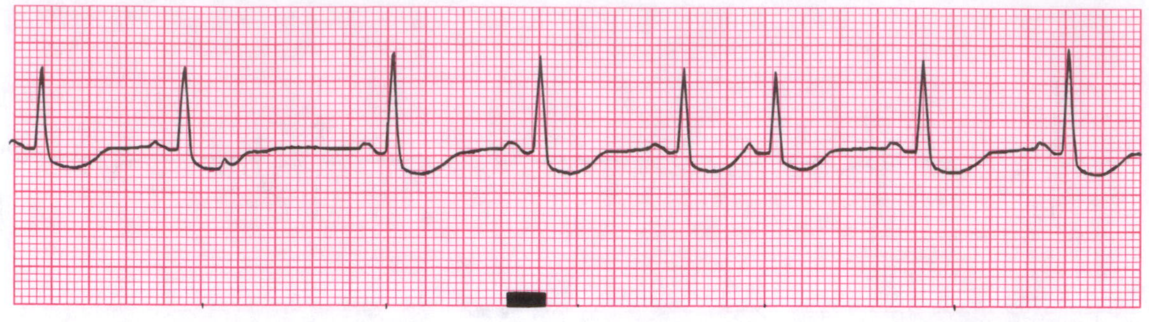

105. QRS complexes ________ Regularity ________ Heart rate ________
P waves ____
PR interval ________ QRS interval ________
Interpretation ____

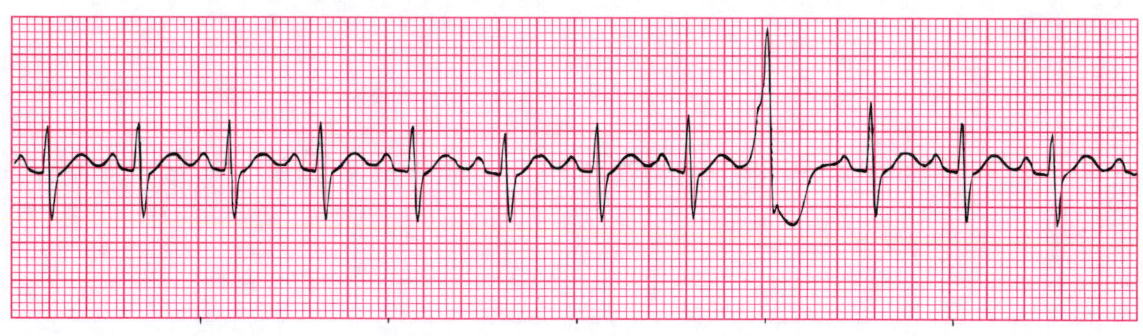

106. QRS complexes ________ Regularity ________ Heart rate ________
P waves ____
PR interval ________ QRS interval ________
Interpretation ____

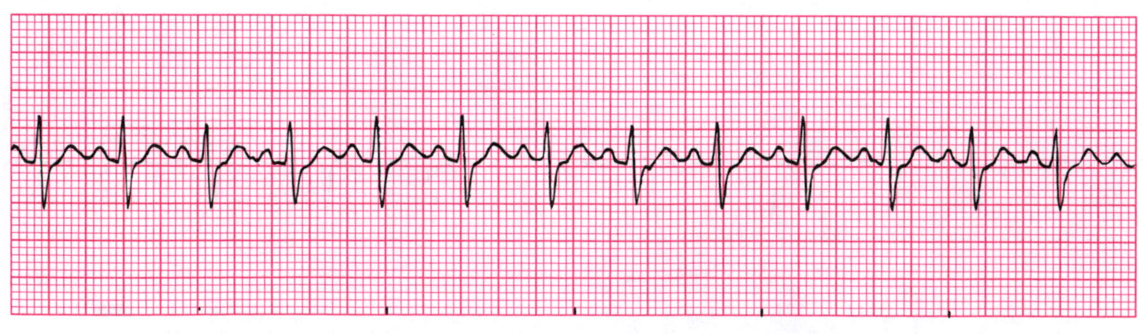

107. QRS complexes ________ Regularity ________ Heart rate ________
P waves ____
PR interval ________ QRS interval ________
Interpretation ____

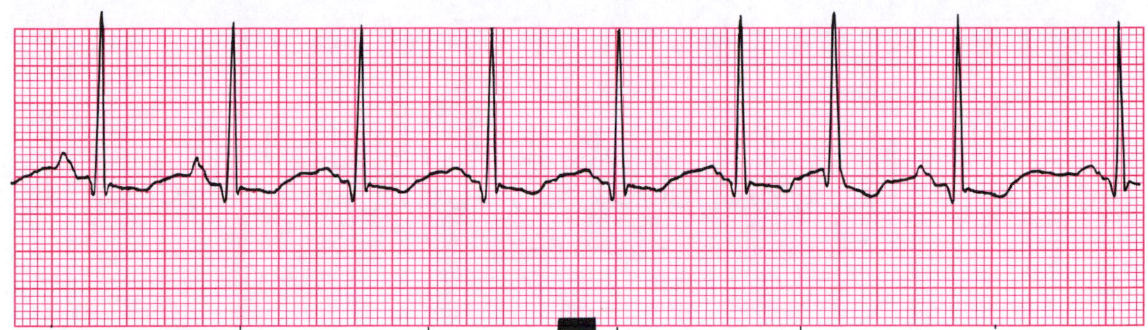

108. QRS complexes ________ Regularity ________ Heart rate ________
P waves ____
PR interval ________ QRS interval ________
Interpretation ____

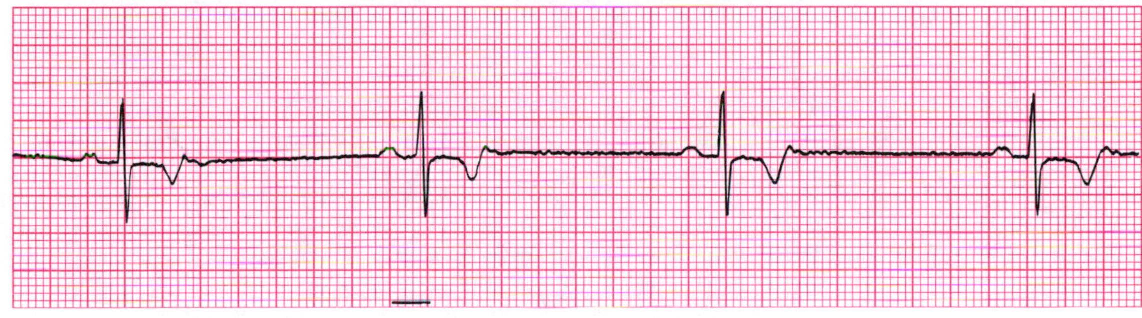

109. QRS complexes ________ Regularity ________ Heart rate ________
P waves ____
PR interval ________ QRS interval ________
Interpretation ____

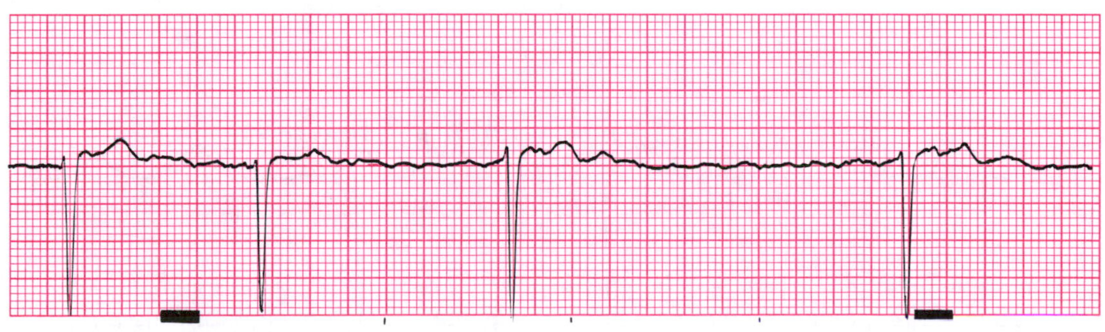

110. QRS complexes ________ Regularity ________ Heart rate ________
P waves ____
PR interval ________ QRS interval ________
Interpretation ____

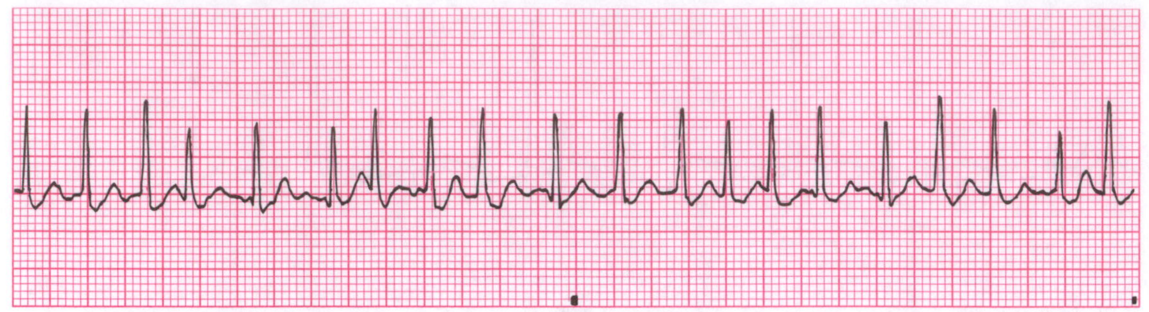

111. QRS complexes ________ Regularity ________ Heart rate ________
P waves ____
PR interval ________ QRS interval ________
Interpretation ____

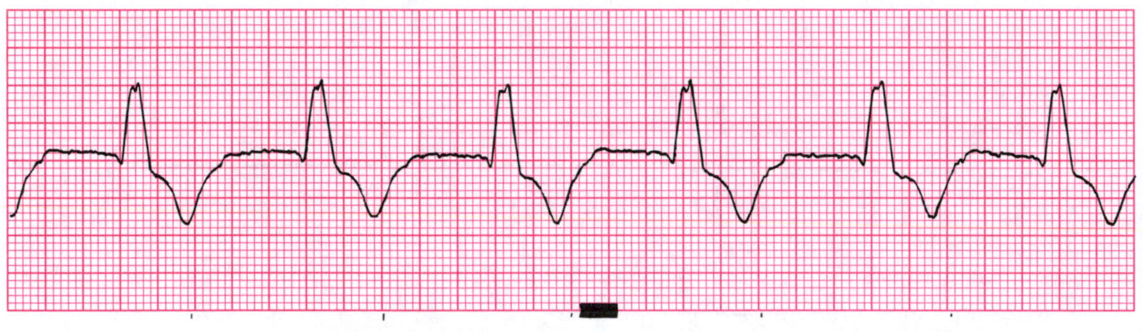

112. QRS complexes ________ Regularity ________ Heart rate ________
P waves ____
PR interval ________ QRS interval ________
Interpretation ____

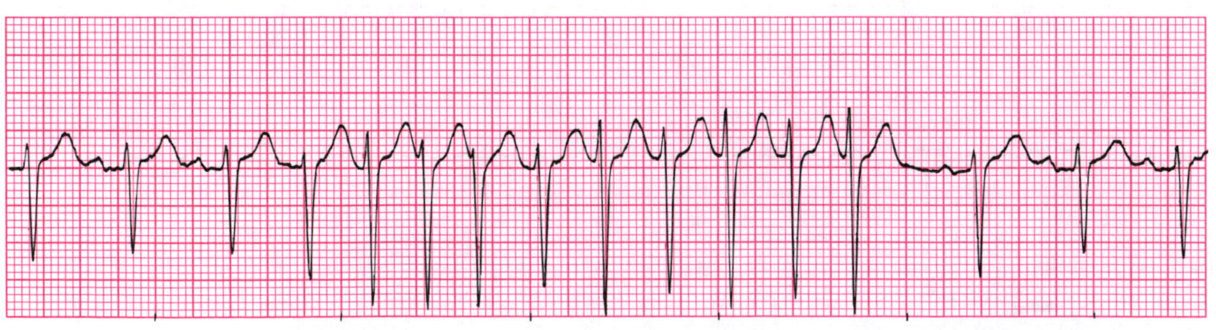

113. QRS complexes ________ Regularity ________ Heart rate ________
P waves ____
PR interval ________ QRS interval ________
Interpretation ____

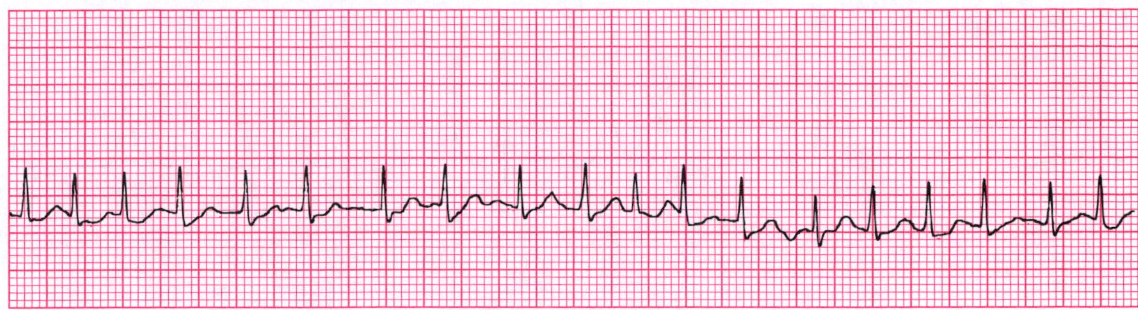

114. QRS complexes ________ Regularity ________ Heart rate ________
P waves ____
PR interval ________ QRS interval ________
Interpretation ____

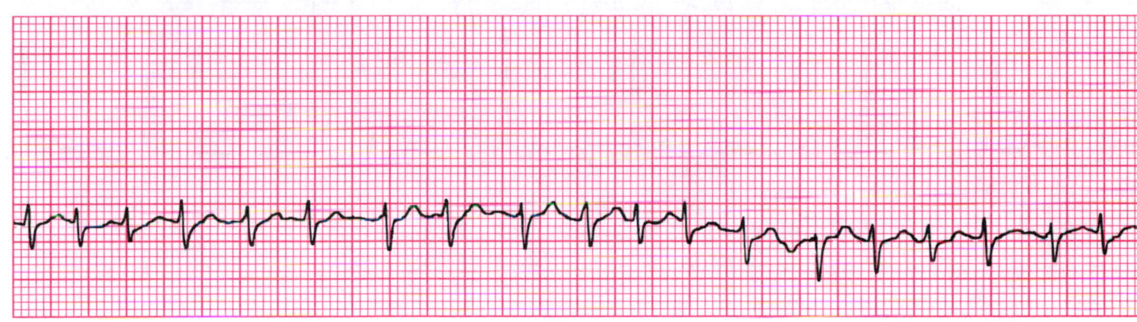

115. QRS complexes ________ Regularity ________ Heart rate ________
P waves ____
PR interval ________ QRS interval ________
Interpretation ____

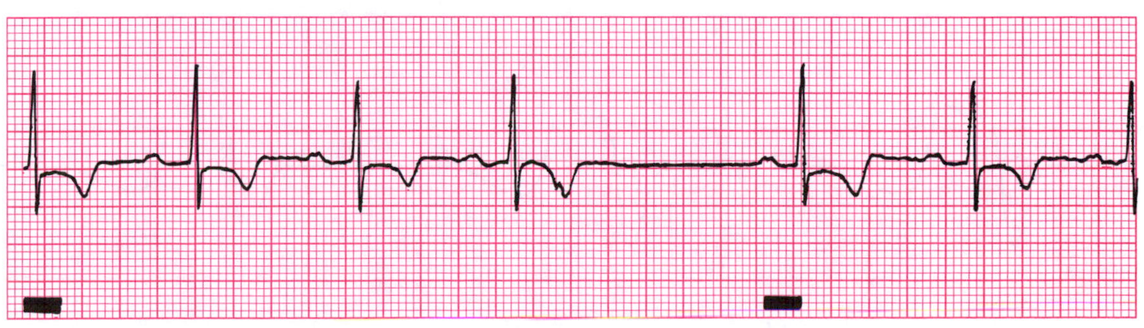

116. QRS complexes ________ Regularity ________ Heart rate ________
P waves ____
PR interval ________ QRS interval ________
Interpretation ____

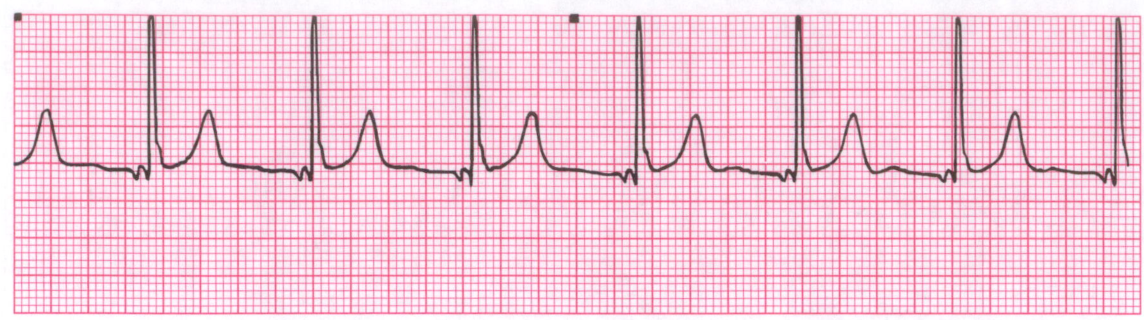

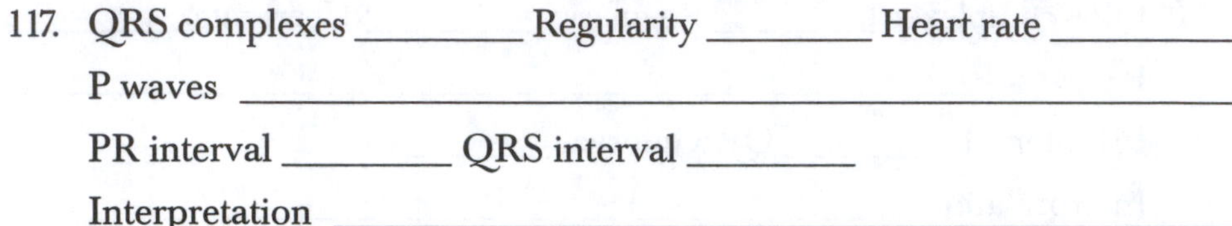

117. QRS complexes ________ Regularity ________ Heart rate ________
P waves ____
PR interval ________ QRS interval ________
Interpretation ____

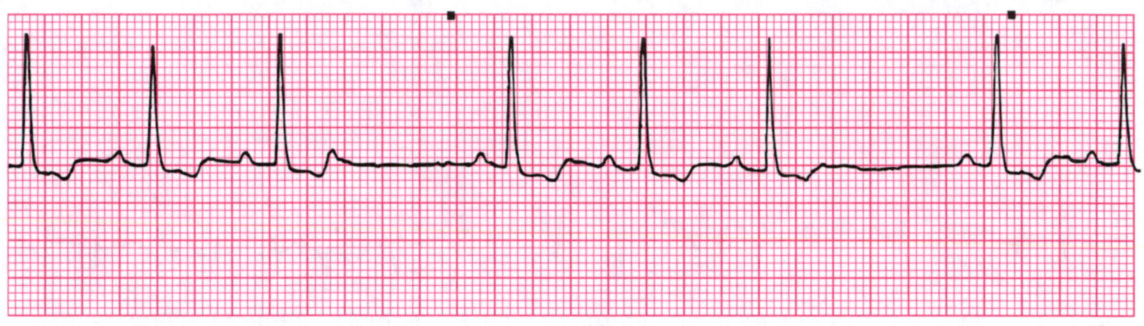

118. QRS complexes ________ Regularity ________ Heart rate ________
P waves ____
PR interval ________ QRS interval ________
Interpretation ____

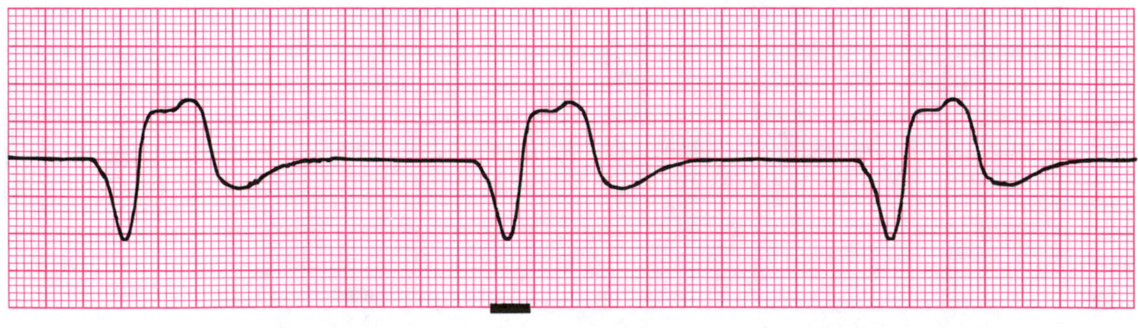

119. QRS complexes ________ Regularity ________ Heart rate ________
P waves ____
PR interval ________ QRS interval ________
Interpretation ____

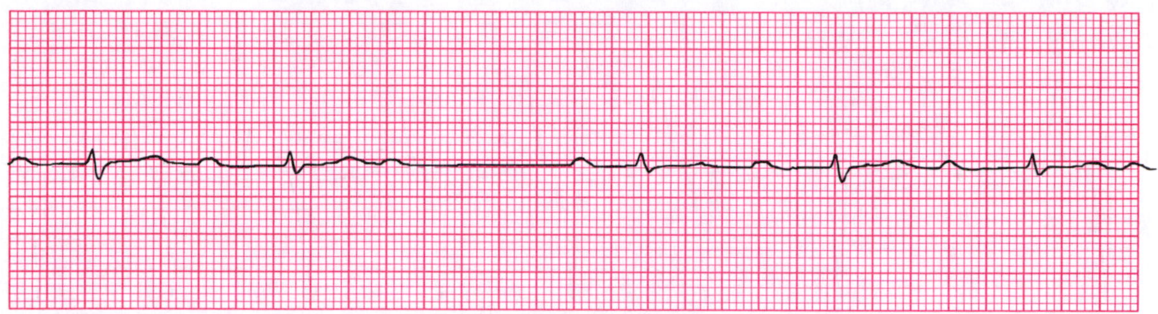

120. QRS complexes ________ Regularity ________ Heart rate ________
P waves ____
PR interval ________ QRS interval ________
Interpretation ____

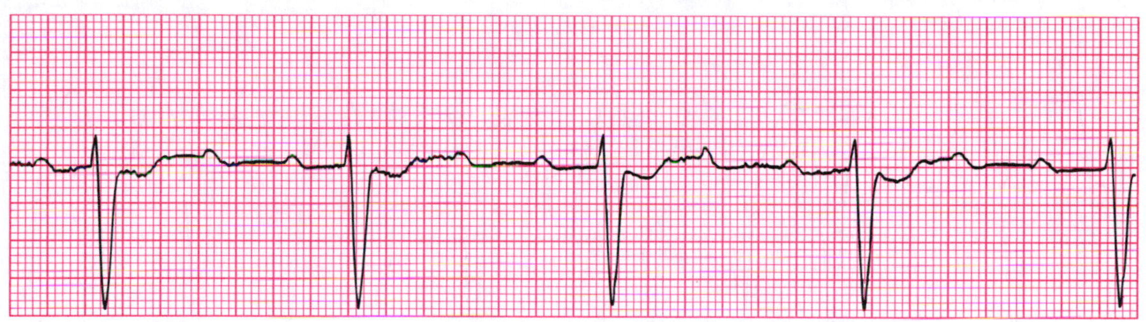

121. QRS complexes ________ Regularity ________ Heart rate ________
P waves ____
PR interval ________ QRS interval ________
Interpretation ____

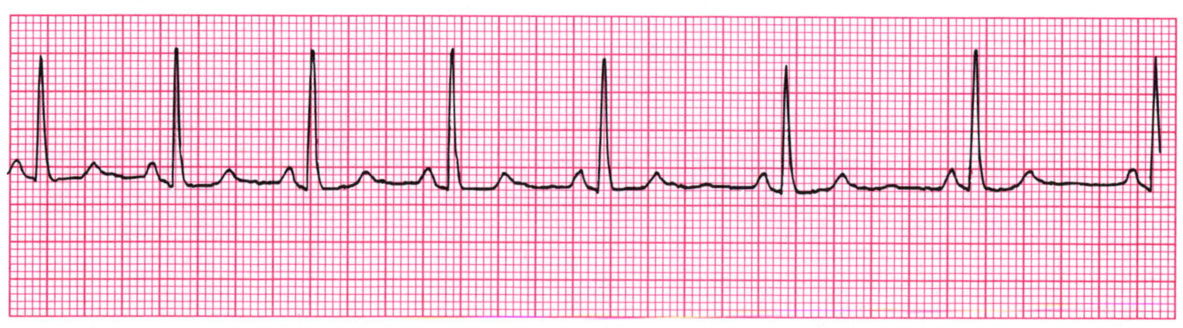

122. QRS complexes ________ Regularity ________ Heart rate ________
P waves ____
PR interval ________ QRS interval ________
Interpretation ____

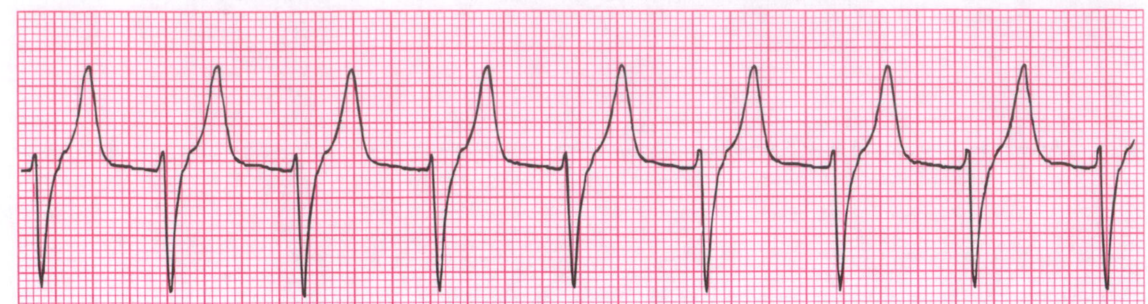

123. QRS complexes ________ Regularity ________ Heart rate ________
P waves ____
PR interval ________ QRS interval ________
Interpretation ____

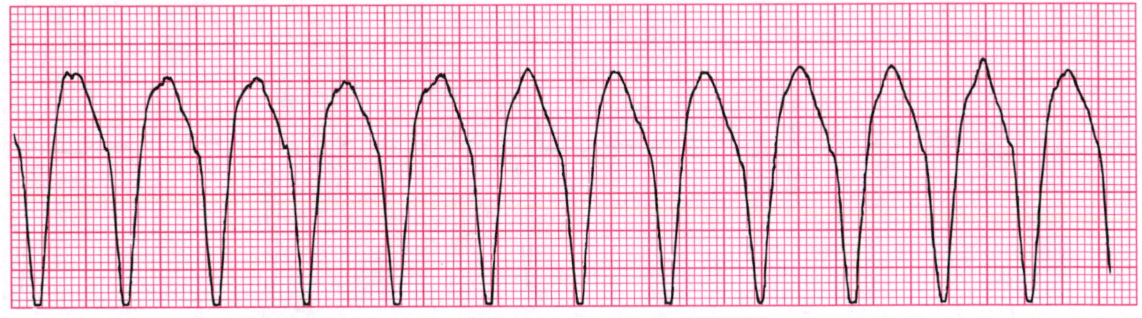

124. QRS complexes ________ Regularity ________ Heart rate ________
P waves ____
PR interval ________ QRS interval ________
Interpretation ____

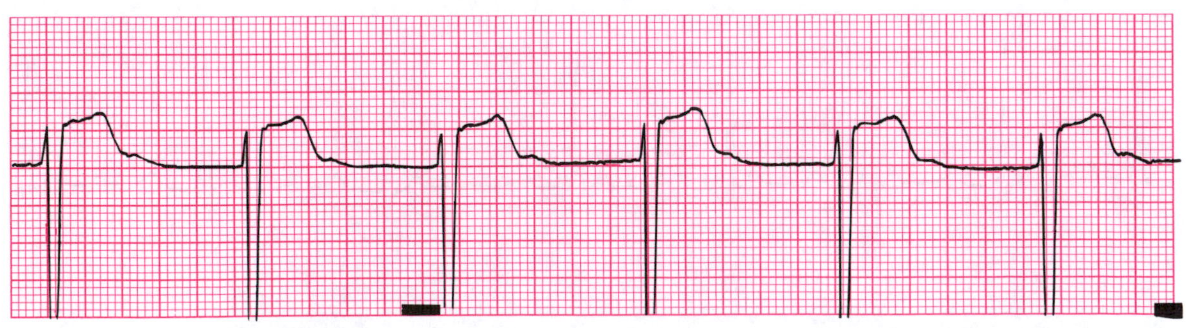

125. QRS complexes ________ Regularity ________ Heart rate ________
P waves ____
PR interval ________ QRS interval ________
Interpretation ____

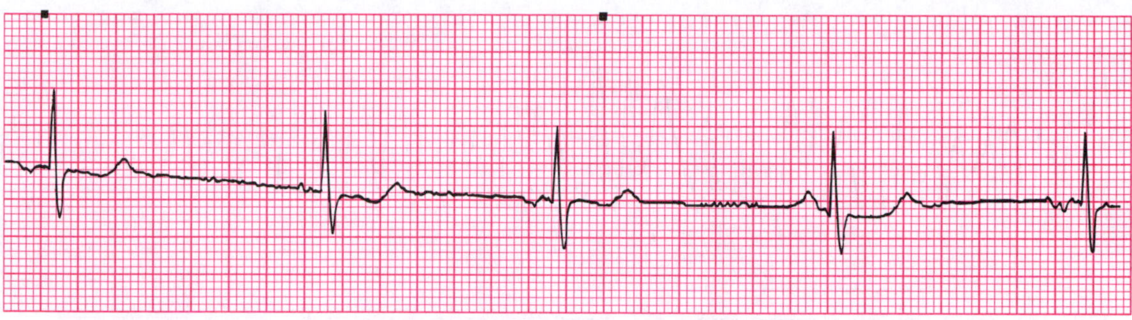

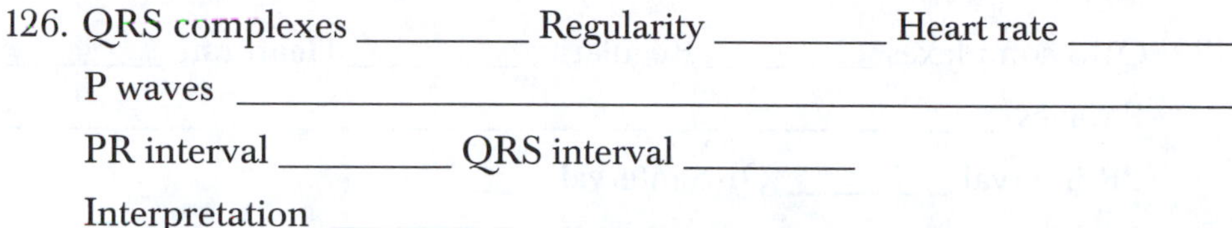

126. QRS complexes ________ Regularity ________ Heart rate ________

P waves ____

PR interval ________ QRS interval ________

Interpretation ____

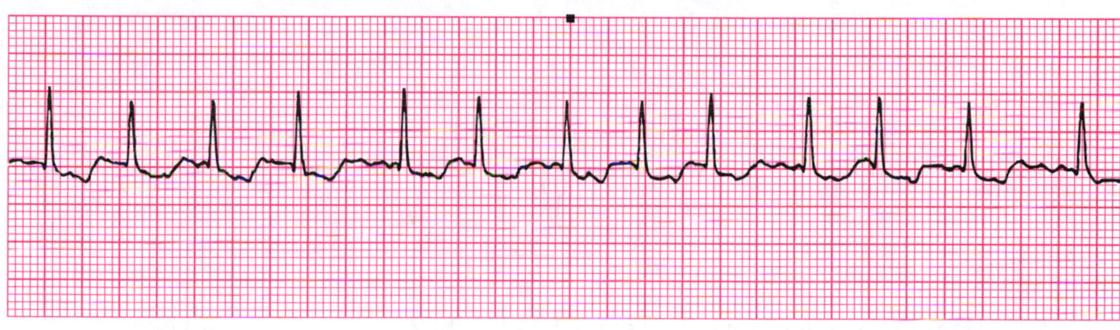

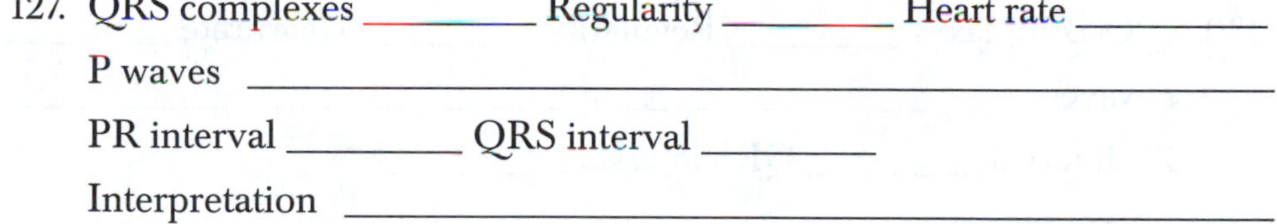

127. QRS complexes ________ Regularity ________ Heart rate ________

P waves ____

PR interval ________ QRS interval ________

Interpretation ____

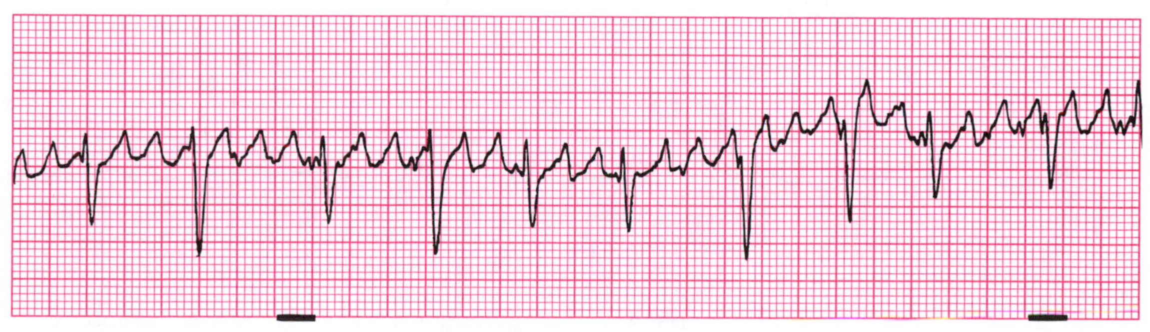

128. QRS complexes ________ Regularity ________ Heart rate ________

P waves ____

PR interval ________ QRS interval ________

Interpretation ____

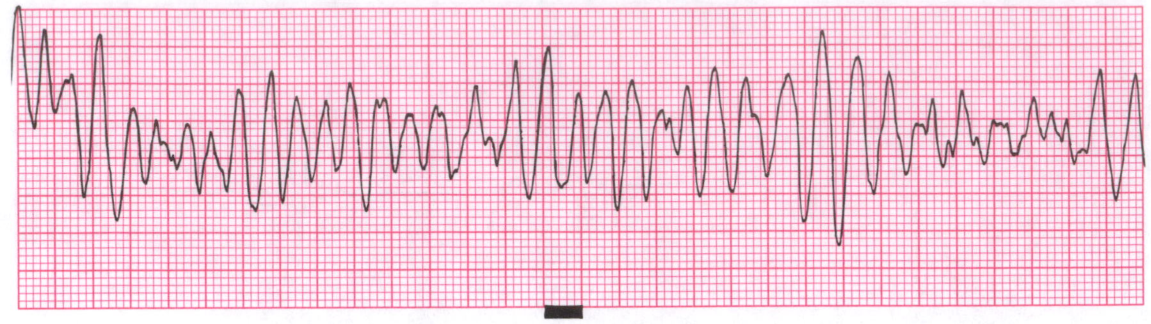

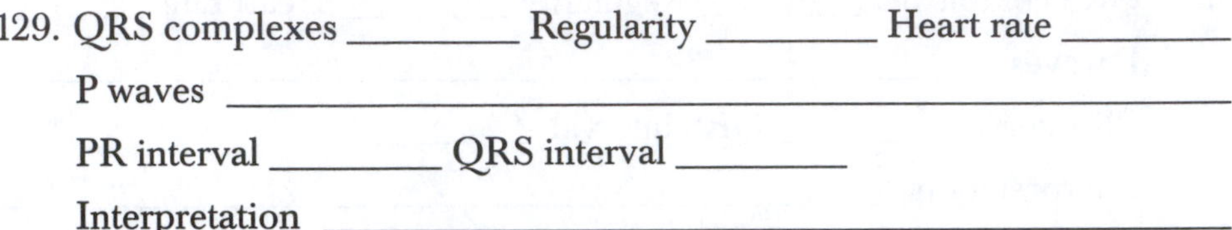

129. QRS complexes ________ Regularity ________ Heart rate ________
P waves ____
PR interval ________ QRS interval ________
Interpretation ____

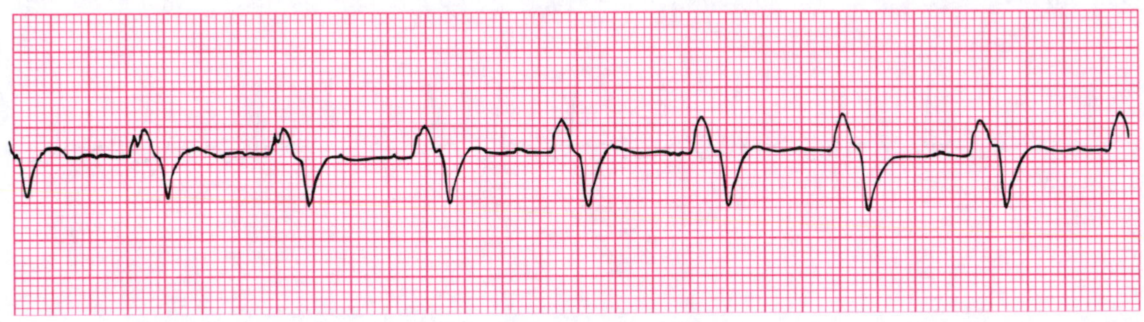

130. QRS complexes ________ Regularity ________ Heart rate ________
P waves ____
PR interval ________ QRS interval ________
Interpretation ____

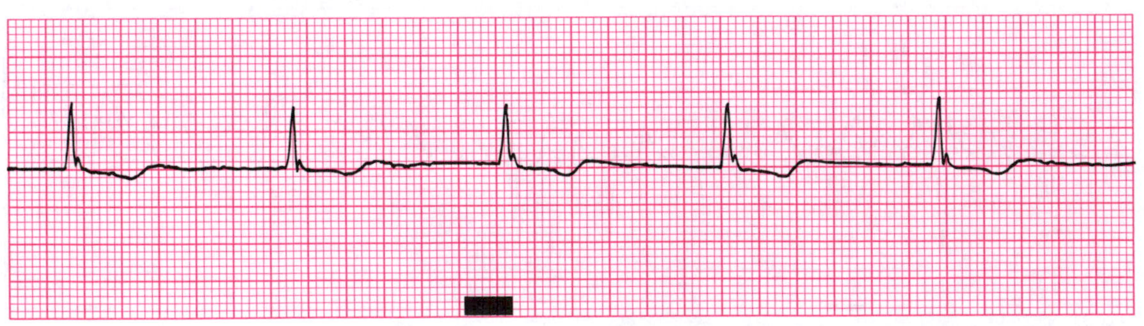

131. QRS complexes ________ Regularity ________ Heart rate ________
P waves ____
PR interval ________ QRS interval ________
Interpretation ____

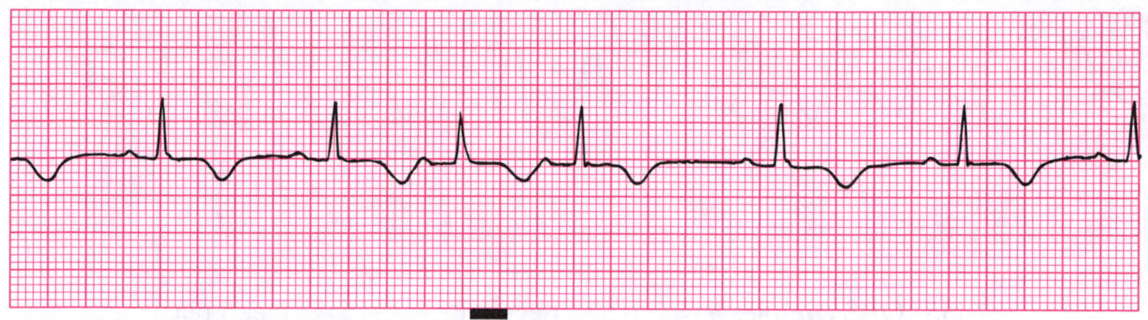

132. QRS complexes ________ Regularity ________ Heart rate ________
P waves ____
PR interval ________ QRS interval ________
Interpretation ____

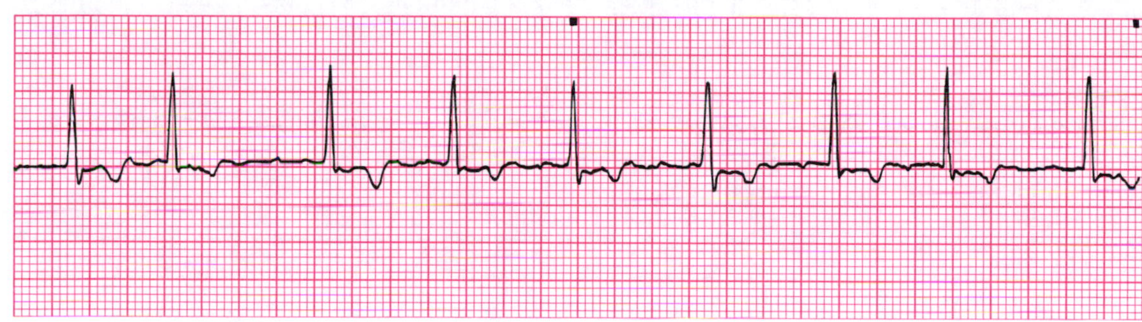

133. QRS complexes ________ Regularity ________ Heart rate ________
P waves ____
PR interval ________ QRS interval ________
Interpretation ____

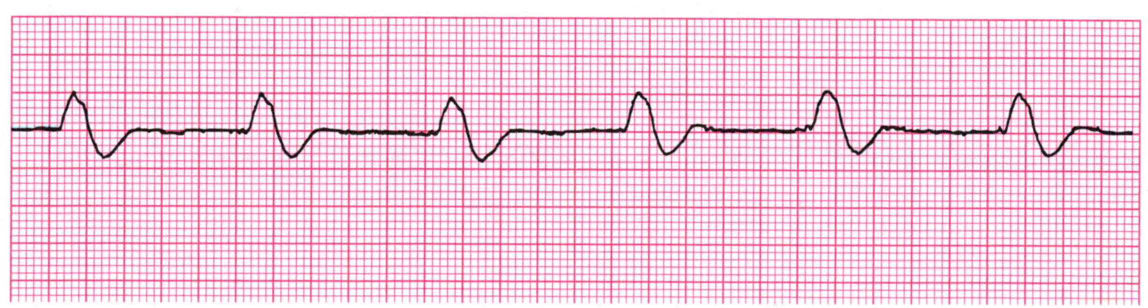

134. QRS complexes ________ Regularity ________ Heart rate ________
P waves ____
PR interval ________ QRS interval ________
Interpretation ____

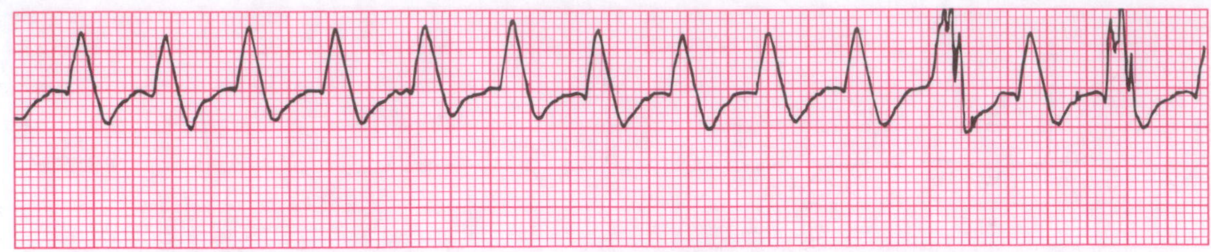

135. QRS complexes ________ Regularity ________ Heart rate __________
P waves ____
PR interval ________ QRS interval ________
Interpretation ____

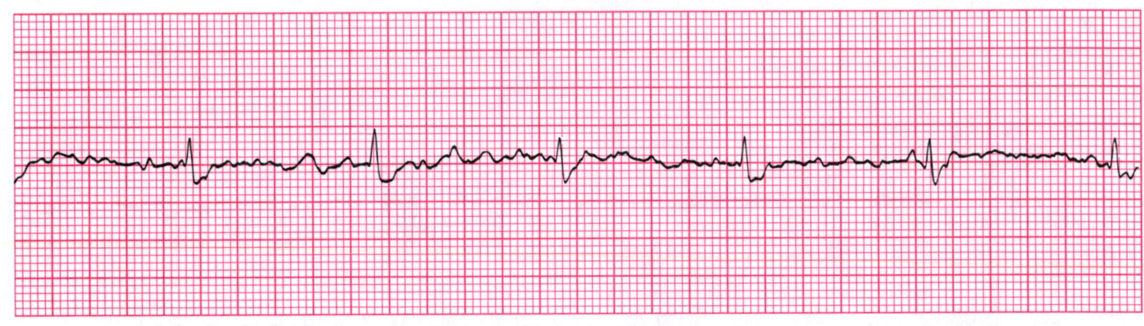

136. QRS complexes ________ Regularity ________ Heart rate __________
P waves ____
PR interval _____ QRS interval _____
Interpretation ____

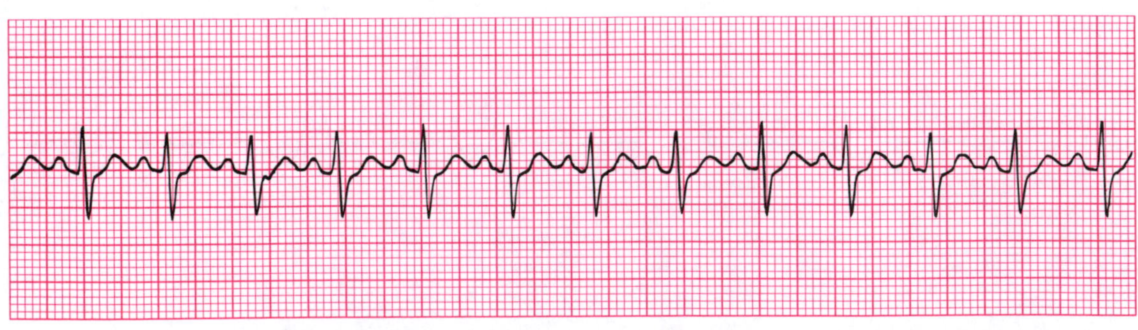

137. QRS complexes ________ Regularity __________ Heart rate __________
P waves ____
PR interval ________ QRS interval ________
Interpretation ____

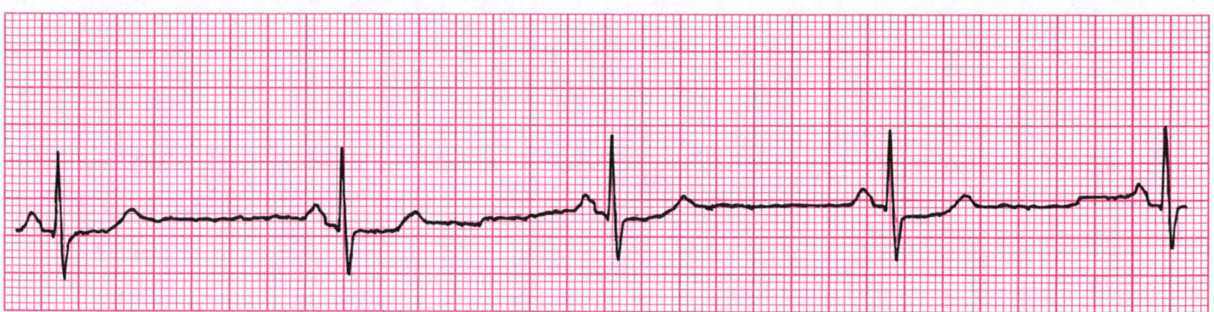

138. QRS complexes ________ Regularity ________ Heart rate ________

P waves ____

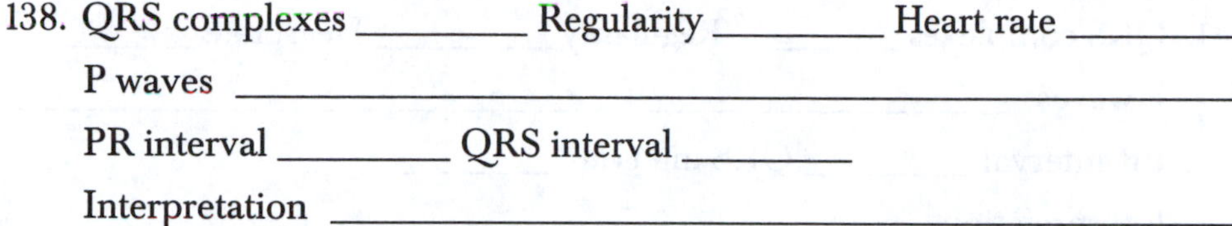

PR interval ________ QRS interval ________

Interpretation ____

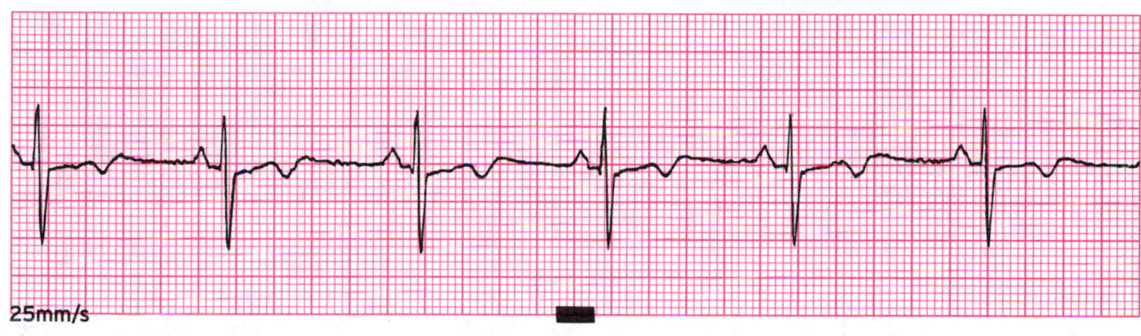

139. QRS complexes ________ Regularity ________ Heart rate ________

P waves ____

PR interval ________ QRS interval ________

Interpretation ____

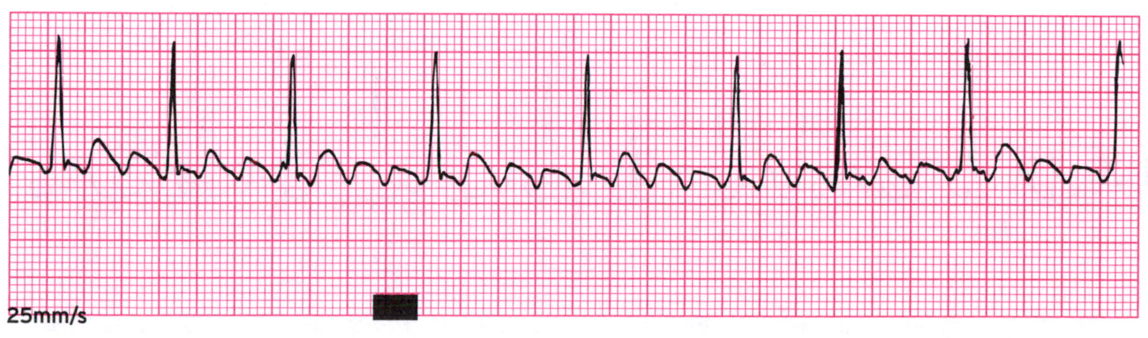

140. QRS complexes ________ Regularity ________ Heart rate ________

P waves ____

PR interval ________ QRS interval ________

Interpretation ____

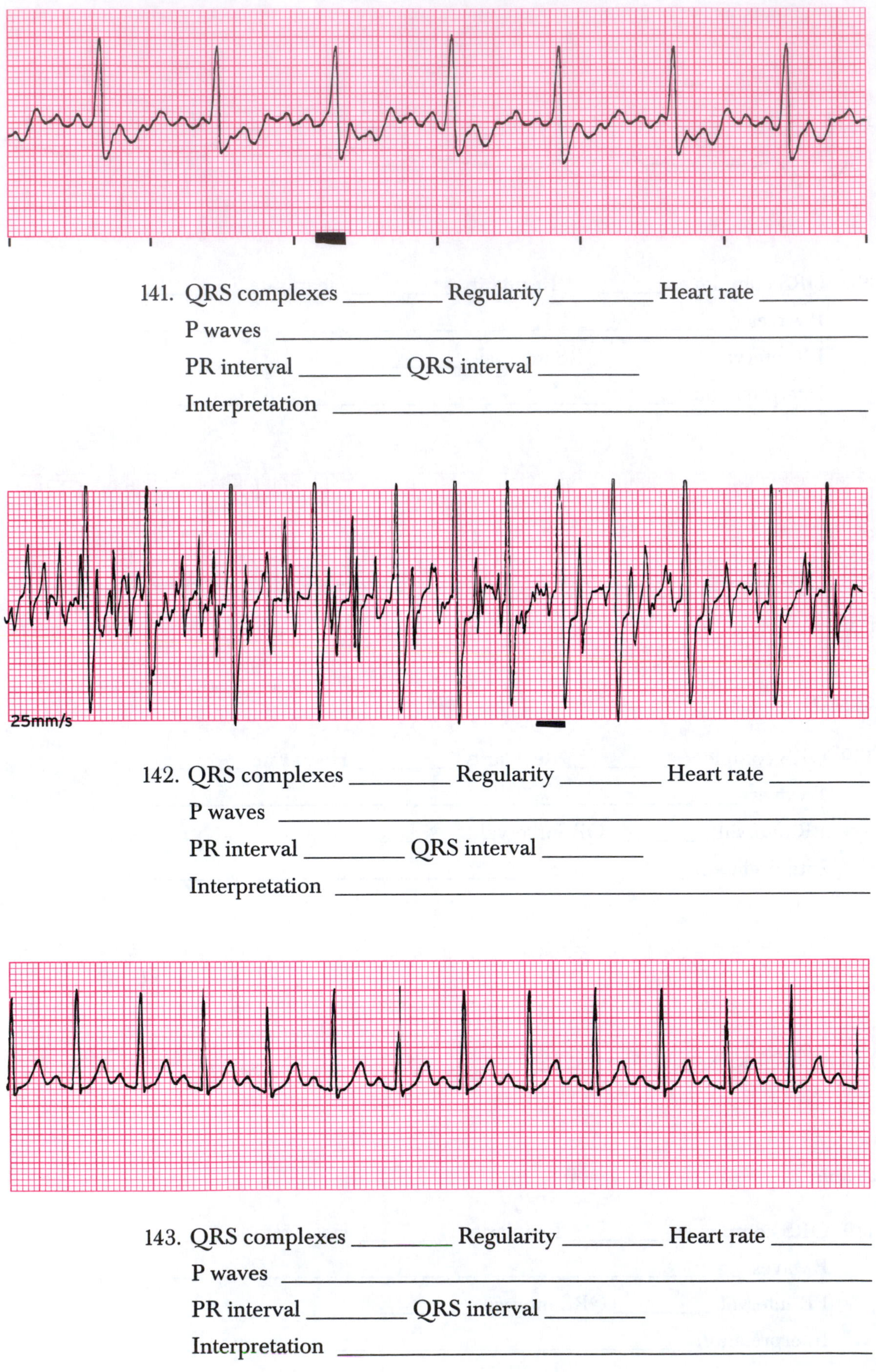

141. QRS complexes ________ Regularity ________ Heart rate ________
P waves ______________________________
PR interval ________ QRS interval ________
Interpretation ______________________________

142. QRS complexes ________ Regularity ________ Heart rate ________
P waves ______________________________
PR interval ________ QRS interval ________
Interpretation ______________________________

143. QRS complexes ________ Regularity ________ Heart rate ________
P waves ______________________________
PR interval ________ QRS interval ________
Interpretation ______________________________

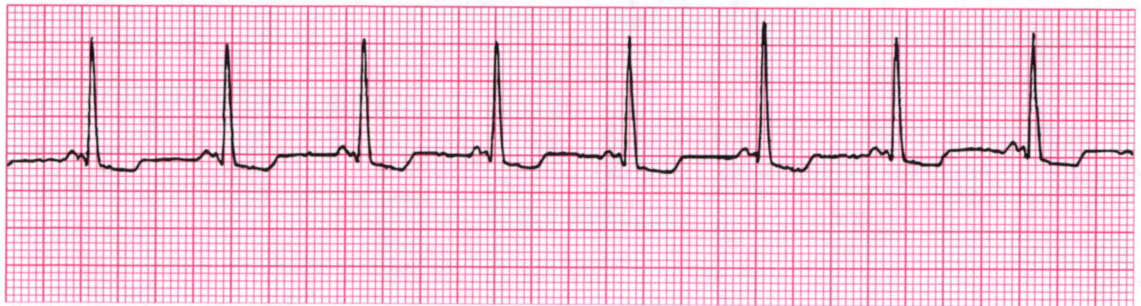

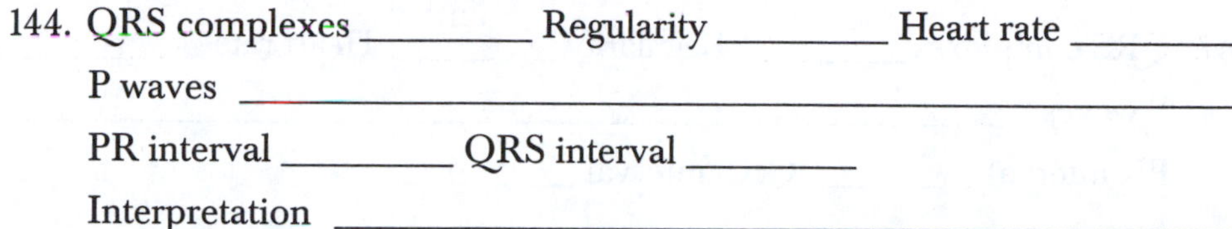

144. QRS complexes ________ Regularity ________ Heart rate ________
P waves ____
PR interval ________ QRS interval ________
Interpretation ____

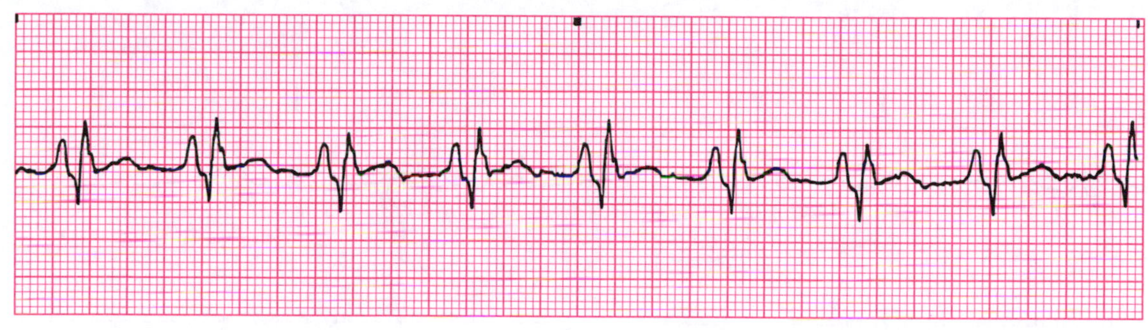

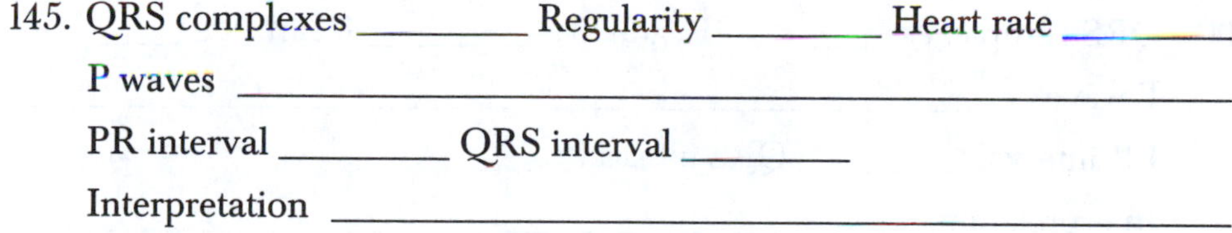

145. QRS complexes ________ Regularity ________ Heart rate ________
P waves ____
PR interval ________ QRS interval ________
Interpretation ____

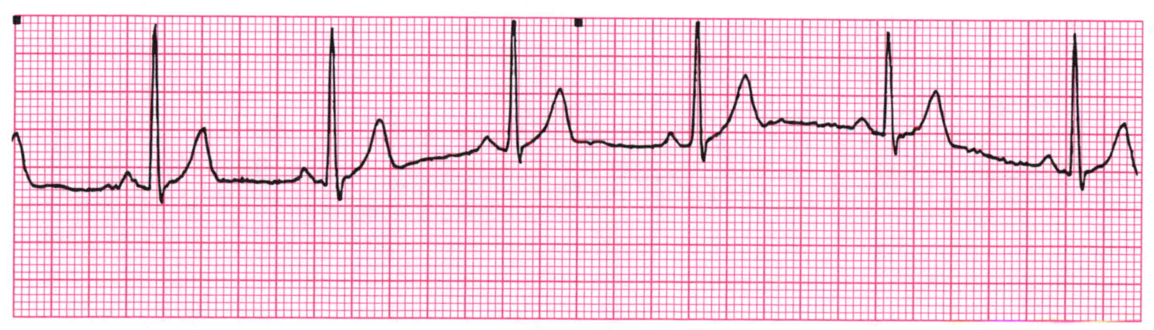

146. QRS complexes ________ Regularity ________ Heart rate ________
P waves ____
PR interval ________ QRS interval ________
Interpretation ____

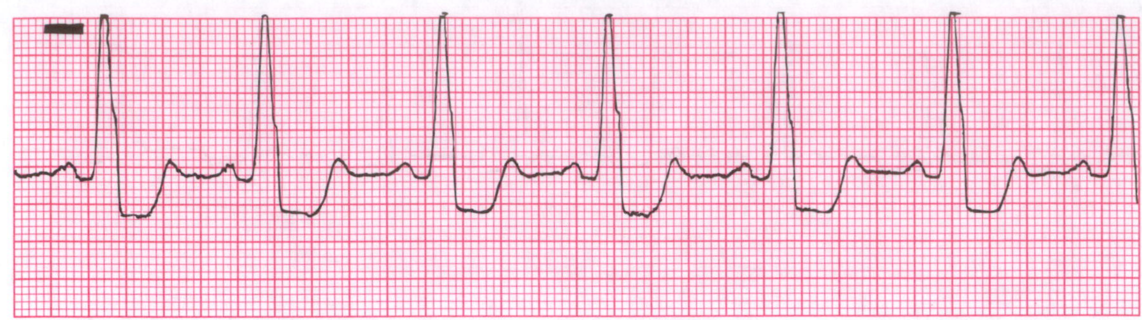

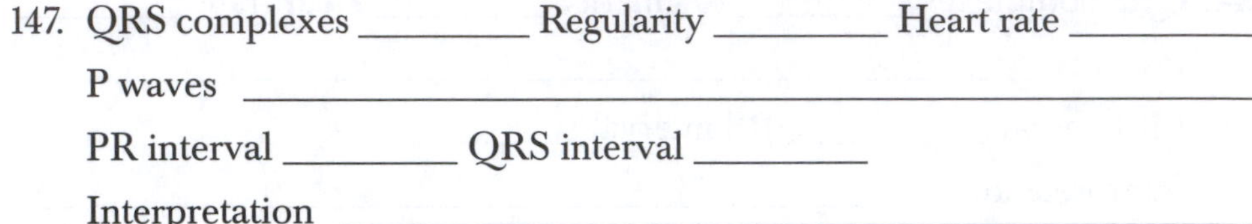

147. QRS complexes ________ Regularity ________ Heart rate ________
P waves ____
PR interval ________ QRS interval ________
Interpretation ____

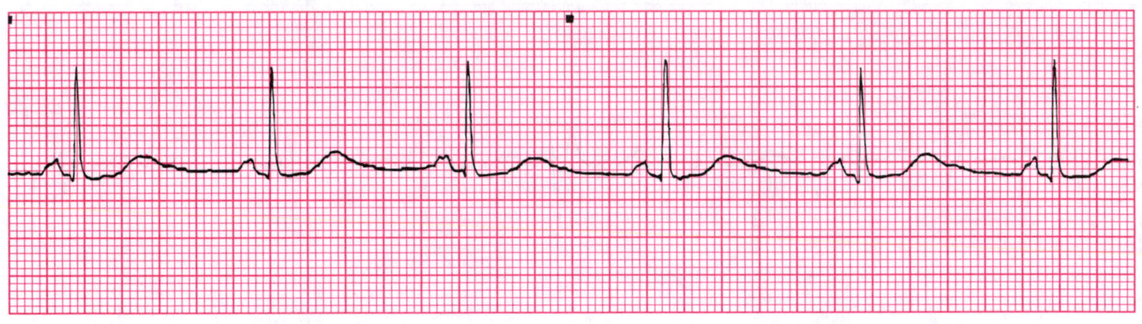

148. QRS complexes ________ Regularity ________ Heart rate ________
P waves ____
PR interval ________ QRS interval ________
Interpretation ____

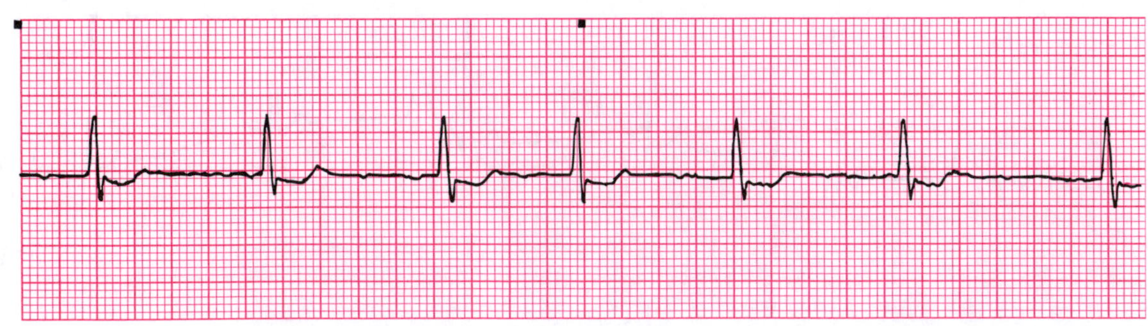

149. QRS complexes ________ Regularity ________ Heart rate ________
P waves ____
PR interval ________ QRS interval ________
Interpretation ____

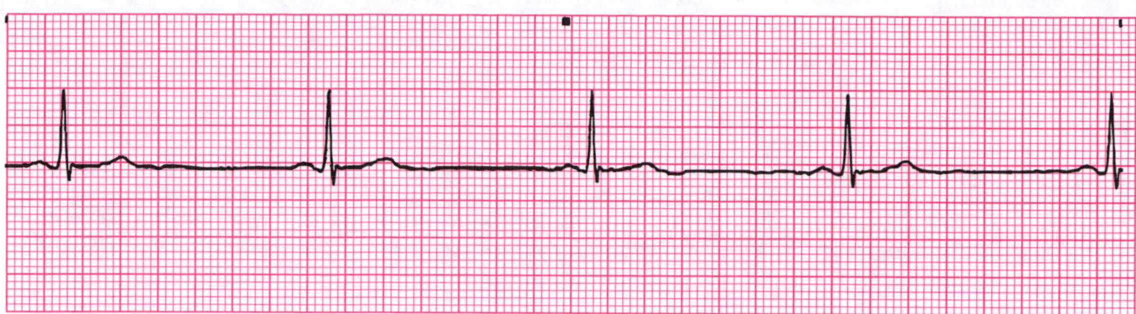

150. QRS complexes ________ Regularity ________ Heart rate ________
P waves ____
PR interval ________ QRS interval ________
Interpretation ____

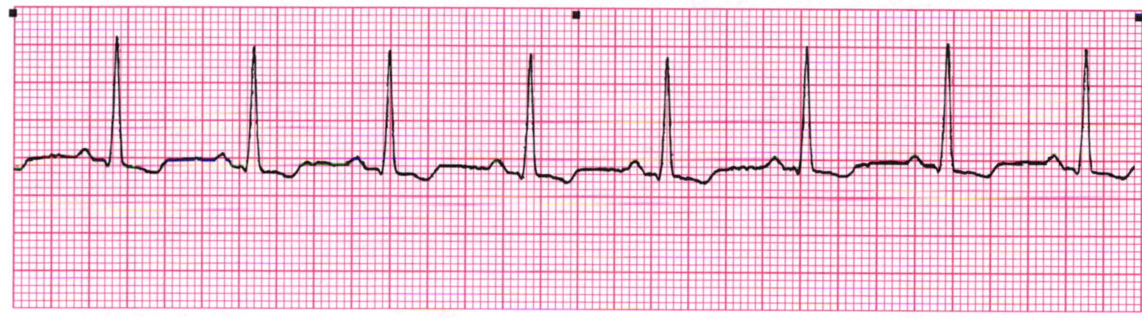

151. QRS complexes ________ Regularity ________ Heart rate ________
P waves ____
PR interval ________ QRS interval ________
Interpretation ____

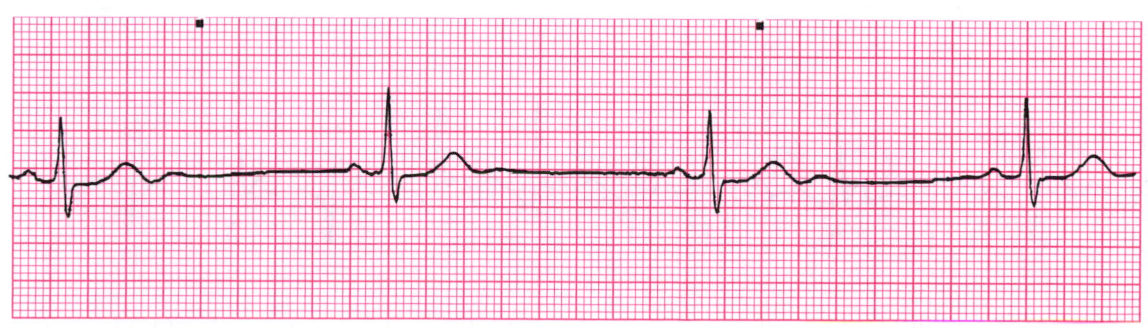

152. QRS complexes ________ Regularity ________ Heart rate ________
P waves ____
PR interval ________ QRS interval ________
Interpretation ____

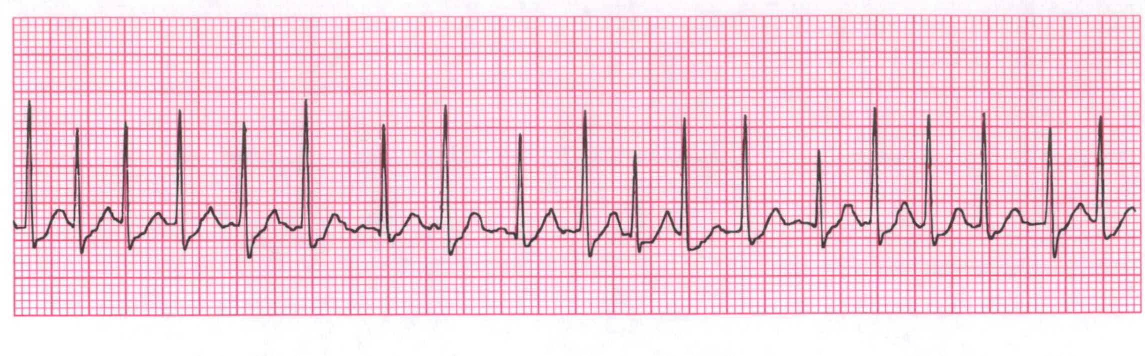

153. QRS complexes ________ Regularity ________ Heart rate ________
P waves ________________________________
PR interval ________ QRS interval ________
Interpretation ________________________________

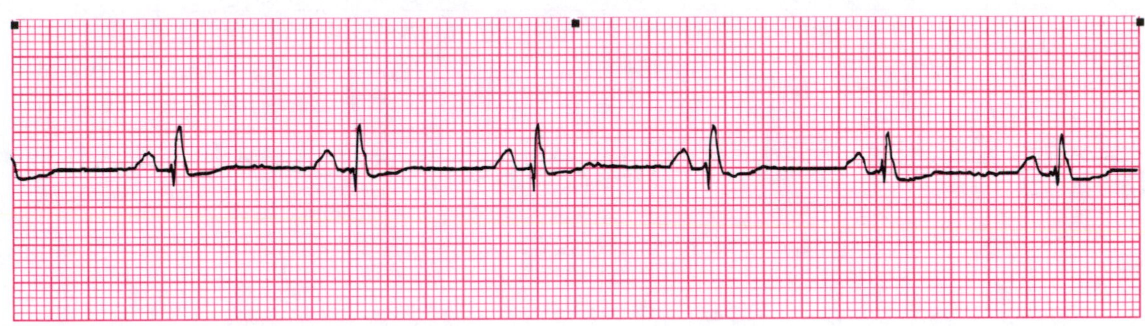

154. QRS complexes ________ Regularity ________ Heart rate ________
P waves ________________________________
PR interval ________ QRS interval ________
Interpretation ________________________________

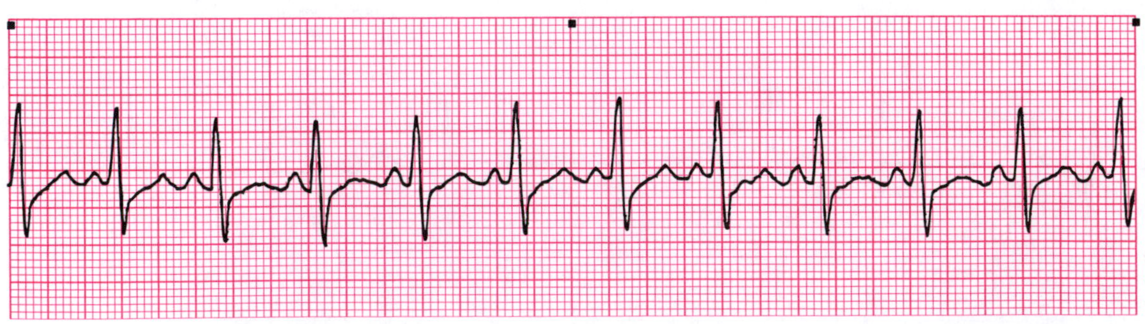

155. QRS complexes ________ Regularity ________ Heart rate ________
P waves ________________________________
PR interval ________ QRS interval ________
Interpretation ________________________________

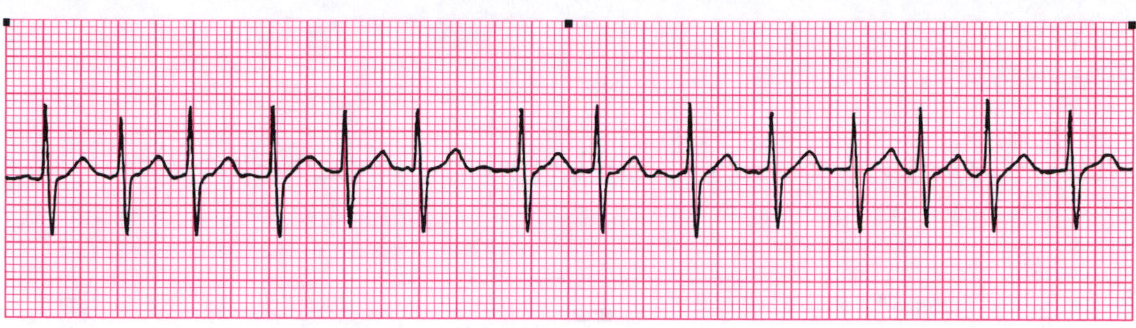

156. QRS complexes ________ Regularity ________ Heart rate ________

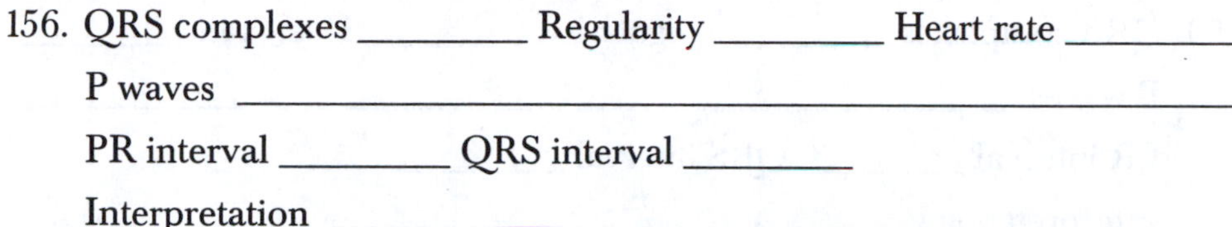

P waves ____

PR interval ________ QRS interval ________

Interpretation ____

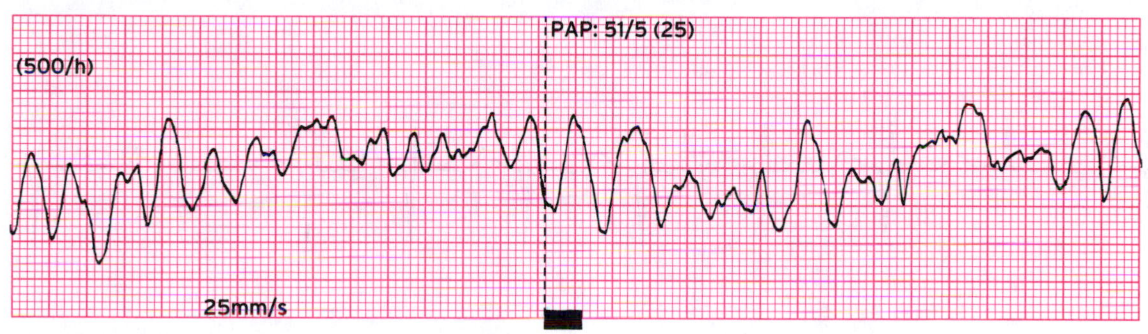

157. QRS complexes ________ Regularity ________ Heart rate ________

P waves ____

PR interval ________ QRS interval ________

Interpretation ____

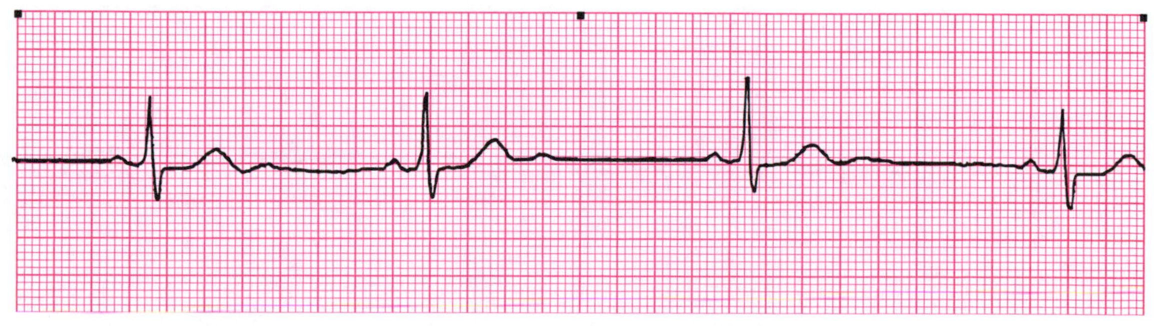

158. QRS complexes ________ Regularity ________ Heart rate ________

P waves ____

PR interval ________ QRS interval ________

Interpretation ____

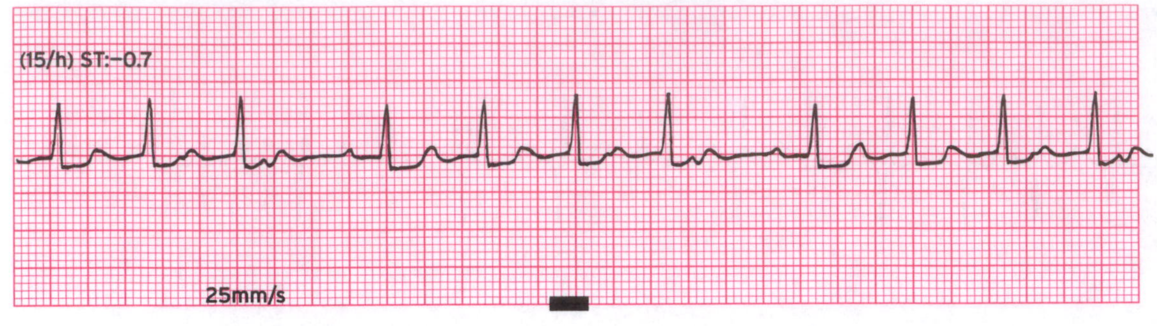

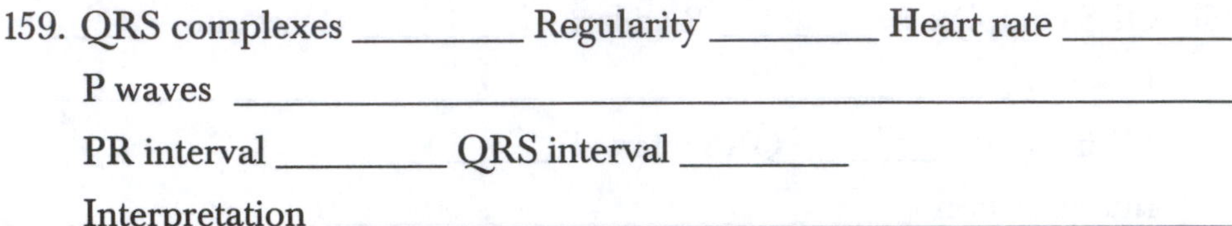

159. QRS complexes ________ Regularity ________ Heart rate ________

P waves ____

PR interval ________ QRS interval ________

Interpretation ____

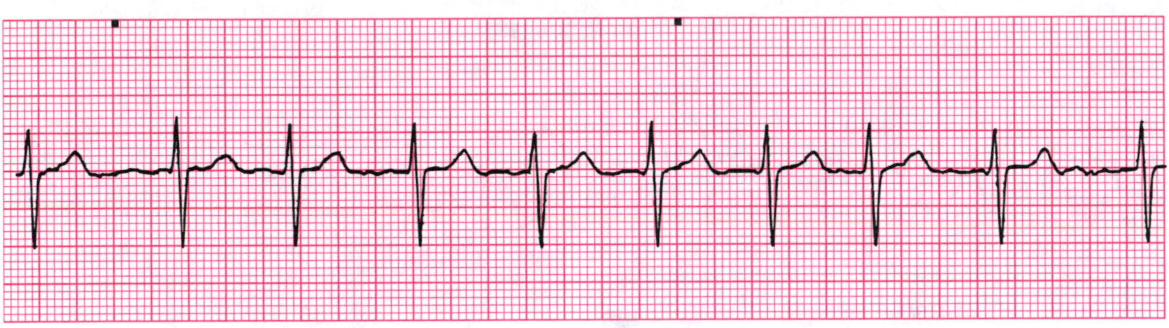

160. QRS complexes ________ Regularity ________ Heart rate ________

P waves ____

PR interval ________ QRS interval ________

Interpretation ____

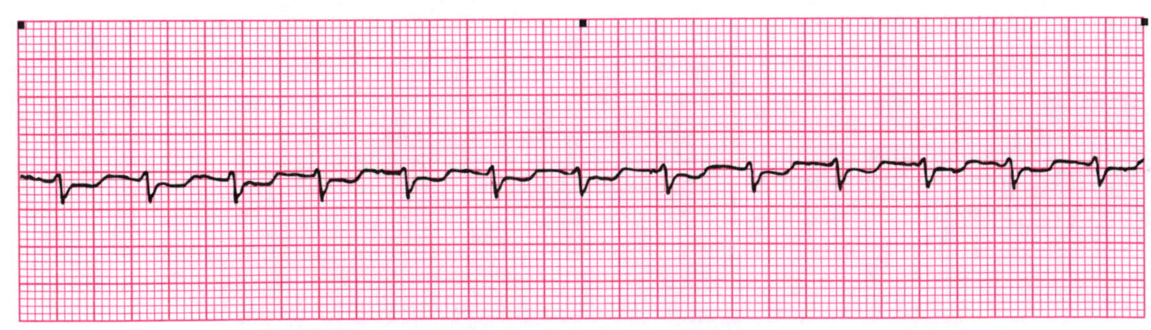

161. QRS complexes ________ Regularity ________ Heart rate ________

P waves ____

PR interval ________ QRS interval ________

Interpretation ____

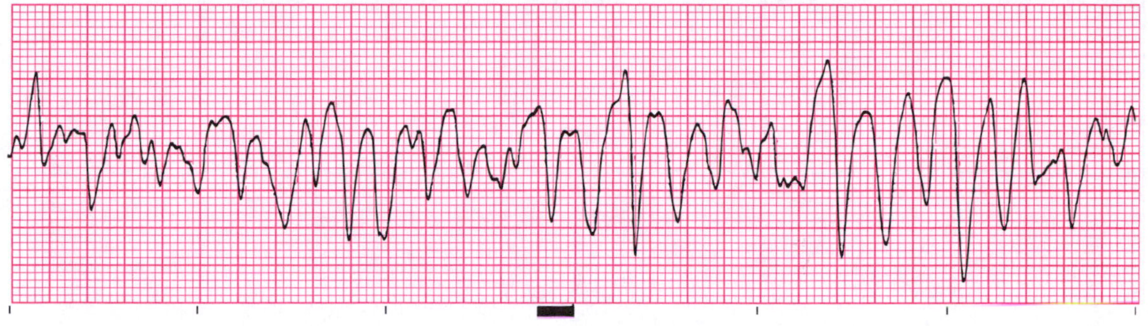

162. QRS complexes ________ Regularity ________ Heart rate ________
P waves ____
PR interval ________ QRS interval ________
Interpretation ____

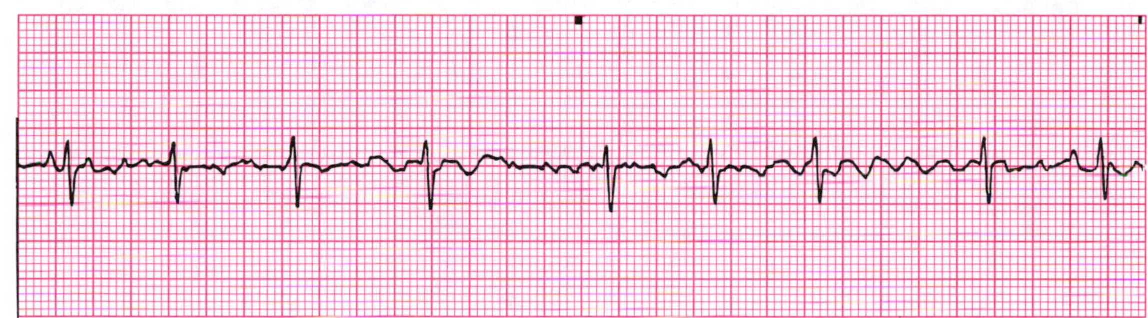

163. QRS complexes ________ Regularity ________ Heart rate ________
P waves ____
PR interval ________ QRS interval ________
Interpretation ____

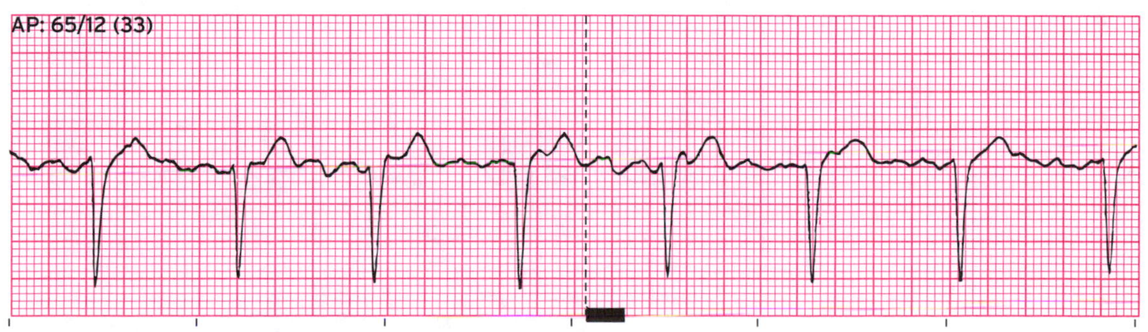

164. QRS complexes ________ Regularity ________ Heart rate ________
P waves ____
PR interval ________ QRS interval ________
Interpretation ____

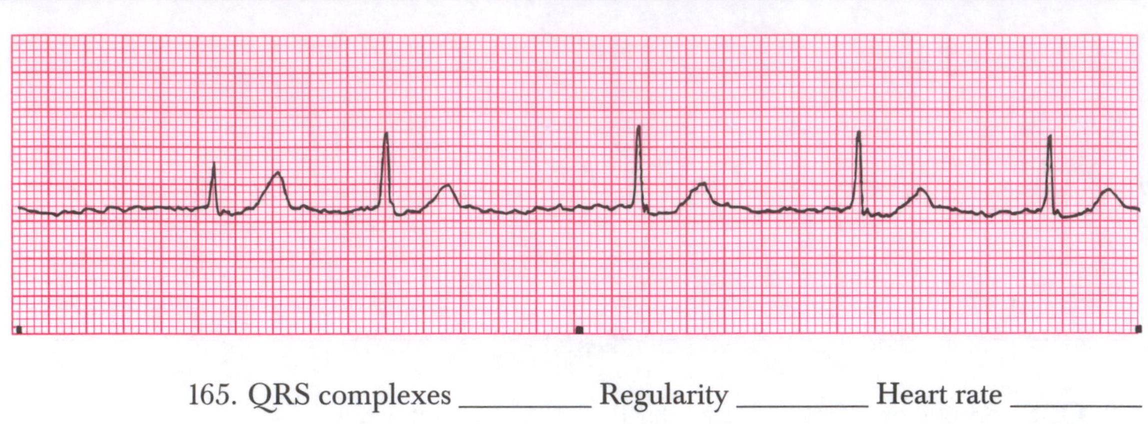

165. QRS complexes ________ Regularity ________ Heart rate ________
P waves ____
PR interval ________ QRS interval ________
Interpretation ____

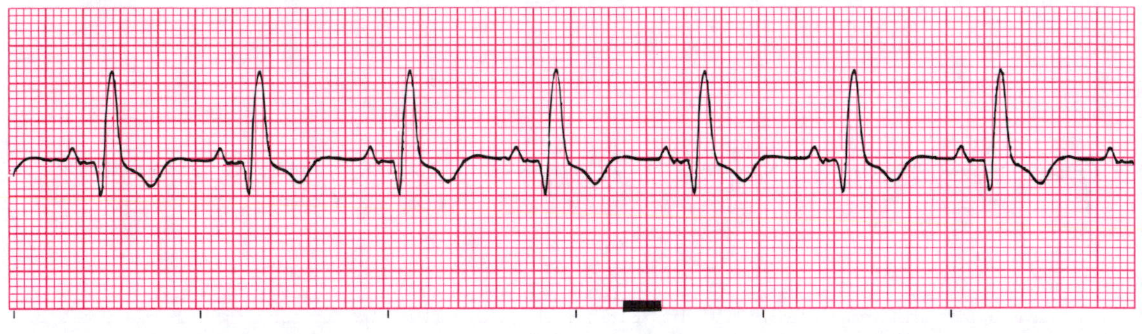

166. QRS complexes ________ Regularity ________ Heart rate ________
P waves ____
PR interval ________ QRS interval ________
Interpretation ____

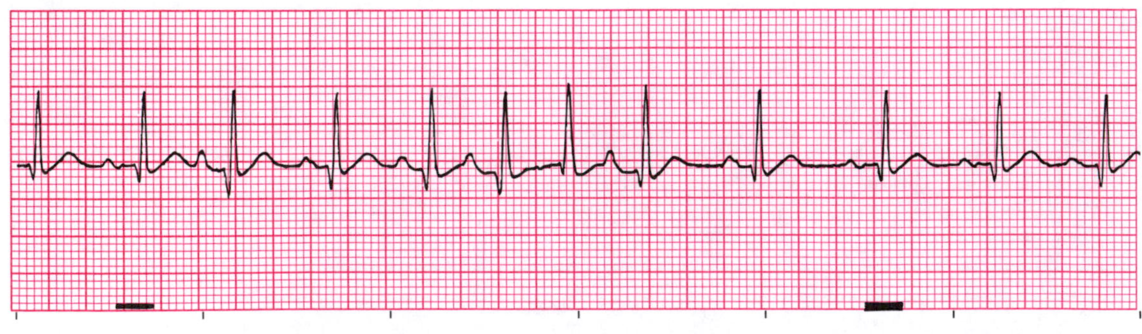

167. QRS complexes ________ Regularity ________ Heart rate ________
P waves ____
PR interval ________ QRS interval ________
Interpretation ____

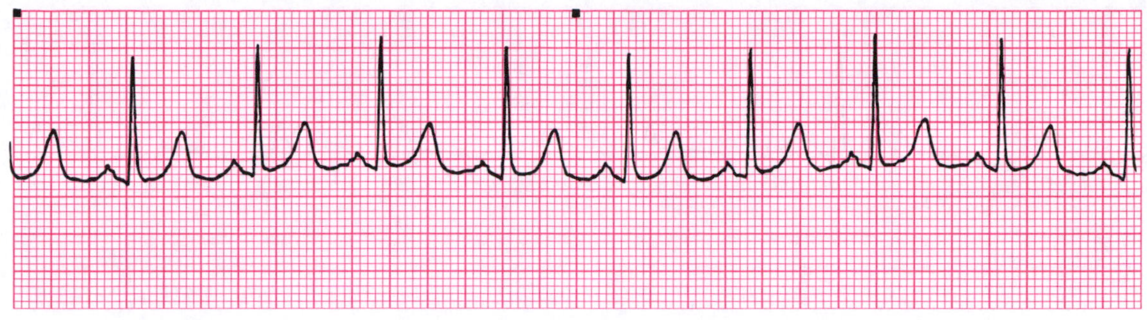

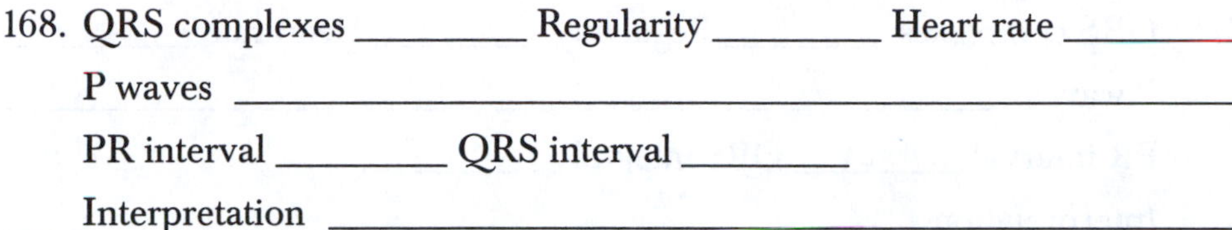

168. QRS complexes ________ Regularity ________ Heart rate ________

P waves ____

PR interval ________ QRS interval ________

Interpretation ____

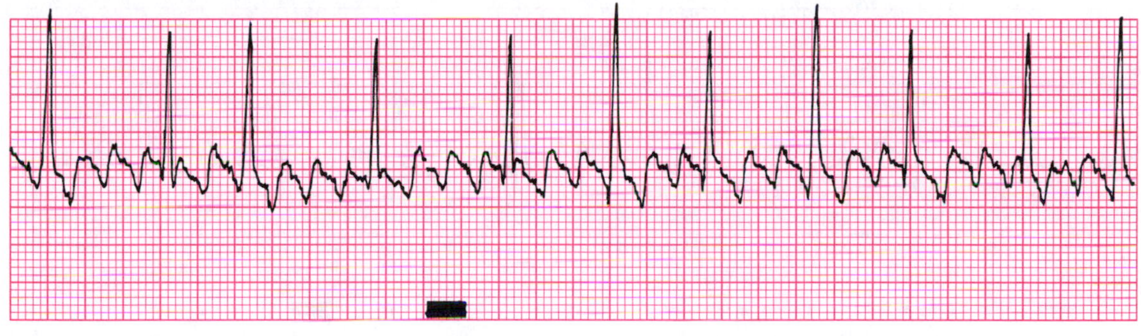

169. QRS complexes ________ Regularity ________ Heart rate ________

P waves ____

PR interval ________ QRS interval ________

Interpretation ____

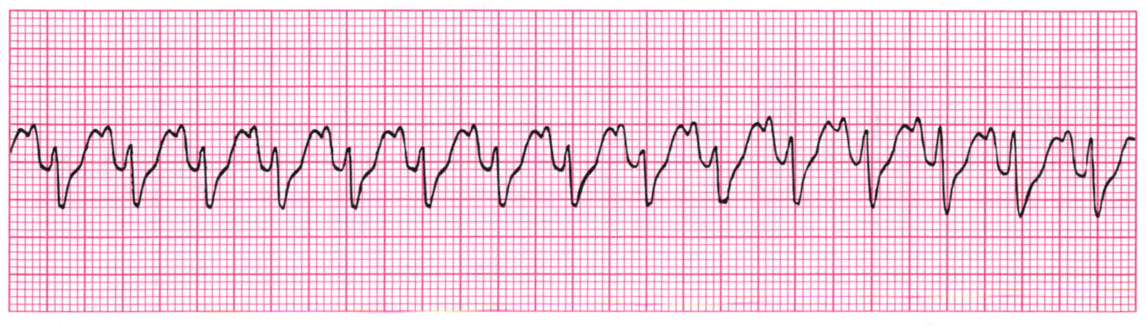

170. QRS complexes ________ Regularity ________ Heart rate ________

P waves ____

PR interval ________ QRS interval ________

Interpretation ____

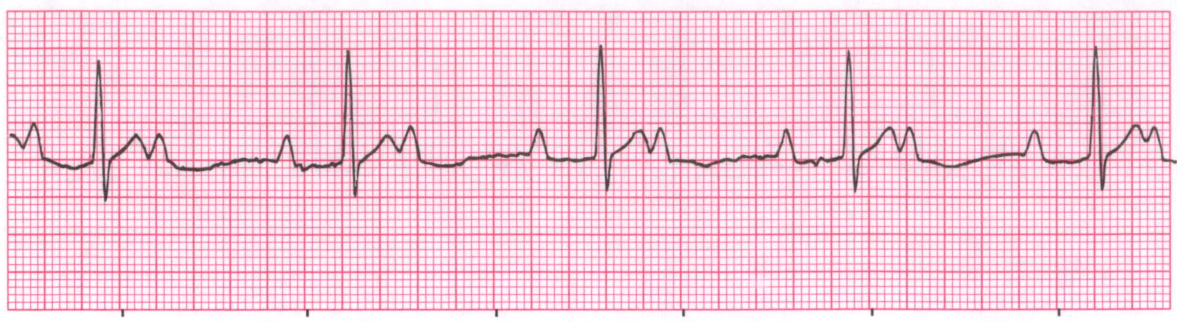

171. QRS complexes ________ Regularity ________ Heart rate ________
P waves ____
PR interval ________ QRS interval ________
Interpretation ____

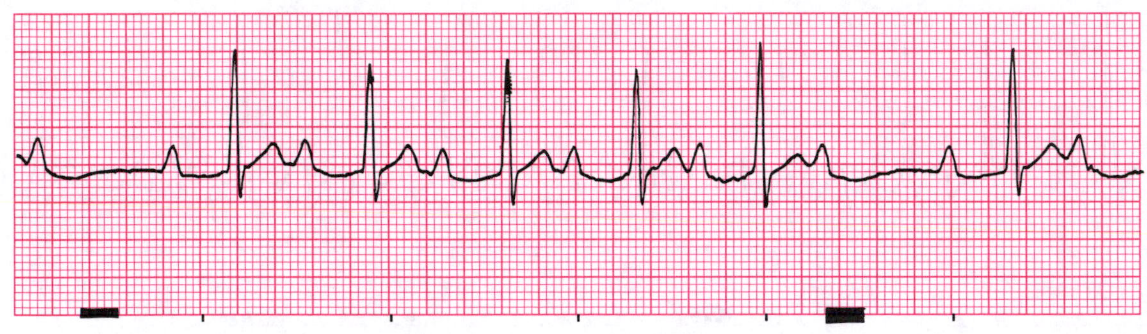

172. QRS complexes ________ Regularity ________ Heart rate ________
P waves ____
PR interval ________ QRS interval ________
Interpretation ____

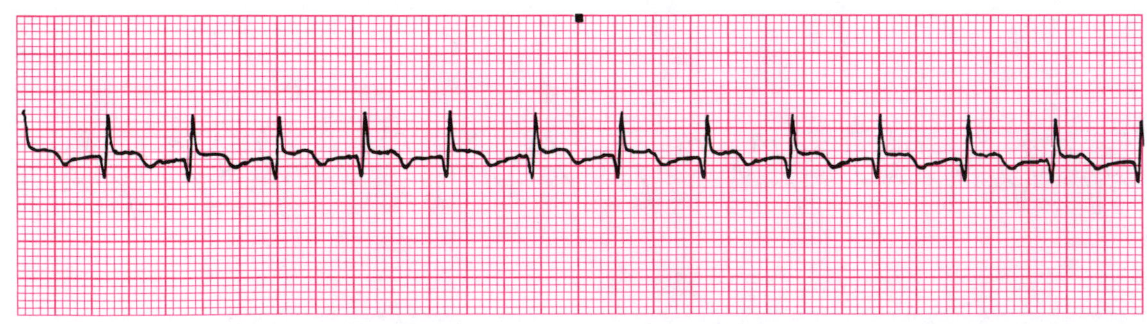

173. QRS complexes ________ Regularity ________ Heart rate ________
P waves ____
PR interval ________ QRS interval ________
Interpretation ____

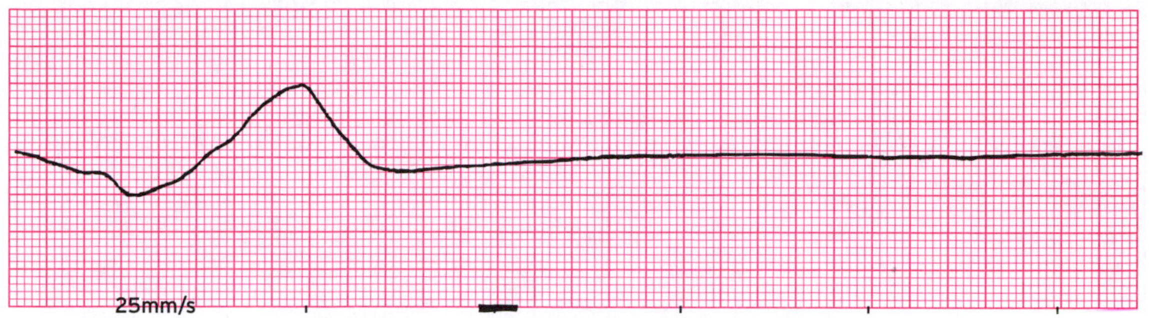

174. QRS complexes ________ Regularity ________ Heart rate ________
P waves ________
PR interval ________ QRS interval ________
Interpretation ________

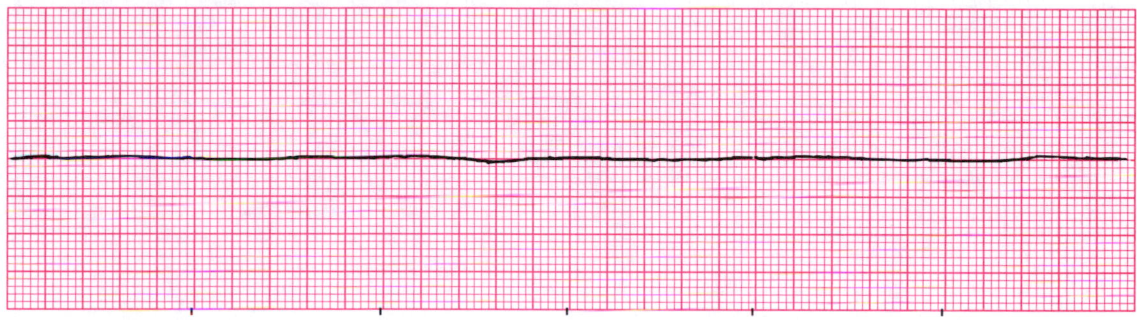

175. QRS complexes ________ Regularity ________ Heart rate ________
P waves ________
PR interval ________ QRS interval ________
Interpretation ________

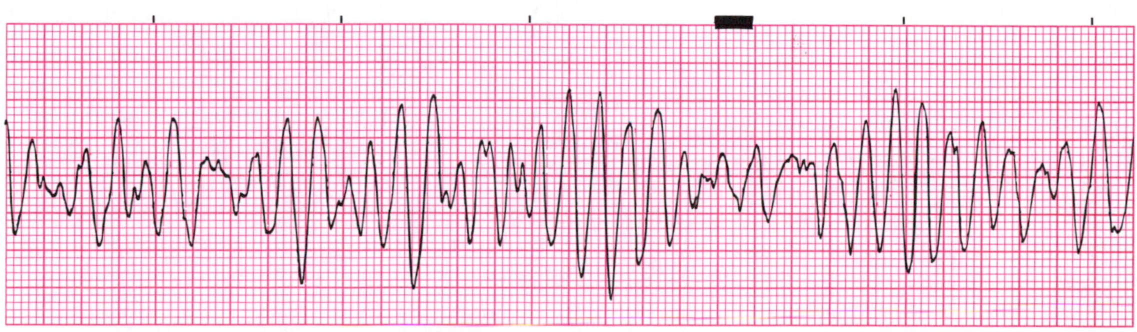

176. QRS complexes ________ Regularity ________ Heart rate ________
P waves ________
PR interval ________ QRS interval ________
Interpretation ________

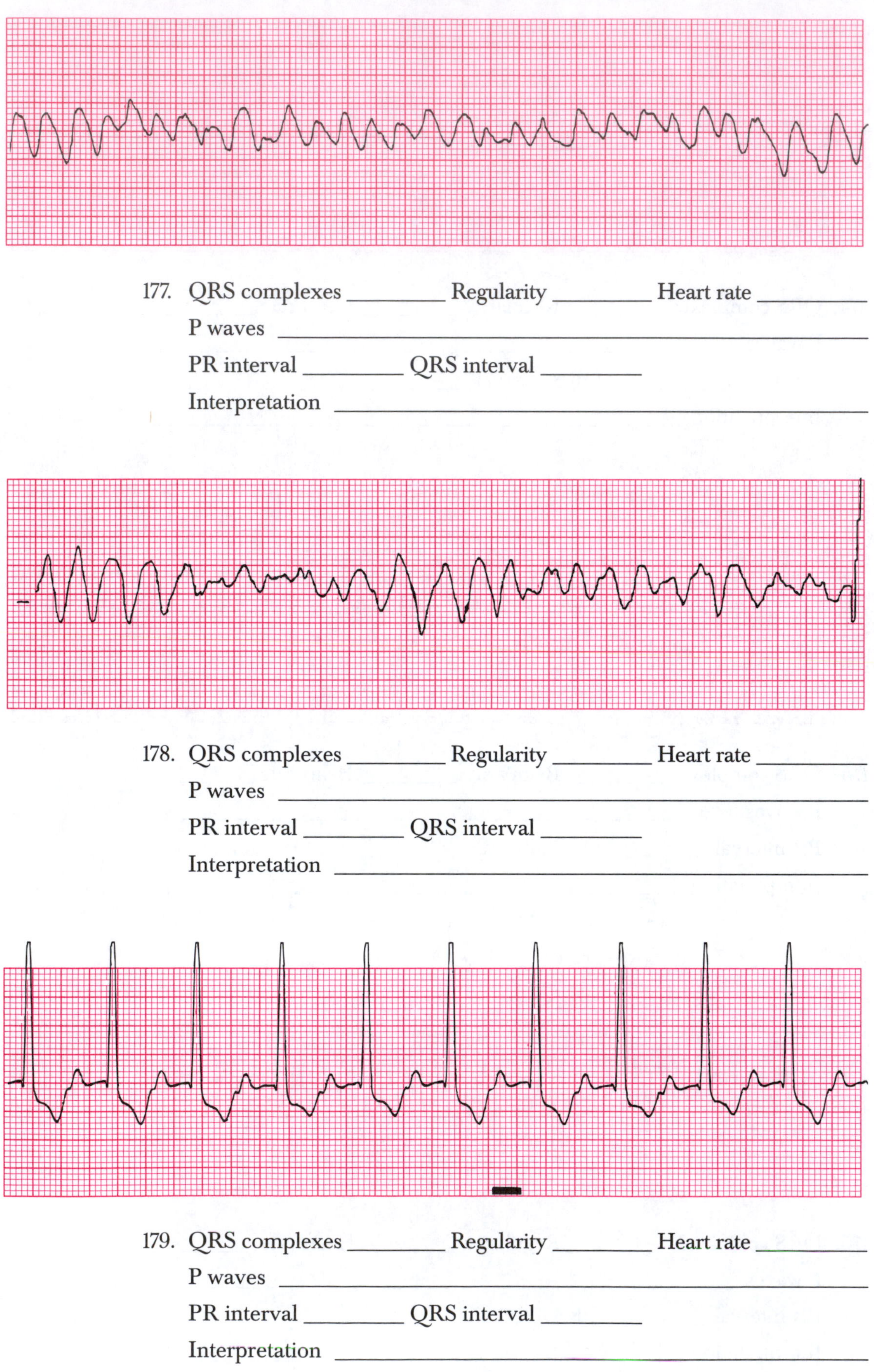

177. QRS complexes ________ Regularity ________ Heart rate ________
P waves ________
PR interval ________ QRS interval ________
Interpretation ________

178. QRS complexes ________ Regularity ________ Heart rate ________
P waves ________
PR interval ________ QRS interval ________
Interpretation ________

179. QRS complexes ________ Regularity ________ Heart rate ________
P waves ________
PR interval ________ QRS interval ________
Interpretation ________

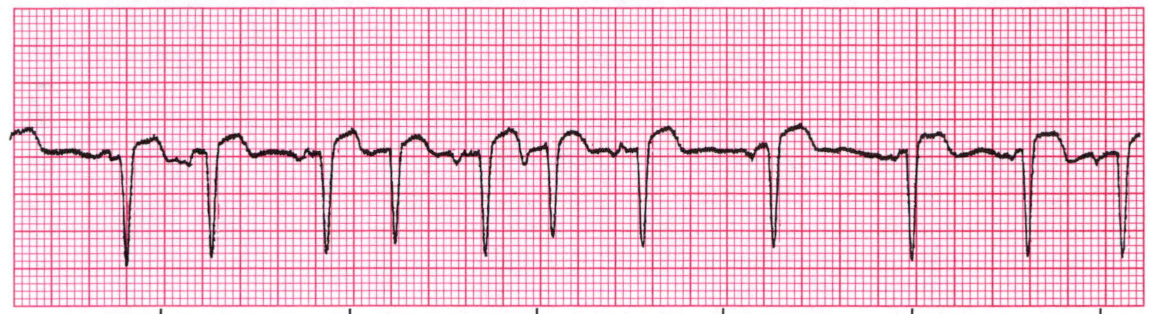

180. QRS complexes ________ Regularity ________ Heart rate ________
P waves ____
PR interval ________ QRS interval ________
Interpretation ____

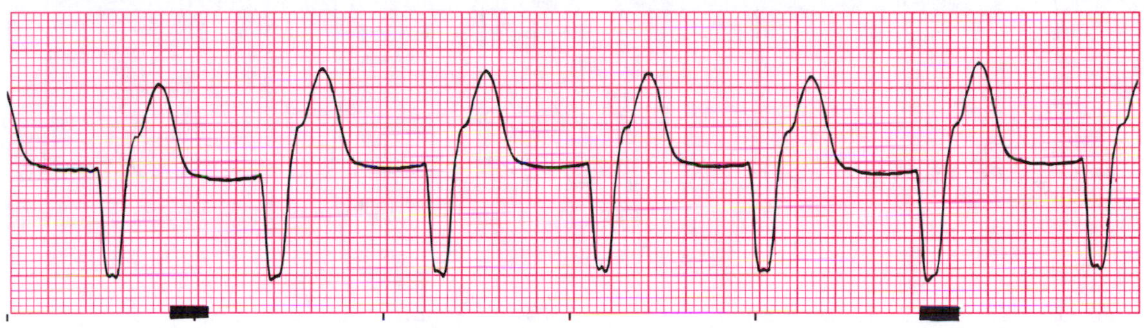

181. QRS complexes ________ Regularity ________ Heart rate ________
P waves ____
PR interval ________ QRS interval ________
Interpretation ____

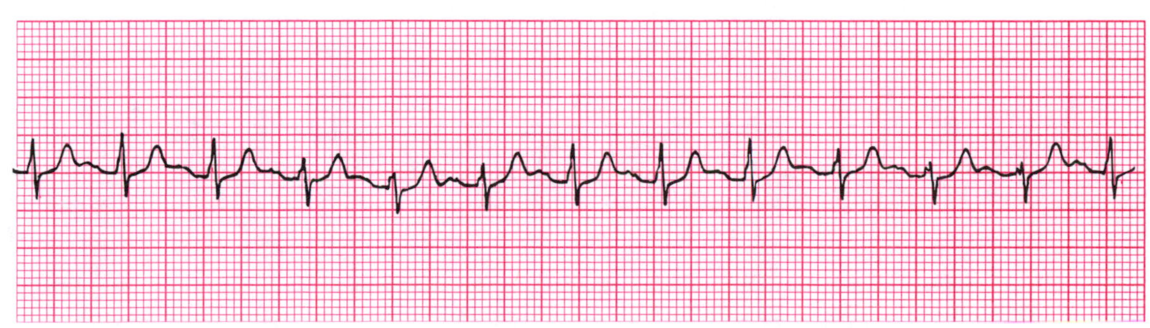

182. QRS complexes ________ Regularity ________ Heart rate ________
P waves ____
PR interval ________ QRS interval ________
Interpretation ____

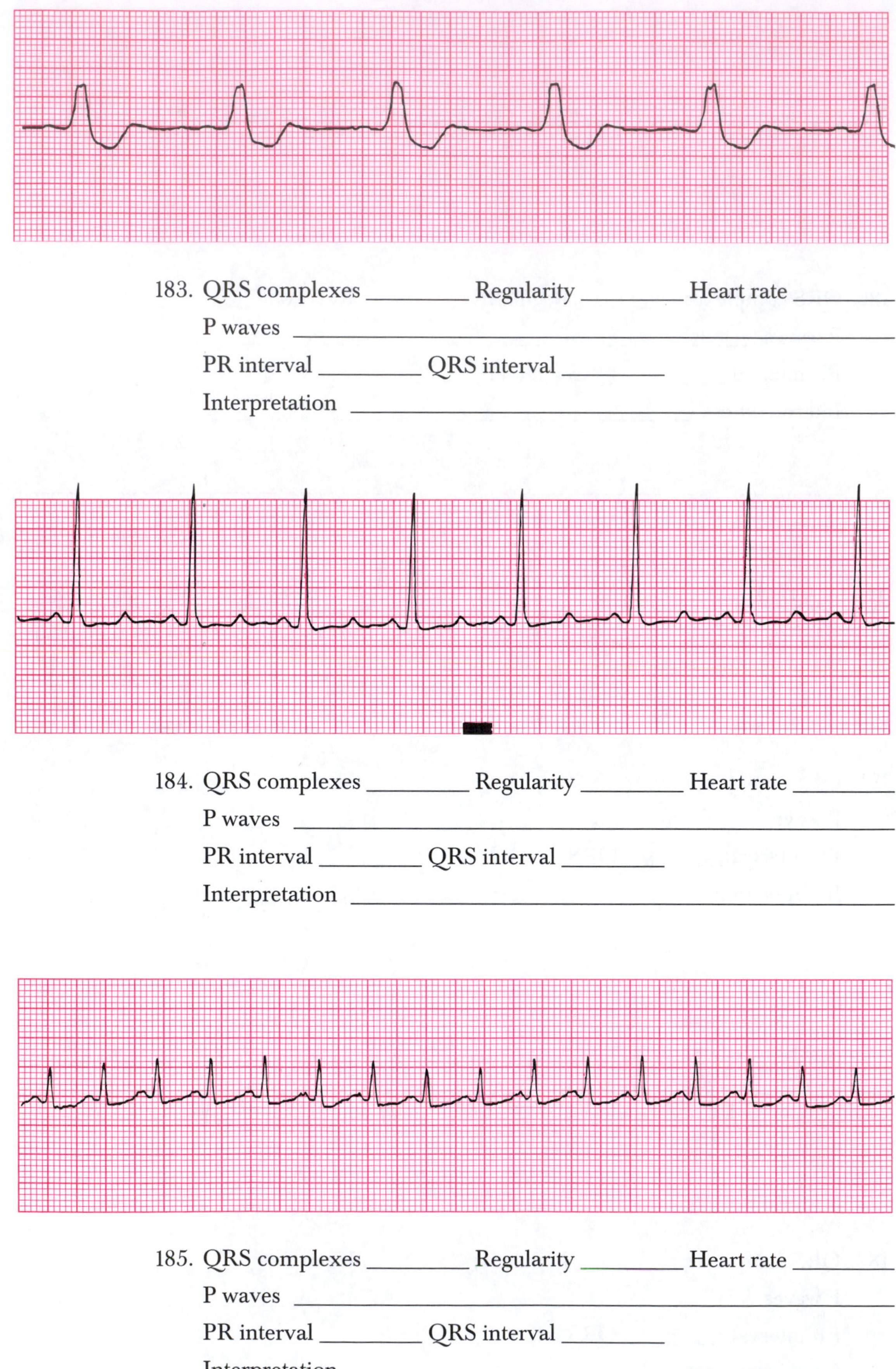

183. QRS complexes ________ Regularity ________ Heart rate ________
P waves ____
PR interval ________ QRS interval ________
Interpretation ____

184. QRS complexes ________ Regularity ________ Heart rate ________
P waves ____
PR interval ________ QRS interval ________
Interpretation ____

185. QRS complexes ________ Regularity ________ Heart rate ________
P waves ____
PR interval ________ QRS interval ________
Interpretation ____

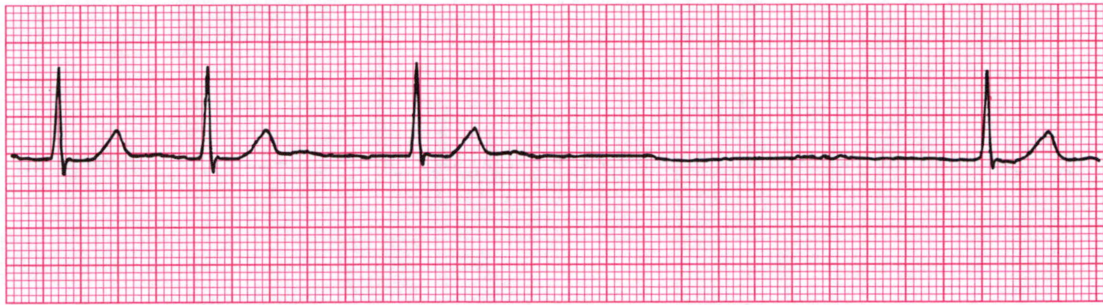

186. QRS complexes ________ Regularity ________ Heart rate ________
P waves ____
PR interval ________ QRS interval ________
Interpretation ____

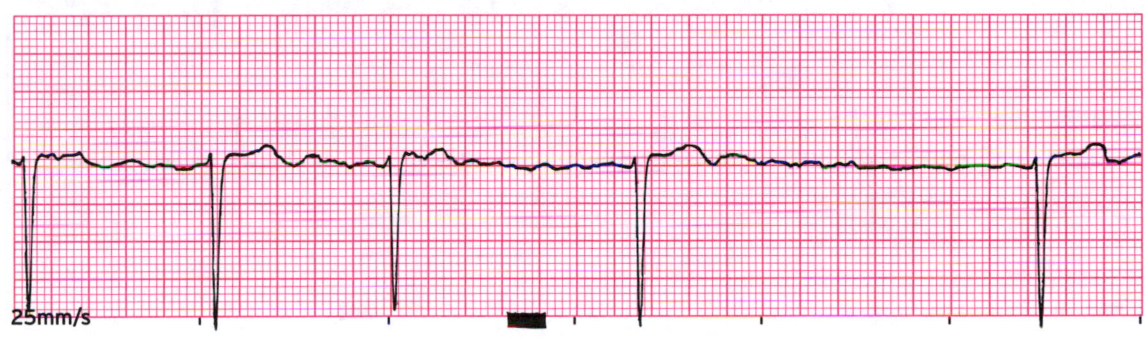

187. QRS complexes ________ Regularity ________ Heart rate ________
P waves ____
PR interval ________ QRS interval ________
Interpretation ____

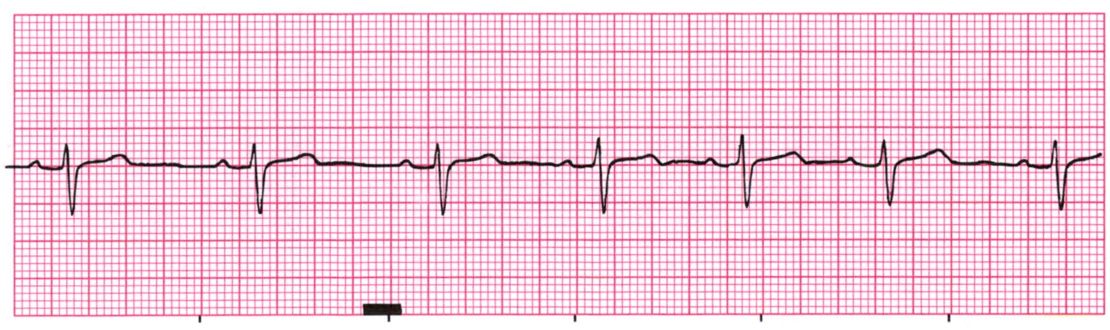

188. QRS complexes ________ Regularity ________ Heart rate ________
P waves ____
PR interval ________ QRS interval ________
Interpretation ____

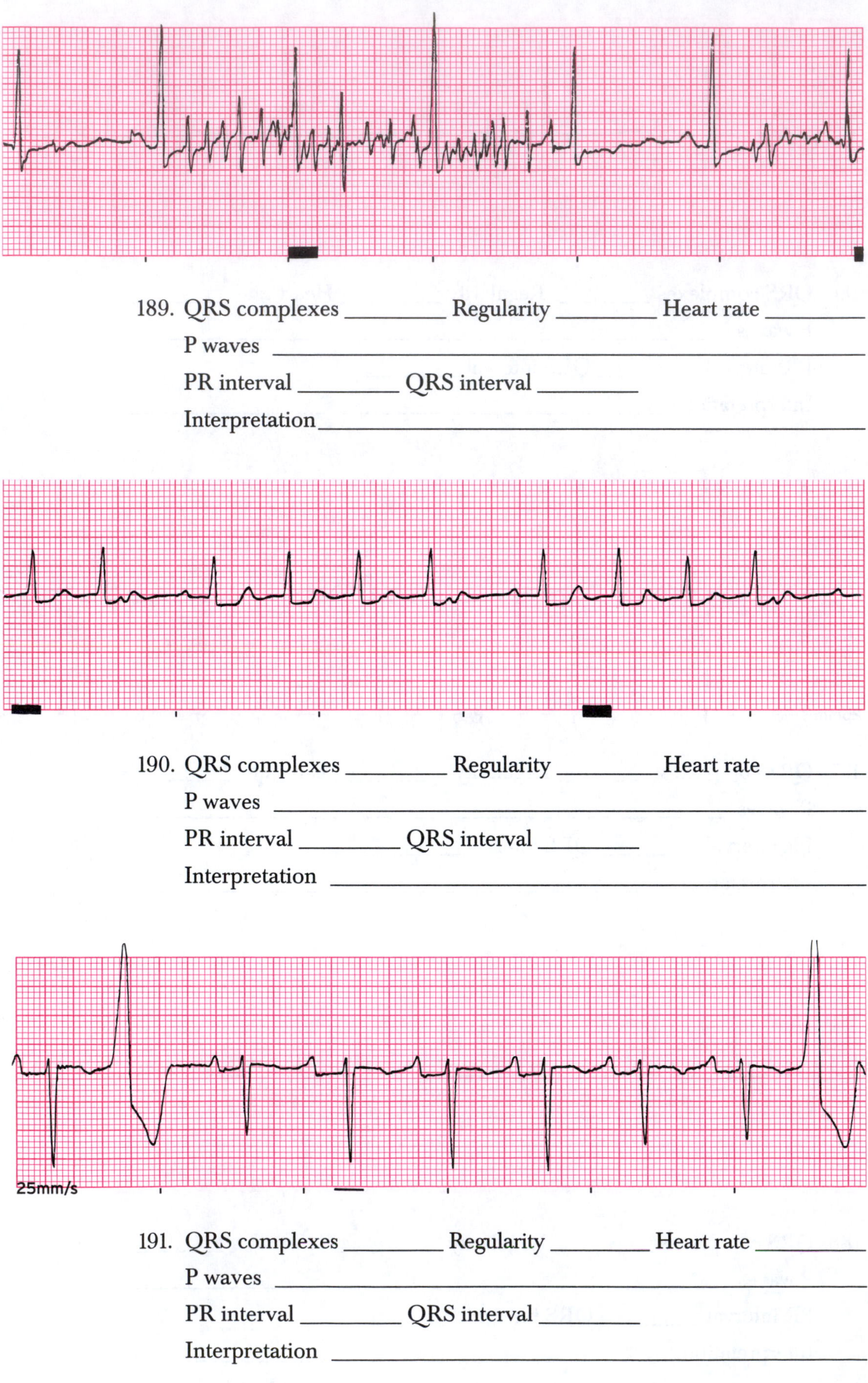

189. QRS complexes ________ Regularity ________ Heart rate ________

P waves ____

PR interval ________ QRS interval ________

Interpretation ____

190. QRS complexes ________ Regularity ________ Heart rate ________

P waves ____

PR interval ________ QRS interval ________

Interpretation ____

191. QRS complexes ________ Regularity ________ Heart rate ________

P waves ____

PR interval ________ QRS interval ________

Interpretation ____

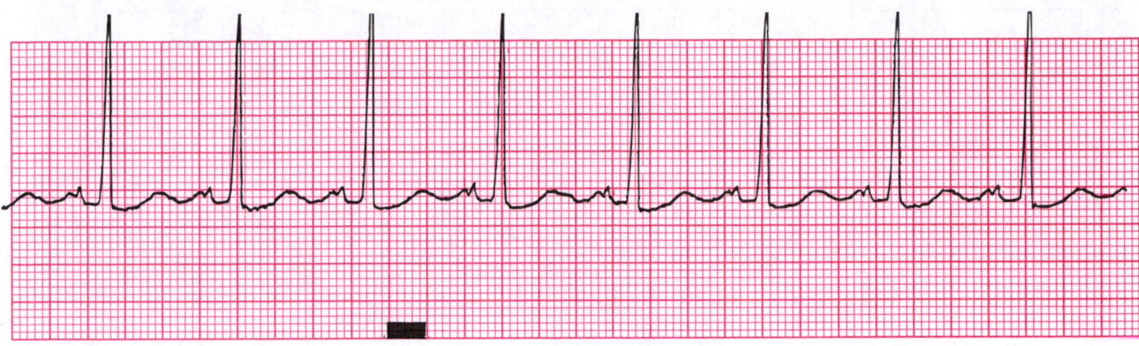

192. QRS complexes ________ Regularity ________ Heart rate ________
P waves ____
PR interval ________ QRS interval ________
Interpretation ____

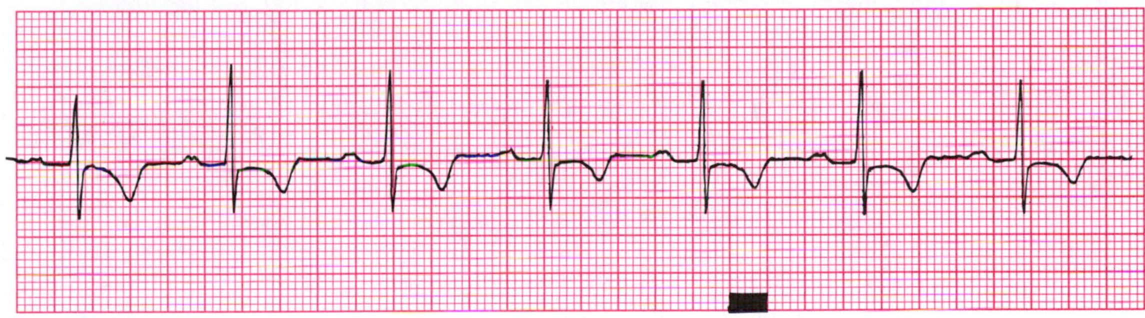

193. QRS complexes ________ Regularity ________ Heart rate ________
P waves ____
PR interval ________ QRS interval ________
Interpretation ____

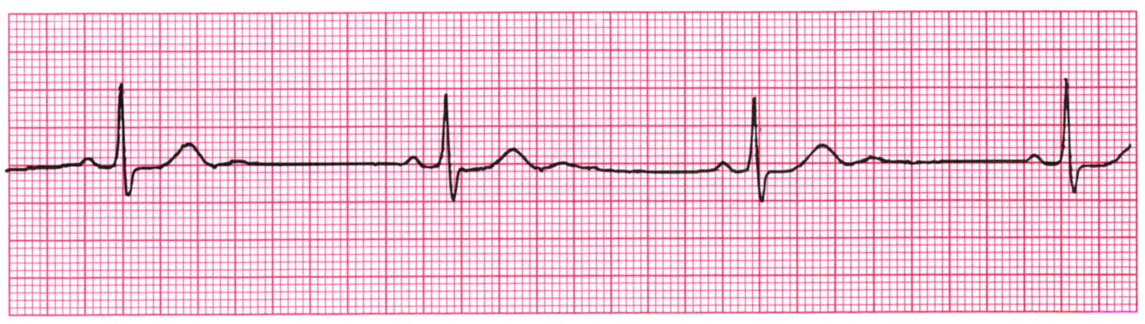

194. QRS complexes ________ Regularity ________ Heart rate ________
P waves ____
PR interval ________ QRS interval ________
Interpretation ____

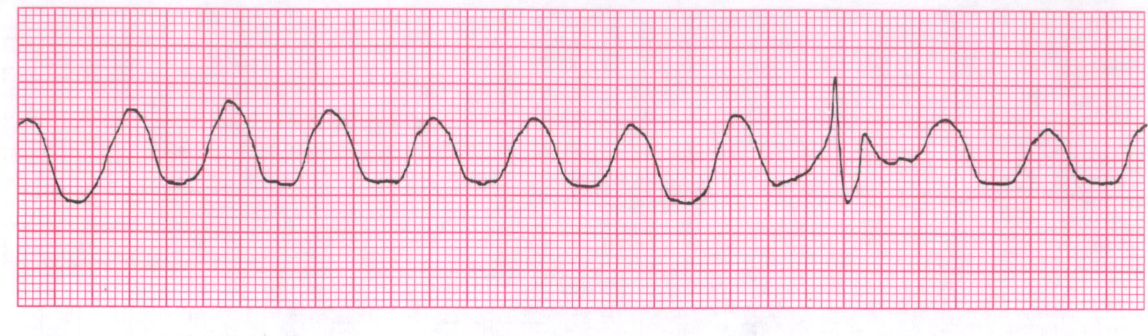

195. QRS complexes ________ Regularity ________ Heart rate ________
P waves ____
PR interval ________ QRS interval ________
Interpretation ____

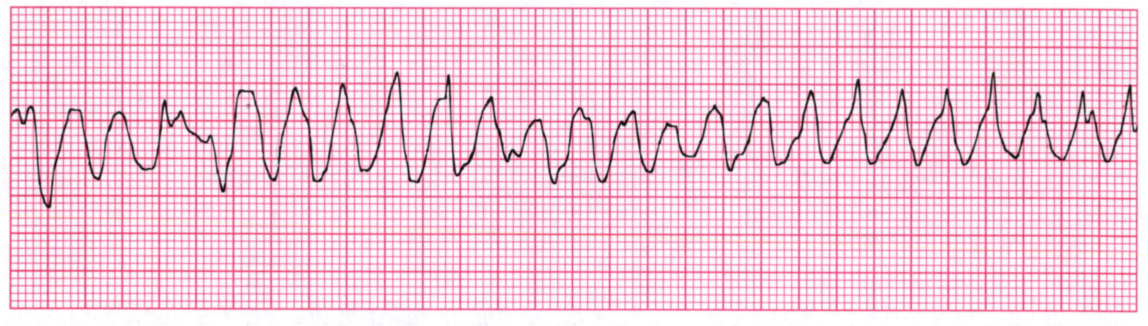

196. QRS complexes ________ Regularity ________ Heart rate ________
P waves ____
PR interval ________ QRS interval ________
Interpretation ____

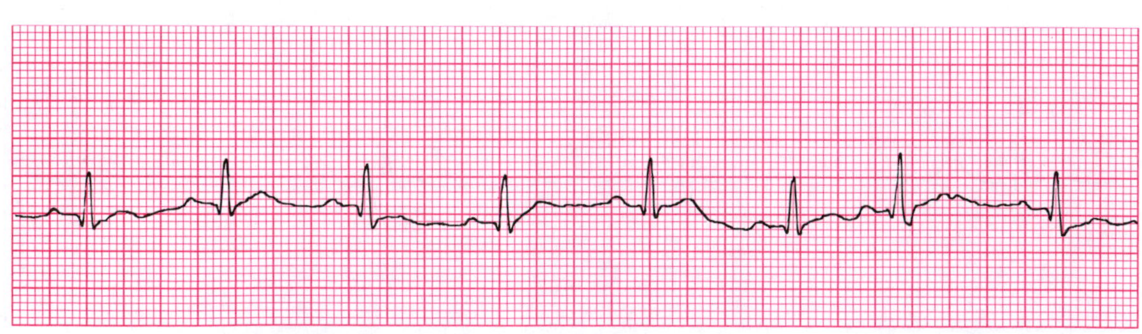

197. QRS complexes ________ Regularity ________ Heart rate ________
P waves ____
PR interval ________ QRS interval ________
Interpretation ____

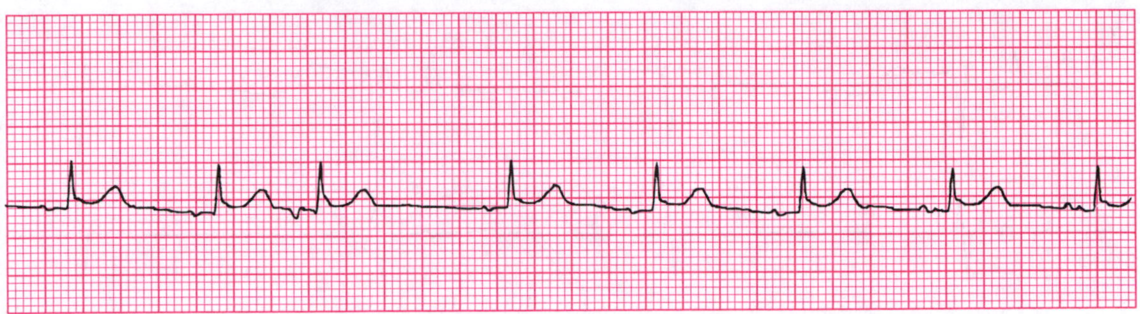

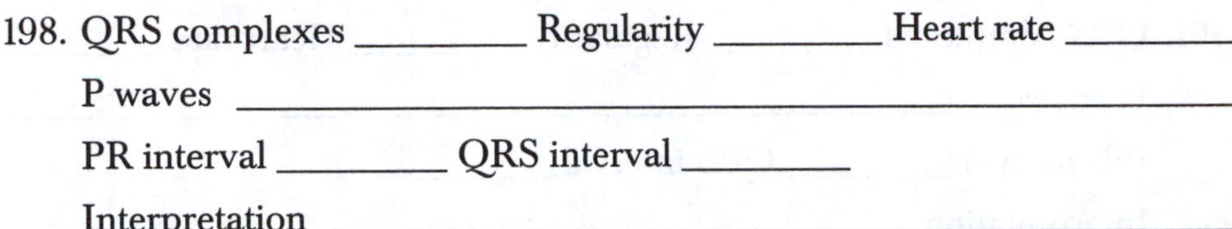

198. QRS complexes ________ Regularity ________ Heart rate ________

P waves ____

PR interval ________ QRS interval ________

Interpretation ____

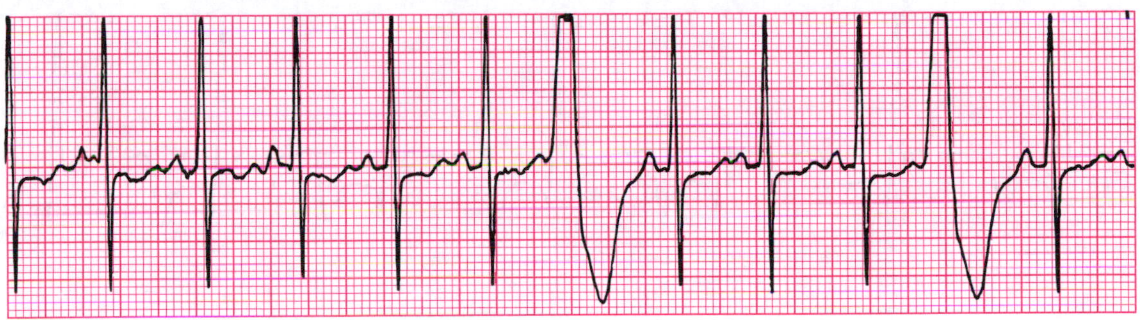

199. QRS complexes ________ Regularity ________ Heart rate ________

P waves ____

PR interval ________ QRS interval ________

Interpretation ____

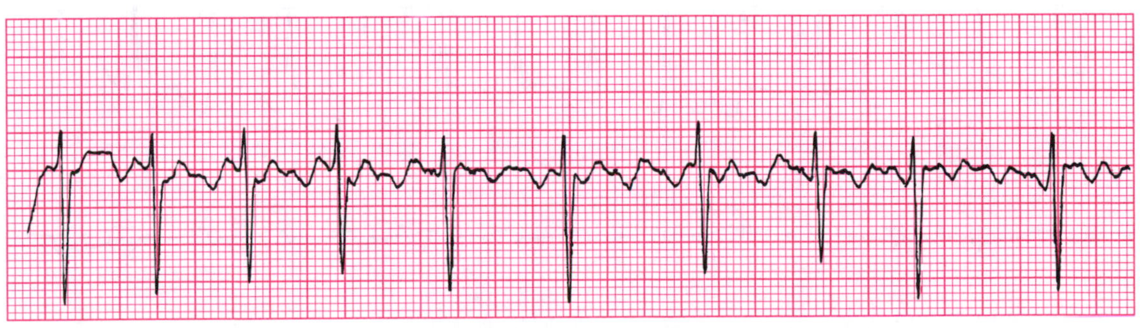

200. QRS complexes ________ Regularity ________ Heart rate ________

P waves ____

PR interval ________ QRS interval ________

Interpretation ____

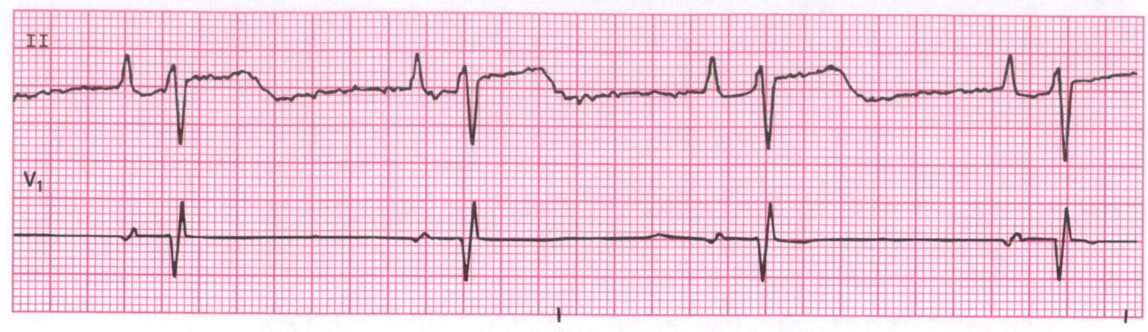

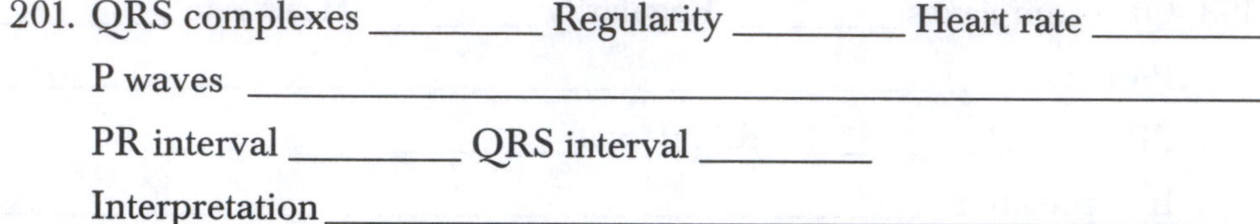

201. QRS complexes ________ Regularity ________ Heart rate ________
P waves ______________________________
PR interval ________ QRS interval ________
Interpretation ______________________________

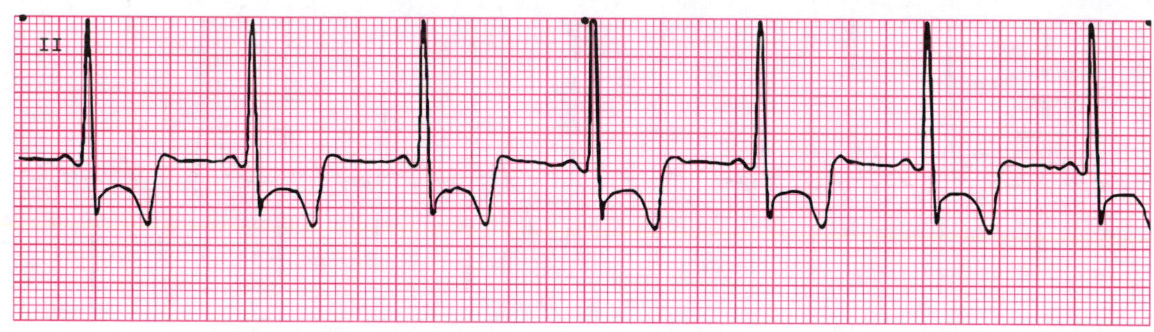

202. QRS complexes ________ Regularity ________ Heart rate ________
P waves ______________________________
PR interval ________ QRS interval ________
Interpretation ______________________________

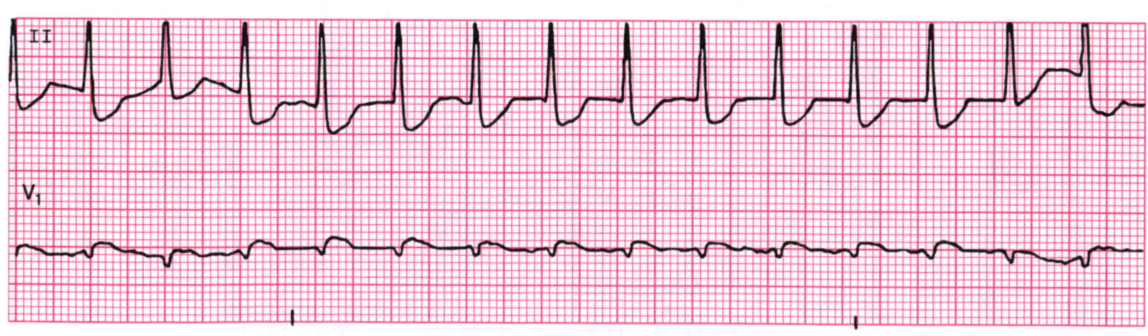

203. QRS complexes ________ Regularity ________ Heart rate ________
P waves ______________________________
PR interval ________ QRS interval ________
Interpretation ______________________________

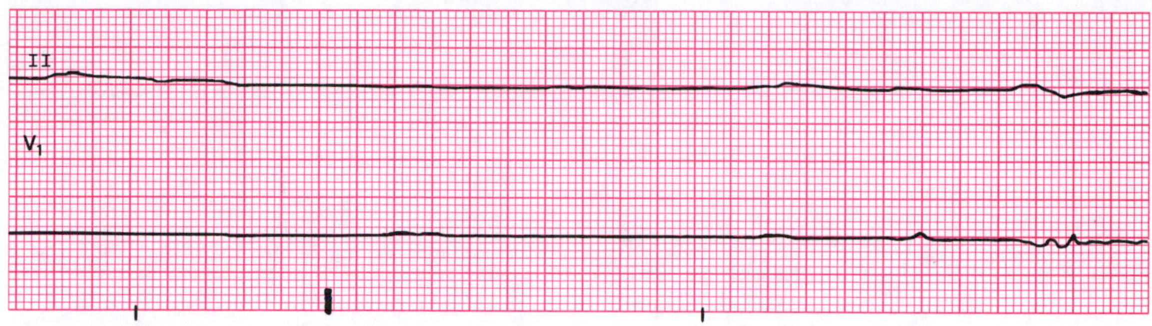

204. QRS complexes ________ Regularity ________ Heart rate ________
P waves ________________________________
PR interval ________ QRS interval ________
Interpretation ________________________________

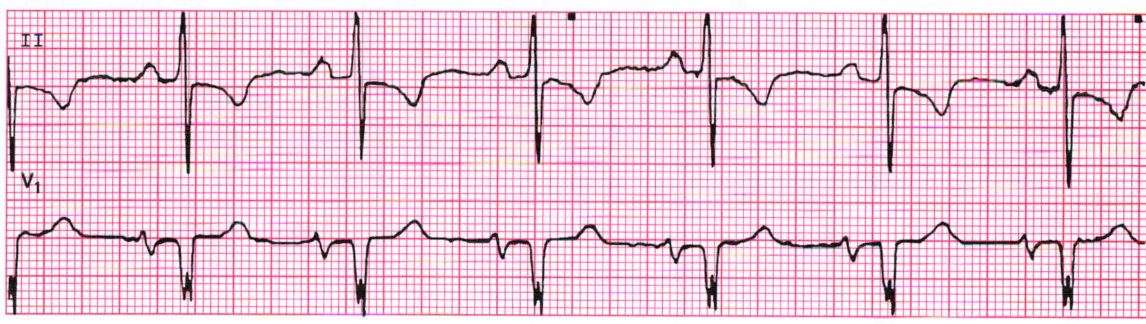

205. QRS complexes ________ Regularity ________ Heart rate ________
P waves ________________________________
PR interval ________ QRS interval ________
Interpretation ________________________________

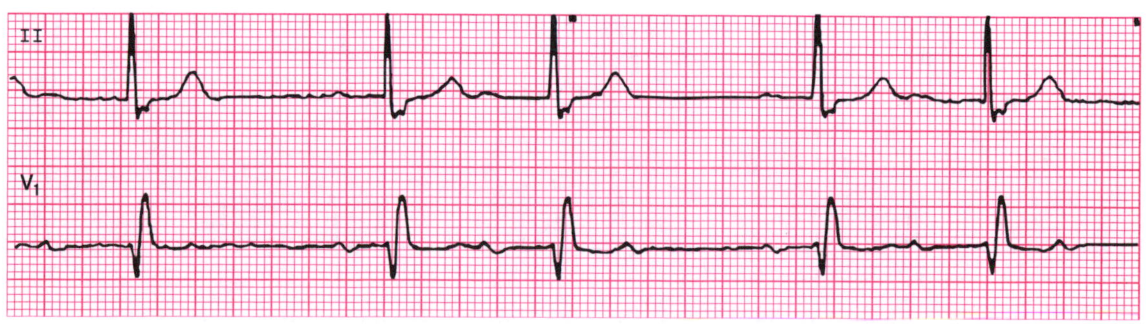

206. QRS complexes ________ Regularity ________ Heart rate ________
P waves ________________________________
PR interval ________ QRS interval ________
Interpretation ________________________________

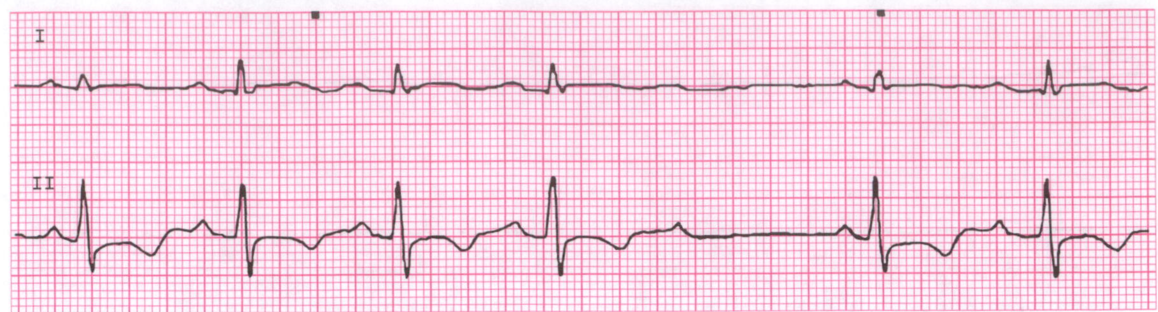

207. QRS complexes ________ Regularity ________ Heart rate ________

P waves ____

PR interval ________ QRS interval ________

Interpretation ____

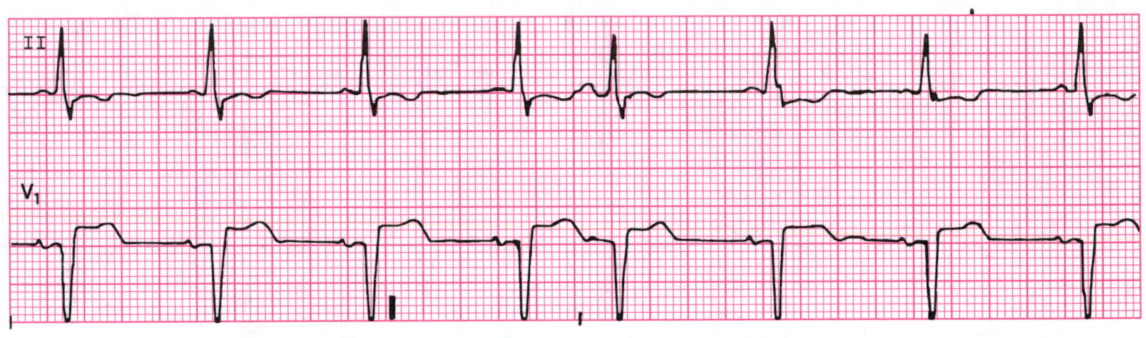

208. QRS complexes ________ Regularity ________ Heart rate ________

P waves ____

PR interval ________ QRS interval ________

Interpretation ____

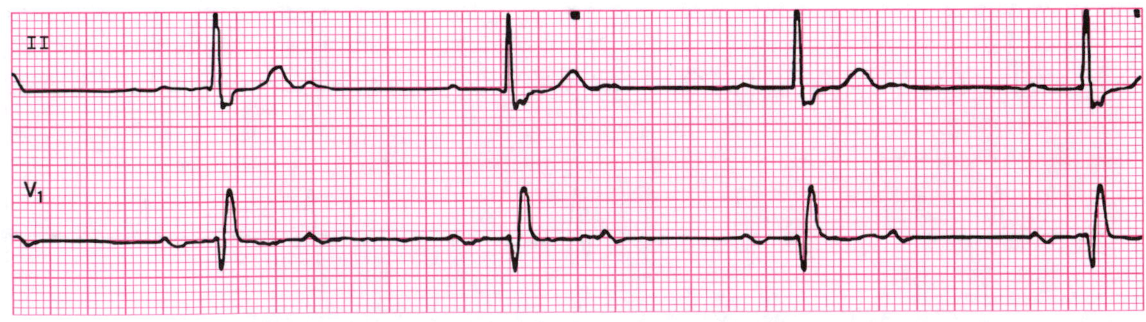

209. QRS complexes ________ Regularity ________ Heart rate ________

P waves ____

PR interval ________ QRS interval ________

Interpretation ____

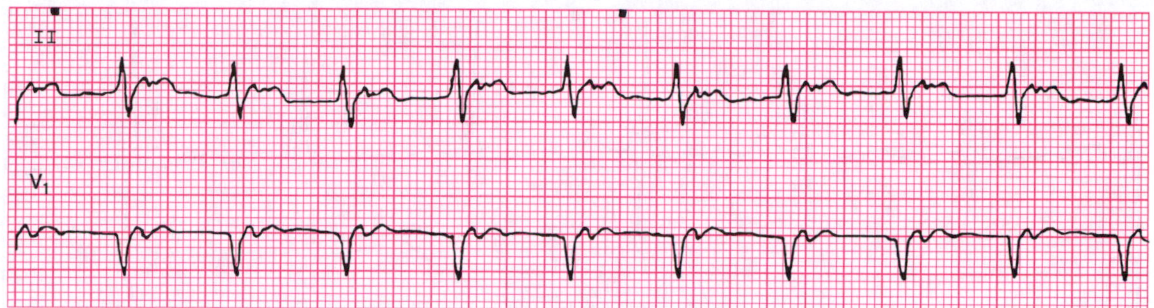

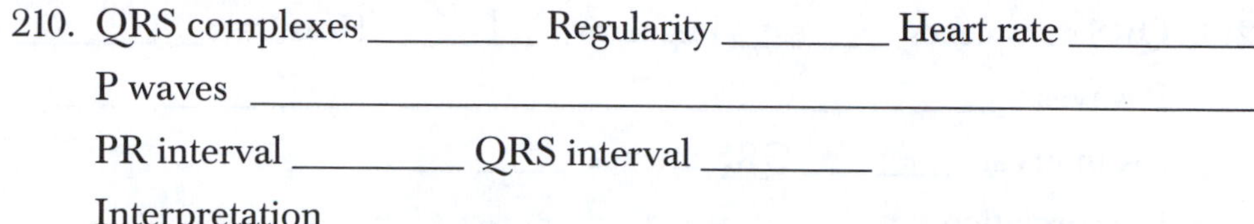

210. QRS complexes ________ Regularity ________ Heart rate ________

P waves ____

PR interval ________ QRS interval ________

Interpretation ____

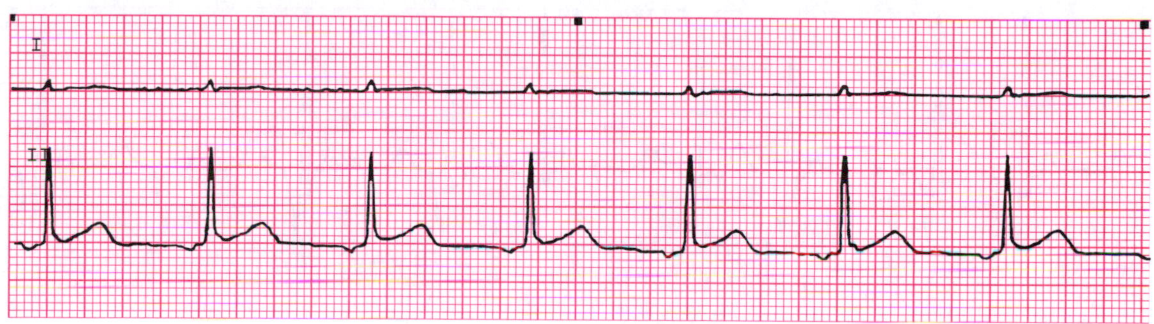

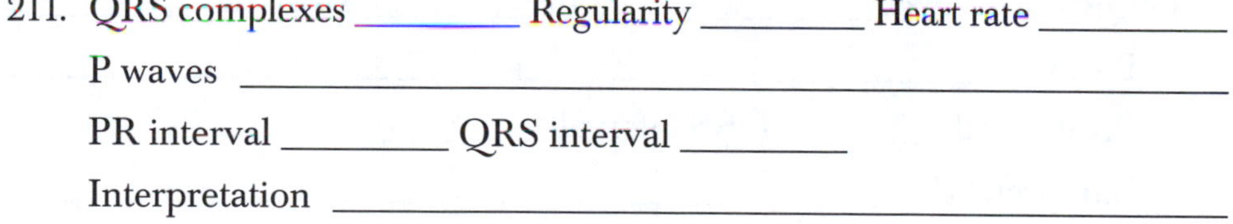

211. QRS complexes ________ Regularity ________ Heart rate ________

P waves ____

PR interval ________ QRS interval ________

Interpretation ____

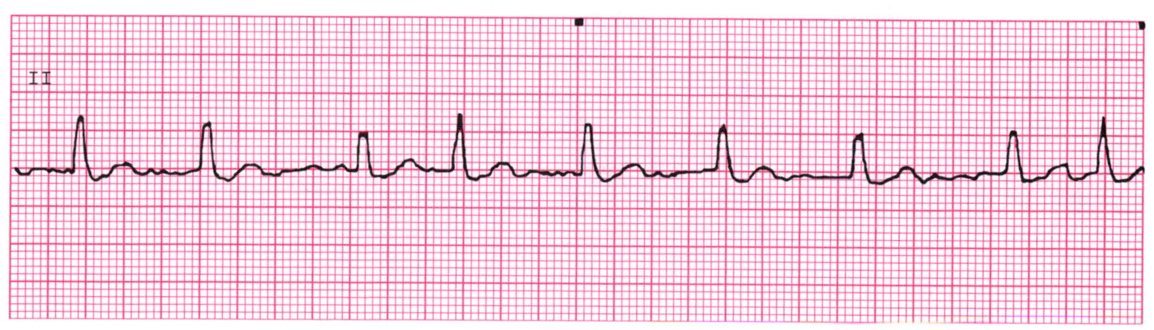

212. QRS complexes ________ Regularity ________ Heart rate ________

P waves ____

PR interval ________ QRS interval ________

Interpretation ____

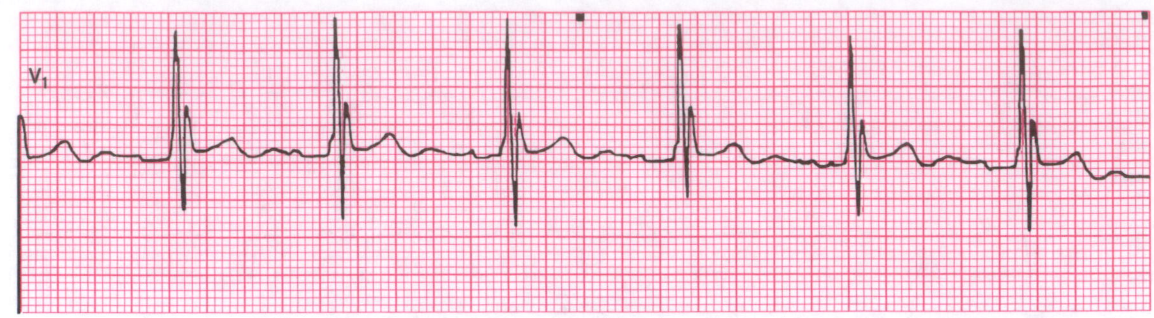

213. QRS complexes ________ Regularity ________ Heart rate ________
P waves ________
PR interval ________ QRS interval ________
Interpretation ________

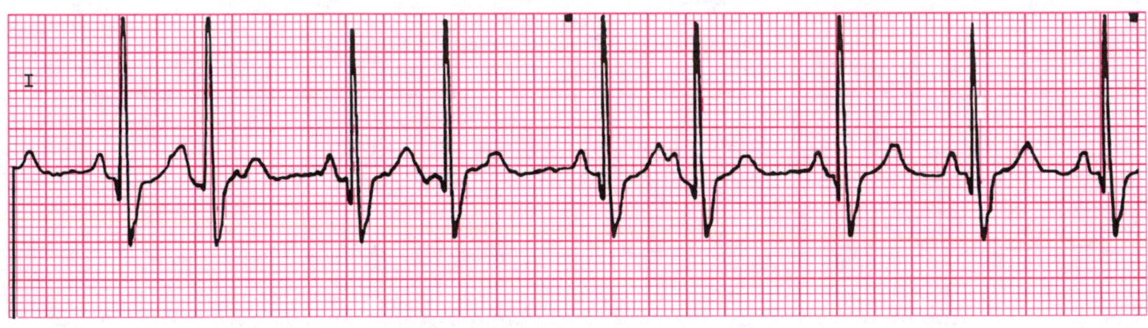

214. QRS complexes ________ Regularity ________ Heart rate ________
P waves ________
PR interval ________ QRS interval ________
Interpretation ________

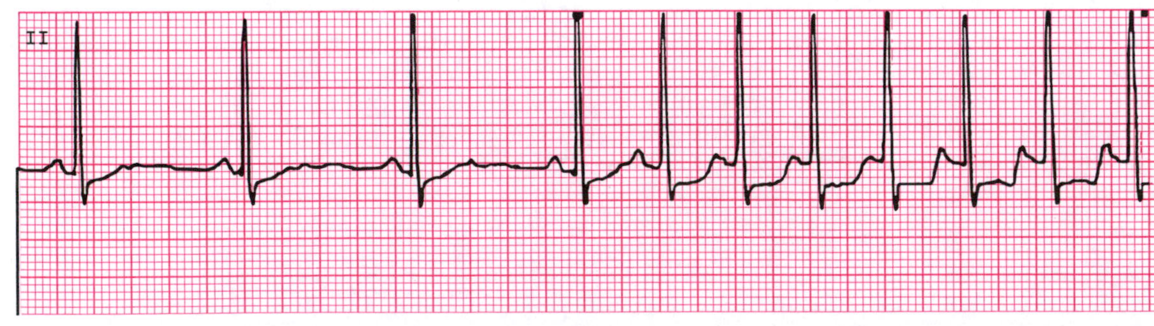

215. QRS complexes ________ Regularity ________ Heart rate ________
P waves ________
PR interval ________ QRS interval ________
Interpretation ________

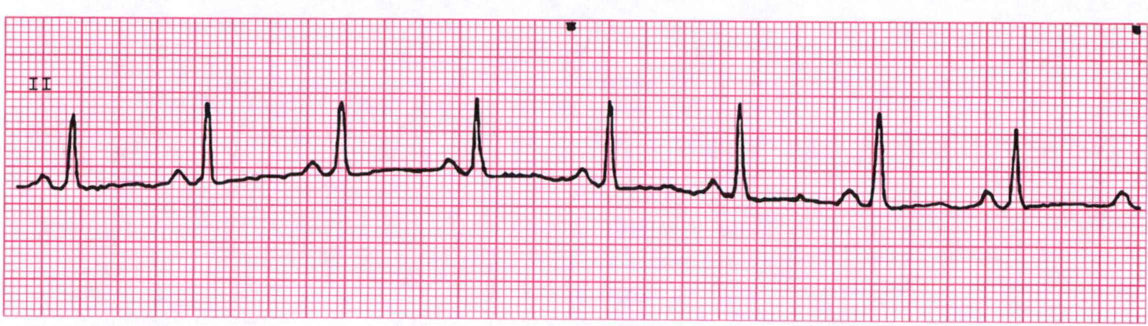

216. QRS complexes ________ Regularity ________ Heart rate __________

P waves ____

PR interval ________ QRS interval ________

Interpretation ______________________________________

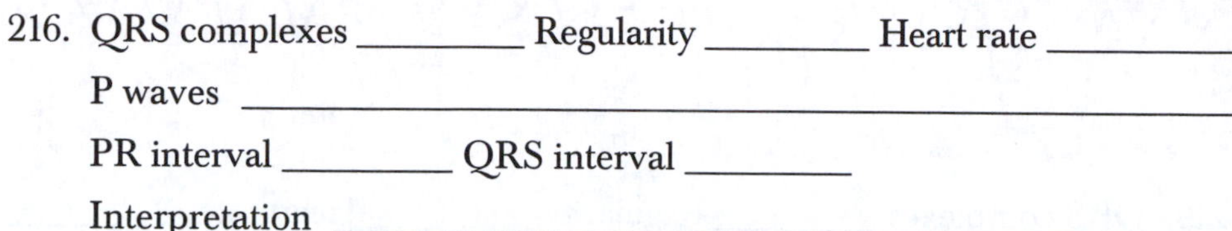

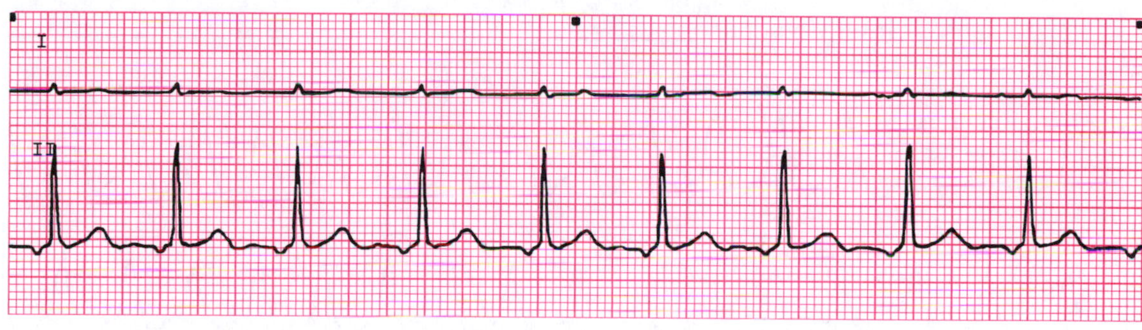

217. QRS complexes ________ Regularity ________ Heart rate __________

P waves ____

PR interval ________ QRS interval ________

Interpretation ______________________________________

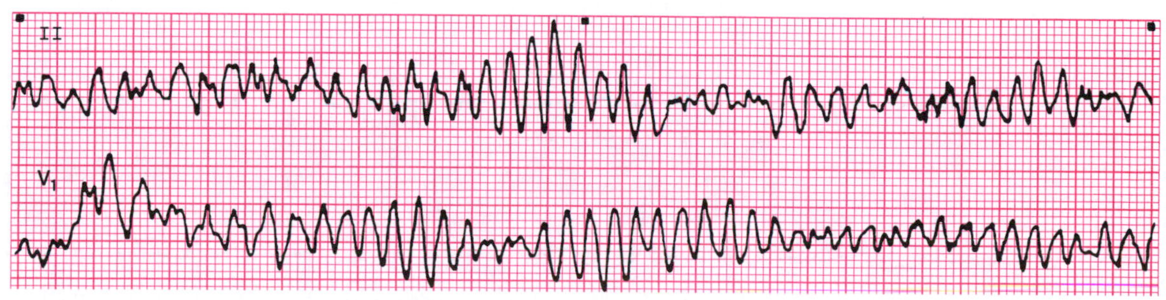

218. QRS complexes ________ Regularity ________ Heart rate __________

P waves ____

PR interval ________ QRS interval ________

Interpretation ______________________________________

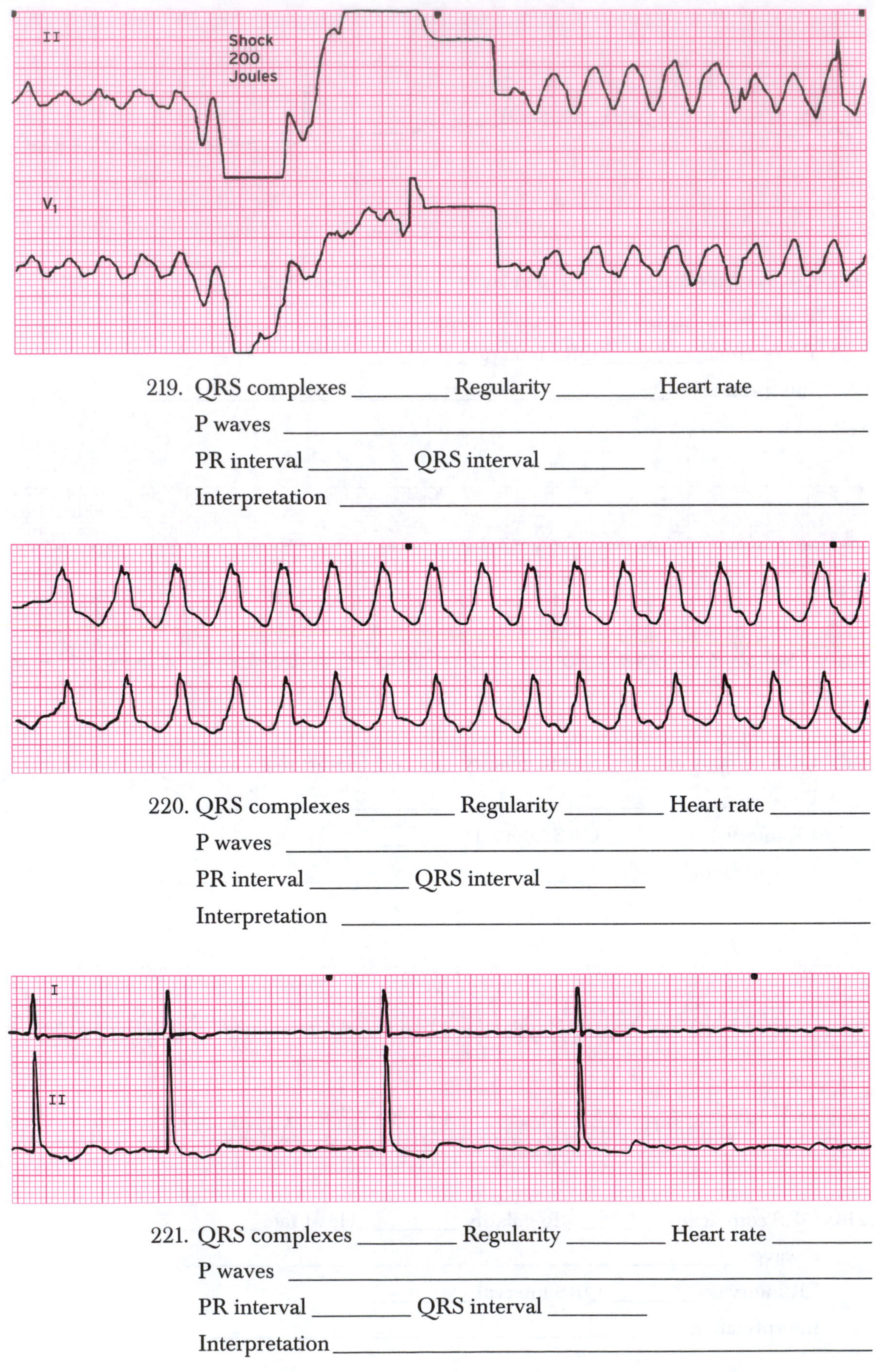

219. QRS complexes ________ Regularity ________ Heart rate ________
P waves ____
PR interval ________ QRS interval ________
Interpretation ____

220. QRS complexes ________ Regularity ________ Heart rate ________
P waves ____
PR interval ________ QRS interval ________
Interpretation ____

221. QRS complexes ________ Regularity ________ Heart rate ________
P waves ____
PR interval ________ QRS interval ________
Interpretation ____

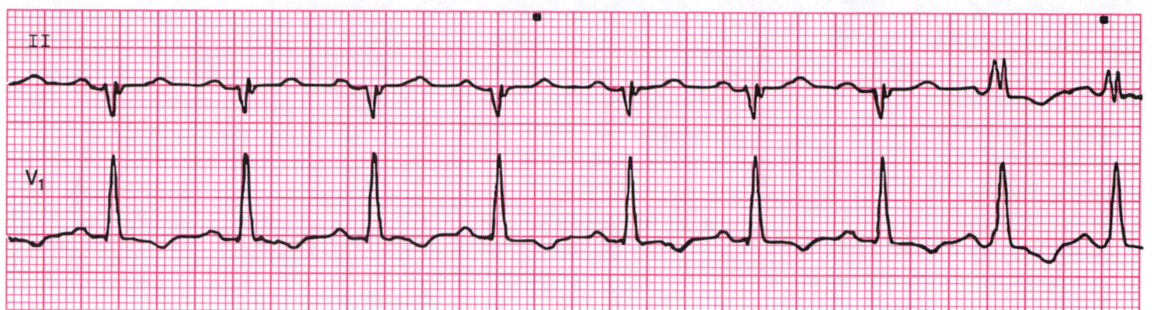

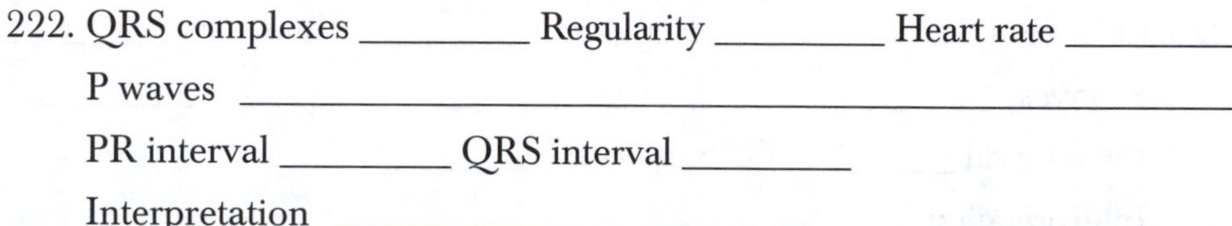

222. QRS complexes ________ Regularity ________ Heart rate ________

P waves ____

PR interval ________ QRS interval ________

Interpretation ____

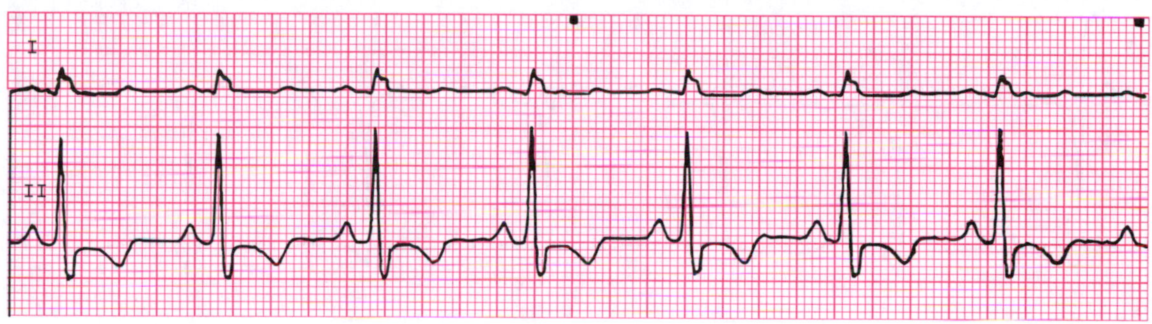

223. QRS complexes ________ Regularity ________ Heart rate ________

P waves ____

PR interval ________ QRS interval ________

Interpretation ____

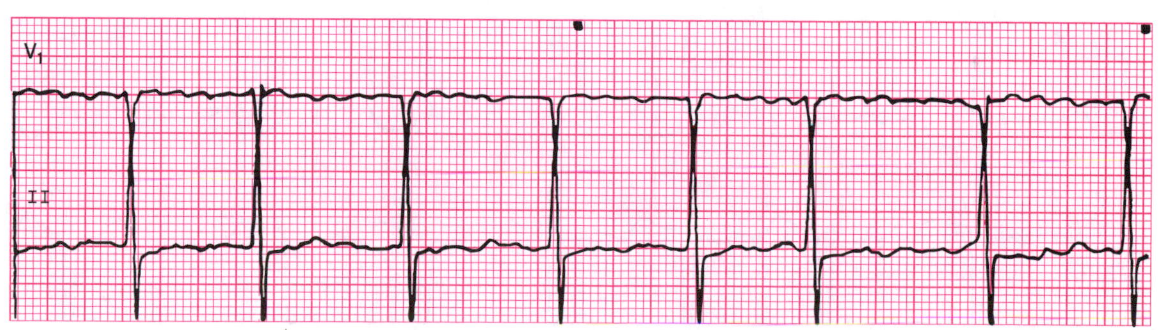

224. QRS complexes ________ Regularity ________ Heart rate ________

P waves ____

PR interval ________ QRS interval ________

Interpretation ____

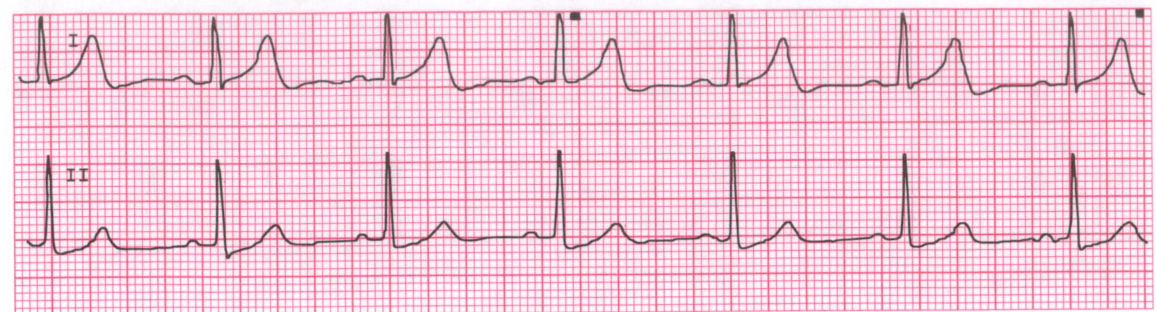

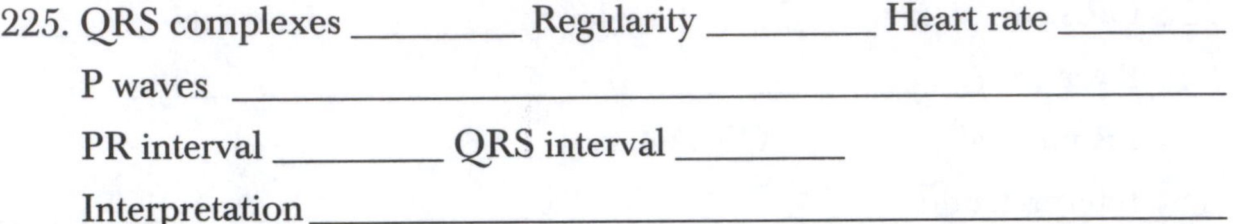

225. QRS complexes ________ Regularity ________ Heart rate ________
P waves ____
PR interval ________ QRS interval ________
Interpretation ____

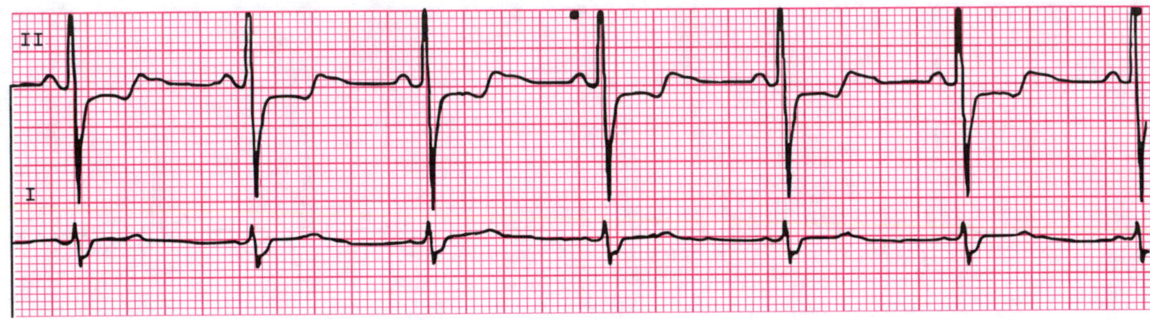

226. QRS complexes ________ Regularity ________ Heart rate ________
P waves ____
PR interval ________ QRS interval ________
Interpretation ____

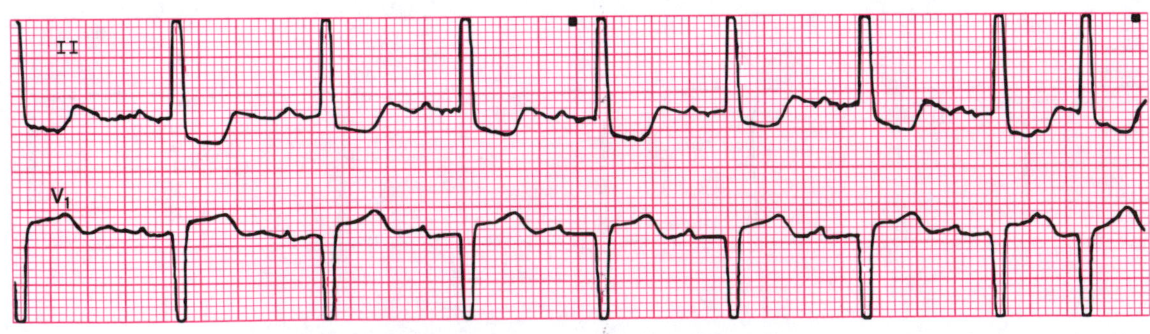

227. QRS complexes ________ Regularity ________ Heart rate ________
P waves ____
PR interval ________ QRS interval ________
Interpretation ____

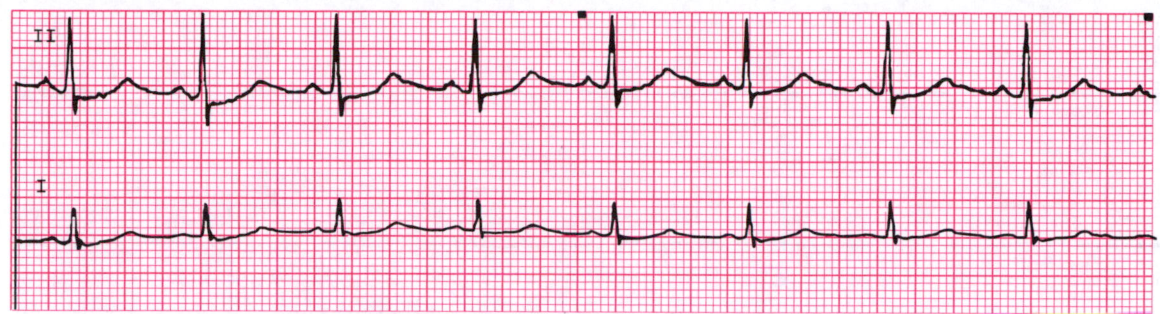

228. QRS complexes ________ Regularity ________ Heart rate ________

P waves ____

PR interval ________ QRS interval ________

Interpretation ____

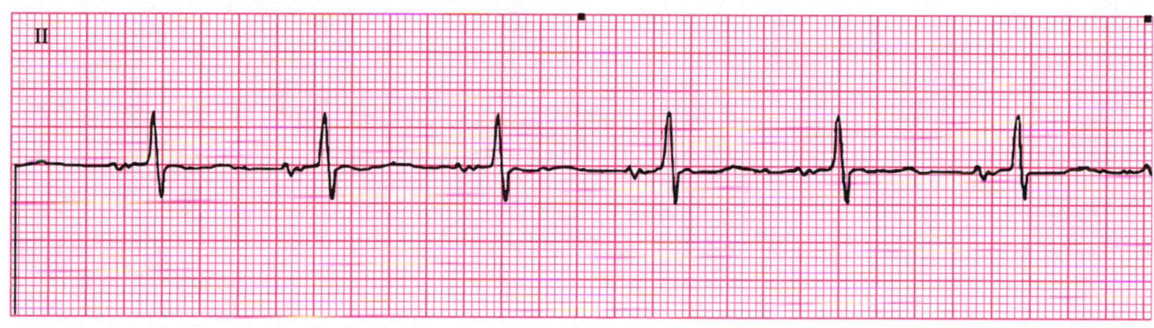

229. QRS complexes ________ Regularity ________ Heart rate ________

P waves ____

PR interval ________ QRS interval ________

Interpretation ____

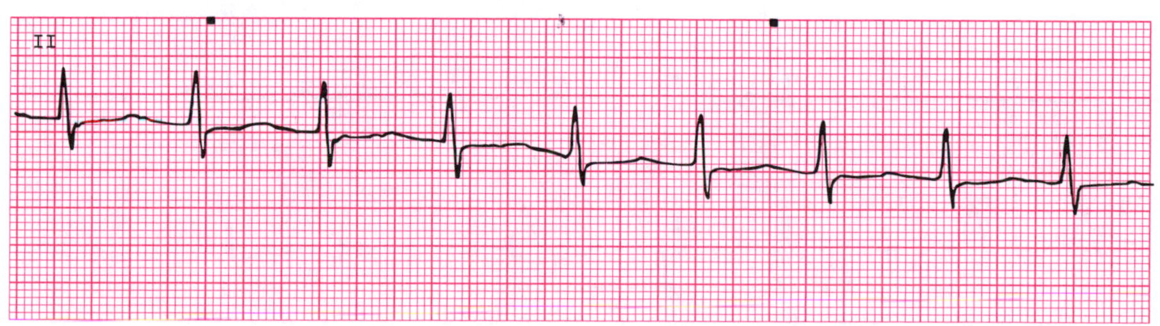

230. QRS complexes ________ Regularity ________ Heart rate ________

P waves ____

PR interval ________ QRS interval ________

Interpretation ____

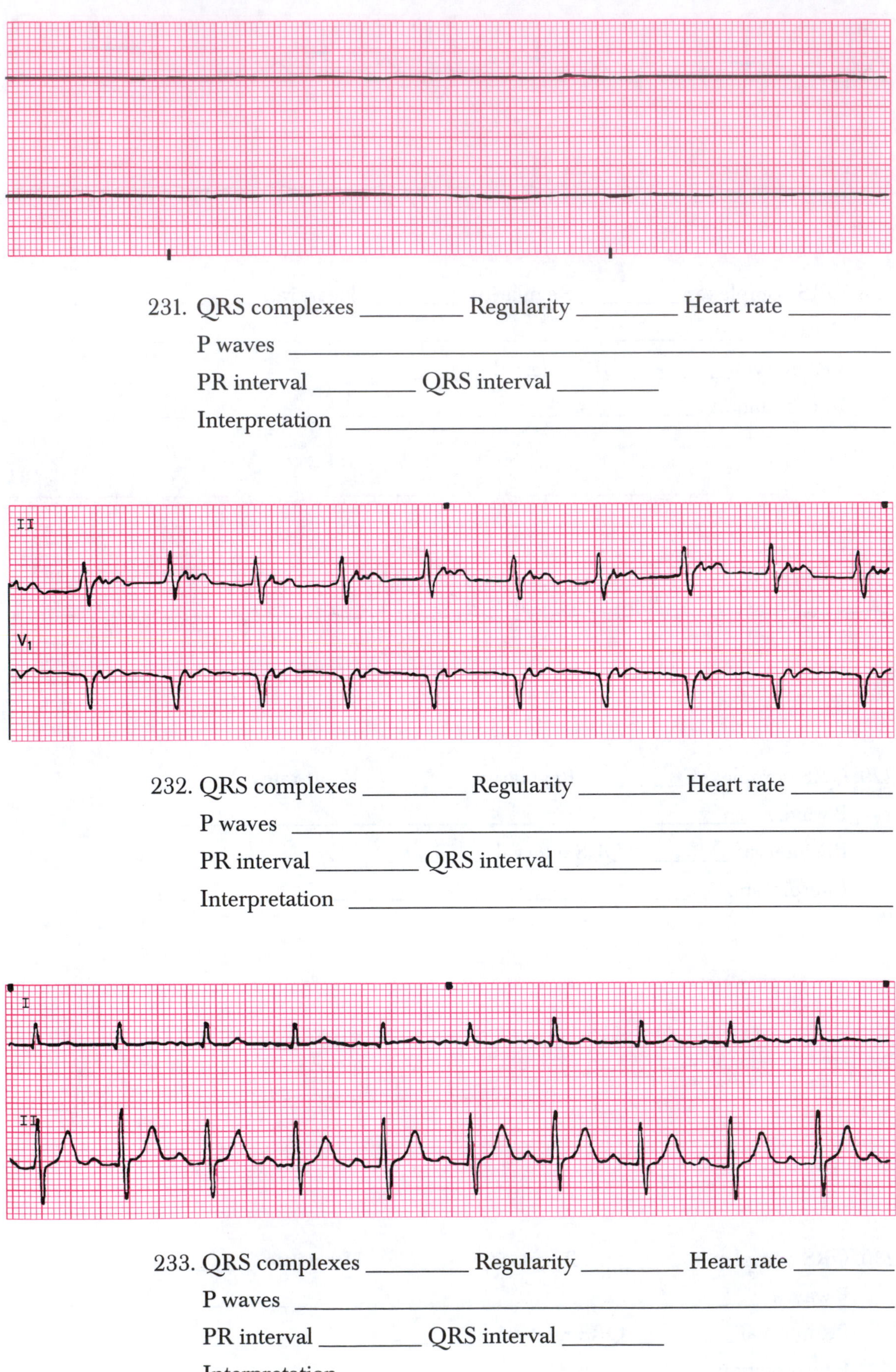

231. QRS complexes _________ Regularity _________ Heart rate _________
P waves ____
PR interval _________ QRS interval _________
Interpretation ____

232. QRS complexes _________ Regularity _________ Heart rate _________
P waves ____
PR interval _________ QRS interval _________
Interpretation ____

233. QRS complexes _________ Regularity _________ Heart rate _________
P waves ____
PR interval _________ QRS interval _________
Interpretation ____

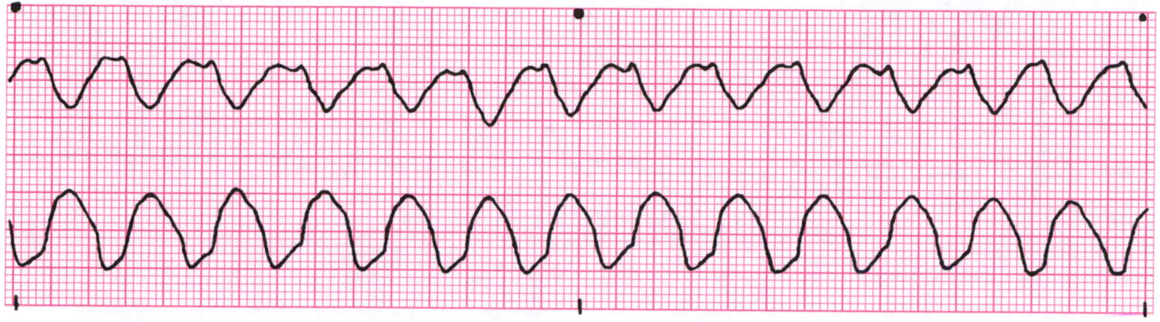

234. QRS complexes ________ Regularity ________ Heart rate ________
P waves ______________________________
PR interval ________ QRS interval ________
Interpretation ______________________________

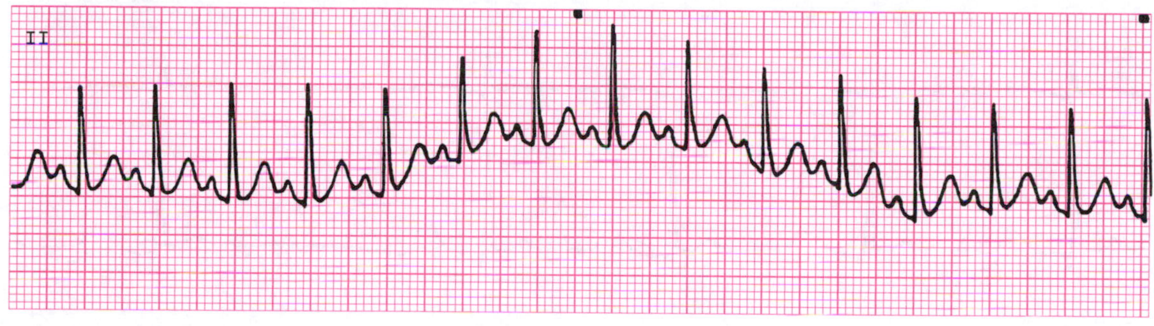

235. QRS complexes ________ Regularity ________ Heart rate ________
P waves ______________________________
PR interval ________ QRS interval ________
Interpretation ______________________________

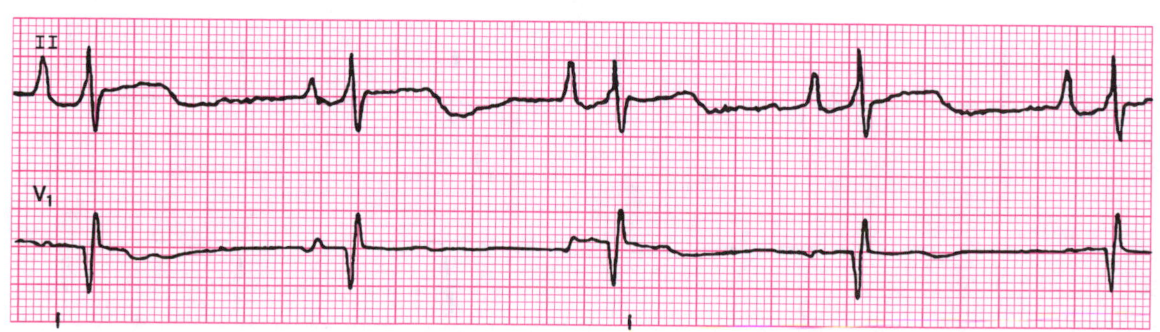

236. QRS complexes ________ Regularity ________ Heart rate ________
P waves ______________________________
PR interval ________ QRS interval ________
Interpretation ______________________________

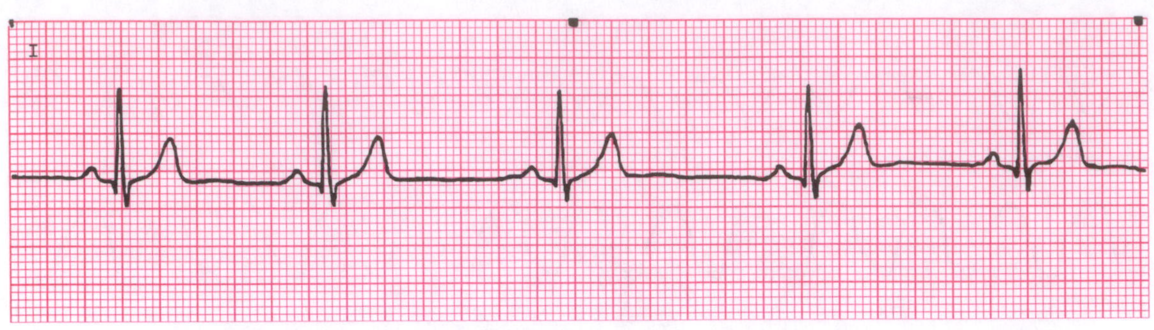

237. QRS complexes ________ Regularity ________ Heart rate ________
P waves ____
PR interval ________ QRS interval ________
Interpretation ____

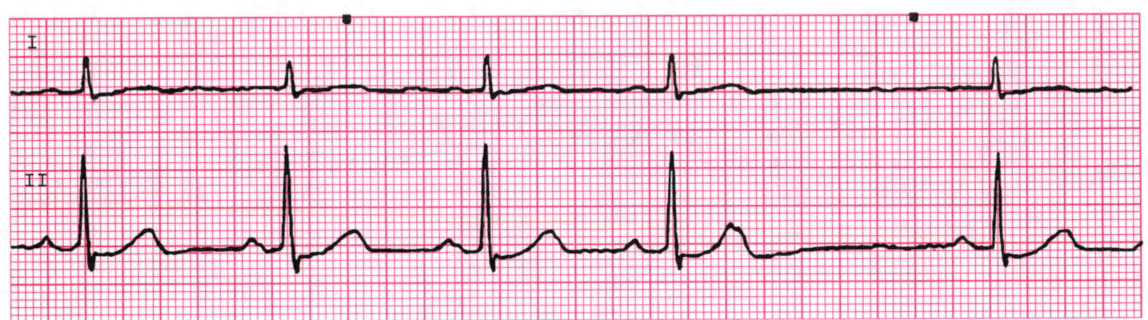

238. QRS complexes ________ Regularity ________ Heart rate ________
P waves ____
PR interval ________ QRS interval ________
Interpretation ____

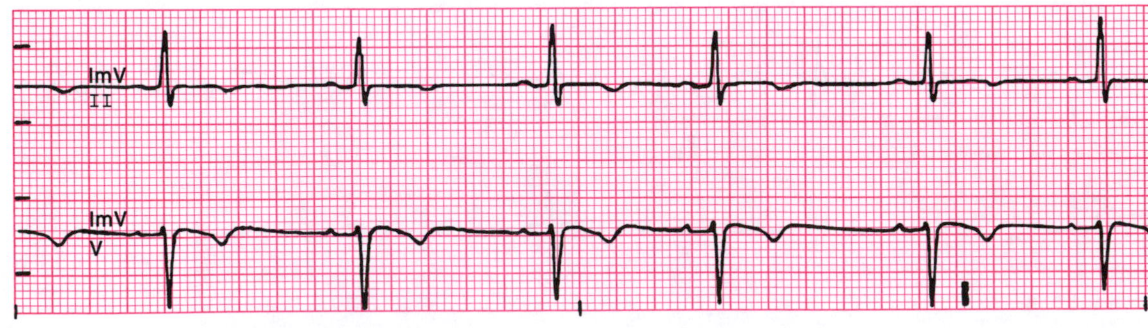

239. QRS complexes ________ Regularity ________ Heart rate ________
P waves ____
PR interval ________ QRS interval ________
Interpretation ____

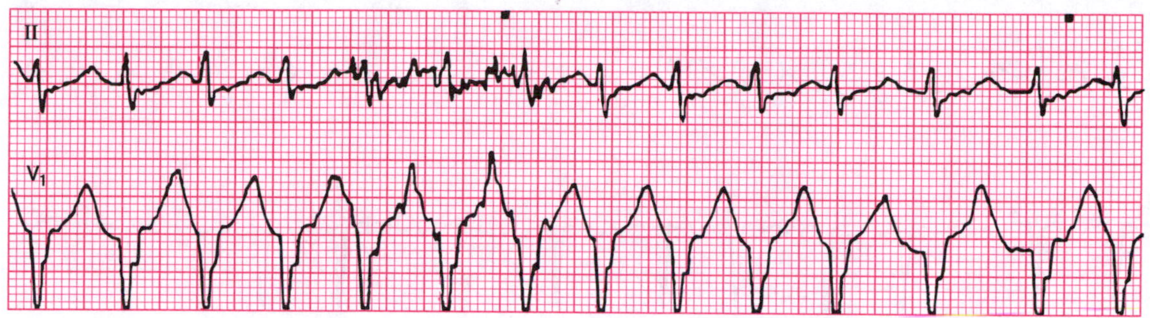

240. QRS complexes ________ Regularity ________ Heart rate ________
P waves ____
PR interval ________ QRS interval ________
Interpretation ____

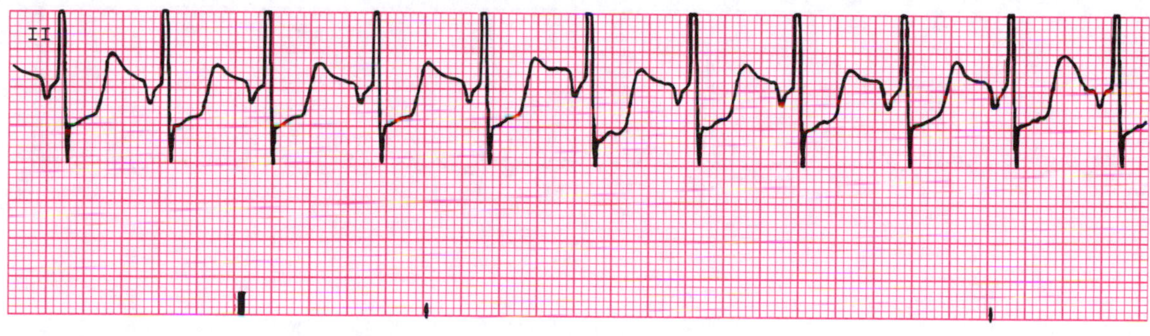

241. QRS complexes ________ Regularity ________ Heart rate ________
P waves ____
PR interval ________ QRS interval ________
Interpretation ____

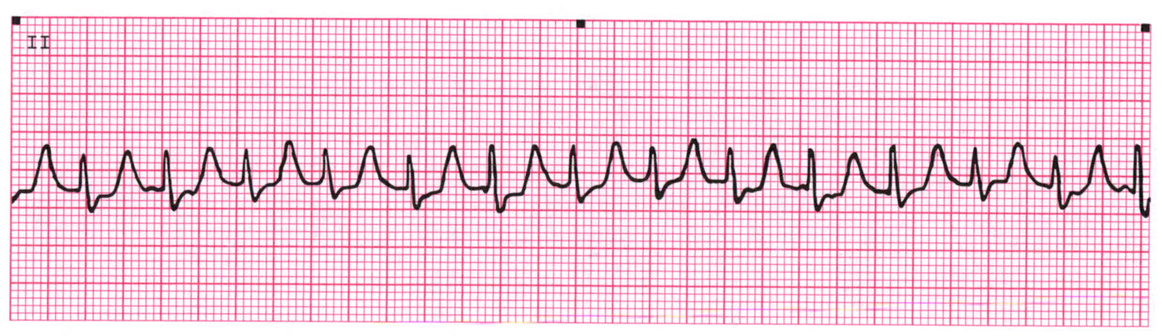

242. QRS complexes ________ Regularity ________ Heart rate ________
P waves ____
PR interval ________ QRS interval ________
Interpretation ____

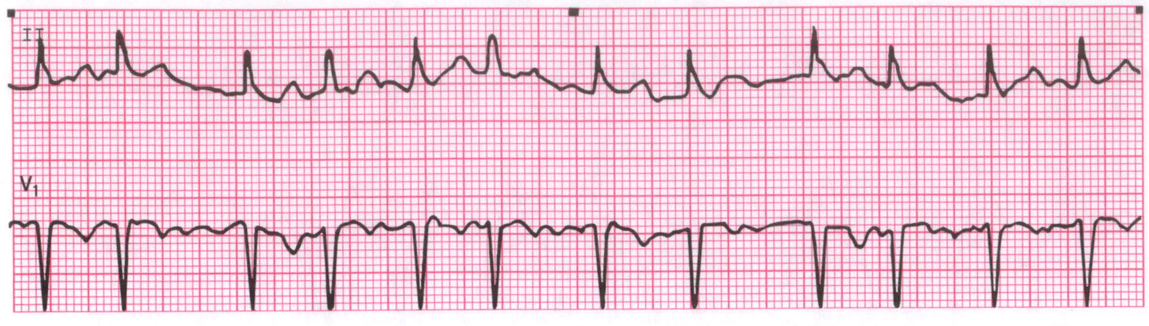

243. QRS complexes ________ Regularity ________ Heart rate ________

P waves ____

PR interval ________ QRS interval ________

Interpretation ____

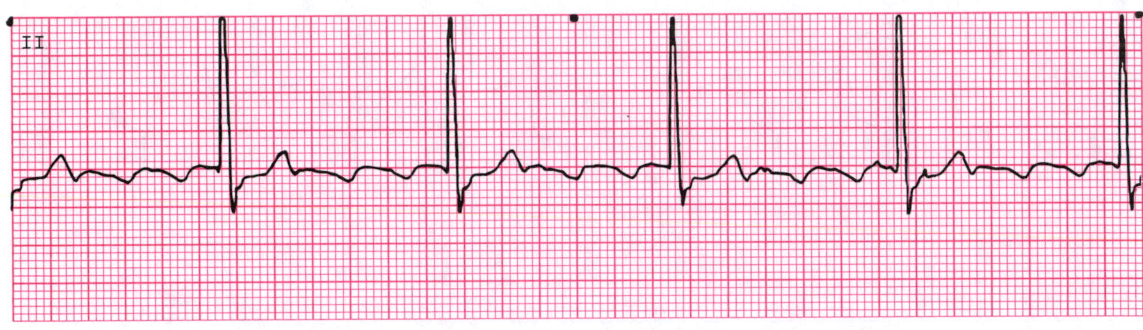

244. QRS complexes ________ Regularity ________ Heart rate ________

P waves ____

PR interval ________ QRS interval ________

Interpretation ____

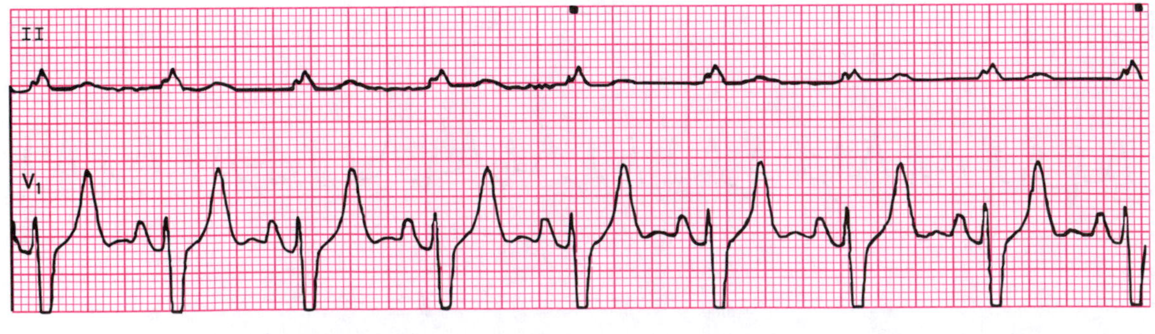

245. QRS complexes ________ Regularity ________ Heart rate ________

P waves ____

PR interval ________ QRS interval ________

Interpretation ____

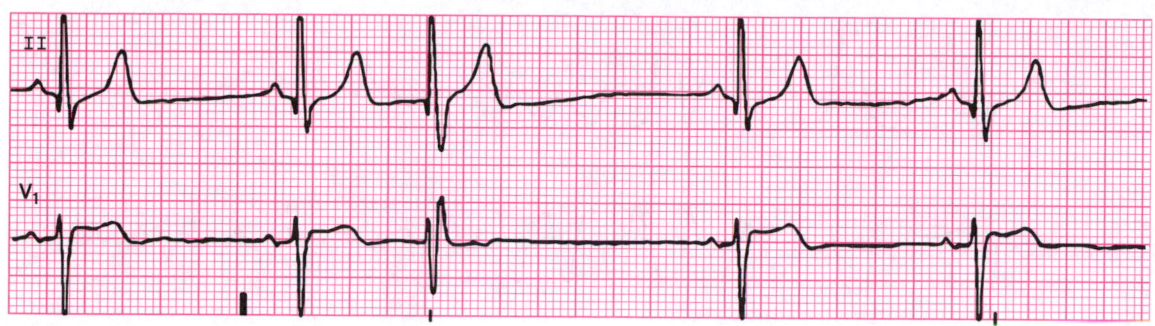

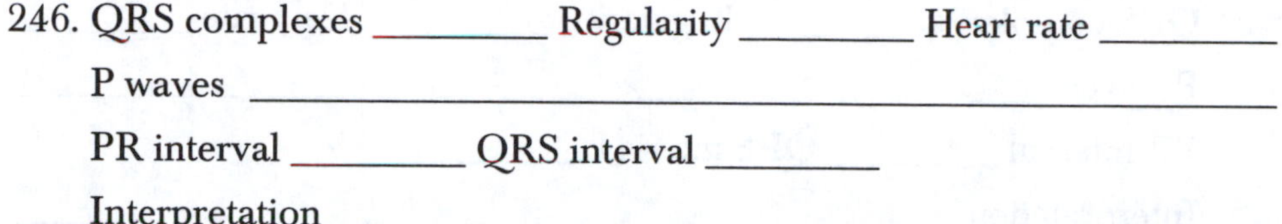

246. QRS complexes ________ Regularity ________ Heart rate ________

P waves ____

PR interval ________ QRS interval ________

Interpretation ____

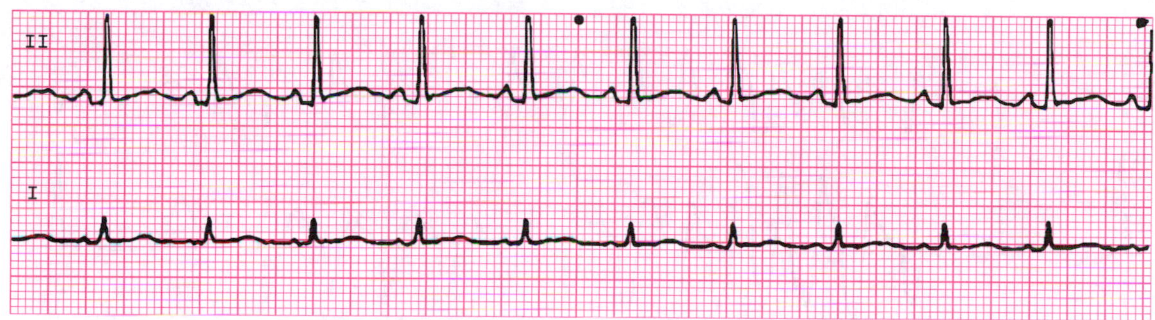

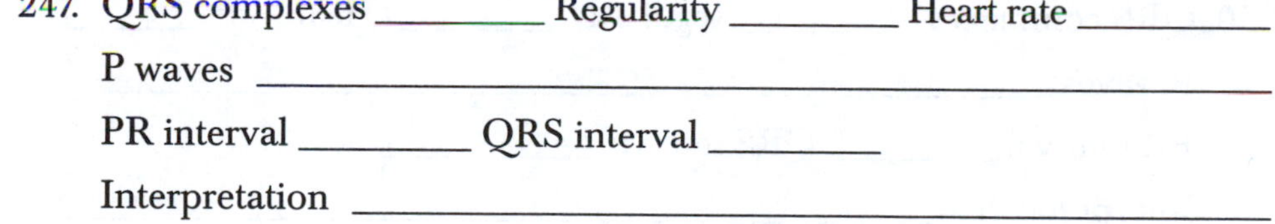

247. QRS complexes ________ Regularity ________ Heart rate ________

P waves ____

PR interval ________ QRS interval ________

Interpretation ____

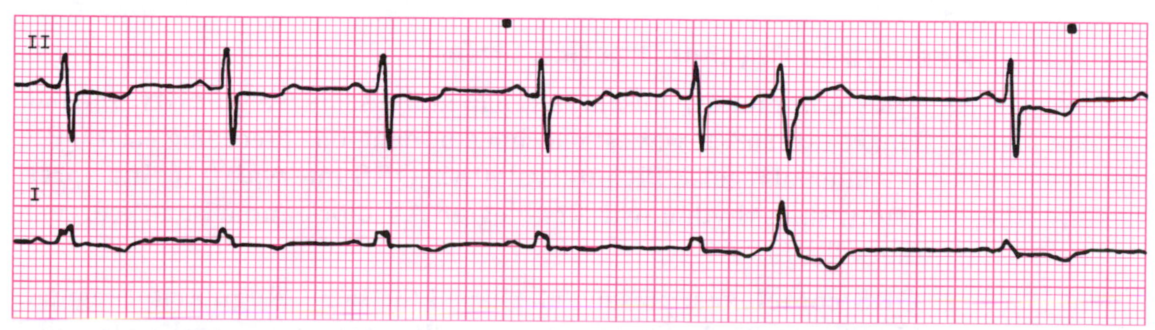

248. QRS complexes ________ Regularity ________ Heart rate ________

P waves ____

PR interval ________ QRS interval ________

Interpretation ____

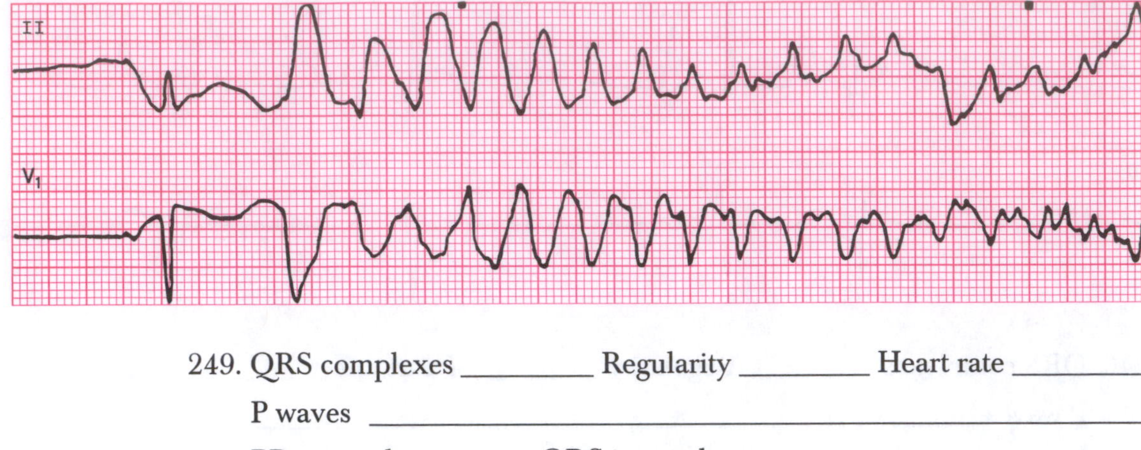

249. QRS complexes ________ Regularity ________ Heart rate ________
P waves ________________________________
PR interval ________ QRS interval ________
Interpretation ________________________________

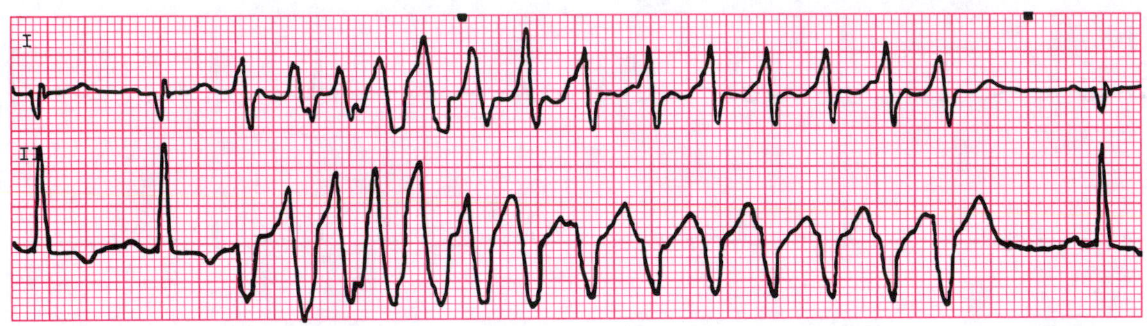

250. QRS complexes ________ Regularity ________ Heart rate ________
P waves ________________________________
PR interval ________ QRS interval ________
Interpretation ________________________________

Answers to Rhythm Practice Strips

1. **QRS complexes:** present, all shaped the same. **Regularity:** regular. **Heart rate:** 68. **P waves:** matching, upright, one preceding each QRS; P-P interval regular. **PR interval:** 0.42. **QRS interval:** 0.16. **Interpretation:** sinus rhythm with first-degree AV block and a bundle branch block (BBB).
2. **QRS complexes:** present, all shaped the same. **Regularity:** regular. **Heart rate:** 37. **P waves:** none seen. **PR interval:** not applicable. **QRS interval:** 0.12 **Interpretation:** junctional bradycardia with BBB.
3. **QRS complexes:** present, all shaped the same. **Regularity:** regular. **Heart rate:** 71. **P waves:** matching, upright, one preceding each QRS; P-P interval regular. **PR interval:** 0.24. **QRS interval:** 0.12. **Interpretation:** sinus rhythm with first-degree AV block and BBB.

4. **QRS complexes:** present, all shaped the same. **Regularity:** regular. **Heart rate:** 125. **P waves:** an occasional dissociated P can be seen. **PR interval:** cannot measure. **QRS interval:** 0.22. **Interpretation:** ventricular tachycardia.

5. **QRS complexes:** present, all shaped the same. **Regularity:** irregular. **Heart rate:** 65 to 94, with a mean rate of 80. **P waves:** none present; wavy, undulating baseline is present. **PR interval:** not applicable. **QRS interval:** 0.06. **Interpretation:** atrial fibrillation.

6. **QRS complexes:** Present, all shaped the same, low voltage. **Regularity:** regular. **Heart rate:** 125. **P waves:** matching, upright, one preceding each QRS, low voltage; P-P interval regular. **PR interval:** 0.16. **QRS interval:** 0.06. **Interpretation:** sinus tachycardia.

7. **QRS complexes:** present, all shaped the same. **Regularity:** regular. **Heart rate:** 32. **P waves:** upright, matching, some nonconducted; P-P interval regular; atrial rate 125. **PR interval:** varies. **QRS interval:** 0.13. **Interpretation:** sinus tachycardia with third-degree AV block and an idioventricular rhythm.

8. **QRS complexes:** present, all shaped the same. **Regularity:** regular. **Heart rate:** 150. **P waves:** none present; regular sawtooth-shaped waves between QRS complexes present instead, two to each QRS; atrial rate about 300. **PR interval:** not applicable. **QRS interval:** 0.06. **Interpretation:** atrial flutter with 2:1 conduction. Were you thinking it was something else? Look at the tail end of the QRS complex. See how it looks rounded at the bottom? That rounded part looks a lot like the other rounded wave that follows it, doesn't it? Those are both flutter waves. You'll notice these flutter waves march out–they're all the same distance from each other. Always be very suspicious when the heart rate is 150–it may be atrial flutter with 2:1 conduction.

9. **QRS complexes:** present, all shaped the same. **Regularity:** regular but interrupted (by two pauses). **Heart rate:** 44 to 75, with a mean rate of 60. **P waves:** upright, one preceding each QRS; shape varies slightly, but not enough to be significant. Don't get too hyper about the P wave shapes. Slight variability can be caused by fine baseline artifact. Different P wave shapes will be much more obvious. If you have to agonize over whether the P waves are shaped the same or are different, they're probably not different enough to be significant in terms of rhythm interpretation. **PR interval:** 0.20 to 0.22. **QRS interval:** 0.08. **Interpretation:** sinus rhythm with two sinus pauses. Why is this not a sinus arrhythmia? Sinus arrhythmia is cyclic, with slow periods, then faster periods. And it's irregular. Here the rhythm is regular, with an R-R interval of about 20 small blocks, except during the pauses. Sinus arrhythmia would be more irregular across the strip. Pay close attention to the regularity and it should lead the way.

10. **QRS complexes:** present, all shaped the same. Say what? They look different, you say? Hold on–the explanation is coming soon. **Regularity:** irregular. **Heart rate:** 100 to 150, with a mean rate of 120. **P waves:**

upright and matching on the first four beats, then changes to flutter waves after that. **PR interval:** 0.16 on the first four beats, not applicable after that. **QRS interval:** 0.08. **Interpretation:** sinus tachycardia converting after four beats to atrial flutter with variable conduction. The QRS complexes in atrial flutter here are distorted by the flutter waves. That's why they look different.

11. **QRS complexes:** present, all shaped the same. **Regularity:** regular. **Heart rate:** 44. **P waves:** upright, matching, some nonconducted; P-P interval regular; atrial rate 150. **PR interval:** varies. **QRS interval:** 0.14. **Interpretation:** sinus tachycardia with third-degree AV block and an accelerated idioventricular rhythm.
12. **QRS complexes:** present, all shaped the same. **Regularity:** regular. **Heart rate:** 125. **P waves:** upright, matching, one preceding each QRS; P-P interval regular. **PR interval:** 0.16. **QRS interval:** 0.06. **Interpretation:** sinus tachycardia.
13. **QRS complexes:** present, all but three shaped the same. Three beats are wide and bizarre in shape. **Regularity:** regular but interrupted (by premature beats). **Heart rate:** 125. **P waves:** upright and matching on the narrow beats, absent on the wide beats. **PR interval:** 0.12. **QRS interval:** 0.08 on the narrow beats, 0.16 on the wide beats. **Interpretation:** sinus tachycardia with unifocal PVCs in quadrigeminy (every fourth beat is a PVC).
14. **QRS complexes:** present, all shaped the same. **Regularity:** regular. **Heart rate:** 137. **P waves:** none seen. **PR interval:** not applicable. **QRS interval:** 0.10. **Interpretation:** SVT.
15. **QRS complex:** present, all shaped the same, very low voltage. **Regularity:** regular. **Heart rate:** about 135. **P waves:** not discernible; they may be present, but can't tell for sure. **PR interval:** cannot measure. **QRS interval:** 0.08. **Interpretation:** junctional tachycardia or SVT. Since there are no P waves, it's safer to call this SVT, as the real origin of this rhythm is not clear.
16. **QRS complex:** present, all shaped the same. **Regularity:** irregular. **Heart rate:** 56 to 71, with a mean rate of 70. **P waves:** upright, matching, one preceding each QRS; P-P interval irregular. **PR interval:** 0.12. **QRS interval:** 0.10. **Interpretation:** sinus arrhythmia. Note the longest R-R interval is between the last two QRS complexes on the strip, ending with the barely–there QRS at the very end. That R-R interval is 27 small blocks. The shortest R-R is between the third and fourth QRS complexes. That R-R is 21 small blocks. Since the rhythm is irregular, the longest R-R exceeds the shortest by four or more small blocks and this is definitely sinus in origin, it's a sinus arrhythmia. If you thought there was a sinus pause here, remember that sinus pause usually interrupts an otherwise regular rhythm. This rhythm is irregular.
17. **QRS complexes:** present, all shaped the same. **Regularity:** slightly irregular. R-R intervals vary from 22 to 25 small blocks. **Heart rate:** 60 to 68, with a mean rate of 60. **P waves:** upright, matching, one preceding

each QRS. **PR interval:** 0.12. **QRS interval:** 0.10. **Interpretation:** sinus rhythm versus sinus arrhythmia. This one is a bit odd. It's really not irregular enough to call it a sinus arrhythmia, since the longest R-R interval does not exceed the shortest by four or more small blocks. On the other hand, it's a bit irregular for the typical sinus rhythm. Since we're in a gray area here, it's OK to call it one versus the other. It would be nice to have a longer rhythm strip to evaluate. If, on the longer strip, the rhythm is an obvious sinus rhythm or an obvious sinus arrhythmia, then this little stretch of the total rhythm is probably also that same rhythm.

18. **QRS complexes:** present, all shaped the same. **Regularity:** regular. **Heart rate:** 75. **P waves:** none seen. **PR interval:** not applicable. **QRS interval:** around 0.20 to 0.28. This is a guesstimate, since it's hard to tell where the QRS ends and the ST segment begins. **Interpretation:** accelerated idioventricular rhythm.

19. **QRS complexes:** present, all shaped the same. **Regularity:** regular. **Heart rate:** 167. **P waves:** occasionally seen hidden in the T waves. Note the T waves between the first and second and eleventh and twelfth QRS complexes. Those T waves reveal the hidden P waves. **PR interval:** cannot measure, as cannot see the beginning of the P wave. **QRS interval:** 0.08. **Interpretation:** atrial tachycardia or SVT. It's probably more correct to call it atrial tachycardia, because the P waves are evident in places, but it's acceptable to say SVT.

20. **QRS complexes:** present, all shaped the same. **Regularity:** regular but interrupted (by premature beats). Remember it's normal to have a short pause following each premature beat. That's why this is not an irregular rhythm. **Heart rate:** about 85. Where did that heart rate come from? The first two beats on the strip are sinus beats with a rate of 85. From then on, every other beat is a PAC, so the heart rate cannot be determined accurately there. **P waves:** upright, two different shapes; almost every other P wave is premature and of a different shape. **PR interval:** 0.12 on the sinus beats, 0.16 on the premature beats. **QRS interval:** 0.08. **Interpretation:** sinus rhythm with frequent PACs, most of it in bigeminy.

21. **QRS complexes:** none present; wavy, static-looking baseline present instead. **Regularity:** not applicable. **Heart rate:** cannot measure, has no QRS complexes. **P waves:** none. **PR interval:** not applicable. **QRS interval:** not applicable. **Interpretation:** ventricular fibrillation.

22. **QRS complexes:** present, two different shapes. Some QRS complexes are narrow, others are wide. **Regularity:** regular but interrupted (by premature beats). **Heart rate:** 94. **P waves:** upright and matching preceding the narrow QRS complexes, and seen in the T wave following the premature beats. **PR interval:** 0.18 on the narrow beats; not calculated on the premature beats, as the P is retrograde. **QRS interval:** 0.08 on the narrow beats, 0.14 on the wide beats. **Interpretation:** sinus rhythm with unifocal PVCs in trigeminy.

23. **QRS complexes:** present, all shaped the same. **Regularity:** irregular. **Heart rate:** 48 to 81, with a mean rate of 60. **P waves:** upright, matching, some nonconducted; P-P interval regular. **PR interval:** varies. **QRS interval:** 0.11. **Interpretation:** sinus rhythm with type I second-degree AV block (Wenckebach). Note how the PR interval gradually prolongs, then a beat is dropped.

24. **QRS complexes:** present, all shaped the same. **Regularity:** regular. **Heart rate:** 79. **P waves:** none present; regular sawtooth-shaped waves present instead. **PR interval:** not applicable. **QRS interval:** 0.08. **Interpretation:** atrial flutter with 4:1 conduction.

25. **QRS complexes:** present, all but one having the same shape. One is very wide compared to the others. **Regularity:** regular but interrupted (by a premature beat). **Heart rate:** 107. **P waves:** upright and matching on the narrow beats, absent on the wide beat. **PR interval:** 0.12 to 0.14. **QRS interval:** 0.08 on the narrow beats, 0.16 on the wide beat. **Interpretation:** sinus tachycardia with one PVC.

26. **QRS complexes:** none. **Regularity:** not applicable, as there are no QRS complexes. **Heart rate:** zero. **P waves:** none. **PR interval:** not applicable. **QRS interval:** not applicable. **Interpretation:** asystole.

27. **QRS complexes:** present, all shaped the same. **Regularity:** regular. **Heart rate:** 50. **P waves:** upright, matching, P-P interval regular; one P wave is hidden inside the last QRS; atrial rate 88. **PR interval:** varies. **QRS interval:** 0.14. **Interpretation:** sinus rhythm with third-degree AV block and an accelerated idioventricular rhythm.

28. **QRS complexes:** present, all shaped the same. **Regularity:** regular. **Heart rate:** 79. **P waves:** matching, upright, one preceding each QRS; P-P interval regular. **PR interval:** 0.28. **QRS interval:** 0.08. **Interpretation:** sinus rhythm with first-degree AV block.

29. **QRS complexes:** present, all shaped the same. **Regularity:** regular. **Heart rate:** 68. **P waves:** none present; regular sawtooth-shaped waves present instead. **PR interval:** not applicable. **QRS interval:** about 0.10. The end of the QRS is distorted by a flutter wave, making the QRS look artificially wide. **Interpretation:** atrial flutter with 4:1 conduction. Two of the flutter waves are hidden inside the QRS and T wave. So how can we tell the flutter waves are even there if we can't see them? We can definitely see two obvious flutter waves between the QRS complexes. Since we know that flutter waves are regular, we simply note the distance between the two flutter waves we see together, then march out where the rest of them should be.

30. **QRS complexes:** present, most shaped the same. An occasional QRS is missing the notch on the downstroke. **Regularity:** regular. **Heart rate:** 187. **P waves:** an occasional dissociated P wave is seen. **PR interval:** not applicable. **QRS interval:** 0.14. **Interpretation:** ventricular tachycardia.

31. **QRS complexes:** present, all shaped the same. **Regularity:** irregular. **Heart rate:** 48 to 60, with a mean rate of 60. **P waves:** all upright, but

there are at least three different shapes; P-P interval irregular. **PR interval:** 0.24 to 0.28. **QRS interval:** 0.10. **Interpretation:** wandering atrial pacemaker.

32. **QRS complexes:** present, all shaped the same. **Regularity:** regular but interrupted (by a prematurely arriving beat). **Heart rate:** 71. **P waves:** none present; regular sawtooth-shaped waves present instead. **PR interval:** not applicable. **QRS interval:** 0.10. **Interpretation:** atrial flutter with 2:1 and 4:1 conduction. The one episode of the 2:1 conduction is responsible for the interruption of this otherwise regular 4:1 conduction. This beat that comes in early because of the conduction ratio change is not per se a premature beat in the way that PVCs are, but nevertheless it does arrive earlier than expected, given the surrounding R-R intervals. For this reason the regularity is called *regular but interrupted* rather than irregular. All R-R intervals except this short one are about the same.
33. **QRS complexes:** present, all shaped the same. **Regularity:** regular but interrupted (by pauses). **Heart rate:** 62 to 107, with a mean rate of 90. **P waves:** upright, matching, some nonconducted, others hidden inside T waves; P-P interval regular; atrial rate about 115. **PR interval:** varies. **QRS interval:** 0.08. **Interpretation:** sinus tachycardia with type I second-degree AV block (Wenckebach).
34. **QRS complexes:** present, all shaped the same. **Regularity:** regular but interrupted (by premature beats). **Heart rate:** 79. **P waves:** biphasic except for the two that are inside the T wave. There are two different shapes of P waves. P-P interval varies. **PR interval:** 0.18 on the normal beats, approximately 0.22 on the premature beats. **QRS interval:** 0.08. **Interpretation:** sinus rhythm with two PACs.
35. **QRS complexes:** present, all shaped the same, one shorter than the rest. **Regularity:** regular but interrupted (by a pause). **Heart rate:** 19 to 54, with a mean rate of 50. **P waves:** upright, matching, none present on the beat ending the pause; P-P interval irregular. **PR interval:** 0.16 to 0.18. **QRS interval:** 0.09. **Interpretation:** sinus bradycardia with a 3.28-second sinus arrest ending with a junctional escape beat. Whenever there is a pause, the length of it must be recorded. If there is a sinus arrest, the beat ending the pause will be an escape beat from a lower pacemaker. Which pacemaker takes over should also be recorded.
36. **QRS complexes:** present, all shaped the same. **Regularity:** regular; the R-R intervals vary only by two small blocks. **Heart rate:** about 50. **P waves:** upright and matching, one preceding each QRS; P-P interval regular. **PR interval:** 0.20. **QRS interval:** 0.08. **Interpretation:** sinus bradycardia. A PR interval of 0.20 is still normal. There's no first-degree AV block.
37. **QRS complexes:** present, all shaped the same. **Regularity:** regular. **Heart rate:** 61. **P waves:** inverted inside ST segment following the QRS complexes. **PR interval:** not applicable. **QRS interval:** 0.12. **Interpretation:** accelerated junctional rhythm with a BBB.

38. **QRS complexes:** present, all shaped the same. **Regularity:** regular. **Heart rate:** 88. **P waves:** upright and matching, one preceding each QRS; P-P interval regular. **PR interval:** 0.24. **QRS interval:** 0.10. **Interpretation:** sinus rhythm with first-degree AV block.
39. **QRS complexes:** present, all shaped the same. **Regularity:** regular. The R-R intervals vary by only two small blocks. **Heart rate:** about 36. **P waves:** upright and matching, one preceding each QRS; P-P interval regular. **PR interval:** 0.16. **QRS interval:** 0.12. **Interpretation:** sinus bradycardia with a BBB; there's a prominent U wave following the T waves.
40. **QRS complexes:** present, all shaped the same. **Regularity:** regular. **Heart rate:** 60. **P waves:** upright, notched, and matching, one preceding each QRS; P-P interval regular. **PR interval:** 0.16. **QRS interval:** 0.08. **Interpretation:** sinus rhythm.
41. **QRS complexes:** present, all shaped the same. **Regularity:** irregular. The R-R intervals vary from 11 to 15 small blocks. **Heart rate:** 100 to 137, with a mean rate of 120. **P waves:** none seen. **PR interval:** not applicable. **QRS interval:** 0.20. **Interpretation:** ventricular tachycardia. Remember v-tach is usually regular, but can be irregular at times.
42. **QRS complexes:** present, all shaped the same. **Regularity:** irregular. **Heart rate:** 39 to 88, with a mean rate of 60. **P waves:** none present; wavy, undulating baseline present instead. **PR interval:** not applicable. **QRS interval:** 0.06. **Interpretation:** atrial fibrillation.
43. **QRS complexes:** present, all shaped the same. **Regularity:** regular. **Heart rate:** 115. **P waves:** upright and matching, one preceding each QRS; P-P interval regular. **PR interval:** 0.12. **QRS interval:** 0.10. **Interpretation:** sinus tachycardia.
44. **QRS complexes:** present, all shaped the same. **Regularity:** irregular. **Heart rate:** 83 to 167, with a mean rate of 140. **P waves:** none present; wavy, undulating baseline present instead. **PR interval:** not applicable. **QRS interval:** 0.04. **Interpretation:** atrial fibrillation.
45. **QRS complexes:** present, all shaped the same. **Regularity:** regular. **Heart rate:** about 52. **P waves:** upright, matching, one preceding each QRS. **PR interval:** 0.18. **QRS interval:** 0.13. **Interpretation:** sinus bradycardia with a BBB.
46. **QRS complexes:** present, all shaped the same. **Regularity:** regular. **Heart rate:** 28. **P waves:** upright, matching, some nonconducted. P-P interval regular. Atrial rate 83. **PR interval:** 0.16. **QRS interval:** 0.06. **Interpretation:** sinus rhythm with type II second-degree AV block.
47. **QRS complexes:** present, all but one shaped the same. **Regularity:** regular. **Heart rate:** 26. **P waves:** matching, upright, some nonconducted; P-P interval regular; atrial rate 75. **PR interval:** varies. **QRS interval:** 0.04 to 0.08. **Interpretation:** sinus rhythm with third-degree AV block and a junctional bradycardia. This heart rate is extremely slow for the junction. Remember, it normally escapes at a rate of 40 to 60.

This patient not only has an AV block, but also a sick AV node in terms of its pacemaking ability. Also of concern is the ventricle as a pacemaker. It normally escapes at a rate of 20 to 40. Where is it? Why didn't it kick in as the pacemaker at a faster rate than we have here? This rhythm indicates a very sick heart.

48. **QRS complexes:** present, all shaped the same. **Regularity:** regular. The R-R intervals vary by only two small blocks. **Heart rate:** 88. **P waves:** biphasic, matching, one preceding each QRS; P-P interval regular. **PR interval:** 0.12. **QRS interval:** 0.10. **Interpretation:** sinus rhythm.

49. **QRS complexes:** present, all shaped the same, though one is shorter than the other. **Regularity:** cannot assess as only two QRS complexes are present (at least three QRS complexes are needed to determine regularity). **Heart rate:** about 11. **P waves:** none present; wavy, undulating baseline present instead. **PR interval:** not applicable. **QRS interval:** 0.12. **Interpretation:** atrial fibrillation with a BBB. This could also be called atrial fib-flutter, as it does look quite fluttery in places. It is best not to call this an outright atrial flutter, though, as the waves dampen out in the middle of the strip, causing the waves to look different throughout the strip. This is a drastic representation of how slow the heart rate can go with atrial fibrillation. This is a 5.6-second pause, erroneously labeled on the strip as 5.52 seconds. This patient was lucky to be asleep and had no problems. A pause this long could easily have caused serious symptoms of low cardiac output.

50. **QRS complexes:** present, all shaped the same. **Regularity:** slightly irregular. The R-R intervals vary by three small blocks. **Heart rate:** 30 to 32. **P waves:** upright, three different shapes, one preceding each QRS; P-P interval slightly irregular. **PR interval:** 0.16 to 0.20. **QRS interval:** 0.10. **Interpretation:** wandering atrial pacemaker.

51. **QRS complexes:** present, all shaped the same. **Regularity:** regular. **Heart rate:** 94. **P waves:** matching, biphasic, two to each QRS; atrial rate 187. **PR interval:** 0.06. **QRS interval:** 0.08. **Interpretation:** atrial tachycardia with 2:1 block. One P wave is easy to see between the QRS complexes. The other is right *on* the QRS, distorting the shape of the QRS and the P a little. It wouldn't be correct to call this atrial flutter, since there is an obvious flat baseline between the P waves. You'll recall atrial flutter has no flat isoelectric line–flutter waves all zigzag one after the other.

52. **QRS complexes:** present, all shaped the same. **Regularity:** regular. **Heart rate:** 68. **P waves:** negative, one preceding each QRS; P-P interval regular. **PR interval:** 0.24. **QRS interval:** 0.20. **Interpretation:** sinus rhythm with first-degree AV block and a BBB. Though the lead is not recorded on this strip, it's probably V_1. Sinus rhythms can have a negative P wave in V_1 This is a very sick heart. The AV node is sick, as evidenced by the first-degree block, but also the bundle branches are sick, as evidenced by the width of the QRS complexes. Many cardiologists feel that to some extent a patient's ventricular function can be predicted

by the QRS interval. This patient was predicted to have a very low functioning heart, and that was borne out by further studies.

53. **QRS complexes:** present, all shaped the same. **Regularity:** regular. **Heart rate:** about 103. **P waves:** upright, matching, one preceding each QRS. **PR interval:** 0.16. **QRS interval:** 0.08. **Interpretation:** sinus tachycardia.
54. **QRS complexes:** present, all shaped the same. **Regularity:** irregular. **Heart rate:** 29 to 83, with a mean rate of 50. **P waves:** none present; *very* low voltage wavy, undulating baseline present instead. **PR interval:** not applicable. **QRS interval:** 0.08. **Interpretation:** atrial fibrillation. This is an example of what's sometimes called *straight-line* atrial fibrillation. There is barely a bobble of the baseline between QRS complexes. The most obvious feature that suggests atrial fibrillation is the irregularity of the rhythm. Then you notice the very fine fibrillatory waves. This patient has probably been in atrial fibrillation for years.
55. **QRS complexes:** present, all shaped the same. **Regularity:** irregular. **Heart rate:** 37 to 52, with a mean rate of 30. The strip starts in the middle of a 2.6-second pause, though, so we know the heart rate actually gets much slower at times. **P waves:** none present. Regular sawtooth-shaped waves present instead. **PR interval:** not applicable. **QRS interval:** 0.08. **Interpretation:** atrial flutter with variable conduction.
56. **QRS complexes:** present, all shaped the same. **Regularity:** regular. **Heart rate:** 94. **P waves:** upright, matching, one preceding each QRS. **PR interval:** 0.16. **QRS interval:** 0.14. **Interpretation:** sinus rhythm with BBB.
57. **QRS complexes:** present, all shaped the same. **Regularity:** irregular. **Heart rate:** about 19 to 23, with a mean rate of 30. **P waves:** none present. **PR interval:** not applicable. **QRS interval:** 0.28. **Interpretation:** dying heart (agonal rhythm). Though the heart rate is a little fast for dying heart, it must be called this because it is so irregular. Idioventricular rhythm is usually more regular.
58. **QRS complexes:** present, all shaped the same. **Regularity:** regular. R-R intervals vary by only one small block. **Heart rate:** 60. **P waves:** upright, matching, one preceding each QRS; P-P interval regular. **PR interval:** 0.12. **QRS interval:** 0.10. **Interpretation:** sinus rhythm.
59. **QRS complexes:** none present; wavy, static-looking baseline present instead. **Regularity:** not applicable. **Heart rate:** cannot measure. **P waves:** none present. **PR interval:** not applicable. **QRS interval:** not applicable. **Interpretation:** ventricular fibrillation.
60. **QRS complexes:** present, all shaped the same. **Regularity:** irregular. The R-R intervals vary by four small blocks. **Heart rate:** about 37 to 40, with a mean rate of 40. **P waves:** upright, matching, one preceding each QRS; P-P interval slightly irregular. **PR interval:** 0.13. **QRS interval:** 0.09. **Interpretation:** sinus arrhythmia.

61. **QRS complexes:** present, all but one having the same shape. One is much wider than the others. **Regularity:** regular but interrupted (by a premature beat). **Heart rate:** 115. **P waves:** upright, matching, one preceding all QRS complexes except the wide one. **PR interval:** 0.14. **QRS interval:** 0.06 on the narrow beats, 0.14 on the wide beat. **Interpretation:** sinus tachycardia with a PVC.

62. **QRS complexes:** none present. **Regularity:** cannot determine since there are no QRS complexes. **Heart rate:** zero. **P waves:** upright and matching; P-P interval irregular. **PR interval:** not applicable. **QRS interval:** not applicable. **Interpretation:** ventricular asystole.

63. **QRS complexes:** present, all shaped the same. **Regularity:** regular. **Heart rate:** about 110. **P waves:** upright, matching, one preceding each QRS; P-P interval regular. **PR interval:** 0.16. **QRS interval:** 0.08. **Interpretation:** sinus tachycardia.

64. **QRS complexes:** present, all but one shaped the same. One is wider than the others. **Regularity:** regular but interrupted (by a premature beat). **Heart rate:** 62. **P waves:** upright, matching, one preceding all QRS complexes except the premature one. There is a P wave in the premature beat's ST segment. **PR interval:** 0.20. **QRS interval:** 0.10 on the narrow beats, 0.18 on the wide beat. **Interpretation:** sinus rhythm with a PVC.

65. **QRS complexes:** present, all shaped the same. **Regularity:** irregular. **Heart rate:** 68 to 125, with a mean rate of 100. **P waves:** upright, matching, some nonconducted; P-P interval regular; atrial rate 115. **PR interval:** varies. **QRS interval:** 0.10. **Interpretation:** sinus tachycardia with type I second-degree AV block (Wenckebach).

66. **QRS complexes:** present, all shaped the same. **Regularity:** regular. **Heart rate:** 65. **P waves:** upright, matching, one preceding each QRS; P-P interval regular. **PR interval:** 0.22. **QRS interval:** 0.10. **Interpretation:** sinus rhythm with first-degree AV block.

67. **QRS complexes:** present, all shaped the same. **Regularity:** irregular. **Heart rate:** 62 to 137, with a mean rate of 110. **P waves:** none present; wavy, undulating baseline present instead. **PR interval:** not applicable. **QRS interval:** 0.08. **Interpretation:** atrial fib-flutter. Though this may indeed be a true atrial flutter, the flutter waves are not as obvious at the beginning of the strip as they are later on, so it's possible this may be a combination of fib and flutter.

68. **QRS complexes:** present, all shaped the same. **Regularity:** regular. **Heart rate:** 44. **P waves:** upright, matching, some nonconducted; P-P interval regular; atrial rate 137. **PR interval:** 0.28 to 0.40. **QRS interval:** 0.14. **Interpretation:** sinus tachycardia with third-degree AV block and accelerated idioventricular rhythm. There are three P waves to each QRS. If you counted only two, look again. Note the distance between two consecutive P waves. Now march out where the rest of them are. There's more here than first meets the eye. Always march out the P waves!

69. **QRS complexes:** present, all shaped the same. **Regularity:** regular. **Heart rate:** 71. **P waves:** upright, matching, one preceding each QRS; P-P interval regular. **PR interval:** 0.28. **QRS interval:** 0.10. **Interpretation:** sinus rhythm with first-degree AV block.
70. **QRS complexes:** present, all shaped the same. **Regularity:** irregular. **Heart rate:** 60 to 94, with a mean rate of 70. **P waves:** none present; wavy, undulating baseline present instead. **PR interval:** not applicable. **QRS interval:** 0.10. **Interpretation:** atrial fibrillation.
71. **QRS complexes:** present, all shaped the same. **Regularity:** regular. **Heart rate:** 56. **P waves:** upright, matching, one preceding each QRS; P-P interval regular. **PR interval:** 0.14. **QRS interval:** 0.10. **Interpretation:** sinus bradycardia.
72. **QRS complexes:** present, all shaped the same. **Regularity:** regular. **Heart rate:** 79. **P waves:** none present; regular, sawtooth-shaped waves present instead. Also note the pacemaker spike preceding each QRS. **PR interval:** not applicable. **QRS interval:** 0.12. **Interpretation:** ventricular pacing with underlying atrial flutter.
73. **QRS complexes:** present, all shaped the same. **Regularity:** regular. **Heart rate:** 94. **P waves:** upright, matching, one preceding each QRS; P-P interval regular. **PR interval:** 0.12. **QRS interval:** 0.08. **Interpretation:** sinus rhythm. Baseline sway artifact is present.
74. **QRS complexes:** present, all shaped the same. **Regularity:** irregular. **Heart rate:** 75 to 107, with a mean rate of 90. **P waves:** none present; regular sawtooth-shaped waves present instead. **PR interval:** not applicable. **QRS interval:** 0.08. **Interpretation:** atrial flutter with variable conduction.
75. **QRS complexes:** present, all shaped the same. **Regularity:** irregular. **Heart rate:** 37 to 62, with a mean rate of 60. **P waves:** upright, matching, one preceding each QRS complex; P-P interval irregular. **PR interval:** 0.12. **QRS interval:** 0.10. **Interpretation:** sinus arrhythmia. If you count out the R-R intervals, you'll note they grow steadily longer throughout the strip.
76. **QRS complexes:** present, all shaped the same. **Regularity:** regular. **Heart rate:** 79. **P waves:** upright, matching, one preceding each QRS complex; P-P interval regular. **PR interval:** 0.14. **QRS interval:** 0.08. **Interpretation:** sinus rhythm.
77. **QRS complexes:** present, all shaped the same. **Regularity:** regular. **Heart rate:** 27. **P waves:** none present. **PR interval:** not applicable. **QRS interval:** 0.08. **Interpretation:** junctional bradycardia.
78. **QRS complexes:** present, all shaped the same. **Regularity:** regular. **Heart rate:** 45. **P waves:** upright, matching, one preceding each QRS; P-P interval regular. **PR interval:** 0.20. **QRS interval:** 0.08. **Interpretation:** sinus bradycardia. Note also a very prominent U wave.
79. **QRS complexes:** present, all shaped the same. **Regularity:** regular. **Heart rate:** 115. **P waves:** upright, matching, one preceding each

QRS; P-P interval regular. **PR interval:** 0.12. **QRS interval:** 0.06. **Interpretation:** sinus tachycardia.

80. **QRS complexes:** present, all shaped the same. **Regularity:** regular. **Heart rate:** 107. **P waves:** biphasic, matching, one preceding each QRS; P-P interval regular. **PR interval:** 0.14. **QRS interval:** 0.10. **Interpretation:** sinus tachycardia.
81. **QRS complexes:** present, all shaped the same. **Regularity:** irregular. **Heart rate:** 137 to 167, with a mean rate of 150. **P waves:** none seen. **PR interval:** not applicable. **QRS interval:** 0.08. **Interpretation:** atrial fibrillation. If you thought it was ventricular tachycardia, look again. The QRS complexes are not wide enough to be ventricular. Since it's irregular, it can't be called SVT. Though there are no obvious fibrillatory waves visible, it's prudent to call this rhythm atrial fibrillation because of its pronounced irregularity and lack of P waves.
82. **QRS complexes:** present, all shaped the same. **Regularity:** regular. **Heart rate:** 60. **P waves:** upright, matching, one preceding each QRS; P-P interval regular. **PR interval:** 0.12. **QRS interval:** 0.10. **Interpretation:** sinus rhythm.
83. **QRS complexes:** present, all shaped the same. **Regularity:** irregular. **Heart rate:** 88 to 115, with a mean rate of 110. **P waves:** none present; regular sawtooth-shaped waves present instead. **PR interval:** not applicable. **QRS interval:** 0.08. **Interpretation:** atrial flutter with variable conduction.
84. **QRS complexes:** present, all shaped the same. **Regularity:** irregular. **Heart rate:** 79 to 137, with a mean rate of 110. **P waves:** none present; way, undulating baseline present instead. **PR interval:** not applicable. **QRS interval:** 0.10. **Interpretation:** atrial fibrillation.
85. **QRS complexes:** present, all shaped the same. **Regularity:** regular. **Heart rate:** 88. **P waves:** upright, matching, one preceding each QRS; P-P interval regular. **PR interval:** 0.22. **QRS interval:** 0.12. **Interpretation:** sinus rhythm with first-degree AV block and BBB.
86. **QRS complexes:** present, all shaped the same. **Regularity:** regular. **Heart rate:** 60. **P waves:** none present; regular sawtooth-shaped waves present instead. **PR interval:** not applicable. **QRS interval:** 0.10. **Interpretation:** atrial flutter with variable conduction. Many of the flutter waves are lost inside the big inverted T wave.
87. **QRS complexes:** present, all shaped the same. **Regularity:** regular. **Heart rate:** 59. **P waves:** upright, matching, two to each QRS. The T wave has a double hump–do you see it? The first hump is the first P wave. The second P is right in front of the QRS. P-P interval regular. Atrial rate 115. **PR interval:** 0.24. **QRS interval:** 0.08. **Interpretation:** sinus tachycardia with 2:1 AV block, probably type I.
88. **QRS complexes:** present, all shaped the same. **Regularity:** irregular. **Heart rate:** 33 to 137, with a mean rate of 50. **P waves:** none present; wavy, undulating baseline present instead. **PR interval:** not applicable. **QRS interval:** 0.08. **Interpretation:** atrial fibrillation.

89. **QRS complexes:** present, all shaped the same. **Regularity:** regular. **Heart rate:** 115. **P waves:** upright, matching, one preceding each QRS; P-P interval regular. **PR interval:** 0.16. **QRS interval:** 0.12. **Interpretation:** sinus tachycardia with a BBB.
90. **QRS complexes:** present, all shaped the same. **Regularity:** regular. **Heart rate:** 75. **P waves:** upright, matching, one preceding each QRS; P-P interval regular. **PR interval:** 0.12. **QRS interval:** 0.06. **Interpretation:** sinus rhythm.
91. **QRS complexes:** present, sawtooth-shaped. **Regularity:** irregular. **Heart rate:** 187 to 300. **P waves:** none seen. **PR interval:** not applicable. **QRS interval:** cannot measure, as cannot tell where QRS ends and T wave begins. **Interpretation:** ventricular flutter.
92. **QRS complexes:** present. **Regularity:** regular but interrupted (by premature beats). **Heart rate:** about 85. **P waves:** inverted, matching, one preceding all the narrow QRS complexes. **PR interval:** 0.16. **Interpretation:** sinus rhythm with a unifocal ventricular couplet and a PVC. Wait a minute. The P wave here is negative. Why is this not a junctional rhythm? This is V_1–see the notation at the top of the strip? Recall the P wave can be normally inverted in V_1. So that doesn't necessarily imply a junctional pacemaker. Also, a junctional rhythm would have had a shorter PR interval, less than 0.12.
93. **QRS complexes:** present, all shaped the same. **Regularity:** irregular. **Heart rate:** 29, then slower. **P waves:** none present. **PR interval:** not applicable. **QRS interval:** 0.24 to 0.28. **Interpretation:** dying heart.
94. **QRS complexes:** present, different shapes. **Regularity:** irregular. **Heart rate:** >300 in places. **P waves:** none seen. **PR interval:** not applicable. **QRS interval:** cannot measure, as cannot tell where QRS ends and T wave begins. **Interpretation:** torsades de pointes. Remember torsades is identified more by its classic shape than by any other criteria.
95. **QRS complexes:** present, all shaped the same. **Regularity:** regular. **Heart rate:** 43. **P waves:** inverted following each QRS complex in the ST segment. **PR interval:** not applicable. **QRS interval:** 0.08. **Interpretation:** junctional rhythm.
96. **QRS complexes:** only one present–at the beginning of the strip. Then a wavy, static-looking baseline is seen. **Regularity:** not applicable. **Heart rate:** zero after that first beat. **P waves:** none present. **PR interval:** not applicable. **QRS interval:** 0.28 on the only QRS complex on the strip. **Interpretation:** one ventricular beat, then ventricular fibrillation.
97. **QRS complexes:** none present; wavy, static-looking baseline present instead. **Regularity:** not applicable. **Heart rate:** cannot measure. **P waves:** none present. **PR interval:** not applicable. **QRS interval:** not applicable. **Interpretation:** ventricular fibrillation.
98. **QRS complexes:** none present. **Regularity:** not applicable, as there are no QRS complexes. **Heart rate:** zero. **P waves:** biphasic, matching;

P-P interval regular. **PR interval:** not applicable. **QRS interval:** not applicable. **Interpretation:** ventricular asystole.

99. **QRS complexes:** present, all shaped the same. **Regularity:** irregular. **Heart rate:** 100 to 177. **P waves:** none present; wavy, undulating baseline present instead. **PR interval:** not applicable. **QRS interval:** 0.12. **Interpretation:** atrial fibrillation with a BBB.

100. **QRS complexes:** present, all shaped the same. **Regularity:** regular. **Heart rate:** 60. **P waves:** none present. **PR interval:** not applicable. **QRS interval:** 0.16 to 0.22. **Interpretation:** accelerated idioventricular rhythm.

101. **QRS complexes:** present, all shaped the same. **Regularity:** regular but interrupted (by a premature beat). **Heart rate:** 68. **P waves:** upright and matching except for the very last beat, which has a tiny inverted P wave. One P wave precedes each QRS. P-P interval is irregular. **PR interval:** 0.14 on all but the last beat. The PR interval of the last beat is 0.12. **QRS interval:** 0.12. **Interpretation:** sinus rhythm with a PJC and BBB.

102. **QRS complexes:** present, all shaped the same. **Regularity:** regular but interrupted (by a premature beat and also a pause). **Heart rate:** 39 to 100, with a mean rate of 70. **P waves:** upright and matching on all but the third beat, which has a tiny upright P wave at the end of the preceding T wave. There is also a tiny upright P wave just before the downstroke of the third T wave (inside the pause). P-P interval is irregular. **PR interval:** 0.18 on the normal beats; 0.22 on the premature beat. **QRS interval:** 0.06. **Interpretation:** sinus rhythm with a PAC and a nonconducted PAC. The third beat is the PAC. The P wave at the downstroke of the third beat's T wave is the nonconducted PAC. If you called this an AV block of some kind, remember that in AV blocks the P-P interval is regular. Here we have two premature P waves.

103. **QRS complexes:** present, all shaped the same. **Regularity:** irregular. **Heart rate:** 28 to 38, with a mean rate of 40. **P waves:** none present; wavy, undulating baseline present instead. **PR interval:** not applicable. **QRS interval:** 0.08. **Interpretation:** atrial fibrillation.

104. **QRS complexes:** present, all shaped the same. **Regularity:** regular but interrupted (by a premature beat). **Heart rate:** 100. **P waves:** biphasic and matching on all but the third beat, which is premature and has a different shape P wave. **PR interval:** 0.14 on the normal beats; 0.12 on the premature beat. **QRS interval:** 0.06. **Interpretation:** sinus rhythm with a PAC.

105. **QRS complexes:** present, all shaped the same. **Regularity:** regular but interrupted (by premature beats and pauses). **Heart rate:** 38 to 125, with a mean rate of 80. **P waves:** upright and matching on all but the P wave following the second QRS and also the P wave preceding the sixth QRS. Those P waves have a different shape. P-P interval is irregular. **PR interval:** 0.14 on the normal beats; 0.12 on the sixth

beat. **QRS interval:** 0.08. **Interpretation:** sinus rhythm with a PAC (the sixth beat) and a nonconducted PAC (the premature P after the second QRS).

106. **QRS complexes:** present, all but one shaped the same. One is wider and taller than the others. **Regularity:** regular but interrupted (by a premature beat). **Heart rate:** 125. **P waves:** upright and matching on all but the wide QRS beat, which has no P wave. **PR interval:** 0.16. **QRS interval:** 0.08 on the normal beats, 0.14 on the premature beat. **Interpretation:** sinus tachycardia with a PVC.

107. **QRS complexes:** present, all shaped the same. **Regularity:** regular. **Heart rate:** about 130. **P waves:** upright, matching, one preceding each QRS; P-P interval regular. **PR interval:** 0.14. **QRS interval:** 0.08. **Interpretation:** sinus tachycardia.

108. **QRS complexes:** present, all shaped the same. **Regularity:** irregular. **Heart rate:** 68 to 125, with a mean rate of 90. **P waves:** at least three different shapes; P-P interval irregular. **PR interval:** varies. **QRS interval:** 0.10. **Interpretation:** wandering atrial pacemaker. Since the mean rate is less than 100, it is better to call this WAP than MAT.

109. **QRS complexes:** present, all shaped the same. **Regularity:** regular. **Heart rate:** 38. **P waves:** upright and matching directly preceding the QRS. There is an extra premature P wave at the end of each T wave. That P has a different shape–it's pointy. **PR interval:** 0.20. **QRS interval:** 0.08. **Interpretation:** sinus bradycardia with bigeminal nonconducted PACs. This was a stinky strip, you say. It just looks like sinus bradycardia. That's right. But do you see the premature P wave now that it's been pointed out? Always be suspicious of T waves with humps on their ends. That hump might just be a P wave.

110. **QRS complexes:** present, all shaped the same. **Regularity:** irregular. **Heart rate:** 29 to 60, with a mean rate of 40. **P waves:** none present; wavy, undulating baseline present instead. **PR interval:** not applicable. **QRS interval:** 0.08. **Interpretation:** atrial fibrillation.

111. **QRS complexes:** present; most but not all shaped the same. **Regularity:** irregular. **Heart rate:** 167 to 250, with a mean rate of 200. **P waves:** none present; wavy, undulating baseline present instead. **PR interval:** not applicable. **QRS interval:** 0.06 to 0.08. **Interpretation:** atrial fibrillation. If you were tempted to call this SVT, remember that SVT is a regular rhythm. This strip is not regular.

112. **QRS complexes:** present, all shaped the same. **Regularity:** regular. **Heart rate:** 62. **P waves:** none seen. **PR interval:** not applicable. **QRS interval:** 0.20. **Interpretation:** accelerated idioventricular rhythm.

113. **QRS complexes:** present, all shaped the same, though some are deeper than others. **Regularity:** regular but interrupted (by a run of premature beats). **Heart rate:** 88 when in sinus tachycardia, about 187 when in atrial tachycardia. **P waves:** upright and matching on

all but the very rapid beats, whose P waves are inside the preceding T wave. **PR interval:** 0.20 on the normal beats, unable to measure on the rapid beats, as the P is inside the T wave. **QRS interval:** 0.08. **Interpretation:** sinus tachycardia with a 10-beat run of PAT. We know this is PAT, as we see that the run of PAT begins with a PAC (the fourth beat).

114. **QRS complexes:** present, all shaped the same. **Regularity:** irregular. **Heart rate:** 150 to 250, with a mean rate of 190. **P waves:** none present; wavy, undulating baseline present instead. **PR interval:** not applicable. **QRS interval:** 0.06. **Interpretation:** atrial fibrillation.

115. **QRS complexes:** present, all shaped the same. **Regularity:** irregular. **Heart rate:** 150 to 250, with a mean rate of 190. **P waves:** none present; wavy, undulating baseline present instead. **PR interval:** not applicable. **QRS interval:** 0.06. **Interpretation:** atrial fibrillation.

116. **QRS complexes:** present, all shaped the same. **Regularity:** regular but interrupted (by a pause). **Heart rate:** 37 to 72. **P waves:** upright and matching except for the premature P wave inside the fourth T wave. **PR interval:** 0.24. **QRS interval:** 0.08. **Interpretation:** sinus rhythm with a nonconducted PAC.

117. **QRS complexes:** present, all shaped the same. **Regularity:** regular. **Heart rate:** 71. **P waves:** tiny inverted P waves present preceding the QRS complexes. **PR interval:** about 0.06. **QRS interval:** 0.10. **Interpretation:** accelerated junctional rhythm.

118. **QRS complexes:** present, all shaped the same. **Regularity:** regular but interrupted (by pauses). **Heart rate:** 48 to 88, with a mean rate of 80. **P waves:** upright and matching except for the premature P waves inside the third and sixth T waves. **PR interval:** 0.18. **QRS interval:** 0.08. **Interpretation:** sinus rhythm with two nonconducted PACs.

119. **QRS complexes:** present, all shaped the same. **Regularity:** regular. **Heart rate:** 29. **P waves:** none present. **PR interval:** not applicable. **QRS interval:** 0.28. **Interpretation:** idioventricular rhythm.

120. **QRS complexes:** present, all shaped the same. **Regularity:** regular but interrupted (by a pause). **Heart rate:** 32 to 58, with a mean rate of 50. **P waves:** upright, matching, sometimes more than one per QRS; atrial rate 60. **PR interval:** varies. **QRS interval:** 0.10. **Interpretation:** sinus rhythm with type I second-degree AV block. (Wenckebach). See how the PR interval gradually prolongs until a P wave is blocked (not followed by a QRS)?

121. **QRS complexes:** present, all shaped the same. **Regularity:** regular. **Heart rate:** 45. **P waves:** upright, matching, some nonconducted; atrial rate 137. **PR interval:** varies. **QRS interval:** 0.16. **Interpretation:** sinus tachycardia with third-degree AV block and an accelerated idioventricular rhythm. Did you think this was type II second-degree AV block? The differentiating factor here is the changing PR intervals. Type II has constant PR intervals. Did you think it was type I second-degree AV

block? Type I does not have regular R-R intervals. So it could only be third-degree AV block.

122. **QRS complexes:** present, all shaped the same. **Regularity:** irregular. **Heart rate:** 60 to 83, with a mean rate of 80. **P waves:** upright, matching, one per QRS. P-P interval irregular. **PR interval:** 0.14. **QRS interval:** 0.08. **Interpretation:** sinus arrhythmia.

123. **QRS complexes:** present, all shaped the same. **Regularity:** regular. **Heart rate:** 83. **P waves:** none noted. **PR interval:** not applicable. **QRS interval:** 0.16. **Interpretation:** accelerated idioventricular rhythm.

124. **QRS complexes:** present, all shaped the same. **Regularity:** regular. **Heart rate:** 125. **P waves:** none seen. **PR interval:** not applicable. **QRS interval:** 0.20. **Interpretation:** ventricular tachycardia.

125. **QRS complexes:** present, all shaped the same. **Regularity:** regular. **Heart rate:** 58. **P waves:** none seen. There's a U wave immediately following the T waves–don't confuse those with P waves. **PR interval:** not applicable. **QRS interval:** 0.10. **Interpretation:** junctional rhythm.

126. **QRS complexes:** present, all shaped the same. **Regularity:** irregular. **Heart rate:** 42 to 47, with a mean rate of 50. **P waves:** at least three different shapes, one preceding each QRS. **PR interval:** varies. **QRS interval:** 0.10. **Interpretation:** wandering atrial pacemaker.

127. **QRS complexes:** present, all shaped the same. **Regularity:** irregular. **Heart rate:** 100 to 150, with a mean ate of 130. **P waves:** none noted; wavy, undulating baseline present instead. **PR interval:** not applicable. **QRS interval:** 0.06. **Interpretation:** atrial fibrillation.

128. **QRS complexes:** present, all shaped the same. **Regularity:** irregular. **Heart rate:** 85 to 137, with a mean rate of 100. **P waves:** none present; sawtooth-shaped waves present between QRS complexes. **PR interval:** not applicable. **QRS interval:** 0.10. **Interpretation:** atrial flutter with variable conduction.

129. **QRS complexes:** present with differing shapes, if indeed those are real QRS complexes and not just spiked fibrillatory waves. **Regularity:** irregular. **Heart rate:** around 300 to 375, but difficult to count as QRS shapes change. **P waves:** none seen. **PR interval:** not applicable. **QRS interval:** cannot measure at times. **Interpretation:** torsades de pointes versus ventricular fibrillation. This is a judgment call, as this rhythm might well be ventricular fibrillation. You will find that torsades and v-fib can be easily mistaken for each other.

130. **QRS complexes:** present, all shaped the same. **Regularity:** regular. **Heart rate:** 79. **P waves:** upright, matching, one preceding each QRS; P-P interval regular. **PR interval:** 0.14. **QRS interval:** 0.12. **Interpretation:** sinus rhythm.

131. **QRS complexes:** present, all shaped the same. **Regularity:** regular. **Heart rate:** 51. **P waves:** none seen. **PR interval:** not applicable. **QRS interval:** 0.10. **Interpretation:** junctional rhythm.

132. **QRS complexes:** present, all shaped the same. **Regularity:** regular but interrupted (by premature beats). **Heart rate:** 65. **P waves:** upright, all except the third and fourth P waves matching. The third and fourth P waves are premature and shaped a bit differently. P-P interval irregular. **PR interval:** 0.16 to 0.20. **QRS interval:** 0.06. **Interpretation:** sinus rhythm with two PACs (the third and fourth beats).

133. **QRS complexes:** present, all shaped the same. **Regularity:** irregular. **Heart rate:** 71 to 110, with a mean rate of 90. **P waves:** none present; wavy, undulating baseline present instead. **PR interval:** not applicable. **QRS interval:** 0.08. **Interpretation:** atrial fibrillation. In places it looks pretty fluttery, doesn't it? You might have been tempted to call this atrial flutter. The problem is that the fluttery pattern is not consistent. Its waves could never be marched out, as the waves dampen out so much in places. It's safer to call this atrial fibrillation.

134. **QRS complexes:** present, all shaped the same. **Regularity:** regular. **Heart rate:** 60. **P waves:** none noted. **PR interval:** not applicable. **QRS interval:** 0.20. **Interpretation:** accelerated idioventricular rhythm.

135. **QRS complexes:** present, all shaped the same, though two are distorted by artifact. **Regularity:** regular. **Heart rate:** 137. **P waves:** none seen. **PR interval:** not applicable. **QRS interval:** 0.18. **Interpretation:** ventricular tachycardia.

136. **QRS complexes:** present, all shaped the same. **Regularity:** regular. **Heart rate:** 60. **P waves:** none seen; wavy, undulating baseline present instead. **PR interval:** not applicable. **QRS interval:** 0.10. **Interpretation:** atrial fibrillation. Though normally atrial fibrillation is a very irregular rhythm, you can see that it may look regular at times. This is not common, but you should be aware it does happen sometimes, typically in individuals who've been in atrial fibrillation for years.

137. **QRS complexes:** present, all shaped the same. **Regularity:** regular. **Heart rate:** 137. **P waves:** upright, matching, one preceding each QRS; P-P interval regular. **PR interval:** 0.16. **QRS interval:** 0.08. **Interpretation:** sinus tachycardia.

138. **QRS complexes:** present, all shaped the same. **Regularity:** regular. **Heart rate:** 42. **P waves:** upright, matching (some a little distorted by artifact), one preceding each QRS; P-P interval regular. **PR interval:** 0.16. **QRS interval:** 0.10. **Interpretation:** sinus bradycardia.

139. **QRS complexes:** present, all shaped the same. **Regularity:** regular. **Heart rate:** 60. **P waves:** upright, matching, one preceding each QRS; P-P interval regular. **PR interval:** 0.14. **QRS interval:** 0.08. **Interpretation:** sinus rhythm.

140. **QRS complexes:** present, all shaped the same. **Regularity:** irregular. **Heart rate:** 71 to 107, with a mean rate of 90. **P waves:** none present; sawtooth waves present instead. **PR interval:** not applicable. **QRS interval:** 0.06. **Interpretation:** atrial flutter with variable conduction.

141. **QRS complexes:** present, all shaped the same. **Regularity:** regular. **Heart rate:** about 73. **P waves:** none noted; sawtooth waves present instead. **PR interval:** not applicable. **QRS interval:** 0.12, though difficult to measure as QRS is distorted by flutter waves. **Interpretation:** atrial flutter with variable conduction and a possible BBB.

142. **QRS complexes:** cannot distinguish. **Regularity:** can't tell. **Heart rate:** can't tell. **P waves:** can't distinguish. **PR interval:** not applicable. **QRS interval:** not applicable. **Interpretation:** unknown rhythm with artifact. Why is this strip even in here if you can't possibly tell what it is? Because it's important for you to know *not to even try to interpret a rhythm this obscured by artifact.* There is no way to tell what the underlying rhythm is here. Check the patient's monitor lead wires and electrode patches or change the lead the patient is being monitored in to get a better tracing, and try again with a clearer strip.

143. **QRS complexes:** present, all shaped the same. **Regularity:** regular. **Heart rate:** about 130. **P waves:** upright, matching, one preceding each QRS; P-P interval regular. **PR interval:** 0.16. **QRS interval:** 0.06. **Interpretation:** sinus tachycardia.

144. **QRS complexes:** present, all shaped the same. **Regularity:** regular. **Heart rate:** 83. **P waves:** upright, matching, one preceding each QRS; P-P interval regular. **PR interval:** 0.10. **QRS interval:** 0.08. **Interpretation:** sinus rhythm with accelerated AV conduction. If the PR interval is this short, we know the impulse blasts through the AV node faster than normal.

145. **QRS complexes:** present, all shaped the same. **Regularity:** regular. **Heart rate:** 88. **P waves:** upright, matching, one preceding each QRS; P-P interval regular. **PR interval:** 0.12. **QRS interval:** 0.12. **Interpretation:** sinus rhythm with BBB.

146. **QRS complexes:** present, all shaped the same. **Regularity:** regular. **Heart rate:** 60. **P waves:** upright, matching, one preceding each QRS; P-P interval regular. **PR interval:** 0.16. **QRS interval:** 0.08. **Interpretation:** sinus rhythm.

147. **QRS complexes:** present, all shaped the same. **Regularity:** regular. **Heart rate:** 68. **P waves:** upright, matching, one preceding each QRS; P-P interval regular. **PR interval:** 0.18. **QRS interval:** 0.14. **Interpretation:** sinus rhythm with a BBB.

148. **QRS complexes:** present, all shaped the same. **Regularity:** regular. **Heart rate:** about 57. **P waves:** upright, matching, one preceding each QRS; P-P interval regular. **PR interval:** 0.16. **QRS interval:** 0.08. **Interpretation:** sinus bradycardia.

149. **QRS complexes:** present, all shaped the same. **Regularity:** irregular. **Heart rate:** 56 to 83, with a mean rate of 70. **P waves:** none noted; wavy, undulating baseline present instead. **PR interval:** not applicable. **QRS interval:** 0.10. **Interpretation:** atrial fibrillation.

150. **QRS complexes:** present, all shaped the same. **Regularity:** regular. **Heart rate:** 43. **P waves:** upright, matching, one preceding each QRS; P-P interval regular. **PR interval:** 0.16. **QRS interval:** 0.08. **Interpretation:** sinus bradycardia.

151. **QRS complexes:** present, all shaped the same. **Regularity:** regular. **Heart rate:** 83. **P waves:** upright, matching, one preceding each QRS; P-P interval regular. **PR interval:** 0.14. **QRS interval:** 0.10. **Interpretation:** sinus rhythm.

152. **QRS complexes:** present, all shaped the same. **Regularity:** regular. **Heart rate:** about 35. **P waves:** upright, matching, one preceding each QRS; P-P interval regular. **PR interval:** 0.16. **QRS interval:** 0.10. **Interpretation:** sinus bradycardia.

153. **QRS complexes:** present, most but not all shaped the same. Some have an S wave, while others do not. **Regularity:** irregular. **Heart rate:** 150 to 250, with a mean rate of 190. **P waves:** none noted; wavy, undulating baseline present instead. **PR interval:** not applicable. **QRS interval:** 0.06 to 0.08. **Interpretation:** atrial fibrillation.

154. **QRS complexes:** present, all shaped the same. **Regularity:** regular. **Heart rate:** 62. **P waves:** upright, matching, one preceding each QRS; P-P interval regular. **PR interval:** 0.20. **QRS interval:** 0.08. **Interpretation:** sinus rhythm.

155. **QRS complexes:** present, all shaped the same. **Regularity:** regular. **Heart rate:** 115. **P waves:** upright, matching, one preceding each QRS; P-P interval regular. **PR interval:** 0.12. **QRS interval:** 0.10. **Interpretation:** sinus tachycardia.

156. **QRS complexes:** present, all shaped the same. **Regularity:** irregular. **Heart rate:** 107 to 167, with a mean rate of 140. **P waves:** none seen; wavy, undulating baseline present instead. **PR interval:** not applicable. **QRS interval:** 0.08. **Interpretation:** atrial fibrillation.

157. **QRS complexes:** one present; wavy, static-looking baseline present instead. **Regularity:** not applicable. **Heart rate:** cannot determine, as there are no QRS complexes. **P waves:** none seen. **PR interval:** not applicable. **QRS interval:** not applicable. **Interpretation:** ventricular fibrillation.

158. **QRS complexes:** present, all shaped the same. **Regularity:** irregular. **Heart rate:** 36 to 42, with a mean rate of 40. **P waves:** upright, matching, one preceding each QRS; P-P interval irregular. **PR interval:** 0.16. **QRS interval:** 0.10. **Interpretation:** sinus arrhythmia.

159. **QRS complexes:** present, all shaped the same. **Regularity:** regular but interrupted (by pauses). **Heart rate:** 75 to 125, with a mean rate of 110. **P waves:** upright, many hidden in T waves. Some P waves are nonconducted. P-P interval regular. Atrial rate 137. **PR interval:** varies. **QRS interval:** 0.06. **Interpretation:** sinus tachycardia with type I second-degree AV block (Wenckebach). This is not a very obvious Wenckebach,

is it? See the pause between the third and fourth QRS complexes? Note the P wave preceding the fourth QRS. Now back up to the T wave of the third beat. See how deformed the shape is? That's because there's a P wave inside it. Note the P-P interval between those two P waves and you can march out where the rest of the P waves are. You'll find the P-P intervals are all regular and the PR intervals gradually prolong until a beat is dropped.

160. **QRS complexes:** present, all shaped the same. **Regularity:** irregular. **Heart rate:** 75 to 107, with a mean rate of 100. **P waves:** none noted; wavy, undulating baseline present instead. **PR interval:** not applicable. **QRS interval:** 0.10. **Interpretation:** atrial fibrillation.

161. **QRS complexes:** present, all shaped the same. **Regularity:** regular. **Heart rate:** about 130. **P waves:** none seen. **PR interval:** not applicable. **QRS interval:** 0.08. **Interpretation:** SVT.

162. **QRS complexes:** can't be sure if there are QRS complexes of varying shapes or if it is just a static-looking baseline without QRS complexes. **Regularity:** irregular. **Heart rate:** 250 to 300. **P waves:** none seen. **PR interval:** not applicable. **QRS interval:** 0.12 or greater. **Interpretation:** either torsades de pointes or ventricular fibrillation. It oscillates like torsades but looks more uncoordinated, like v-fib. The treatment for these is very similar, thankfully, so calling it either torsades or v-fib would still get appropriate treatment for the patient.

163. **QRS complexes:** present, all shaped the same. **Regularity:** irregular. **Heart rate:** 60 to 107, with a mean rate of 90. **P waves:** none seen; wavy, undulating baseline present instead. **PR interval:** not applicable. **QRS interval:** 0.06. **Interpretation:** atrial fibrillation.

164. **QRS complexes:** present, all shaped the same. **Regularity:** regular. **Heart rate:** about 80. **P waves:** none seen; wavy, undulating baseline present instead. **PR interval:** not applicable. **QRS interval:** 0.10. **Interpretation:** atrial fibrillation. This is another example of a regular spell of atrial fibrillation.

165. **QRS complexes:** present, all but one shaped the same. One is shorter than the rest. **Regularity:** irregular. **Heart rate:** 45 to 65, with a mean rate of 50. **P waves:** none noted; wavy, undulating baseline present instead. **PR interval:** not applicable. **QRS interval:** 0.08. **Interpretation:** atrial fibrillation.

166. **QRS complexes:** present, all shaped the same. **Regularity:** regular. **Heart rate:** 75. **P waves:** upright, matching, one preceding each QRS; P-P interval regular. **PR interval:** 0.16. **QRS interval:** 0.14. **Interpretation:** sinus rhythm with a BBB.

167. **QRS complexes:** present, all shaped the same. **Regularity:** irregular. **Heart rate:** 88 to 187, with a mean rate of 120. **P waves:** present, at least three different shapes; P-P interval irregular. **PR interval:** varies. **QRS interval:** 0.08. **Interpretation:** multifocal atrial tachycardia.

168. **QRS complexes:** present, all shaped the same. **Regularity:** regular. **Heart rate:** around 90. **P waves:** upright, matching, one preceding each QRS; P-P interval regular. **PR interval:** 0.14. **QRS interval:** 0.08. **Interpretation:** sinus rhythm.

169. **QRS complexes:** present, all shaped the same. **Regularity:** irregular. **Heart rate:** 83 to 137, with a mean rate of 110. **P waves:** none noted; sawtooth waves present instead. **PR interval:** not applicable. **QRS interval:** 0.08. **Interpretation:** atrial flutter with variable conduction.

170. **QRS complexes:** present, all shaped the same. **Regularity:** regular. **Heart rate:** 150. **P waves:** upright, matching, one preceding each QRS; P-P interval regular. **PR interval:** 0.10. **QRS interval:** 0.10. **Interpretation:** sinus tachycardia with accelerated AV conduction.

171. **QRS complexes:** present, all shaped the same. **Regularity:** regular. **Heart rate:** 45. **P waves:** upright, matching, two preceding each QRS; P-P interval regular; atrial rate 88. **PR interval:** 0.36. **QRS interval:** 0.08. **Interpretation:** sinus rhythm with 2:1 AV block.

172. **QRS complexes:** present, all shaped the same. **Regularity:** regular but interrupted (by pauses). **Heart rate:** 44 to 83, with a mean rate of 60. **P waves:** upright, matching, some nonconducted; P-P interval regular; atrial rate 88. **PR interval:** 0.36. **QRS interval:** 0.08. **Interpretation:** sinus rhythm with type II second-degree AV block.

173. **QRS complexes:** present, all shaped the same. **Regularity:** regular. **Heart rate:** 137. **P waves:** none seen. **PR interval:** not applicable. **QRS interval:** 0.06. **Interpretation:** SVT.

174. **QRS complexes:** only one mammoth QRS on the strip. Believe it or not, that huge wave at the beginning of the strip is a QRS and T wave. **Regularity:** cannot determine. **Heart rate:** cannot determine. **P waves:** none seen. **PR interval:** not applicable. **QRS interval:** about 0.60, but that's a guesstimate. **Interpretation:** dying heart (agonal rhythm). It is unusual for dying heart's QRS complexes to be this wide. It's likely this patient has an *extremely elevated* potassium level in his or her bloodstream, which can cause the QRS to widen out more than usual.

175. **QRS complexes:** none seen. **Regularity:** not applicable. **Heart rate:** zero. **P waves:** none seen. **PR interval:** not applicable. **QRS interval:** not applicable. **Interpretation:** asystole.

176. **QRS complexes:** present, differing shapes. **Regularity:** irregular. **Heart rate:** about 375. **P waves:** none seen. **PR interval:** not applicable. **QRS interval:** 0.12 or greater. **Interpretation:** torsades de pointes.

177. **QRS complexes:** none; wavy, static-looking baseline present instead. **Regularity:** not applicable. **Heart rate:** cannot measure. **P waves:** none seen. **PR interval:** not applicable. **QRS interval:** not applicable. **Interpretation:** ventricular fibrillation.

178. **QRS complexes:** none; wavy, static-looking baseline present instead. **Regularity:** not applicable. **Heart rate:** cannot measure. **P waves:**

none seen. **PR interval:** not applicable. **QRS interval:** not applicable. **Interpretation:** ventricular fibrillation.

179. **QRS complexes:** present, all shaped the same. **Regularity:** regular. **Heart rate:** just a hair over 100. **P waves:** upright, matching, one preceding each QRS; P-P interval regular. **PR interval:** 0.22. **QRS interval:** 0.10. **Interpretation:** sinus tachycardia with a first-degree AV block.

180. **QRS complexes:** present, all shaped the same. **Regularity:** irregular. **Heart rate:** 80 to 167, with a mean rate of 110. **P waves:** present, at least three different shapes. **PR interval:** not applicable. **QRS interval:** 0.06. **Interpretation:** multifocal atrial tachycardia. If you thought it was atrial fibrillation, remember that *atrial fibrillation has no P waves.* There are obvious P waves on this strip.

181. **QRS complexes:** present, all shaped the same. **Regularity:** regular. **Heart rate:** 68. **P waves:** none seen. **PR interval:** not applicable. **QRS interval:** 0.18. **Interpretation:** accelerated idioventricular rhythm.

182. **QRS complexes:** present, all shaped the same. **Regularity:** regular. **Heart rate:** 125. **P waves:** upright, matching, one preceding each QRS; P-P interval regular. **PR interval:** 0.16. **QRS interval:** 0.06. **Interpretation:** sinus tachycardia. You may recognize this strip. It's the same as number 6. Did you come up with the same answer on this strip as on number 6? You should have.

183. **QRS complexes:** present, all shaped the same. **Regularity:** regular. **Heart rate:** 56. **P waves:** upright, matching, one preceding each QRS; P-P interval regular; P waves are very small. **PR interval:** 0.16. **QRS interval:** 0.16. **Interpretation:** sinus bradycardia with a BBB. Look again at this strip if you thought this was atrial fibrillation. There are obvious, though tiny, P waves. And if you thought this was a ventricular rhythm of some kind because of the QRS width, note the matching upright P waves. Ventricular rhythms don't have that. Remember–the width of the QRS does not determine whether a rhythm can be sinus. The P waves are the key criterion.

184. **QRS complexes:** present, all shaped the same. **Regularity:** regular. **Heart rate:** 83. **P waves:** upright, matching, one preceding each QRS; P-P interval regular. **PR interval:** 0.13. **QRS interval:** 0.10. **Interpretation:** sinus rhythm. Did you think this was a 2:1 AV block? The T wave does look an awful lot like the P wave, doesn't it? Remember AV blocks have regular P-P intervals. If this T wave were hiding a P wave, the P-P intervals would not be regular. So it's not an AV block.

185. **QRS complexes:** present, all shaped the same. **Regularity:** regular. **Heart rate:** 167. **P waves:** upright, matching, one preceding each QRS; P-P interval regular. **PR interval:** 0.12. **QRS interval:** 0.06. **Interpretation:** atrial tachycardia. Remember, the sinus node does not usually fire at rates above 160 in supine resting adults. Since this rate is above 160, we must call it atrial tachycardia.

186. **QRS complexes:** present, all shaped the same. **Regularity:** irregular. **Heart rate:** 20 to 75, with a mean rate of 50. **P waves:** none seen; very fine wavy, undulating baseline present instead. **PR interval:** not applicable. **QRS interval:** 0.08. **Interpretation:** atrial fibrillation.

187. **QRS complexes:** present, all shaped the same. **Regularity:** irregular. **Heart rate:** 28 to 62, with a mean rate of 50. **P waves:** none seen; wavy, undulating baseline present instead. **PR interval:** not applicable. **QRS interval:** 0.10. **Interpretation:** atrial fibrillation.

188. **QRS complexes:** present, all shaped the same. **Regularity:** irregular. **Heart rate:** 60 to 79, with a mean rate of 70. **P waves:** upright, matching, one preceding each QRS; P-P interval regular. **PR interval:** 0.18. **QRS interval:** 0.08. **Interpretation:** sinus arrhythmia.

189. **QRS complexes:** present, all shaped the same. **Regularity:** regular. **Heart rate:** 60. **P waves:** upright, matching (the ones that can be seen), one preceding each QRS; P-P interval regular, as far as can be seen. **PR interval:** 0.18. **QRS interval:** 0.08. **Interpretation:** sinus rhythm partially obscured by artifact. Unlike strip number 142, which had so much artifact that the underlying rhythm could not be determined, this strip has measurable waves and complexes. Since we can pick out the QRS complexes throughout the strip, we can deduce that the P waves continue as well during the artifact spells. Even so, it would be better not to mount a strip like this in the patient's chart, since one cannot be entirely sure what is happening during the periods of artifact.

190. **QRS complexes:** present, all shaped the same. **Regularity:** regular but interrupted (by pauses). **Heart rate:** 75 to 125. **P waves:** upright, some hidden in T waves, some nonconducted; P-P interval regular; atrial rate 137. **PR interval:** varies. **QRS interval:** 0.06. **Interpretation:** sinus tachycardia with type I second-degree AV block.

191. **QRS complexes:** present, all but two shaped the same (two are taller and wider). **Regularity:** regular but interrupted (by premature beats). **Heart rate:** 88. **P waves:** upright and matching on the narrow beats, none on the wide beats; P-P regular. **PR interval:** 0.24. **QRS interval:** 0.08 on the narrow beats, 0.14 on the wide beats. **Interpretation:** sinus rhythm with PVCs and a first-degree AV block.

192. **QRS complexes:** present, all shaped the same. **Regularity:** regular. **Heart rate:** 88. **P waves:** notched, matching, one preceding each QRS; P-P interval regular. **PR interval:** 0.20. **QRS interval:** 0.08. **Interpretation:** sinus rhythm.

193. **QRS complexes:** present, all shaped the same. **Regularity:** regular. **Heart rate:** 71. **P waves:** upright, matching, one preceding each QRS; P-P interval regular. **PR interval:** 0.22. **QRS interval:** 0.08. **Interpretation:** sinus rhythm with a first-degree AV block.

194. **QRS complexes:** present, all shaped the same. **Regularity:** regular. **Heart rate:** 36. **P waves:** upright, matching, one preceding each QRS; P-P interval regular. **PR interval:** 0.16. **QRS interval:** 0.10. **Interpretation:** sinus bradycardia.

195. **QRS complexes:** only one seen on the strip. **Regularity:** cannot determine. **Heart rate:** cannot determine from just one QRS complex. **P waves:** cannot distinguish due to artifact. **PR interval:** not applicable. **QRS interval:** cannot measure, as it's distorted by artifact. **Interpretation:** probably agonal rhythm obscured by CPR artifact. This strip looks a lot like the example of CPR artifact, doesn't it? In order to know for sure what this rhythm is, CPR would need to be stopped briefly to allow a strip without artifact to be analyzed.

196. **QRS complexes:** none present; wavy, static-looking baseline present instead. **Regularity:** not applicable. **Heart rate:** not applicable. **P waves:** none seen. **PR interval:** not applicable. **QRS interval:** not applicable. **Interpretation:** ventricular fibrillation.

197. **QRS complexes:** present, all shaped the same. **Regularity:** regular but interrupted (by a premature beat). **Heart rate:** 71 to 107. **P waves:** upright and matching except for the premature P wave on the seventh beat; P-P interval irregular because of this premature beat. **PR interval:** 0.16. **QRS interval:** 0.10. **Interpretation:** sinus rhythm with a PAC.

198. **QRS complexes:** present, all shaped the same. **Regularity:** regular but interrupted (by a premature beat). **Heart rate:** about 77. **P waves:** tiny, biphasic and matching except for the third beat, which is premature. The P-P interval is irregular because of this premature beat. **PR interval:** 0.14 to 0.16. **QRS interval:** 0.06. **Interpretation:** sinus rhythm with a PAC. This premature beat is not a PJC because the PR interval of that beat is greater than 0.12.

199. **QRS complexes:** present, two different shapes. **Regularity:** regular but interrupted (by premature beats). **Heart rate:** 115. **P waves:** upright and matching on the narrow beats, none on the wide beats. **PR interval:** 0.14. **QRS interval:** 0.08 on the narrow beats, 0.16 on the wide beats. **Interpretation:** sinus tachycardia with two PVCs.

200. **QRS complexes:** present, all shaped the same. **Regularity:** irregular. **Heart rate:** 79 to 125, with an atrial rate of 100. **P waves:** none present; sawtooth waves present instead. **PR interval:** not applicable. **QRS interval:** 0.08. **Interpretation:** atrial flutter with variable conduction.

201. **QRS complexes:** present, all shaped the same within each lead. **Regularity:** regular. **Heart rate:** 38. **P waves:** upright in lead II, biphasic in V_1, matching within each lead. **PR interval:** 0.26. **QRS interval:** 0.10. **Interpretation:** sinus bradycardia with 1st degree AVB.

202. **QRS complexes:** present, all shaped the same. **Regularity:** regular. **Heart rate:** 65. **P waves:** upright, matching. **PR interval:** 0.10. **QRS interval:** 0.10. **Interpretation:** sinus rhythm.

203. **QRS complexes:** present, all shaped the same within each lead. **Regularity:** regular. **Heart rate:** 150. **P waves:** none noted. **PR interval:** not applicable. **QRS interval:** 0.06. **Interpretation:** SVT.

204. **QRS complexes:** absent. **Regularity:** not applicable. **Heart rate:** 0. **P waves:** none present. **PR interval:** not applicable. **QRS interval:** not applicable. **Interpretation:** asystole.

205. **QRS complexes:** present, all shaped the same within each lead. **Regularity:** regular. **Heart rate:** 65. **P waves:** upright in lead II, biphasic in V_1, matching within each lead. **PR interval:** 0.20. **QRS interval:** 0.10. **Interpretation:** sinus rhythm with borderline 1st degree AVB.

206. **QRS complexes:** present, all shaped the same within each lead. **Regularity:** irregular. **Heart rate:** 41 to 68, with an mean rate of 50. **P waves:** upright in lead II, biphasic in V1, matching within each lead. P-P interval regular. Atrial rate 79. **PR interval:** varies. **QRS interval:** 0.14. **Interpretation:** Type I second degree AVB (Wenckebach) with BBB.

207. **QRS complexes:** present, all shaped the same within each lead. **Regularity:** regular but interrupted by a pause. **Heart rate:** 36 to 79, with a mean rate of 50. **P waves:** upright,matching. P-P interval regular. Atrial rate 75. **PR interval:** varies. **QRS interval:** 0.10. **Interpretation:** sinus rhythm with type I second degree AVB (Wenckebach).

208. **QRS complexes:** present, all shaped the same within each lead. **Regularity:** regular but interrupted by a premature beat. The fifth QRS complex is premature. **Heart rate:** 75. **P waves:** upright in lead II, biphasic in V_1, matching within each lead except for the fifth P wave, which is shaped differently and is premature. **PR interval:** 0.12. **QRS interval:** 08. **Interpretation:** sinus rhythm with PAC.

209. **QRS complexes:** present, all shaped the same within each lead. **Regularity:** regular. **Heart rate:** 38. **P waves:** upright in lead II, biphasic in V_1, matching within each lead. P-P interval regular. Atrial rate 79. **PR interval:** 0.28. **QRS interval:** 0.14. **Interpretation:** 2:1 AVB with BBB.

210. **QRS complexes:** present, all shaped the same within each lead. **Regularity:** regular. **Heart rate:** 102. **P waves:** matching, inverted following the QRS in both leads. **PR interval:** not applicable. **QRS interval:** 0.08. **Interpretation:** Junctional tachycardia. See the blips following the QRS complexes? Those are the inverted P waves.

211. **QRS complexes:** present, all shaped the same within each lead. **Regularity:** regular. **Heart rate:** 71. **P waves:** cannot see in lead II, inverted in V_1. **PR interval:** 0.11. **QRS interval:** 0.06. **Interpretation:** Accelerated junctional rhythm.

212. **QRS complexes:** present, all shaped the same. **Regularity:** irregular. **Heart rate:** 71 to 125, with a mean rate of 90. **P waves:** none noted. Wavy baseline present between QRS complexes. **PR interval:** not applicable. **QRS interval:** 0.10 **Interpretation:** atrial fibrillation.

213. **QRS complexes:** present, all shaped the same. **Regularity:** regular. **Heart rate:** 65. **P waves:** matching, upright. **PR interval:** 0.20. **QRS**

interval: 0.12. **Interpretation:** Sinus rhythm with borderline 1st degree AVB. And BBB.

214. **QRS complexes:** present, all shaped the same. **Regularity:** regular but interrupted by premature beats.. **Heart rate:** 88. **P waves:** matching on all but the second, forth, and sixth beats–those P waves are shaped differently. **PR interval:** 0.13. **QRS interval:** 0.14. **Interpretation:** Sinus rhythm with three PACs.

215. **QRS complexes:** present, all shaped the same. **Regularity:** regular but interrupted by a run of rapid beats. **Heart rate:** 68, then 150. **P waves:** upright and matching on the first four beats, then shaped differently during the tachycardia. **PR interval:** 0.16. **QRS interval:** 0.10. **Interpretation:** Sinus rhythm, then atrial tachycardia (the fifth beat is a PAC, which starts off a run of PACs–this run of PACs is cald atrial tachycardia).

216. **QRS complexes:** present, all shaped the same. **Regularity:** regular. **Heart rate:** 83. **P waves:** upright, matching, one preceding each QRS. **PR interval:** 0.16. **QRS interval:** 0.08. **Interpretation:** Sinus rhythm.

217. **QRS complexes:** present, all shaped the same within each lead. **Regularity:** regular. **Heart rate:** 94. **P waves:** cannot see in lead I, inverted preceding the QRS in lead II. **PR interval:** 0.08 **QRS interval:** 0.06. **Interpretation:** Accelerated junctional rhythm.

218. **QRS complexes:** present, all different shapes. **Regularity:** irregular. **Heart rate:** up to 500. **P waves:** none seen. **PR interval:** not applicable. **QRS interval:** 0.04–0.08 (hard to measure). **Interpretation:** Torsades de pointes. Note the characteristic oscillating (bigger-smaller- bigger) pattern.

219. **QRS complexes:** None present–chaotic, wavy baseline noted instead. **Regularity:** not applicable as no QRS complexes. **Heart rate:** cannot measure. **P waves:** none. **PR interval:** not applicable. **QRS interval:** not applicable. **Interpretation:** ventricular fibrillation. Note the sudden wild change in baseline on the strip along with the notation of a shock delivered to the heart. This was an attempt to defibrillate the heart. Note that the v-fib continues even after the shock.

220. **QRS complexes:** present, all shaped the same within each lead. **Regularity:** regular. **Heart rate:** 187. **P waves:** an occasional dissociated P wave is noted. See the blip following the 5th, 8th, 10th, 12th, and 14th QRS complexes? Those are P waves. **PR interval:** not applicable. **QRS interval:** 0.14. **Interpretation:** Ventricular tachycardia.

221. **QRS complexes:** present, all shaped the same within each lead. **Regularity:** irregular. **Heart rate:** from less than 30 to 62, with a mean rate of 40. **P waves:** none seen. Wavy baseline noted between QRS complexes. **PR interval:** not applicable. **QRS interval:** 0.06. **Interpretation:** atrial fibrillation.

222. **QRS complexes:** present, all shaped the same within each lead. **Regularity:** regular. **Heart rate:** 88. **P waves:** matching and upright in both

leads. **PR interval:** 0.18. **QRS interval:** 0.10. **Interpretation:** sinus rhythm.

223. **QRS complexes:** present, all shaped the same within each lead. **Regularity:** regular. **Heart rate:** 75. **P waves:** matching, upright in both leads. **PR interval:** 0.16. **QRS interval:** 0.12. **Interpretation:** sinus rhythm with BBB.
224. **QRS complexes:** present, all shaped the same within each lead. **Regularity:** irregular. **Heart rate:** 68 to 94, with a mean rate of 80. **P waves:** none present. Wavy baseline noted between QRS complexes. **PR interval:** not applicable. **QRS interval:** 0.09. **Interpretation:** atrial fibrillation
225. **QRS complexes:** present, all shaped the same within each lead. **Regularity:** regular. **Heart rate:** 68. **P waves:** matching, upright in both leads. **PR interval:** 0.14. **QRS interval:** 0.06. **Interpretation:** sinus rhythm.
226. **QRS complexes:** present, all shaped the same within each lead. **Regularity:** regular. **Heart rate:** 62. **P waves:** matching, right in both leads. **PR interval:** 0.12. **QRS interval:** 0.10. **Interpretation:** sinus rhythm.
227. **QRS complexes:** present, all shaped the same within each lead. **Regularity:** regular but interrupted by a premature beat. **Heart rate:** 75. **P waves:** matching, upright in both leads. **PR interval:** 0.22. **QRS interval:** 0.08. **Interpretation:** sinus rhythm with 1st degree AVB.
228. **QRS complexes:** present, all shaped the same within each lead. **Regularity:** regular. **Heart rate:** 83. **P waves:** matching, upright in both leads. **PR interval:** 0.12. **QRS interval:** 0.08. **Interpretation:** sinus rhythm.
229. **QRS complexes:** present, all shaped the same. **Regularity:** regular. **Heart rate:** 62. **P waves:** matching, M-shaped. **PR interval:** 0.20. **QRS interval:** 0.10. **Interpretation:** sinus rhythm with borderline 1st degree AVB.
230. **QRS complexes:** present, all shaped the same within each lead. **Regularity:** regular. **Heart rate:** 88. **P waves:** none seen. **PR interval:** not applicable. **QRS interval:** 0.08. **Interpretation:** Accelerated junctional rhythm.
231. **QRS complexes:** none noted **Regularity:** not applicable. **Heart rate:** 0. **P waves:** none. **PR interval:** not applicable. **QRS interval:** not applicable. **Interpretation:** asystole.
232. **QRS complexes:** present, all shaped the same within each lead. **Regularity:** regular. **Heart rate:** 107. **P waves:** matching, inverted following the QRS in both leads. **PR interval:** not applicable. **QRS interval:** 0.08. **Interpretation:** Junctional tachycardia. See the blips following the QRS complexes? Those are the inverted P waves.
233. **QRS complexes:** present, all shaped the same within each lead. **Regularity:** regular. **Heart rate:** 100. **P waves:** matching, upright in both

leads. **PR interval:** 0.20. **QRS interval:** 0.08. **Interpretation:** sinus rhythm.

234. **QRS complexes:** present, all shaped the same within each lead. **Regularity:** regular. **Heart rate:** 137. **P waves:** none seen. **PR interval:** not applicable. **QRS interval:** 0.hard to measure, but probably about 0.20. **Interpretation:** ventricular tachycardia.

235. **QRS complexes:** present, all shaped the same. **Regularity:** regular. **Heart rate:** 150. **P waves:** matching, upright. **PR interval:** 0.12. **QRS interval:** 0.08. **Interpretation:** inus tachycardia.

236. **QRS complexes:** present, all shaped the same within each lead. **Regularity:** regular. **Heart rate:** 43. **P waves:** upright and matching in lead II, biphasic and matching in V_1. **PR interval:** 0.26. **QRS interval:** 0.10. **Interpretation:** sinus bradycardia with 1st degree AVB.

237. **QRS complexes:** present, all shaped the same. **Regularity:** irregular. **Heart rate:** 45 to 54, with a mean rate of 50. **P waves:** matching, upright. **PR interval:** 0.18. **QRS interval:** 0.10. **Interpretation:** sinus bradycardia.

238. **QRS complexes:** present, all shaped the same within each lead. **Regularity:** irregular. **Heart rate:** 35 to 60, with mean rate of 50. **P waves:** upright and matching in both leads. The fourth QRS has a P wave at the top of its T wave. P-P interval regular. Atrial rate 60. **PR interval:** 0.24. **QRS interval:** 0.08. **Interpretation:** sinus rhythm with type II second degree AVB.

239. **QRS complexes:** present, all shaped the same within each lead. **Regularity:** irregular. **Heart rate:** 54 to 68, with a mean rate of 60. **P waves:** matching, upright in both leads. **PR interval:** 0.16. **QRS interval:** 0.08. **Interpretation:** sinus arrhythmia (bradycardia).

240. **QRS complexes:** present, all shaped the same within each lead. **Regularity:** irregular. **Heart rate:** 100 to 150, with a mean rate of 140. **P waves:** none noted. **PR interval:** not applicable. **QRS interval:** 0.12. **Interpretation:** ventricular tachycardia.

241. **QRS complexes:** present, all shaped the same within each lead. **Regularity:** regular. **Heart rate:** 107. **P waves:** matching, inverted preceding the QRS. **PR interval:** 0.09. **QRS interval:** 0.08. **Interpretation:** Junctional tachycardia.

242. **QRS complexes:** present, all shaped the same within each lead. **Regularity:** regular. **Heart rate:** 137. **P waves:** none noted. **PR interval:** not applicable. **QRS interval:** 0.10. **Interpretation:** SVT.

243. **QRS complexes:** present, all shaped the same within each lead. **Regularity:** irregular. **Heart rate:** 86 to 150, with a mean rate of 120. **P waves:** none seen. Wavy baseline noted between QRS complexes. **PR interval:** not applicable. **QRS interval:** 0.08. **Interpretation:** atrial fibrillation.

244. **QRS complexes:** present, all shaped the same. **Regularity:** regular. **Heart rate:** 102. **P waves:** none noted. Sawtooth-shaped waves noted

between QRS complexes. **PR interval:** not applicable. **QRS interval:** 0.08. **Interpretation:** atrial flutter.

245. **QRS complexes:** present, all shaped the same. **Regularity:** regular. **Heart rate:** 79. **P waves:** matching, upright in lead II, cannot see Ps in V_1. **PR interval:** 0.14. **QRS interval:** 0.12. **Interpretation:** sinus rhythm with BBB.

246. **QRS complexes:** present, all shaped the same within each lead except for beat number three, which is a different shape. **Regularity:** regular but interrupted by a premature beat. **Heart rate:** 50. **P waves:** matching, upright in lead II, biphasic in V_1. The third QRS has no P wave. **PR interval:** 0.14. **QRS interval:** 0.08. **Interpretation:** sinus bradycardia with a PJC. The PJC beat has a BBB (its QRS is wide).

247. **QRS complexes:** present, all shaped the same within each lead. **Regularity:** regular. **Heart rate:** 107. **P waves:** matching, upright in both leads. **PR interval:** 0.14. **QRS interval:** 0.08. **Interpretation:** sinus tachycardia.

248. **QRS complexes:** present, all but the sixth shaped the same. The sixth QRS is wider. **Regularity:** regular but interrupted by a premature beat. **Heart rate:** 71. **P waves:** upright and matching, in both leads. **PR interval:** 0.14. **QRS interval:** 0.08. **Interpretation:** sinus rhythm with PVC.

249. **QRS complexes:** only one present, then chaotic, spiked, wavy baseline. **Regularity:** not applicable. **Heart rate:** unable to calculate, as only one QRS. **P waves:** none noted. **PR interval:** not applicable **QRS interval:** 0.06 on the one QRS. **Interpretation:** one sinus beat, then v-fib.

250. **QRS complexes:** present, the first two and the last one shaped the same. In between is a run of differently shaped beats. **Regularity:** irregular. **Heart rate:** 94 for the first two beats, then 187 on the run of beats. **P waves:** matching and upright on the first two and the last one beat. No Ps on the other beats. **PR interval:** 0.16. **QRS interval:** 0.10 on the narrow beats, 0.12 on the other beats. **Interpretation:** sinus rhythm with a run of v-tach.

PART **TWO**

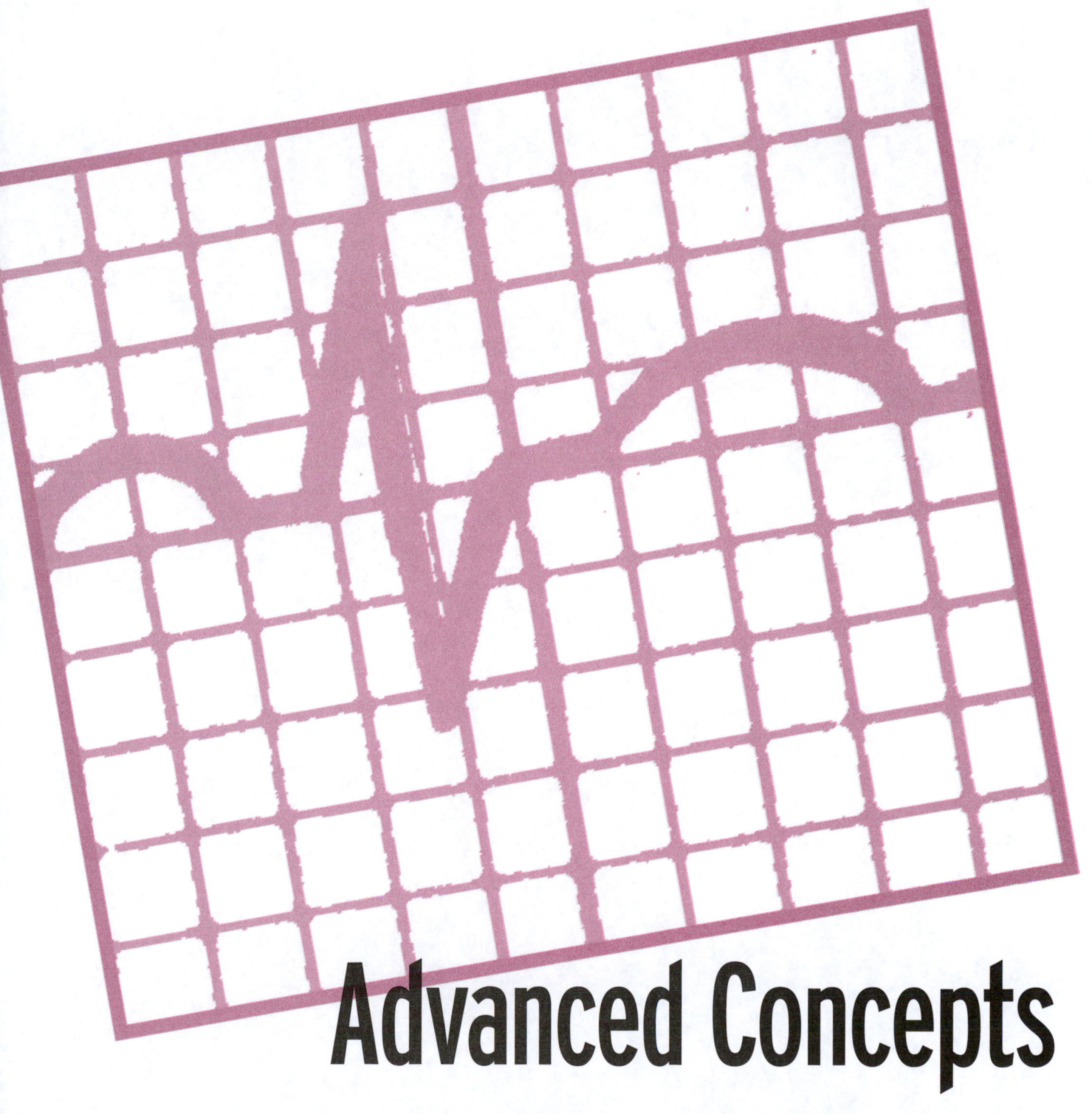

Advanced Concepts

CHAPTER **13**

How to Interpret a 12-Lead EKG

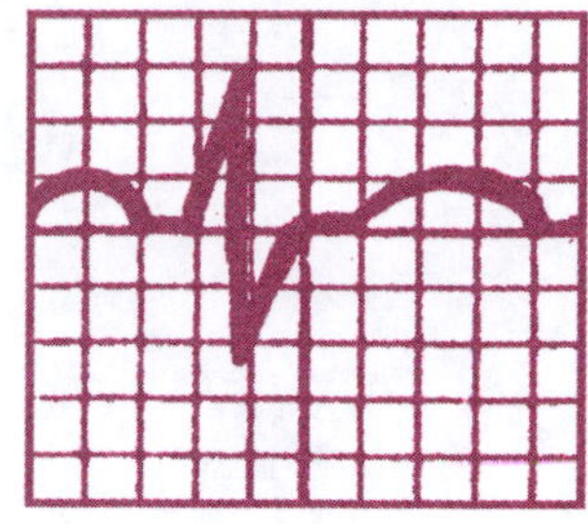

Chapter 13 Objectives

Upon completion of this chapter, the student will be able to:

- **List the six steps to 12-lead EKG interpretation.**
- **Determine the axis quadrant on a variety of practice EKGs.**
- **Determine if right or left bundle branch blocks exist.**
- **Identify right and left ventricular hypertrophy.**
- **Determine if any miscellaneous effects are present.**

Introduction

The 12-lead EKG is a diagnostic test done primarily to identify the presence of myocardial infarction or ischemia, but it is also useful in identifying dysrhythmias, electrolyte imbalances, drug toxicities, and other conditions. It is done with the patient at rest, usually in the supine (back-lying) position. As with rhythm interpretation, it is important to use a systematic method of assessing 12-lead EKGs.

The Six Steps to 12-Lead EKG Interpretation

Use these steps in order:

1. *Interpret the basics–rhythm, heart rate, and intervals (PR, QRS, QT).* These were covered in Part I of the text. If the EKG has a rhythm strip at the bottom, assess the basics here. Otherwise, pick any lead (leads II and V_1 are the best ones to evaluate for rhythm.) Do the intervals fall within normal limits or are they abnormally shortened or prolonged?
2. *Determine the axis quadrant.* Is it normal or is there axis deviation? *Axis* is simply a method of determining the mean direction of current flow in the heart.
3. *Check for bundle branch blocks.*
4. *Check for ventricular hypertrophy (overgrowth of myocardial tissue).* Use V_1 and V_{5-6} to check the QRS complexes for signs of ventricular hypertrophy.
5. *Determine the presence of miscellaneous effects.* Examine all leads for disturbances in calcium or potassium levels in the bloodstream and for digitalis effects.
6. *Check for myocardial infarction/ischemia.* For this you'll look at all leads except aVR. You'll look for ST elevation or depression, inverted T waves, and significant Q waves. You'll also note R wave progression in the precordial leads. This will be covered in depth in chapter 14.

OK, let's get started.

Axis Determination

The electrical axis is a method of determining the direction of the heart's electrical current flow. Recall that the heart's current starts normally in the sinus node and travels downward toward the left ventricle. If we drew an arrow depicting this current flow, it would point downward to the left. In abnormal hearts or abnormal rhythms, this current may travel in an unusual direction, resulting in an **axis deviation** (the arrow would point in a different direction).

Causes of Axis Deviations

- **Normal variant.** It may be normal for some individuals to have an abnormal axis. In these patients, tests have ruled out any pathology as a cause.
- **Myocardial infarction.** Infarcted (dead) tissue does not conduct electrical current, so the current travels away from this dead tissue, shifting the axis away.
- **Ventricular hypertrophy.** Hypertrophied tissue needs more current to depolarize it, so the current shifts toward the hypertrophied area.
- **Dysrhythmias.** Dysrhythmias can cause axis deviation. Ventricular rhythms, for example, start in the ventricle and send their current upward toward the atria. The axis would then point upward rather than downward.
- **Advanced pregnancy or obesity.** Either condition or both physically pushes the diaphragm and the heart upward, causing the axis to shift upward to the left.
- **Chronic lung disease and pulmonary embolism.** These conditions cause a rightward axis shift because they enlarge the right ventricle.

Determining the Axis Quadrant

Since the axis is concerned with direction, axis calculation requires a compass. On a compass there are lines delineating north, south, east, and west. In axis calculation, our compass is the hexiaxial diagram superimposed on the heart, as seen in Figure 13-1. Review chapter two if you need a refresher on the leads. On the hexiaxial diagram are lines depicting the frontal leads– I, II, III, aVR, aVL, and aVF. Lead I runs right to left, and aVF runs up and down. The other leads are points in between. The leads are separated from each other by 30° increments. The **axis circle** is made by joining the ends of these lead lines. Note the degree markings in Figure 13-1. Current of the heart flowing from the sinus node to the left ventricle would yield an axis of about 60°. That's a normal axis.

If we use leads I and aVF to divide the axis circle into four quadrants, **normal axis** would be between 0 to +90°. **Left axis deviation** is between 0 to −90°. **Right axis deviation** is between +90 to ±180°. **Indeterminate axis** (so-called because it cannot be determined whether it is an extreme left axis deviation or an extreme right axis deviation) is between −90 and ±180°. Note the axis quadrants in Figure 13-1.

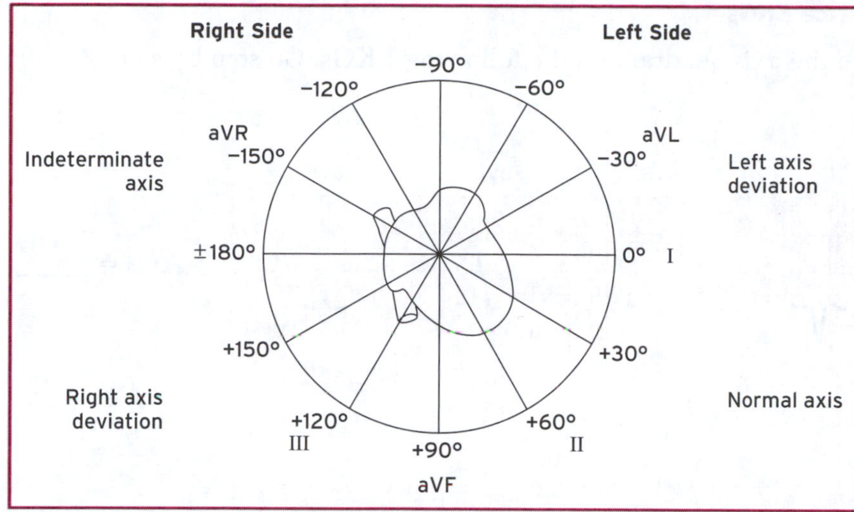

Figure 13-1 Axis circle and quadrants.

Look at the QRS in leads I and aVF to determine the axis quadrant. Since lead I connects right and left arms, it tells us whether the heart's current is traveling to the right or left. AVF is located on the foot, so it tells us whether the heart's current is traveling upward or downward. If the QRS in both lead I and aVF are positive (upright), the axis is normal. If lead I is positive and aVF is negative, it's left axis deviation (LAD). If lead I and aVF are both negative, it's indeterminate axis. If lead I is negative but aVF is positive, it's right axis deviation (RAD). See Figure 13-2.

If leads I and aVF are both upright, you could say they're "on the up and up" and that's always good. (normal).

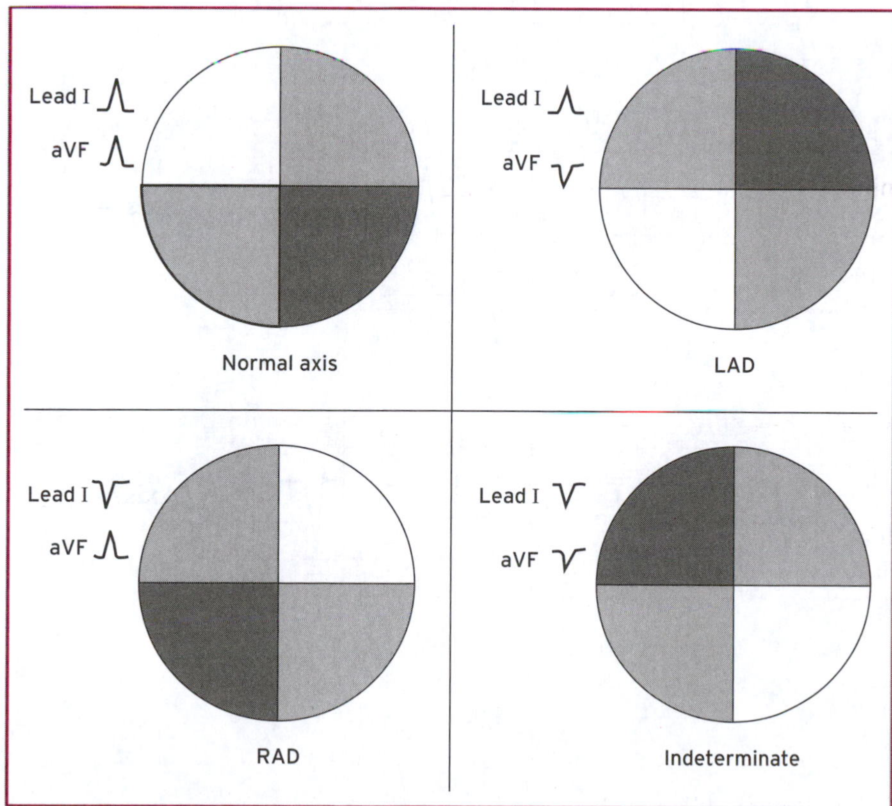

Figure 13-2 Determining the axis quadrant.

Axis Practice EKGs

Determine the axis quadrant on the following EKGs. Go step by step.

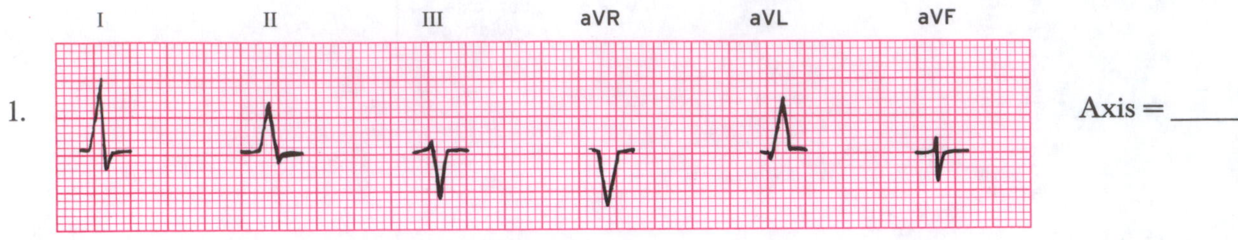

1. Axis = _____

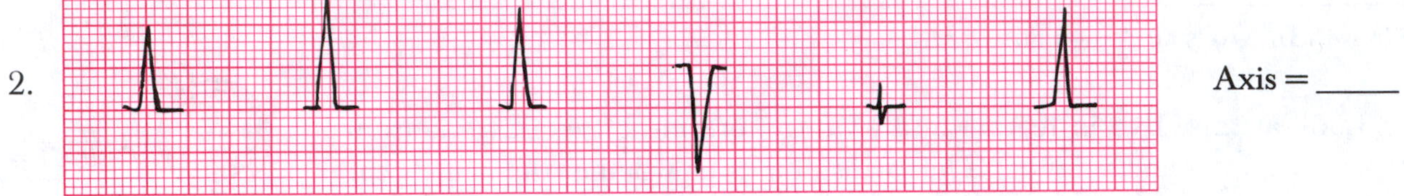

2. Axis = _____

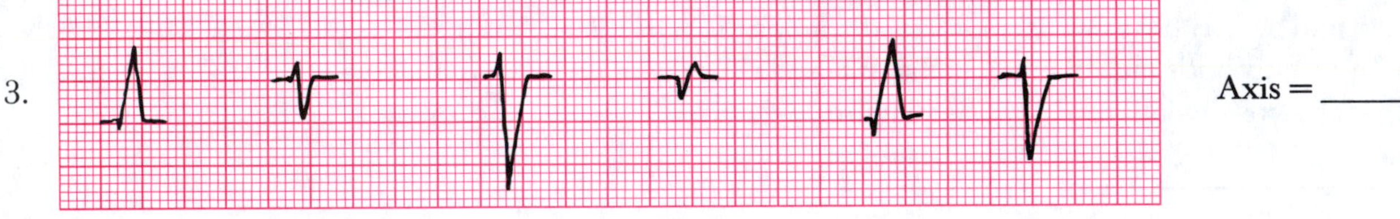

3. Axis = _____

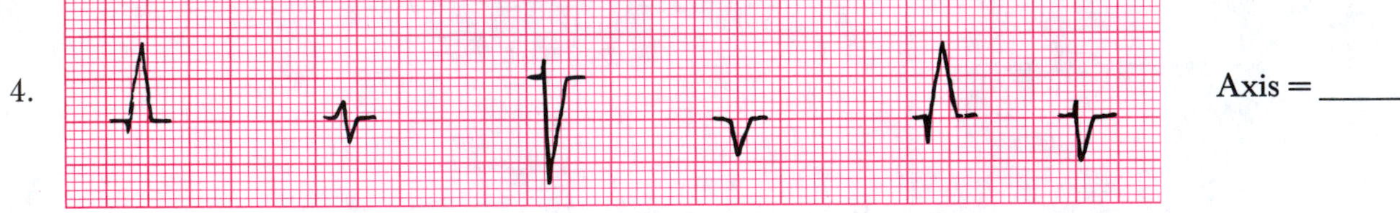

4. Axis = _____

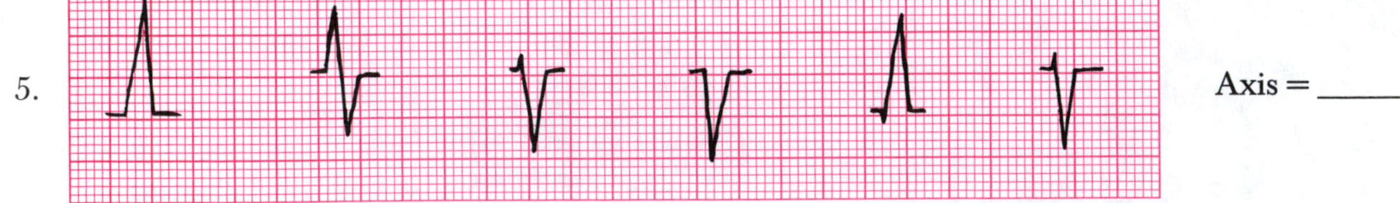

5. Axis = _____

6.

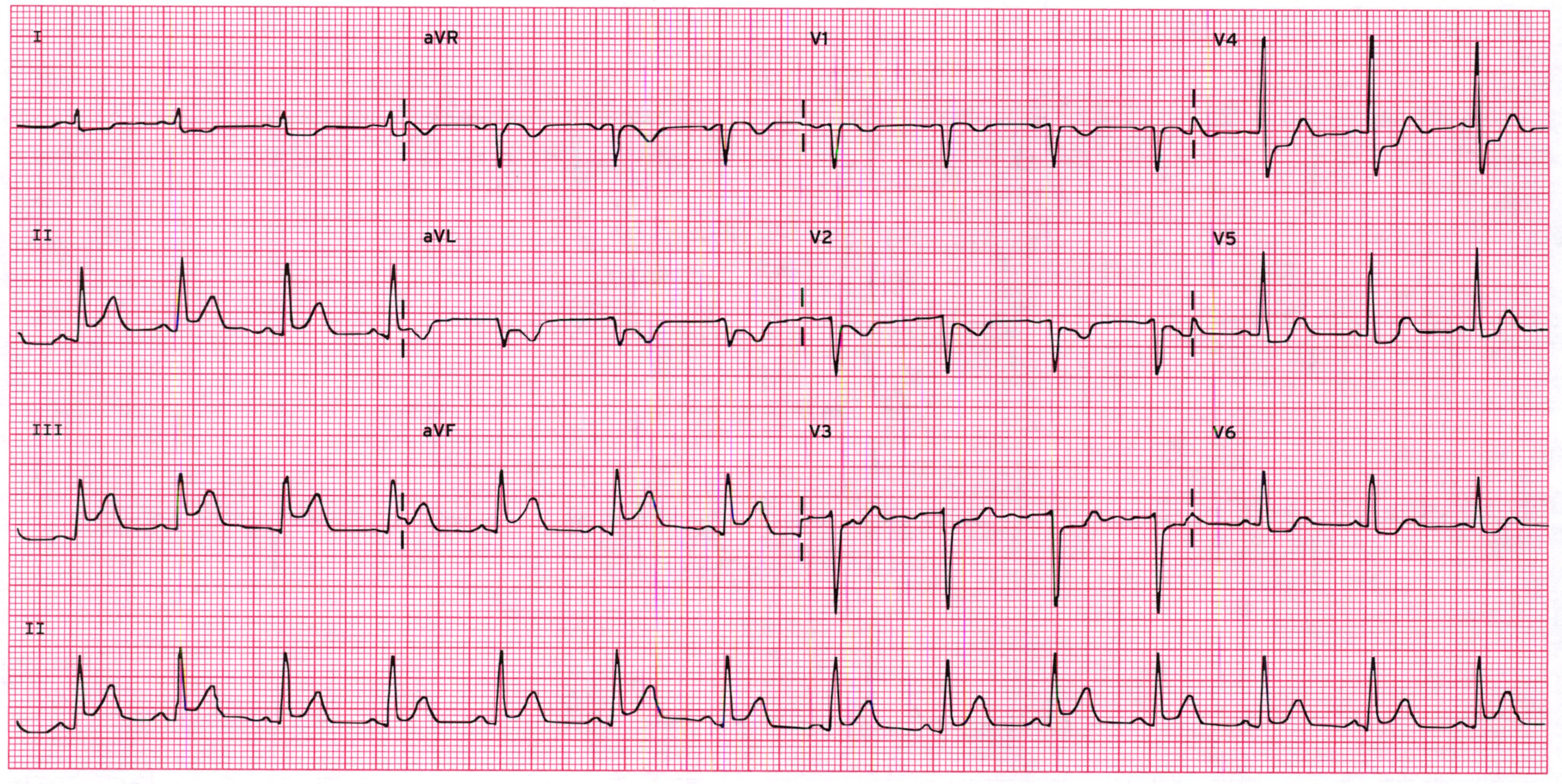

Axis = _____

7.

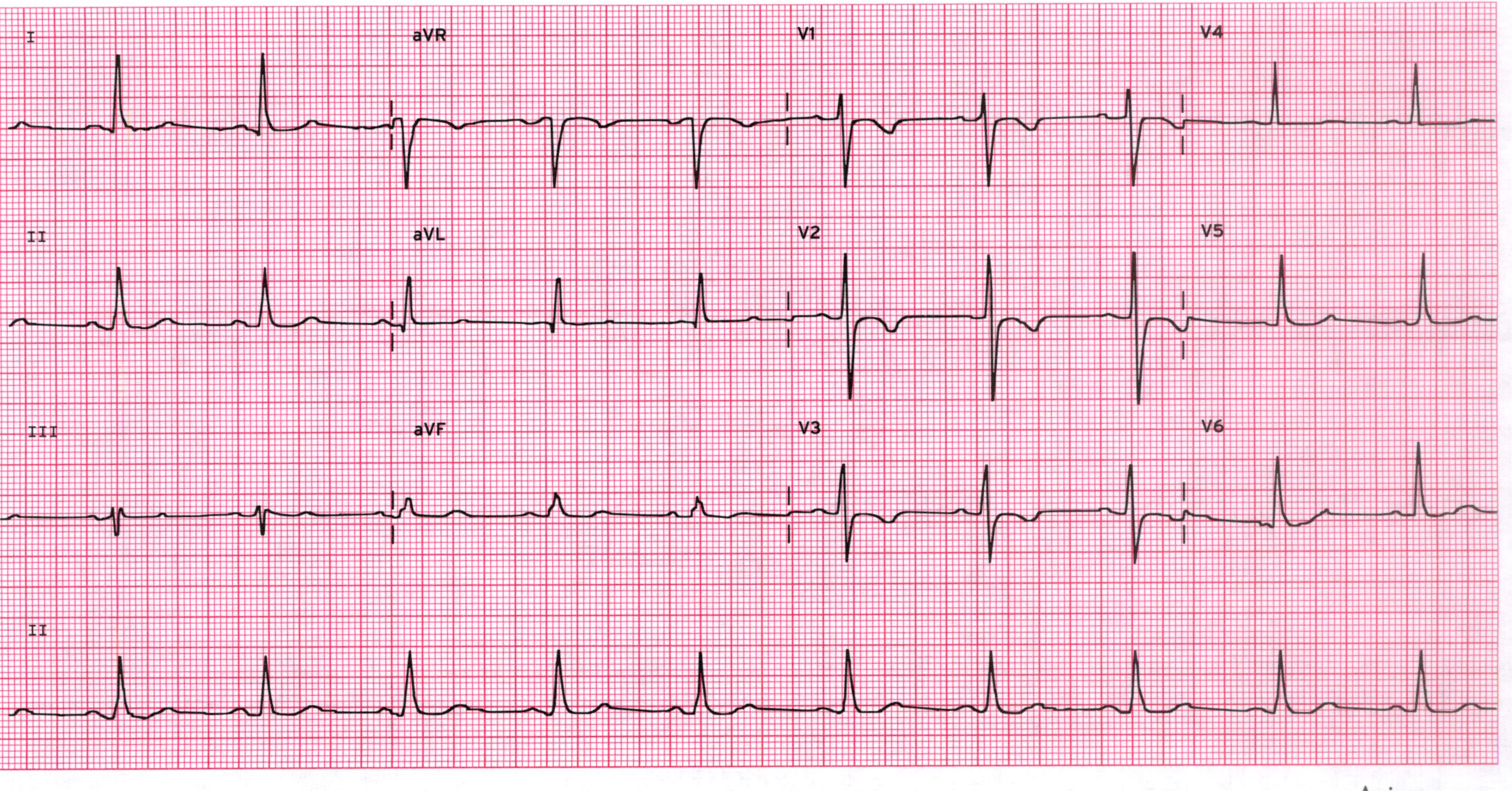

Axis = ____

Answers to Axis Practice EKGs

1. **Left axis deviation.** Lead I is positive and aVF is negative, so there is a left axis deviation.
2. **Normal axis.** Lead I and aVF are both positive, so the axis is in the normal quadrant.
3. **Indeterminate.** Lead I and aVF are both negative, so we have indeterminate axis.
4. **Left axis deviation.** Lead I is positive and aVF is negative, giving us a left axis deviation.
5. **Right axis deviation.** Lead I is negative and aVF is positive, so there is a right axis deviation.
6. **Normal axis.** Lead I and aVF are both positive, so axis is in the normal quadrant.
7. **Normal axis.** Again, lead I and aVF both are positive, so axis is normal.

Bundle Branch Blocks

Bundle branch blocks occur when either the right or left bundle branch becomes blocked and unable to conduct impulses, often as a result of disease. The impulse travels rapidly down the healthy bundle branch, then must trudge very slowly, cell by cell, through the affected ventricle. This difference in impulse conduction in the two ventricles causes the ventricles to depolarize consecutively instead of simultaneously, causing a widened QRS complex with a characteristic QRS configuration. Bundle branch blocks are seen only in supraventricular (sinus, atrial, or junctional) rhythms, since only these rhythms require conduction through the bundle branches. Ventricular rhythms are formed in the ventricular tissue below the bundle branch system and do not use the bundle branches for impulse conduction. Therefore, **ventricular rhythms cannot exhibit bundle branch blocks.**

In Figure 13-3, note the normal anatomy of the bundle branch system. The right bundle branch is located on the right side of the interventricular septum. The left bundle branch is on the left side of the septum. In order to understand the QRS complexes produced by bundle branch blocks, let's first review normal conduction through the bundle branch system. We'll look at lead V_1 since this lead is the best for interpreting bundle branch blocks. See Figure 13-4.

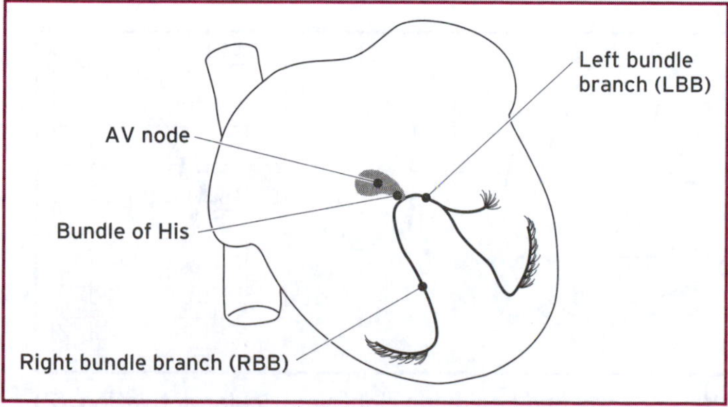

Figure 13-3 Bundle branch system anatomy.

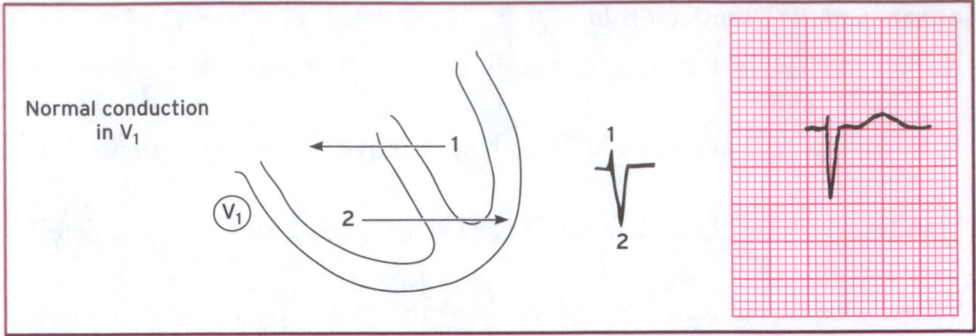

Figure 13-4 Normal conduction in V_1: (1) Septal and beginning right ventricular activation, (2) left ventricular activation.

You'll recall that the heart's normal current starts in the sinus node and travels toward the left ventricle–top to bottom, right to left. Since V_1's electrode sits to the right of the heart, it sees a little current traveling toward it (across the septum toward the right ventricle), then the bulk of the current traveling away from it toward the left ventricle. You'll recall that an impulse traveling away from a positive electrode writes a negative deflection. V_1's QRS complex is therefore primarily negative, showing a small R wave and then a deeper S wave.

Right Bundle Branch Block (RBBB)

See Figure 13-5. In right bundle branch block (RBBB), the QRS complex typically starts out looking normal–primarily negative–indicating initial normal travel through the heart via the healthy left bundle branch. But then the QRS has an extra R wave at the end, signifying the current that's slogging very slowly, cell by cell, through the right ventricle toward V_1's electrode. Thus, V_1 has an R wave, an S wave, then another R wave. This second R wave is called **R′** and is written Ŕ. Occasionally a RBBB will lose its initial R wave and will instead have a small Q wave and then a prominent R wave.

All bundle branch blocks will have a QRS interval of $\geq$*0.12 seconds and a T wave that slopes off opposite the terminal wave of the QRS complex.* If the terminal wave of the QRS is upward, for example, the T wave will be inverted. If the terminal wave of the QRS is downward, the T wave will be upright. See Figure 3-5. In V_1, the QRS interval is 0.14 second and the terminal wave of the QRS is upright, so the T wave is inverted. It is important to recognize these bundle-related T waves so as not to misinterpret them as signs of ischemia. See Figure 13-6 for a RBBB on a 12-lead EKG.

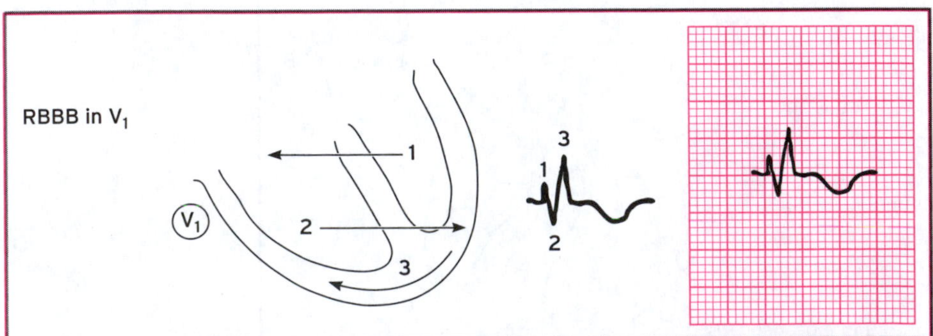

Figure 13-5 RBBB in V_1: (1) Septal and beginning right ventricular activation, (2) left ventricular activation, (3) final right ventricular activation.

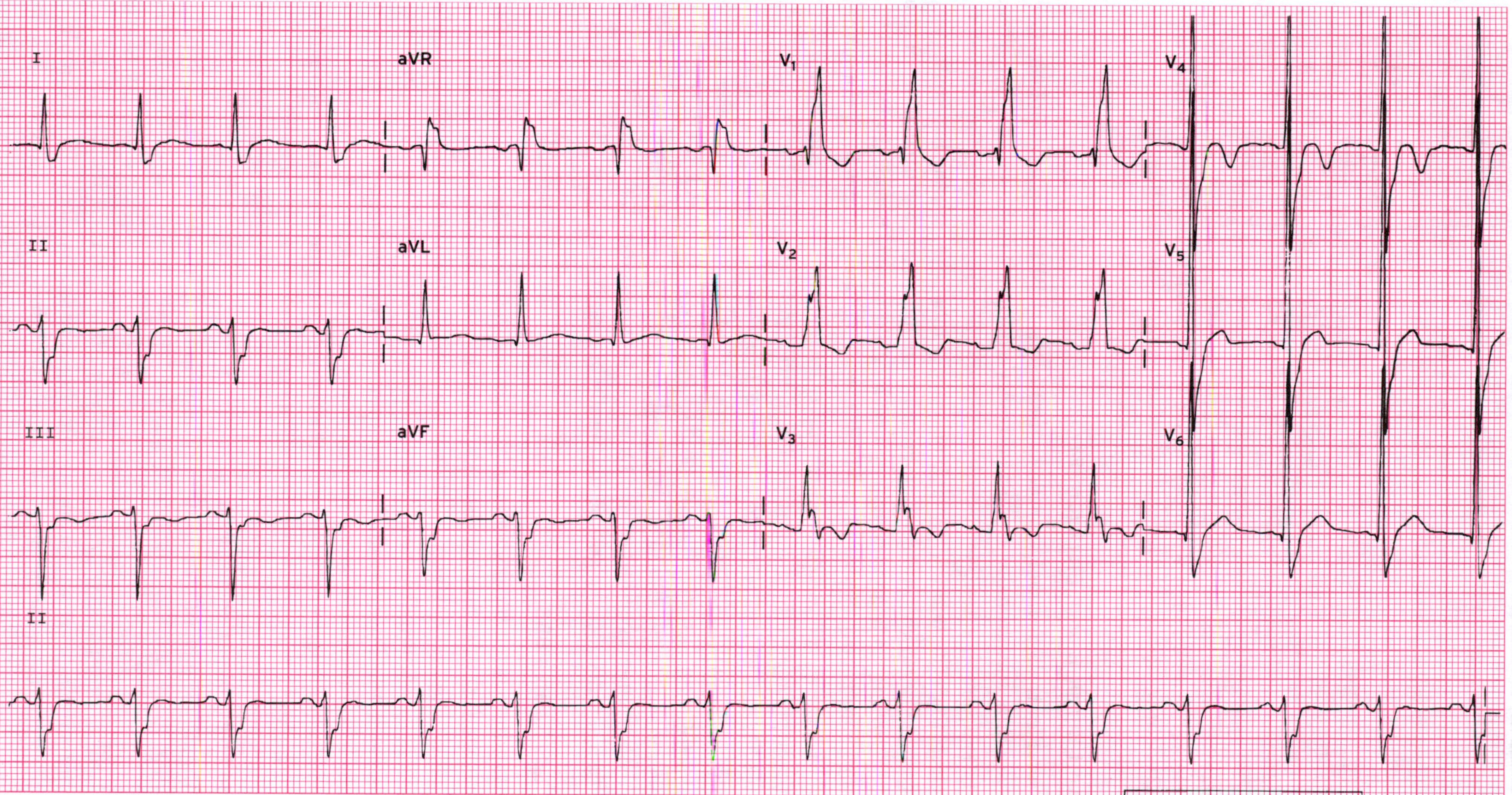

Figure 13-6 Right bundle branch block. Note the RSR′ in V_1 along with the QRS interval $\geq$ 0.12 second and the T waves opposite the terminal QRS wave.

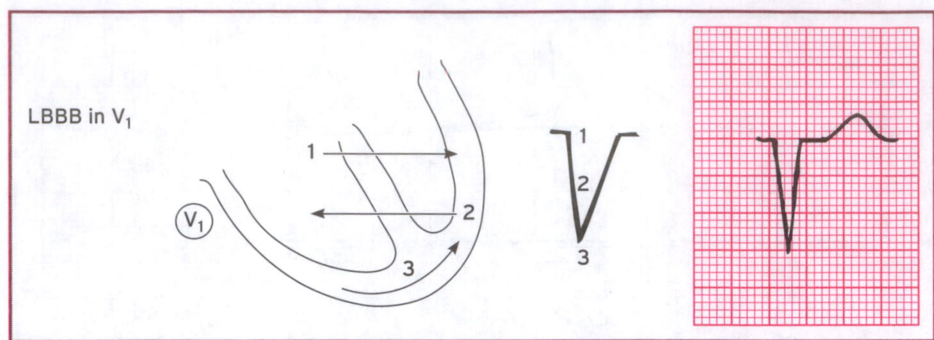

Figure 13-7 LBBB in V_1: (1) Septal and beginning left ventricular activation, (2) right ventricular activation, (3) final left ventricular activation.

Left Bundle Branch Block (LBBB)

See Figure 13-7. In left bundle branch block (LBBB), septal depolarization cannot occur normally. It must go backward, right to left, sending its current away from V_1's positive electrode. When the current reaches the left ventricle, it finds the bundle branch blocked and must traverse the left ventricular tissue very slowly, one cell at a time. Meanwhile, right ventricular activation is occurring normally through the healthy right bundle branch. In Figure 13-7, numbers 1 and 2 are swallowed up inside number 3, as the huge amount of current required to activate the left ventricle dwarfs the current traveling to the septum and right ventricle. The slowed travel through the left ventricle results in a wider-than-normal S wave. LBBB in V_1 thus presents as a large, deep QS complex in V_1. On occasion, there may be a small R wave preceding the deep S wave. As with an RBBB, the QRS interval of an LBBB will be ≥0.12 second, and the T wave will be opposite the terminal wave of the QRS complex. See Figure 13-8 for a LBBB on a 12-lead EKG. See Figure 13-9 for a summary of the criteria for bundle branch blocks.

Rate Related BBB

Bundle branch blocks seen only at certain heart rates are known as **rate-related bundle branch blocks,** and the rate at which the BBB appears is called the **critical rate.** In this disorder, conduction through the bundle branches is normal at heart rates below the critical rate. Once the critical rate is reached, however, one of the bundle branches becomes incapable of depolarizing rapidly enough to allow normal conduction, and a BBB results. When the heart rate falls below the critical rate, bundle branch depolarization returns to normal and the BBB disappears.

Clinical Implications of BBB

Bundle branch blocks do not cause symptoms. In fact, they *are* a symptom that the conduction system is impaired. The question is, what's causing the BBB? See Table 13-1. Though RBBB can be seen in normal healthy hearts, LBBB almost always implies extensive cardiac disease. Patients with bundle branch block are at risk for developing severe AV blocks (for example, if both bundle branches become blocked simultaneously), so it is important to observe their rhythm closely for further signs of conduction disturbance,

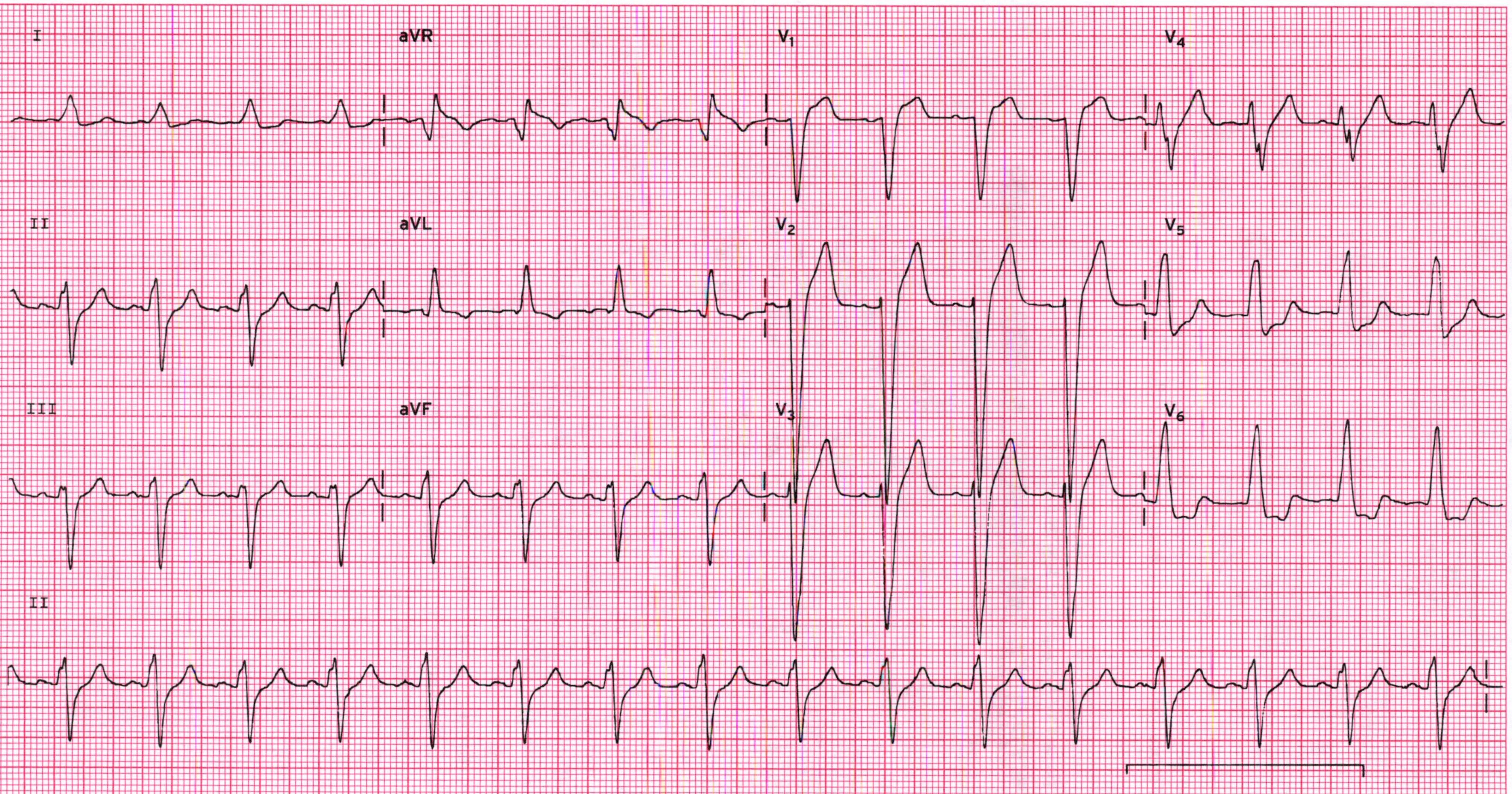

Figure 13-8 Left bundle branch block. Note the RS configuration in V_1 along with the widened QRS interval ($\geq$ 0.12 s) and the T wave opposite the terminal wave of the QRS.

	QRS configuration in V_1	QRS interval	T wave
RBBB	RSR′	≥0.12 s	Opposite the terminal QRS
LBBB	QS or RS	≥0.12 s	Opposite the terminal QRS

Figure 13-9 Summary of criteria for bundle branch blocks.

Table 13-1 Causes of RBBB and LBBB

TYPE OF BBB	CAUSES
RBBB	• Coronary artery disease • Conduction system lesion • Normal variant • Right ventricular hypertrophy • Congenital heart disease • Right ventricular dilatation
LBBB	• Coronary artery disease • Conduction system lesion • Hypertension • Other organic heart disease

such as a new first-degree AV block. *A new bundle branch block should prompt an immediate assessment of the patient.* A 12-lead EKG should be done in an effort to determine the cause of the BBB. Remember–the BBB is a symptom of another problem. For example, the BBB might be a result of an MI in progress. Also remember that BBBs cause T wave changes that can be misinterpreted as ischemia. Certain kinds of MIs (myocardial infarctions–heart attacks) usually cannot be diagnosed in the presence of an LBBB, as the bundle-related changes mask the MI.

BBB Practice

1. Type of BBB (if any): ______________________

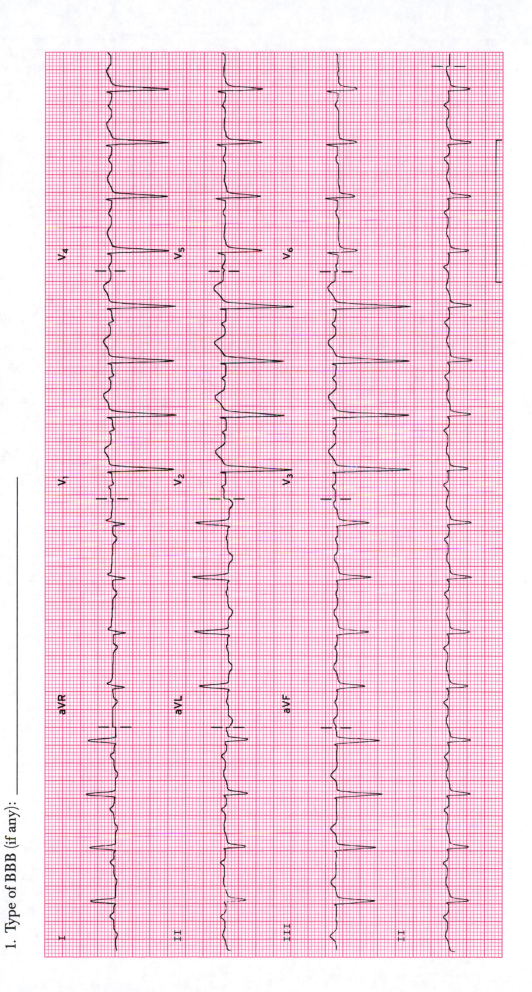

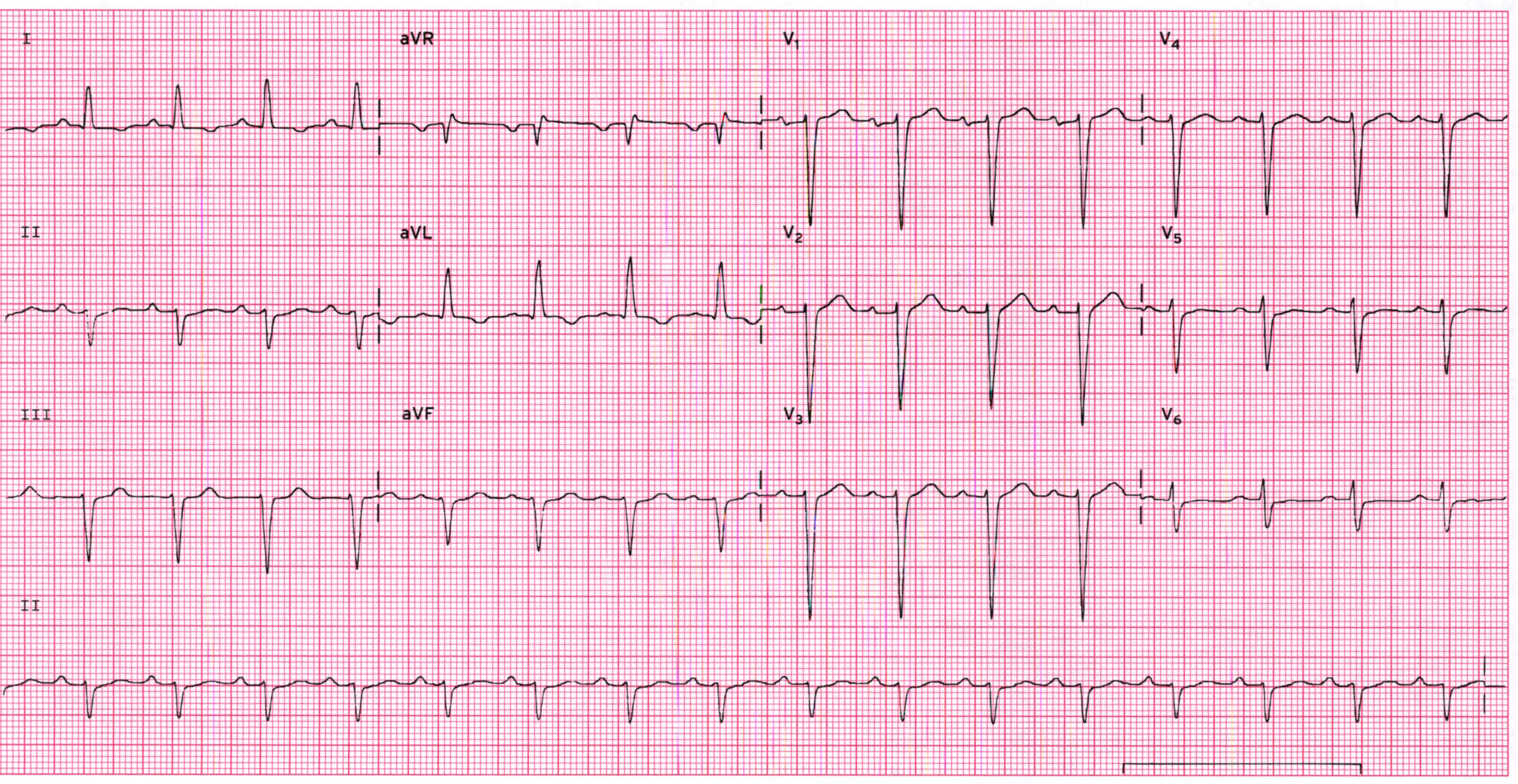

2. Type of BBB (if any): ______________________

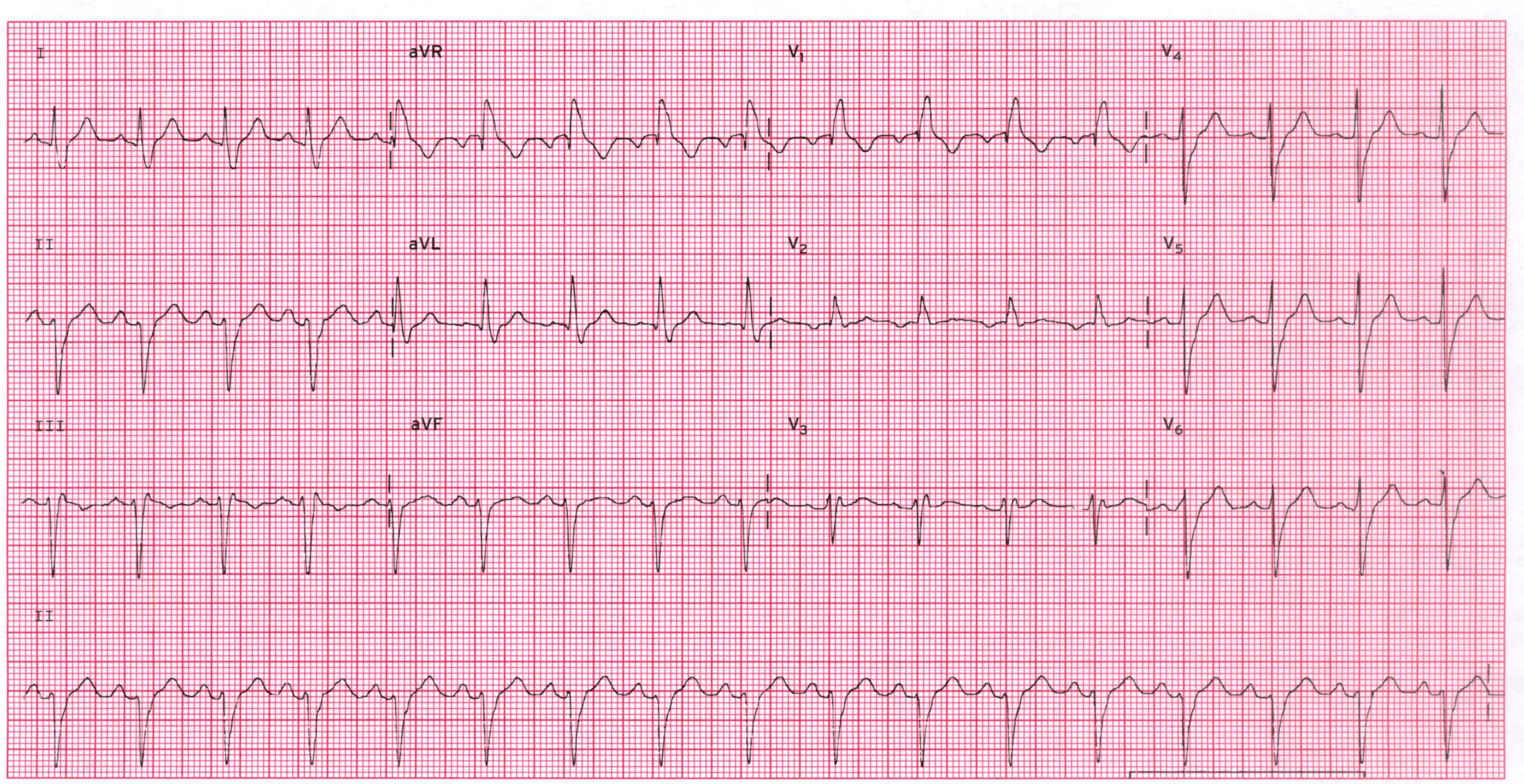

3. Type of BBB (if any): ______________________________

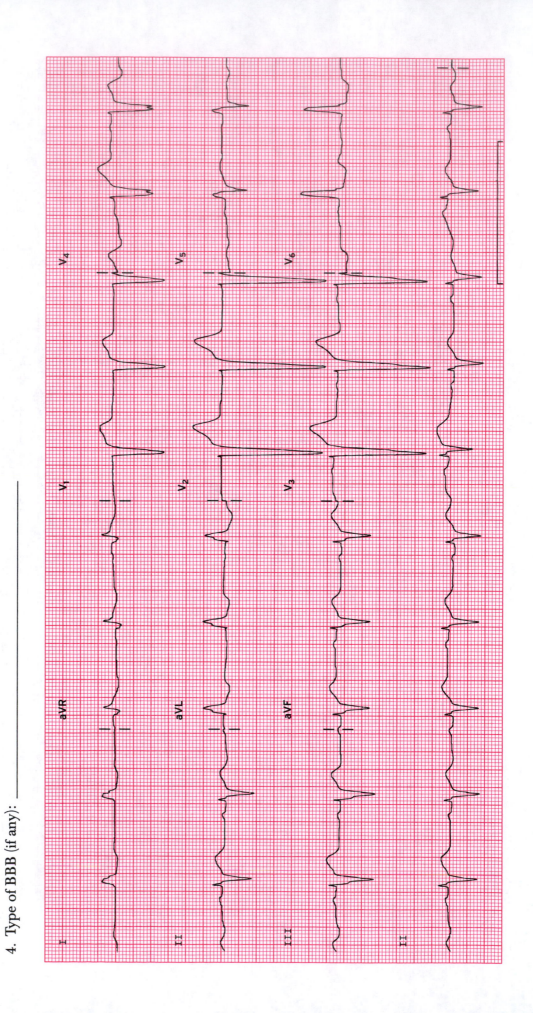

4. Type of BBB (if any): ____________________

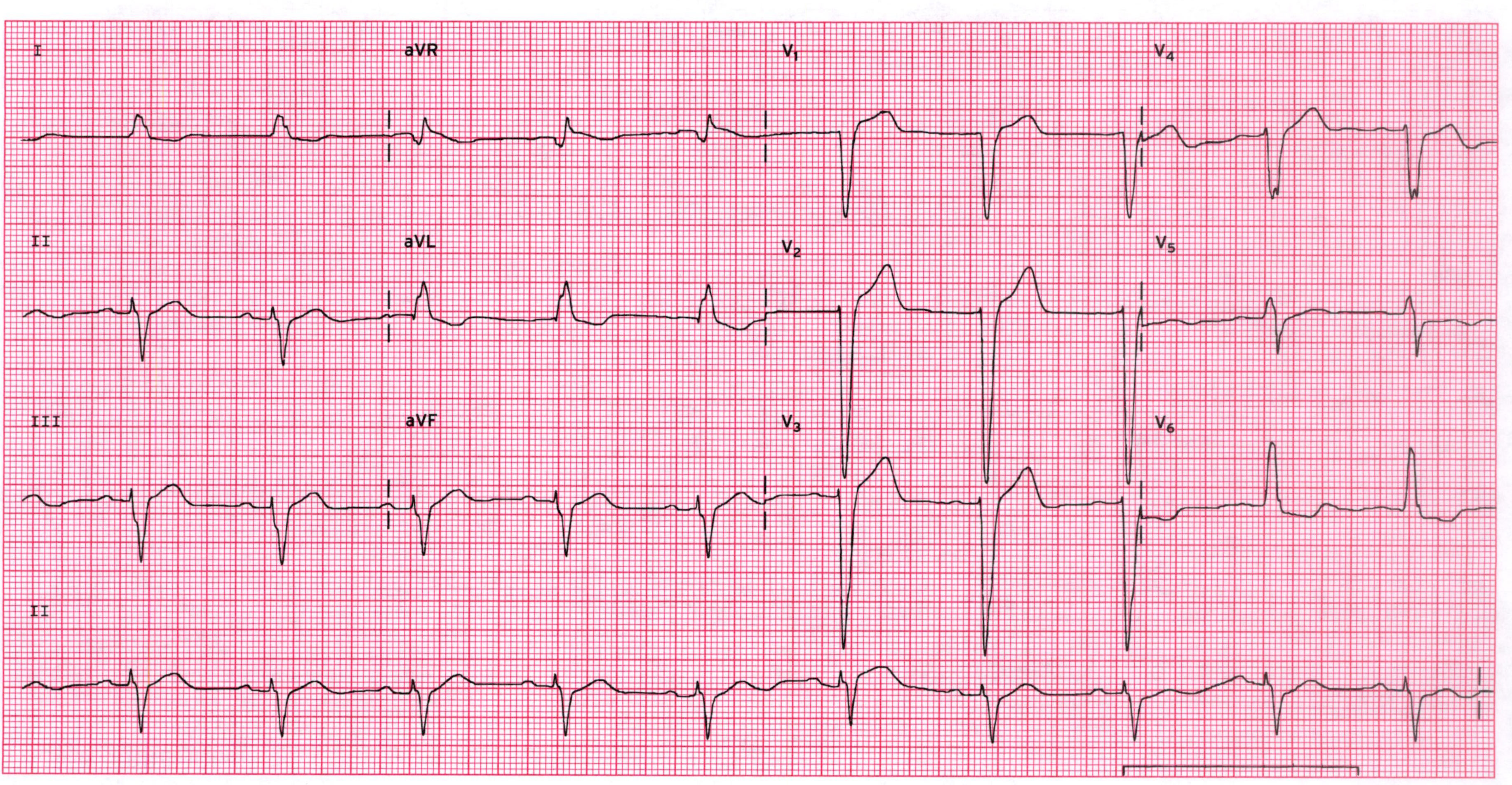

5. Type of BBB (if any): ________________________

I aVR V_1 V_4

II aVL V_2 V_5

III aVF V_3 V_6

II

6. Type of BBB (if any): ______________________

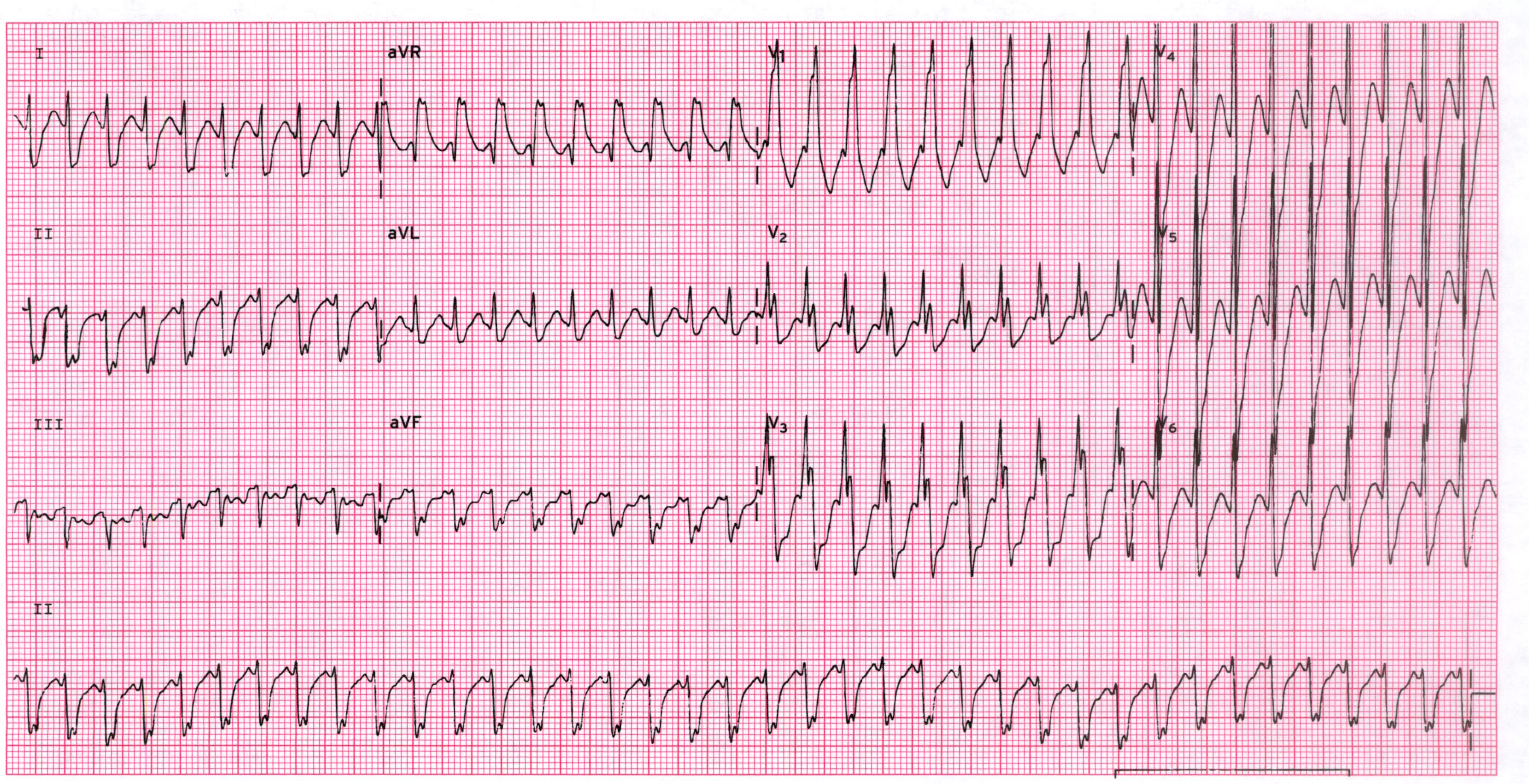

7. Type of BBB (if any): ______________________________

I aVR V_1 V_4

II aVL V_2 V_5

III aVF V_3 V_6

II

8. Type of BBB (if any): ____________________

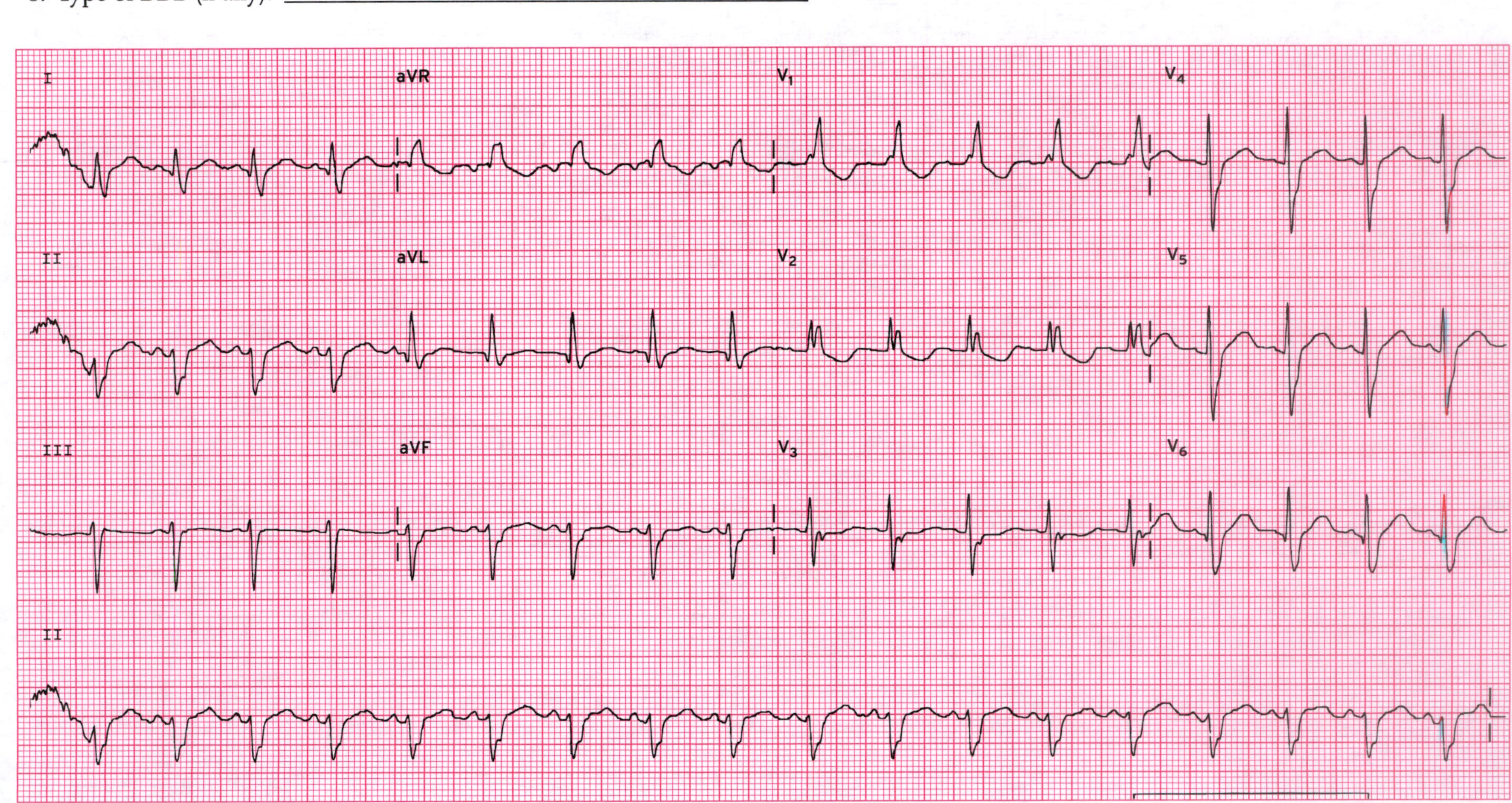

9. Type of BBB (if any): ______________________________

10. Type of BBB (if any): ______________________

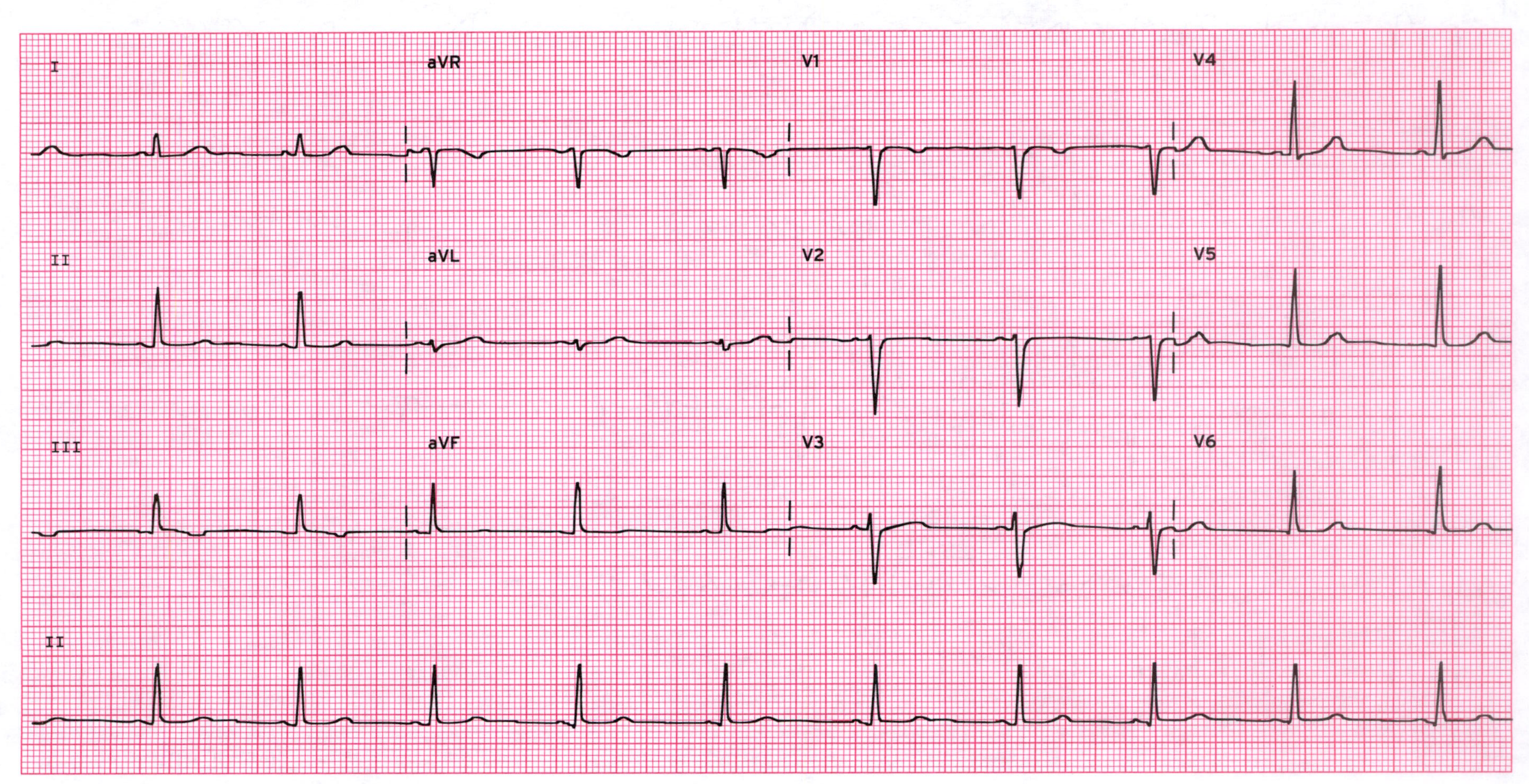

Answers to BBB Practice

1. **No BBB**. The QRS interval is normal (about 0.10 s), so there is no BBB.
2. **RBBB**. There is not the typical RSR' configuration in V_1–the initial R wave is missing–but it is still a RBBB. The QRS is wide (about 0.12 s) and the T wave slopes off opposite the final wave of the QRS complex.
3. **LBBB**. There is a wide QRS (about 0.14 s), and a QS complex in V_1. The T wave is opposite the final part of the QRS.
4. **LBBB**. Again, there is a wide QRS of about 0.13 second, a QS in V_1. The T wave is opposite the final wave of the QRS complex.
5. **RBBB**. There is a wide QRS with a QR configuration in V_1.
6. **RBBB**. Note the RSR′ configuration in V_1, along with the QRS interval of 0.12 seconds and the T wave opposite the terminal wave of the QRS.
7. **LBBB**. Note the QS configuration in V_1 with the QRS interval of 0.14 seconds and the T wave opposite the terminal QRS wave.
8. **RBBB**. Note the RR′ configuration in V_1 along with a QRS interval of about 0.12 seconds and a T wave opposite the terminal QRS wave.
9. **RBBB**. There's an RSR′ in V_1, the QRS interval is 0.16 seconds, and the T wave is opposite the terminal QRS wave.
10. **No BBB**. The QRS interval is normal, about 0.08 seconds.

Ventricular Hypertrophy

Hypertrophy refers to excessive growth of tissue. In ventricular hypertrophy, the muscle mass of the right or left ventricle (or both) is thickened, usually as a result of disease. This thickened tissue requires more current to depolarize it and thus causes greater-than-normal amplitude (voltage) of the QRS complexes in the leads over the hypertrophied ventricle. Let's look at an example of normal QRS amplitude. See Figure 13-10. **The normal QRS complex should be no taller or deeper than 13 mm high (13 small blocks) in any lead.**

Right Ventricular Hypertrophy (RVH)

RVH is evidenced on the EKG by a tall R wave in V_1 (greater than or equal to the size of the S wave), accompanied by a right axis deviation and, often, T wave inversion. Since the R wave in V_1 represents depolarization of the right ventricle, it will be taller than normal if the right ventricle is enlarged. The most common cause of RVH is chronic lung disease, which forces the right ventricle to bulk up in order to force its blood out into the now-high-pressure lung system. See Figure 13-11 for an example of the typical QRST configuration in right ventricular hypertrophy in V_1.

Now let's see what RVH looks like on a 12-lead EKG. See Figure 13-12.

Left Ventricular Hypertrophy (LVH)

LVH is most commonly caused by hypertension (high blood pressure), which causes the left ventricle to bulk up in order to expel its blood against the great resistance of the abnormally high blood pressure.

LVH has several possible criteria but the one most commonly used is the following:

R wave in V_5 or V_6 (whichever is taller) + the S wave in $V_1 \geq 35$ mm

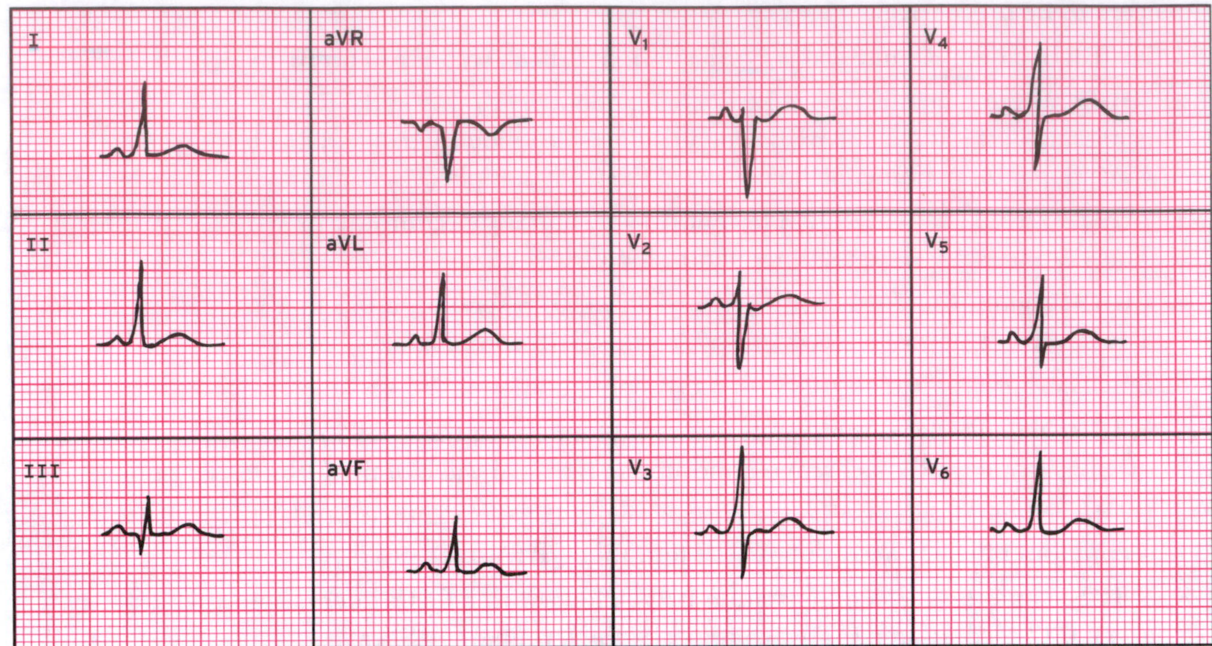

Figure 13-10 Normal QRS amplitude (voltage).

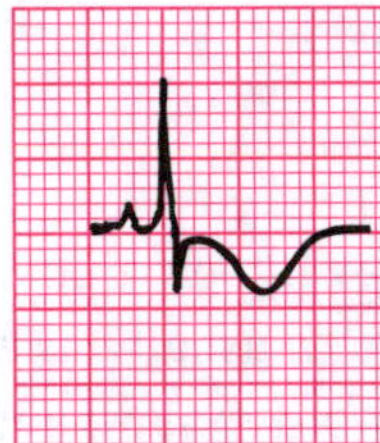

Figure 13-11 QRST configuration typical of RVH in V_1.

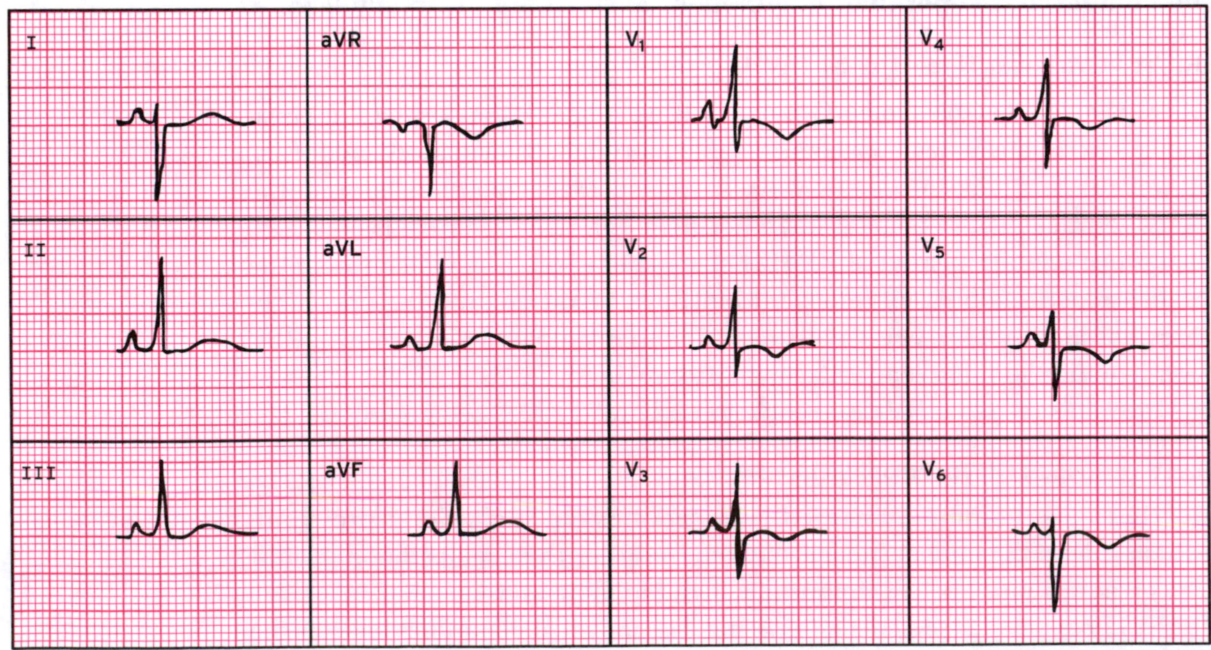

Figure 13-12 Right ventricular hypertrophy. Note that the R wave in V_1 is taller than the S wave is deep; there is right axis deviation and T wave inversion.

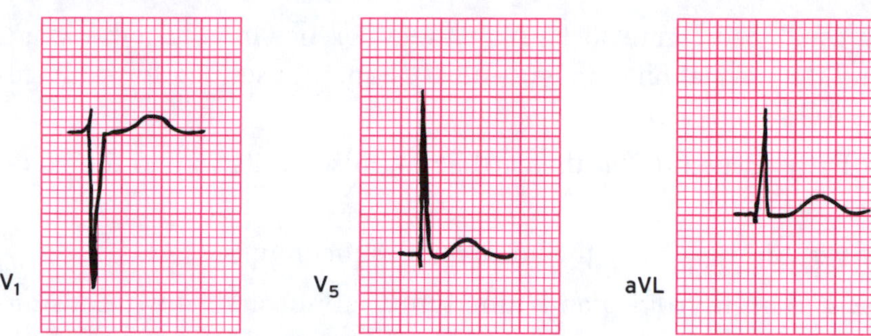

Figure 13-13 LVH by voltage criteria.

In LVH, Leads I, aVL, and V_5 and V_6 will have taller-than-normal R waves as the current travels toward their positive electrodes; leads V_1 and V_2 will have deeper-than-normal S waves as the current travels away from their positive electrode. See Figure 13-13. Add the height of the R wave in V_5 to the depth of the S wave in V_1. The result is ≥35 mm. This is LVH as evidenced by adding the voltages. See Figure 13-14 for a 12-lead EKG example of LVH.

Ventricular hypertrophy does not usually prolong the QRS interval beyond normal limits.

Low-Voltage EKGs

It should be immediately obvious, when checking for hypertrophy, whether there is abnormally **low voltage** of the QRS complexes. Some people have abnormally low-voltage EKGs, in which the waves and complexes are

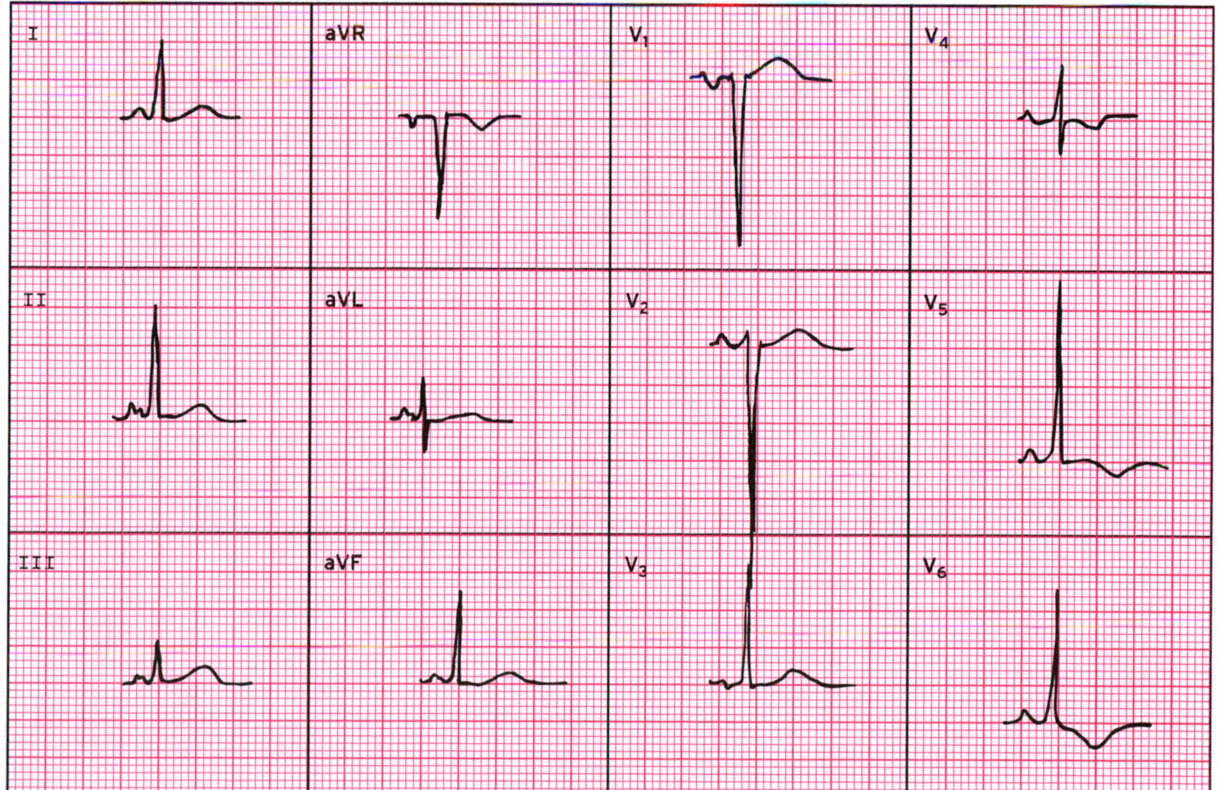

Figure 13-14 Left ventricular hypertrophy. Note the S wave in V_1 is 22 mm deep, and the R wave in V_5 is 24 mm tall, for a total voltage of 46 mm. This meets and exceeds the criteria for LVH.

shorter than usual. See Figure 13-15. Note the difference in voltage between this EKG and the normal one in Figure 13-10. Some causes of a low-voltage EKG are the following:

- *Obesity.* Fatty tissue muffles the cardiac impulse on its way to the electrodes on the skin.
- *Emphysema.* Air trapping in the lungs muffles the impulse.
- *Myxedema.* The thyroid gland function is abnormally low, causing decreased voltage.
- *Pericardial effusion.* In this condition, excessive fluid inside the pericardial sac surrounding the heart muffles the impulse on its way to the skin.

Clinical Implications of Hypertrophy

Hypertrophy is the heart's way of attempting to meet a contractile demand that cannot be met by normal-size heart muscle. Unfortunately, hypertrophy also places increased demands on the coronary circulation to feed that extra muscle bulk. When that increased blood and oxygen demand cannot be adequately met, ischemia results. Hypertrophy increases the likelihood of ischemia and infarction simply by increasing the amount of muscle to be nourished by the coronary arteries.

Ventricular dilatation, a stretching of the myocardial fibers that results from overfilling of the ventricles or inadequate pumping of blood out of the ventricles, can also result in a hypertrophy pattern on the EKG. Low-voltage EKGs, contrary to what may seem logical, do not imply that the heart is smaller than normal, or that it is generating less current than normal. It is usually caused by an outside influence that affects the heart's current on its way to the electrodes on the skin.

Let's practice.

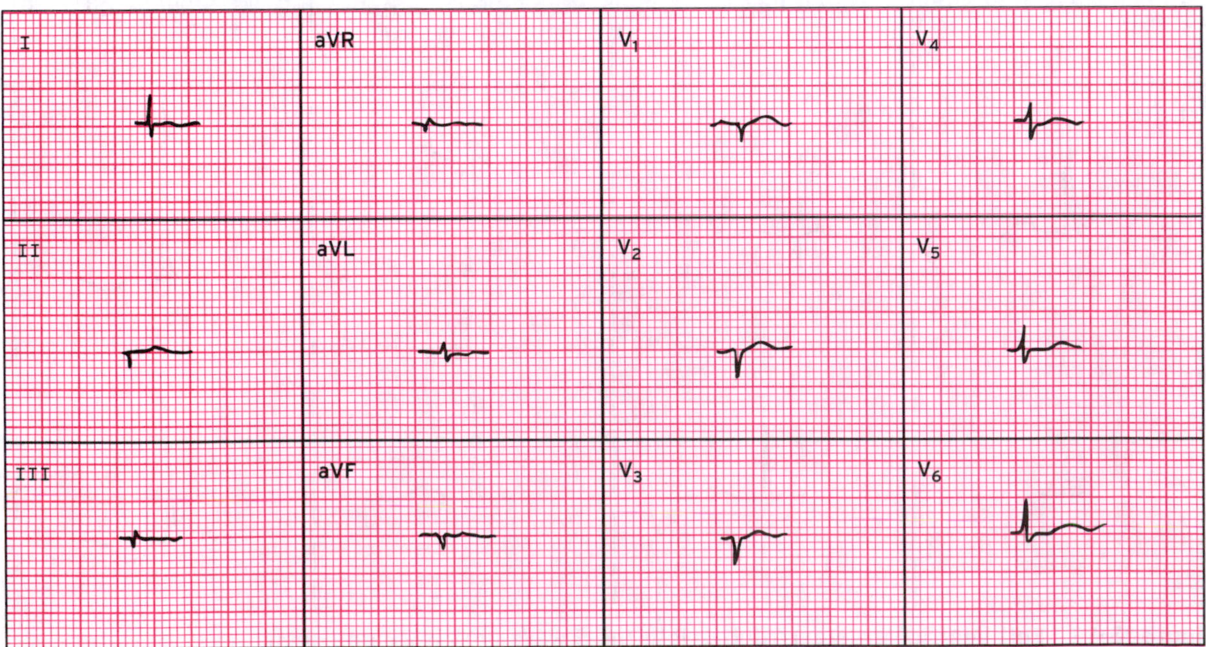

Figure 13-15 Low-voltage EKG.

Hypertrophy Practice

Look for hypertrophy and low voltage on the following EKGs. Your answer will be one of these: RVH, LVH, low voltage, or normal.

1. Answer = ______________________________

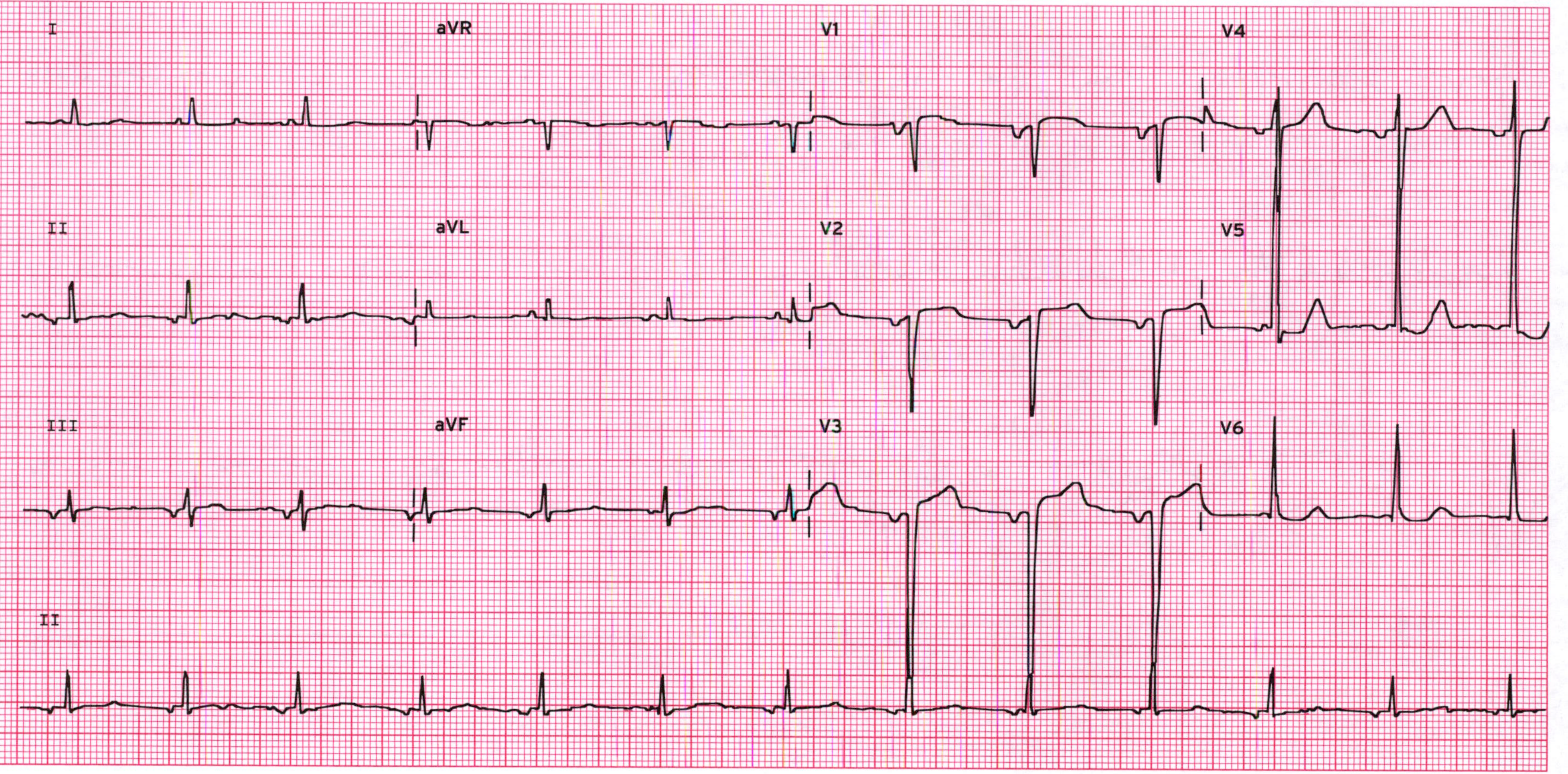

2. Answer = ______________________________

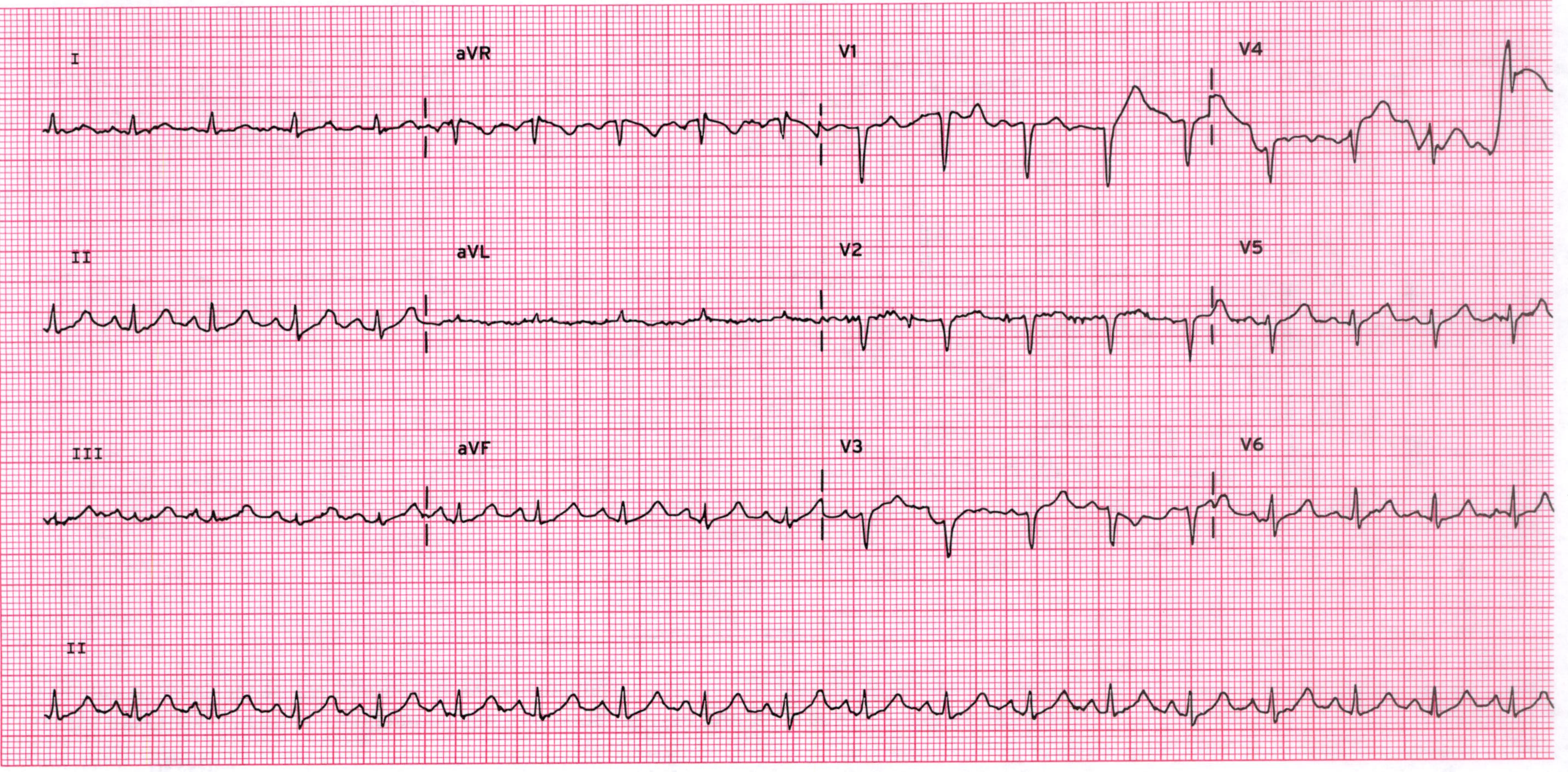

3. Answer = ____________________

I aVR V1 V4

II aVL V2 V5

III aVF V3 V6

II

4. Answer = ______________________________

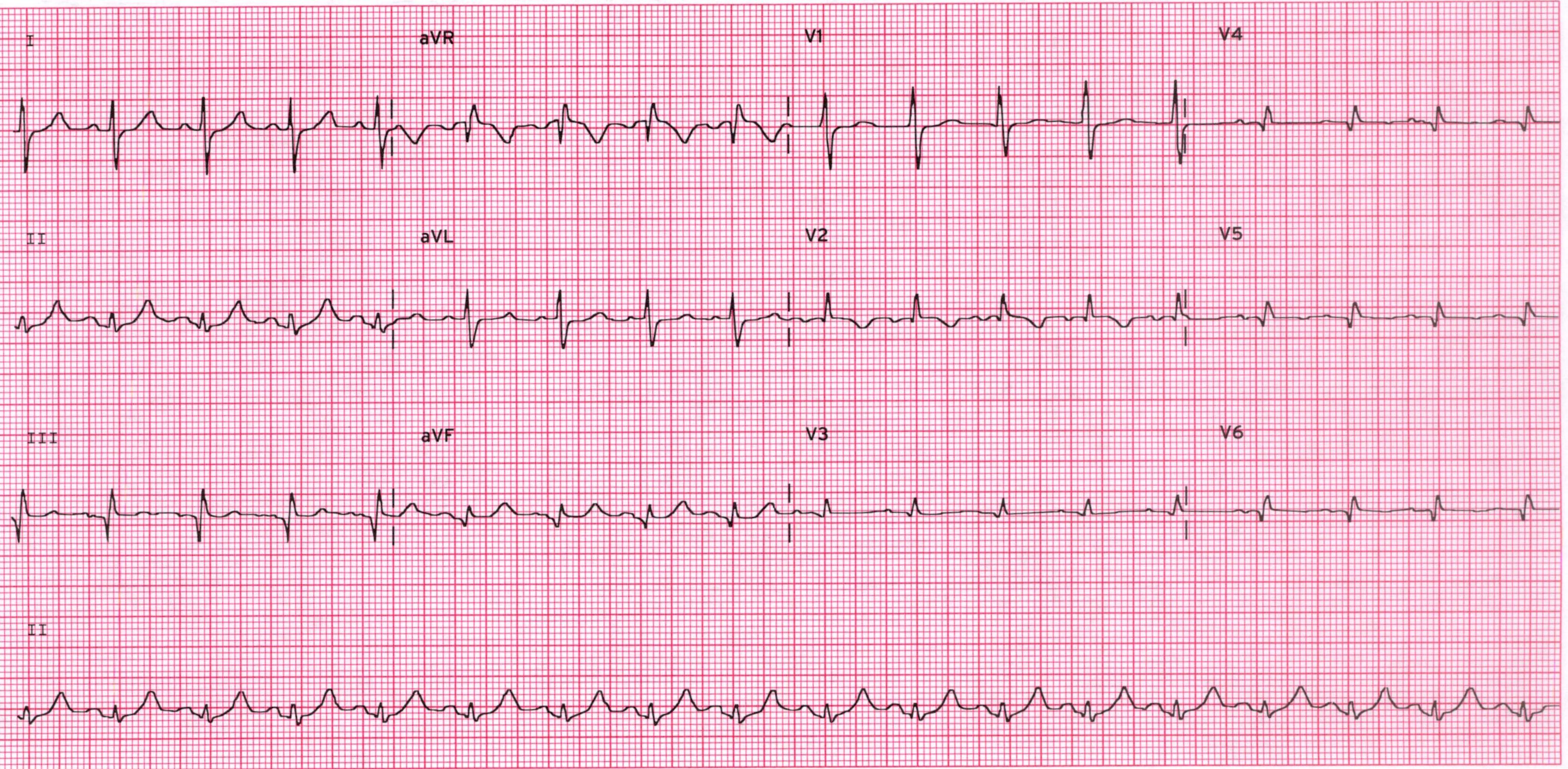

5. Answer = ______________________________

Hypertrophy Practice Answers

1. **LVH.** The QRS in V_1 is about 8 mm deep, and the R wave in V_5 is 41 mm tall (it extends up beyond the QRS in V_4). Total is greater than 35 mm, so this EKG meets and exceeds the criteria for LVH.
2. **Low voltage.** The QRS complexes are short in all leads, especially aVL, which is tiny.
3. **Normal.** There is no hypertrophy or low voltage.
4. **RVH.** The R wave in V_1 is as tall as, if not slightly taller than, the S wave is deep and there is right axis deviation. The T wave is not inverted here as it often is, but that is not an absolute requirement for RVH.
5. **LVH.** The QRS in V_1 is 23 mm deep and in V_5 is 15 mm tall, for a total of 38 mm, more than enough to meet the voltage criteria for LVH.

Miscellaneous Effects

Electrolyte abnormalities and certain medications can affect the EKG. Let's look at some of these effects.

Digitalis Effect

Digitalis is a medication given to increase the force of myocardial contraction in patients with heart failure, or to slow the heart rate in patients with tachycardias. Digitalis medications are notorious for causing sagging ST segment depression (also called a **scooping** ST segment) that is easily misinterpreted as ischemia. The cause of this ST segment change is still not understood. Digitalis also prolongs the PR interval because it slows conduction through the AV node. These effects are not necessarily indicative of **digitalis toxicity** (excessive digitalis in the bloodstream), as they also occur at normal therapeutic levels. See Figure 13-16. See the sagging, very rounded ST segments and prolonged PR interval? This is typical of the digitalis effect.

Electrolyte Abnormalities

Hyperkalemia

A high potassium level in the bloodstream has two main EKG effects. First, at potassium levels of about 6, it causes tall, pointy, narrow T waves. Normal blood potassium level is 3.5 to 5. As the potassium level rises to around 8, the tall T wave is replaced by a very widened QRS complex. This widened QRS is a sign that cardiac arrest may be imminent if the potassium level is

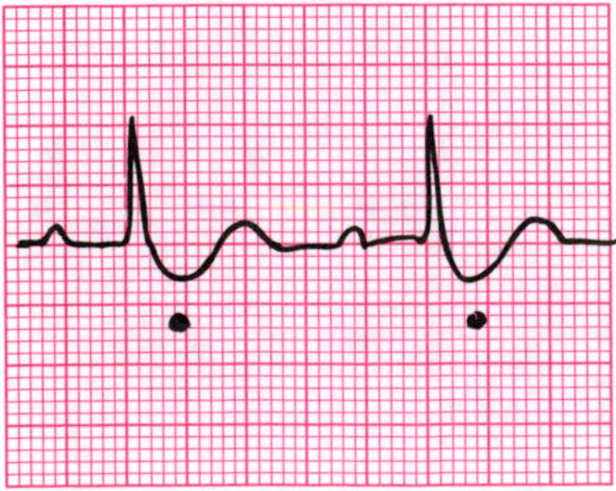

Figure 13-16 Digitalis effect.

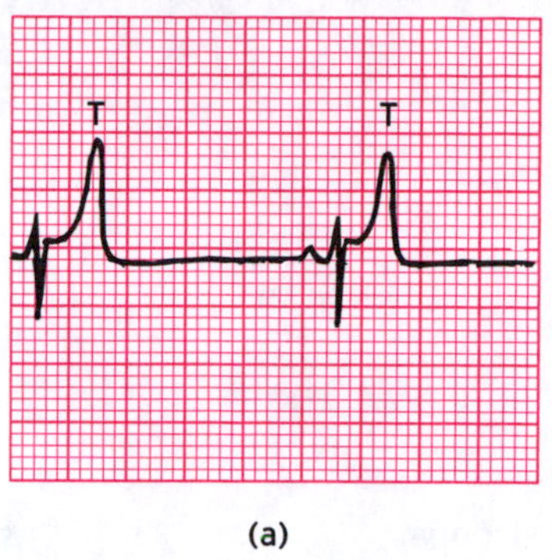

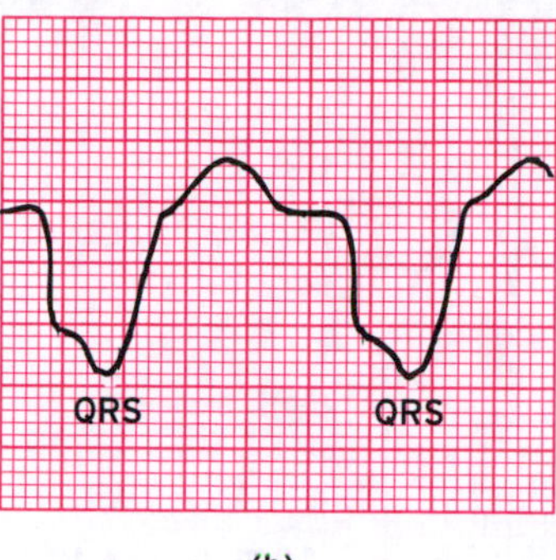

(a) (b)

Figure 13-17 Hyperkalemia.

not lowered quickly. These EKG effects are due to potassium's effect on depolarization and repolarization, and will return to normal once the potassium level is normalized. One way to remember potassium's effect on the T wave is to think of the T wave as a tent containing potassium. The more potassium, the taller the tent. See Figure 13-17. In Figure 13-17(a), note the tall, pointy T waves. In Figure 13-17(b), note the widened QRS complex.

Hypokalemia

A low potassium level in the bloodstream results in a prominent U wave and flattened T waves. The potassium tent is almost empty, so it flattens out. These effects are due to the fact that repolarization, especially phase 3 of the action potential, is disturbed by the potassium deficit. See Figure 13-18.

Note the flattened T wave and the prominent U wave in Figure 13-18. Recall the U wave is not usually seen on the EKG, but if it is present it follows the T wave. T waves always follow QRS complexes. *If there are no obvious T waves on the strip, be sure the QRS complexes are really QRS complexes and not artifact.* Then, if you still can't really see T waves following those QRS complexes, you can be reasonably sure the potassium level is quite low, usually around a blood level of 2.0. T waves will improve after supplemental potassium is given.

Hypercalcemia

An elevated blood calcium level causes the ST segment to shorten to such an extent that the T wave seems to be almost on top of the QRS. This effect occurs because the elevated calcium level shortens the repolarization phase of the action potential. See Figure 13-19.

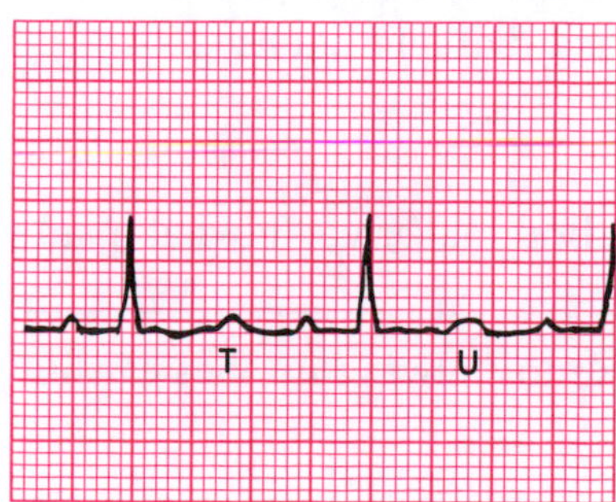

Figure 13-18 Hypokalemia.

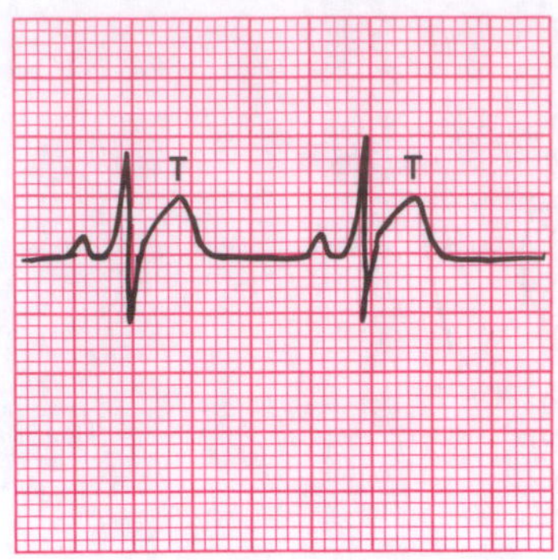

Figure 13-19 Hypercalcemia.

In Figure 13-19, note the extremely short ST segment, which in turn causes a very short QT interval. The ST segment and QT interval will return to normal once the calcium level is normalized.

Hypocalcemia

Low calcium levels in the bloodstream prolong repolarization and cause a very prolonged ST segment, thus prolonging the QT interval. See Figure 13-20.

In Figure 13-20, note how far the T wave is from the QRS complex. This demonstrates a very prolonged ST segment and QT interval.

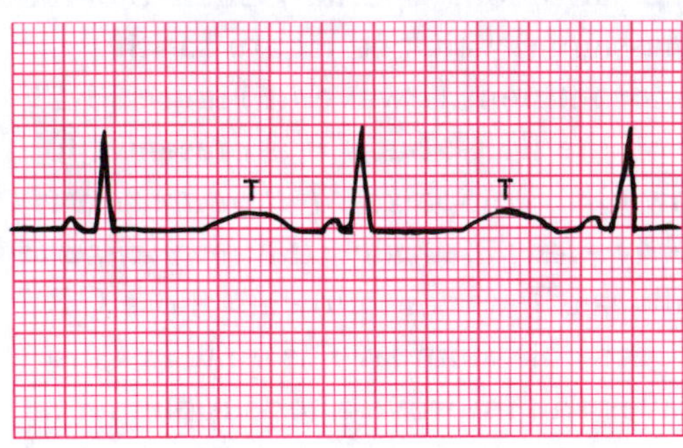

Figure 13-20 Hypocalcemia.

Summary of Miscellaneous Effects

See Figure 13-21 for a summary of miscellaneous effects.

In Summary

We now can evaluate **almost all** of a 12-lead EKG with one very important exception—we need to know if our patient is having a heart attack. Let's move on to the next chapter to learn about myocardial infarctions.

Practice Quiz

1. If the QRS complex in leads I and aVF are both negative, in what quadrant is the axis? ______________________
2. True or False. Right bundle branch block almost always implies cardiovascular disease.

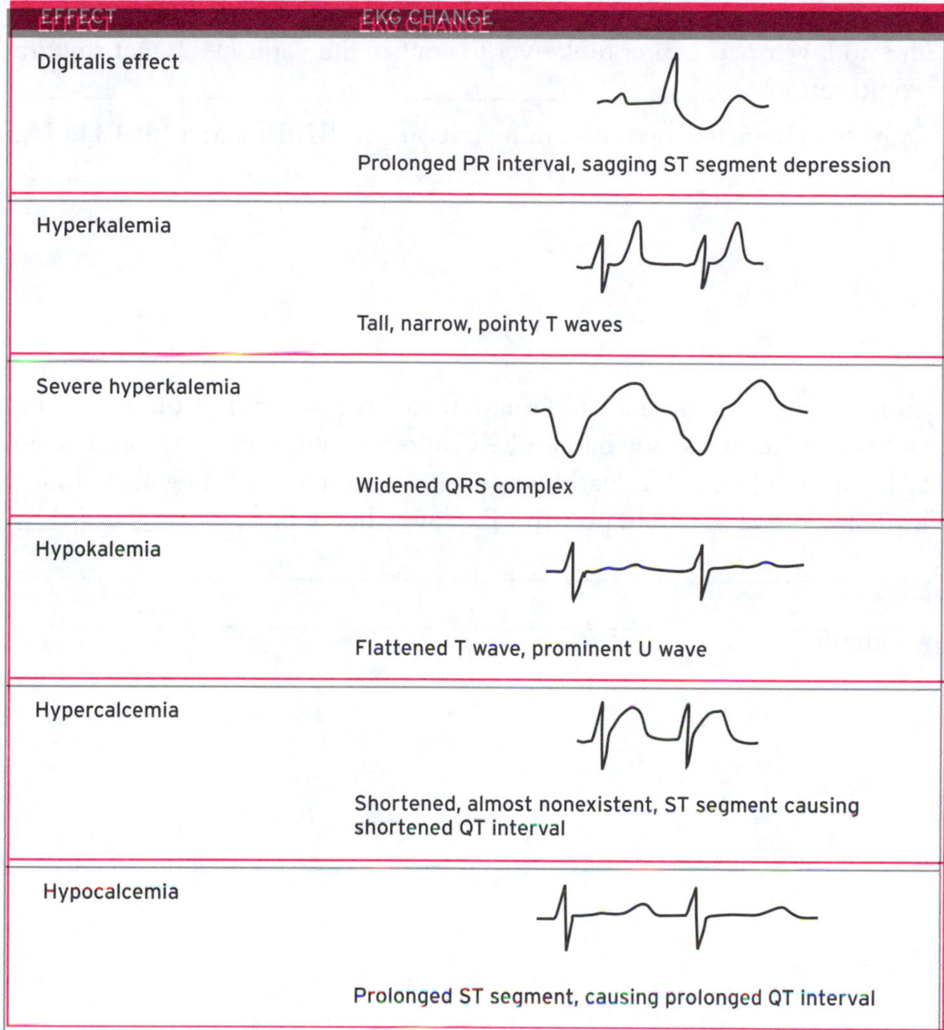

EFFECT	EKG CHANGE
Digitalis effect	Prolonged PR interval, sagging ST segment depression
Hyperkalemia	Tall, narrow, pointy T waves
Severe hyperkalemia	Widened QRS complex
Hypokalemia	Flattened T wave, prominent U wave
Hypercalcemia	Shortened, almost nonexistent, ST segment causing shortened QT interval
Hypocalcemia	Prolonged ST segment, causing prolonged QT interval

Figure 13-21 Miscellaneous Effects Summary.

3. Sagging ST segments are associated with what miscellaneous effect? ______
4. True or False. Tall pointy T waves are typical of RBBB.
5. Name three causes of axis deviations. ______
6. Write the voltage criteria for LVH. ______
7. True or False. RVH is always associated with an inverted T wave.
8. Define hypertrophy. ______
9. Hypokalemia has what effect on the T wave? ______
10. In a BBB, the QRS interval must be at least ______ seconds.

Putting It All Together—Critical Thinking Exercises

These exercises may consist of diagrams to label, scenarios to analyze, brain-stumping questions to ponder, or other challenging exercises to boost your understanding of the chapter material.

1. If both the right and left bundle branches became blocked simultaneously and no lower pacemaker took over to control the ventricles, what rhythm would result? ______________________________

2. Draw the characteristic QRS configuration of a RBBB and a LBBB in V_1.

3. Your patient is a 29-year old female who has a six-month old baby and eight-year old twins. She had an EKG about seven months ago and again today. In the first EKG, lead I was positive and aVF was negative. Today leads I and aVF are both positive. Explain what happened. ______________

____

____

CHAPTER **14**

Myocardial Infarction

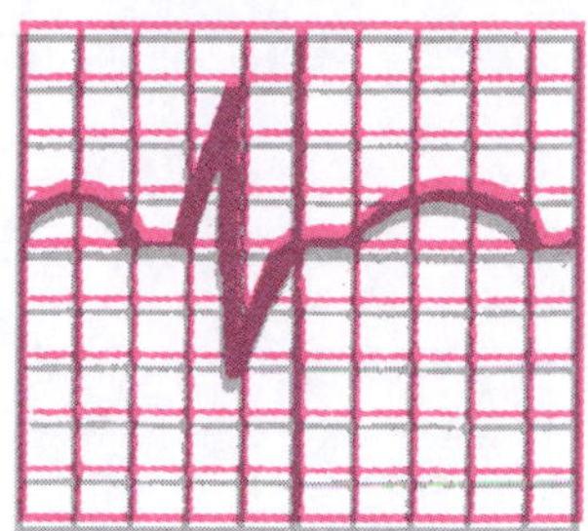

Chapter 14 Objectives

Upon completion of this chapter, the student will be able to:

- Describe the difference between Q wave myocardial infarction (MI) and non–Q wave MI.
- Describe the three Is of infarction.
- Describe what EKG changes are associated with ischemia, injury, and infarction.
- Draw the different kinds of ST segment abnormalities and explain what each implies.
- Draw the different T wave abnormalities and explain what each implies.
- Describe how a significant Q wave differs from a normal Q wave.
- Describe normal R wave progression.
- Identify the transition zone in a variety of EKGs.
- Describe where the transition zone is for clockwise and counterclockwise rotation.
- Describe the EKG changes associated with MI evolution and give the timeline associated with each change.
- Explain how to determine the age of an MI.
- Name the four walls of the left ventricle.
- Name the leads that look at each of the four walls of the left ventricle.
- Describe an easy way to find posterior MIs.
- Name the coronary artery that feeds each of the four walls of the left ventricle.
- Describe how to determine if a right ventricular infarction is present.
- Describe precordial lead placement for a right-sided EKG.
- Describe how pericarditis and early repolarization mimic an MI.

Introduction

Myocardial infarctions (MIs) involve death of myocardial tissue in an area deprived of blood flow by an **occlusion** (blockage) of a coronary artery. Actual death of tissue is the end of a process that begins with ischemia and injury.

There are two types of myocardial infarctions: **Q wave MIs** and **non–Q wave MIs**.

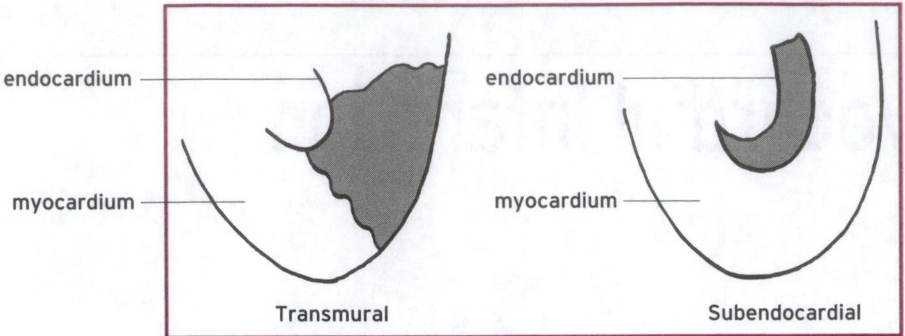

Figure 14-1 Transmural and subendocardial MIs.

- Q wave MIs tend to be **transmural** (i.e., they usually, though not always, damage the entire thickness of the myocardium in a certain area of the heart). Q wave MIs result in ST segment elevation, T wave inversion, and significant Q waves, along with the usual symptoms of an MI.
- The non–Q wave MI tends to be **subendocardial** or **incomplete**, damaging only the innermost layer of the myocardium just beneath the endocardium. This kind of MI typically does less damage than a Q wave MI and does not result in the typical EKG changes associated with Q wave MIs. Non–Q wave MIs can be difficult to diagnose. They sometimes present with widespread ST segment depression and T wave inversion. At other times the MI is diagnosed only by patient history, ST segment changes, and elevated lab values that indicate myocardial damage. With non–Q wave MIs, the patient will have the usual symptoms of an MI, and will typically go on to have a Q wave MI within a few months if treatment for the coronary artery blockage is not rendered. Non–Q wave MIs are less common than Q wave MIs. See Figure 14-1.

The Three Is of Infarction

The sequence of events that occurs when a coronary artery becomes occluded is known as the *three Is of infarction.*

- **Ischemia**. Experiments on dogs have shown that almost immediately after a coronary artery becomes occluded, the *T wave inverts* in the EKG leads overlooking the occluded area. This indicates that myocardial tissue is ischemic, starving for blood and oxygen due to the lack of blood flow. Myocardial tissue becomes pale and whitish in appearance.
- **Injury**. Soon, as the coronary occlusion continues, the once-ischemic tissue becomes injured by the continued lack of perfusion. The tissue becomes bluish in appearance. The *ST segment rises,* indicating a current of injury and the beginning of an acute MI.
- **Infarction**. If occlusion persists, the jeopardized myocardial tissue **necroses** (dies) and turns black. *Significant Q waves develop* (in Q wave MIs) on the EKG. In time, the dead tissue will become scar tissue.

Ischemia and injury to myocardial tissue cause repolarization changes, so the ST segments and the T waves will be abnormal. Infarction causes

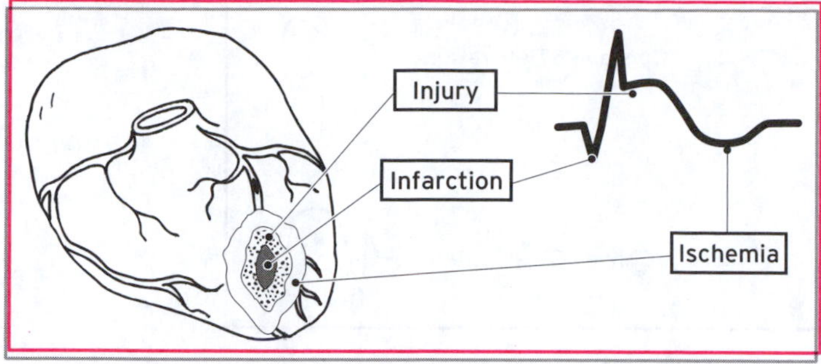

Figure 14-2 The three Is of infarction.

depolarization changes, so the QRS complex on the EKG will show telltale signs of permanent damage. See Figure 14-2.

In Figure 14-2, an occlusion in a coronary artery is blocking the blood flow to the portion of myocardium fed by that artery. This creates three distinct zones. The innermost zone is the infarcted zone. It is the area that has been deprived of oxygen the longest, as it's the deepest layer and thus farthest away from the blood supply. Immediately surrounding that area is the injured zone, and surrounding that is the ischemic zone.

Ischemia and injury are reversible if circulation is restored. Once the tissue has infarcted, however, the tissue is permanently dead. Myocardial cells do not regenerate.

To determine if an MI is present, we look at the ST segments, the T waves, and the QRS complexes. Let's look at each of those separately.

ST Segment

The normal ST segment should be on the baseline at the same level as the PR segment. (Think of the PR segment as the baseline for ST segment evaluation purposes.) Abnormal ST segments can be elevated or depressed. To see if the ST segment is elevated or depressed, draw a straight line extending from the PR segment out past the QRS. An elevated ST segment is one that is above this line. A depressed ST segment is one that is below this line. *ST segment elevation implies myocardial injury.* ST elevation can be either concave or convex. Convex ST segment elevation (also called a **coved ST segment**) is most often associated with an MI in progress. Concave ST elevation is often associated with **pericarditis**, an inflammation of the pericardium and the myocardium immediately beneath it, but it can also be seen in MIs. *ST depression implies ischemia or reciprocal changes opposite the area of infarct.* See Figure 14-3.

In Figure 14-3, note how the ST segment is right on line with the PR segment in the normal ST example.

T Wave

The normal T wave should be rounded with an amplitude less than or equal to 5 mm in the frontal leads and should be upright in all leads except aVR and V_1. aVR's T wave should be negative. V_1's T wave can be flat, inverted, or upright. See Figure 14-4.

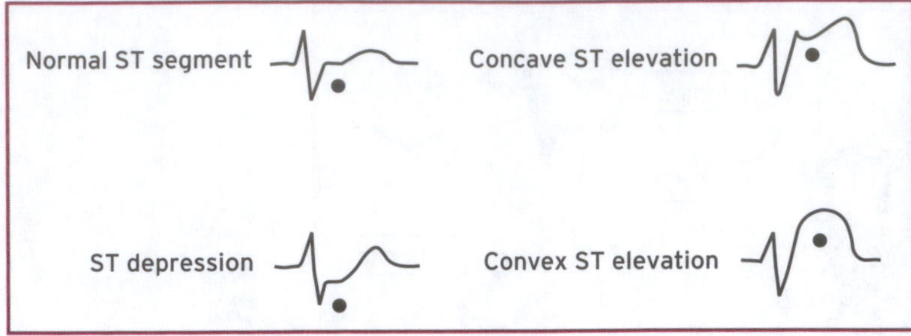

Figure 14-3 ST segment abnormalities.

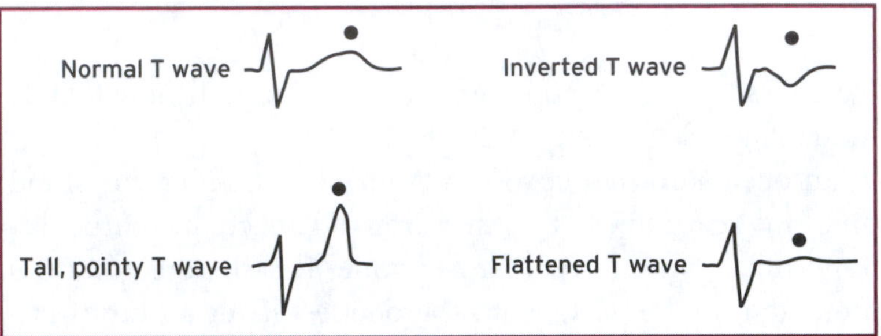

Figure 14-4 T wave abnormalities.

All the abnormal T waves in Figure 14-4 can imply myocardial ischemia. The tall, pointy T can also signal hyperkalemia or **hyperacute** changes of an MI in progress. Hyperacute changes are those that accompany an MI in its earliest stages.

QRS Complexes

We look for significant Q waves and poor R wave progression as clues to an MI. Normal Q waves imply septal and right ventricular depolarization. A significant (i.e., pathological) Q wave implies myocardial necrosis. For a Q wave to be significant, it must be *either* 0.04 second (one small block) wide *or* at least one-fourth the size of the R wave. In Figure 14-5, see the difference between a normal Q and a significant Q.

R Wave Progression and Transition

In the precordial leads, you'll recall that the QRS starts out primarily negative in V_1 and goes through a transition around V_3 or V_4, where the QRS is isoelectric. The QRS then ends up primarily positive by V_6. This means that, accordingly, the R waves progress from very small in V_1 to very large in V_6. If the R waves do not get progressively larger in the precordial leads, as they should, this can imply myocardial infarction. Sometimes, poor R wave progression is the only electrocardiographic evidence of an MI.

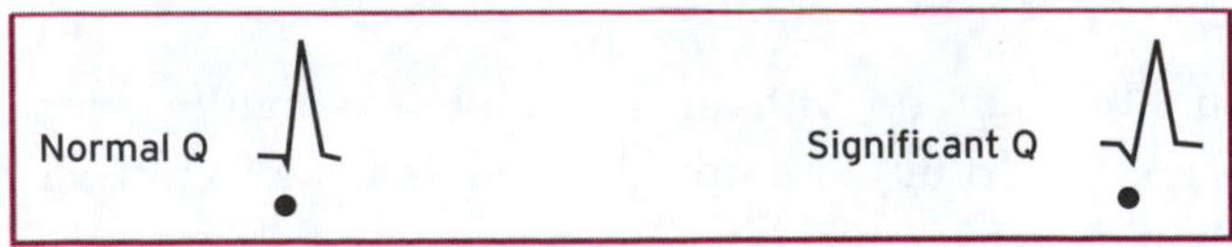

Figure 14-5 Normal versus significant Q waves.

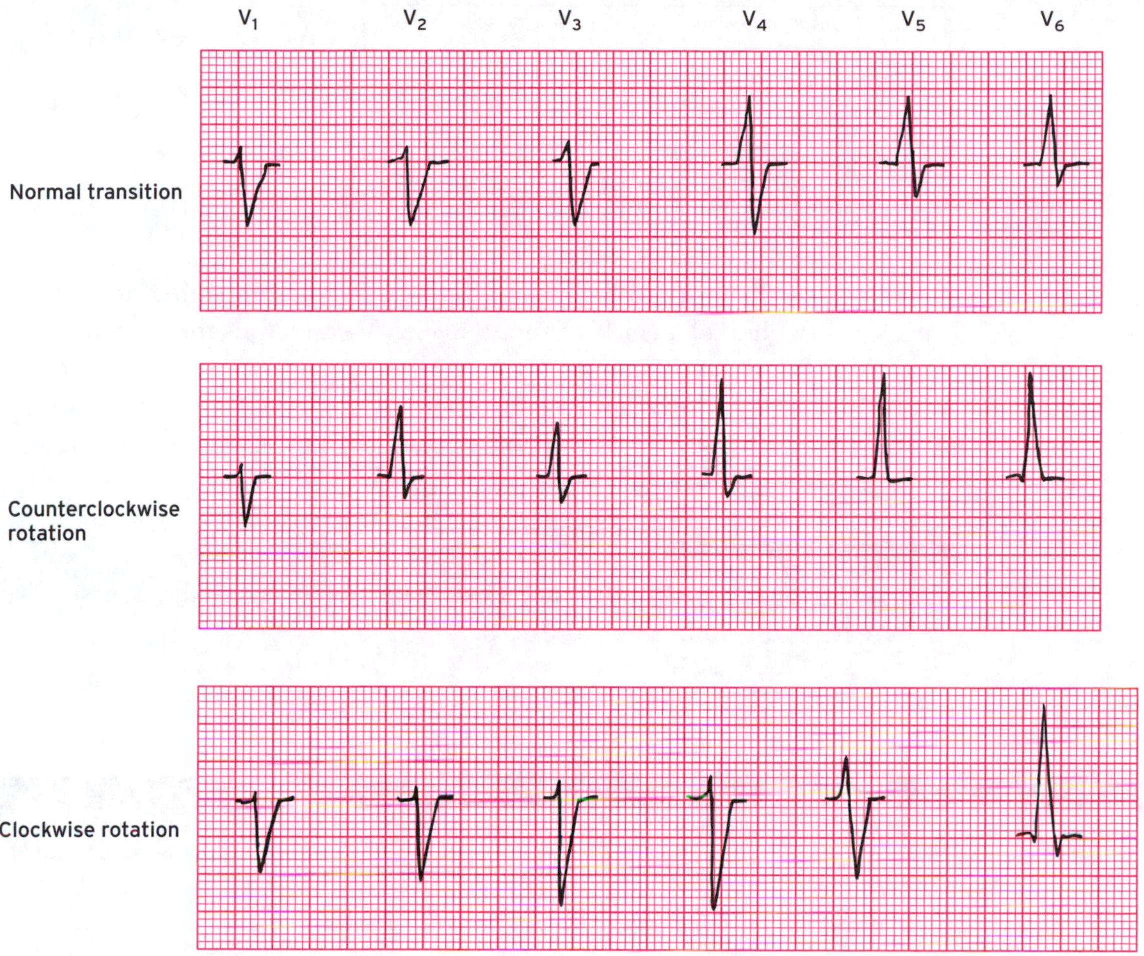

Figure 14-6 R wave progression and transition zones in the precordial leads.

The transition zone is the lead in which the QRS becomes isoelectric. This transition zone can help determine the heart's rotation in the chest cavity. Imagine looking up at the heart from under the diaphragm. If the front of the heart rotates toward the left, it's considered to have **clockwise rotation**. If the front of the heart rotates toward the right, it's **counterclockwise rotation**. A transition in V_1 or V_2 is counterclockwise; a transition in V_5 or V_6 is clockwise. Rotation in the precordial leads is like axis in the frontal leads. See Figure 14-6.

In Figure 14-6, look at the R wave progression in the normal transition example. The R waves grow progressively taller across the precordium, and the transition zone is in V_4. See how V_4's QRS complex is mostly isoelectric? Here, V_1 through V_3 are mostly negative, V_5 and V_6 are positive, and V_4 is where the transition from negative to positive occurs.

In the counterclockwise example, the transition zone is between V_1 and V_2. There is no real isoelectric complex. V_1 is negative and V_2 is already positive, so the transition zone would have to be between the two. The R wave progression is abnormal. The R waves progress from very small in V_1 to unusually large in V_2.

In the clockwise example, the transition zone is between V_5 and V_6. R wave progression is abnormal–the R wave is small in V_5 and very tall in V_6.

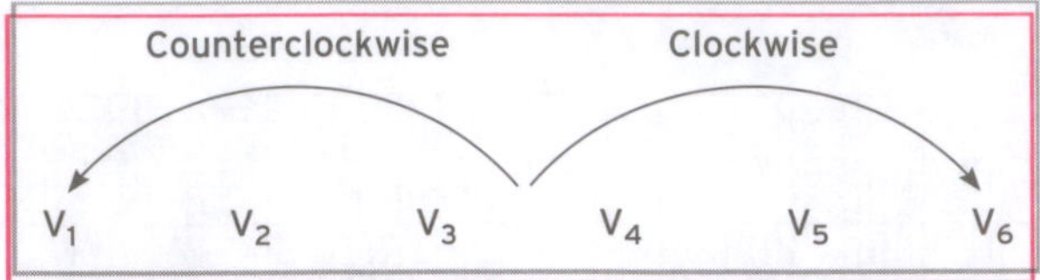

Figure 14-7 Clockwise versus counterclockwise rotation.

Here's a quick way to determine the heart's rotation: Imagine leads V_3 and V_4 as the hub of a clock's hand. Between V_3 and V_4 is the normal transition zone. If the transition is in V_1 or V_2, draw a rounded arrow from V_3 and V_4 to V_1 and V_2. The arrow is going counterclockwise. If the transition is in V_5 or V_6 draw a rounded arrow from V_3 and V_4 to V_5 and V_6. This arrow is going clockwise. See Figure 14-7.

Evolution of an MI

MIs occur over a period of time. The EKG changes over the course of an MI are its **evolution**. See Figure 14-8.

TIMELINE	AGE OF MI	EKG CHANGE	IMPLICATION
Immediately before the actual MI starts		T wave inversion	Cardiac tissue is ischemic, as evidenced by the newly inverted T waves.
Within hours after the MI's start	Acute	Marked ST elevation + upright T wave	Acute MI has begun, starting with myocardial injury.
Hours later	Acute	Significant Q + ST elevation + upright T	Some of the injured myocardial tissue has died, while other tissue remains injured.
Hours to a day or two later	Acute	Significant Q + less ST elevation + marked T inversion	Infarction is almost complete. Some injury and ischemia persist at the infarct edges.
Days to weeks later (in some cases this stage may last up to a year)	Age indeterminate	Significant Q + T wave inversion	Infarction is complete. Though there is no more ischemic tissue (it has either recovered or died), the T wave inversion persists.
Weeks, months, years later	Old	Significant Q only	The significant Q wave persists, signifying permanent tissue death.

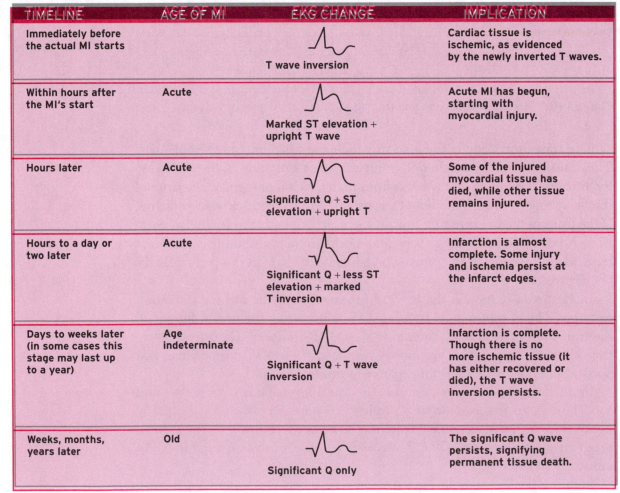

Figure 14-8 Evolution of an MI.

Determining the Age of an MI

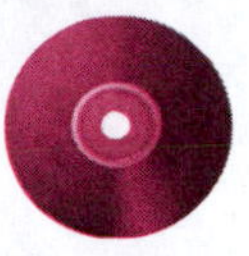

When an EKG is interpreted, the interpreter does not necessarily know the patient's clinical status and therefore must base determination of the MI's age on the indicative changes present on the EKG. The age of an MI is determined as follows (see CD-ROM for a video on the topic of heart attacks):

- An MI that has ST segment elevation is **acute** (one to two days old or less).
- An MI with significant Q waves, baseline (or almost back to baseline) ST segments, and inverted T waves is of **age indeterminate** (several days old, up to a year in some cases). Some authorities call this a **recent MI.**
- The MI with significant Q waves, baseline ST segments, and upright T waves is **old** (weeks to years old).

Walls of the Left Ventricle

Though it is possible to have an infarction of the right ventricle, infarctions occur mostly in the left ventricle, since it has the greatest oxygen demand and thus is impacted more adversely by poor coronary artery flow. MIs can affect any of the four walls of the left ventricle (see Figure 14-9):

- **Anterior wall.** The front wall–fed by the left anterior descending coronary artery.
- **Inferior wall.** The bottom wall–fed by the right coronary artery.
- **Lateral wall.** The left side wall of the heart–fed by the circumflex coronary artery.
- **Posterior wall.** The back wall–fed by the right coronary artery.

Each of these left ventricular walls can be "seen" by our EKG electrodes. You'll recall that the positive pole of leads II, III, and aVF sit on the left foot. They look at the heart from the bottom. Which wall of the heart would they see? Good for you if you said the inferior wall.

What about leads I, aVL, and V_5 and V_6? They sit on the heart's left side, so they look at the lateral wall.

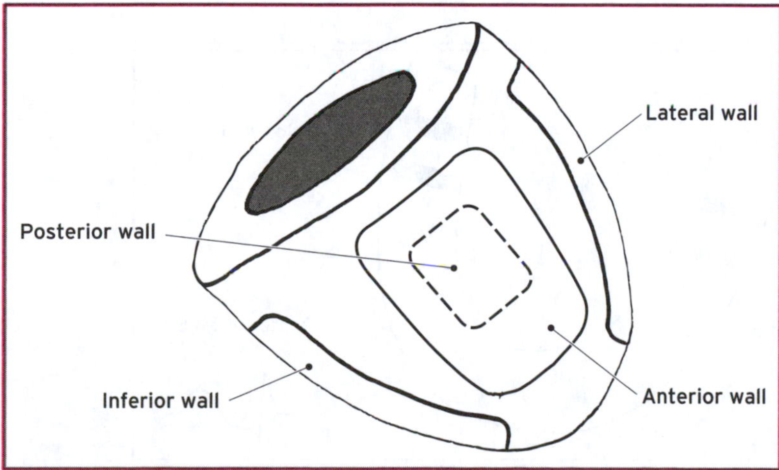

Figure 14-9 Walls of the left ventricle.

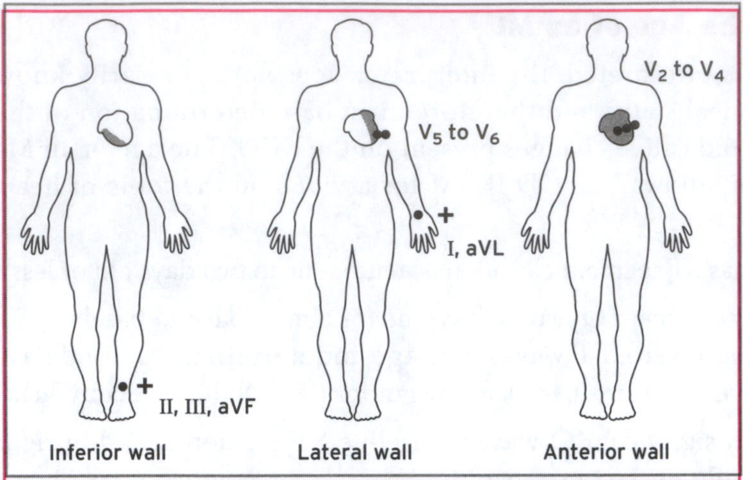

Figure 14-10 Leads looking at the anterior, inferior, and lateral walls of the left ventricle.

Leads V_2 through V_4 sit right in the front of the heart, looking at the anterior wall. See Figure 14-10.

What about the posterior wall? Unlike the other infarct locations, there are no leads looking directly at the posterior wall because we do not put EKG electrodes on the patient's back for a routine 12-lead EKG. Therefore, the only way to look at the posterior wall is to look *through* the anterior wall. See Figure 14-11.

The ventricles depolarize from endocardium to epicardium (from inside to outside). You'll note on Figure 14-11 that the vectors (arrows) representing depolarization of the anterior and posterior walls are opposite each other. Therefore, *the only way to diagnose a posterior MI is to look for changes opposite those that would be seen with an anterior MI.* We use leads V_1 and V_2 since they sit almost directly opposite the posterior wall. What's the opposite of a Q wave? An R wave. What's opposite ST elevation? ST depression. What's opposite T wave inversion? Upright T wave. Those are what we look for with a posterior infarct.

An easy way to find posterior MIs is to turn the EKG upside down and look at V_1 and V_2 from the back of the EKG. This mimics what the EKG would look like if

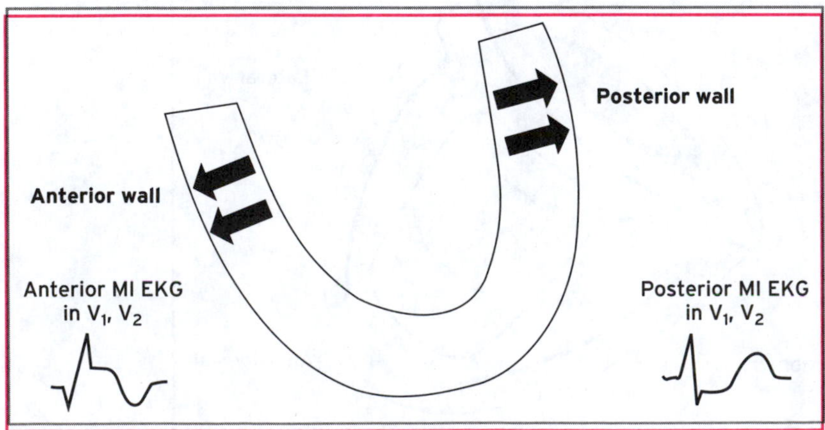

Figure 14-11 Posterior wall MI changes.

we had leads directly over the posterior wall. If there is a significant Q wave and T wave inversion in V_1 and V_2 in this upside-down reverse approach, there is a posterior MI. The ST segment may be elevated or at baseline, depending on the age of the MI. Also keep in mind that posterior MIs almost always accompany an inferior MI, so always look for a posterior MI when an inferior MI is present.

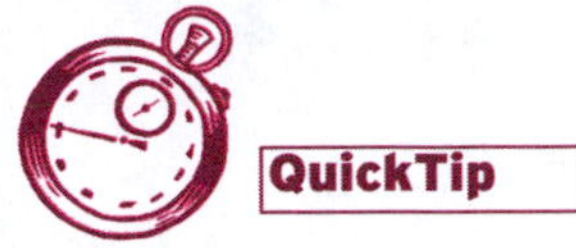

If there is significant ST segment elevation in the indicative leads, there will be significant ST depression in the reciprocal leads. Likewise, if there is only a little ST elevation in the indicative leads, there will be only a little depression in the reciprocal leads.

Myocardial Infarct Locations

A Q wave MI is diagnosed on the EKG by **indicative changes** (i.e., ST elevation, T wave inversion, and significant Q waves) in the leads for that area. Depending on the age of the infarct, not all of those indicative changes will be present.

In the area electrically opposite the infarct area are **reciprocal changes** (i.e., ST depression). Reciprocal ST depression is seen only when there is ST elevation in the indicative leads.

Let's look at the EKG changes associated with the different infarct locations. It is not necessary to have every single change listed in order to determine the kind of infarct, but most of the criteria should be met. Note the coronary artery involved. See Table 14-1.

Indicative changes are so named because they indicate in which leads the MI is located.

The MIs in Table 14-1 involve only one wall of the left ventricle. MIs can extend across into other walls as well. For example, a patient might have an

Table 14-1 Infarct Locations

LOCATION OF MI	EKG CHANGES	CORONARY ARTERY
Anterior	Indicative changes in V_2 to V_4 Reciprocal changes in II, III, aVF	Left anterior descending (LAD)
Inferior	Indicative changes in II, III, aVF Reciprocal changes in I, aVL, and V leads	Right coronary artery (RCA)
Lateral	Indicative changes in I, aVL, V_5 to V_6 May see reciprocal changes in II, III, aVF	Circumflex
Posterior	No indicative changes, since no leads look directly at posterior wall Diagnosed by reciprocal changes in V_1 and V_2 (large R wave, upright T wave, and possibly ST . depression)Seen as a mirror image of an anterior MI.	RCA or circumflex
Extensive anterior (sometimes called *extensive anterior-lateral*)	Indicative changes in I, aVL, V_1 to V_6 Reciprocal changes in II, III, aVF	LAD or left main
Anteroseptal	Indicative changes in V_1 plus any of leads V_2-V_4 Usually no reciprocal changes	LAD

inferior-lateral MI, which would involve the inferior leads as well as the lateral leads. Combination MIs such as this do not always involve every one of the usual leads. For example, an inferior-lateral MI might involve the inferior leads and only a few lateral leads. An anterior-lateral MI might include the anterior leads and only a few lateral leads.

On the next several pages, you will find helpful ways of determining the kind of MI you're seeing. First you will find infarction squares, then a pictorial of the different MI types, and finally an MI algorithm. Let's take a look.

Infarction Squares

In Table 14-2, each lead square is labeled with the wall of the heart at which it looks. When you analyze an EKG, note which leads have ST elevation and/or significant Q waves. Then use the infarction squares to determine the type of infarction. For example, if there were ST elevation in leads II, III, aVF, and V_5 and V_6, you would note that the MI involves inferior and lateral leads. The MI would be inferior-lateral.

Next let's look at some MI pictorials. Ignore the QRS width in these pictorials–the drawings are just to illustrate what these types of MIs look like.

Table 14-2 Infarction Squares

I Lateral	aVR Ignore this lead when looking for MIs	V_1 Septal (posterior if mirror image)	V_4 Anterior
II Inferior	aVL Lateral	V_2 Anterior (posterior if mirror image)	V_5 Lateral
III Inferior	aVF Inferior	V_3 Anterior	V_6 Lateral

MI Pictorials

Anterior MI

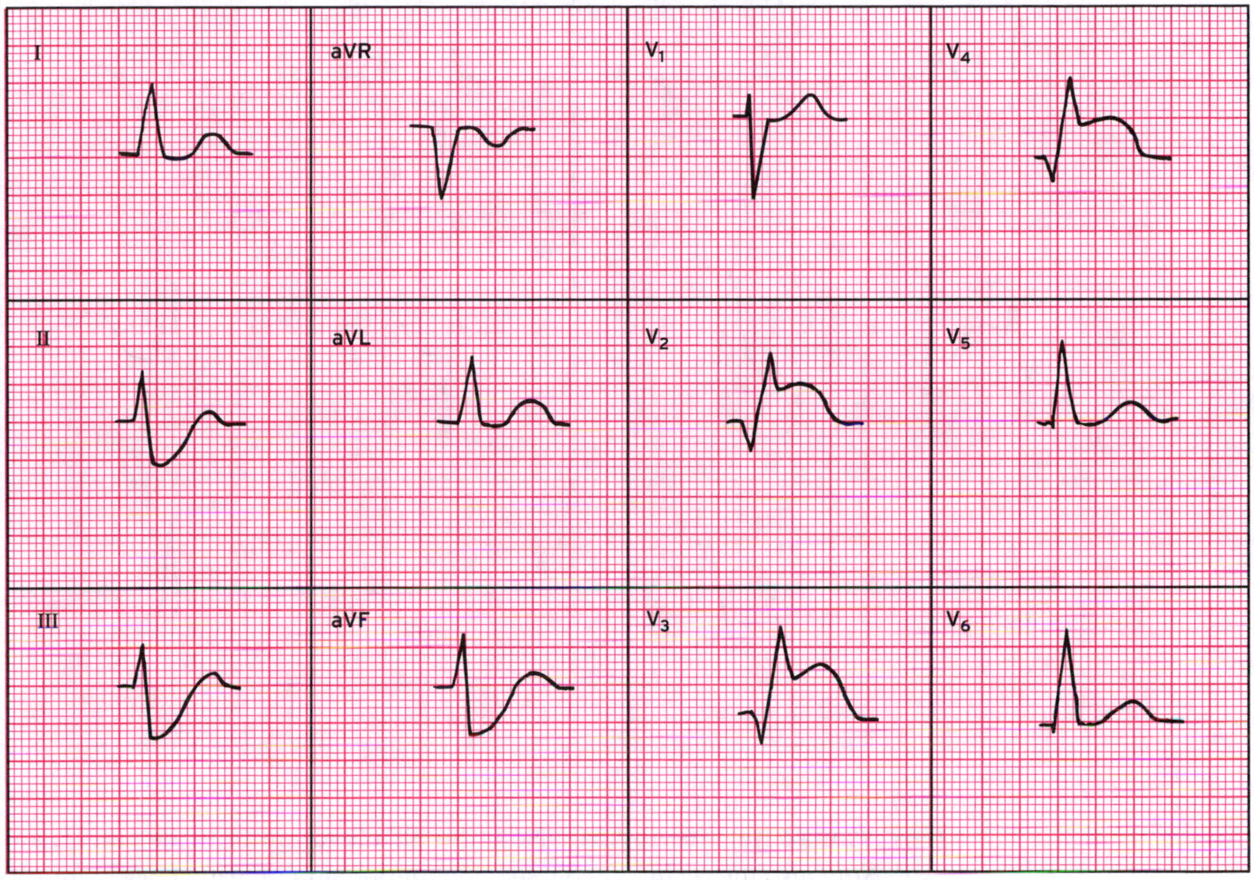

This is an **acute anterior MI**, as evidenced by the ST elevation in V_2 to V_4. Also note the reciprocal ST depression in leads II, III, and aVF.

If this MI were **age indeterminate**, it would have more normal ST segments, significant Q waves, and T wave inversions in V_1 to V_4.

If this MI were **old**, it would have only the significant Q wave remaining. The ST segment would be back at baseline and the T wave would be upright.

Inferior MI

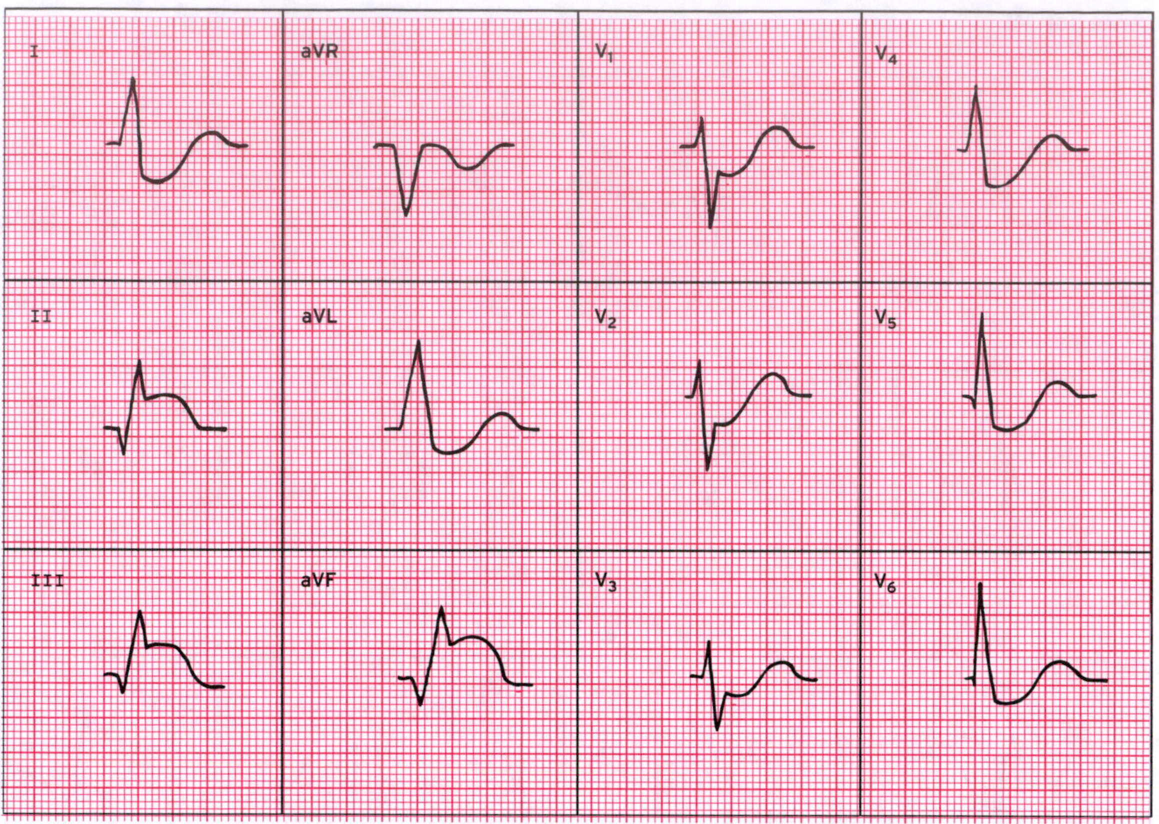

This is an **acute inferior MI**. Note the ST elevation in leads II, III, and aVF. Note also the reciprocal ST segment depression in leads I, aVL, and V_1 to V_6.

The **age indeterminate inferior MI** would have more normal ST segments along with significant Q waves and inverted T waves in leads II, III, and aVF.

The **old inferior MI** would have only significant Q waves in II, III, and aVF. The ST segments would be at baseline and T waves would be upright.

Lateral Wall MI

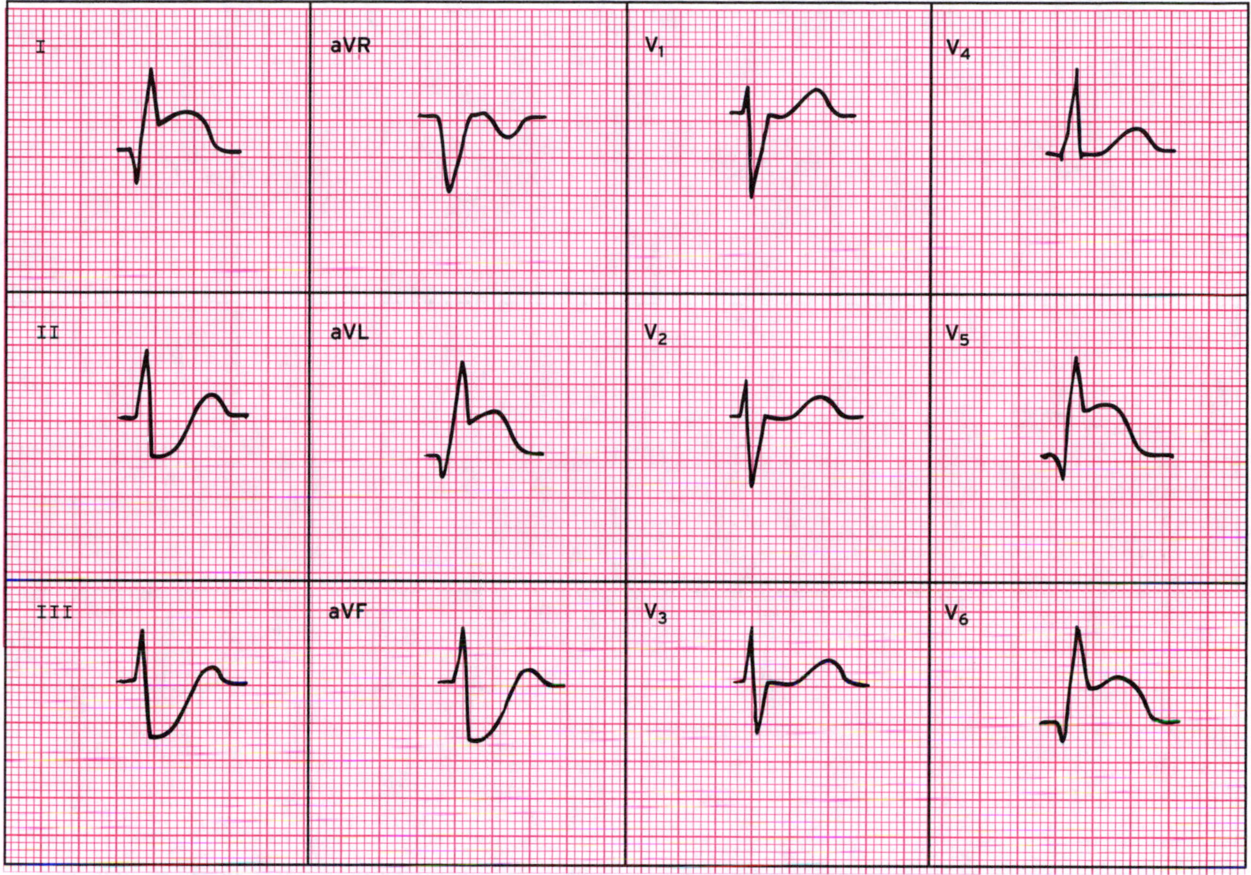

This is an **acute lateral wall MI**, as evidenced by the ST elevation in leads I, aVL, and V_5 to V_6. Note also the reciprocal ST depression in leads II, III, and aVF.

If this were an **age indeterminate lateral MI**, there would be more normal ST segments along with significant Q waves and inverted T waves in I, aVL, and V_5 to V_6.

An **old lateral wall MI** would have baseline ST segments, significant Q waves, and upright T waves in I, aVL, and V_5 to V_6.

Posterior MI

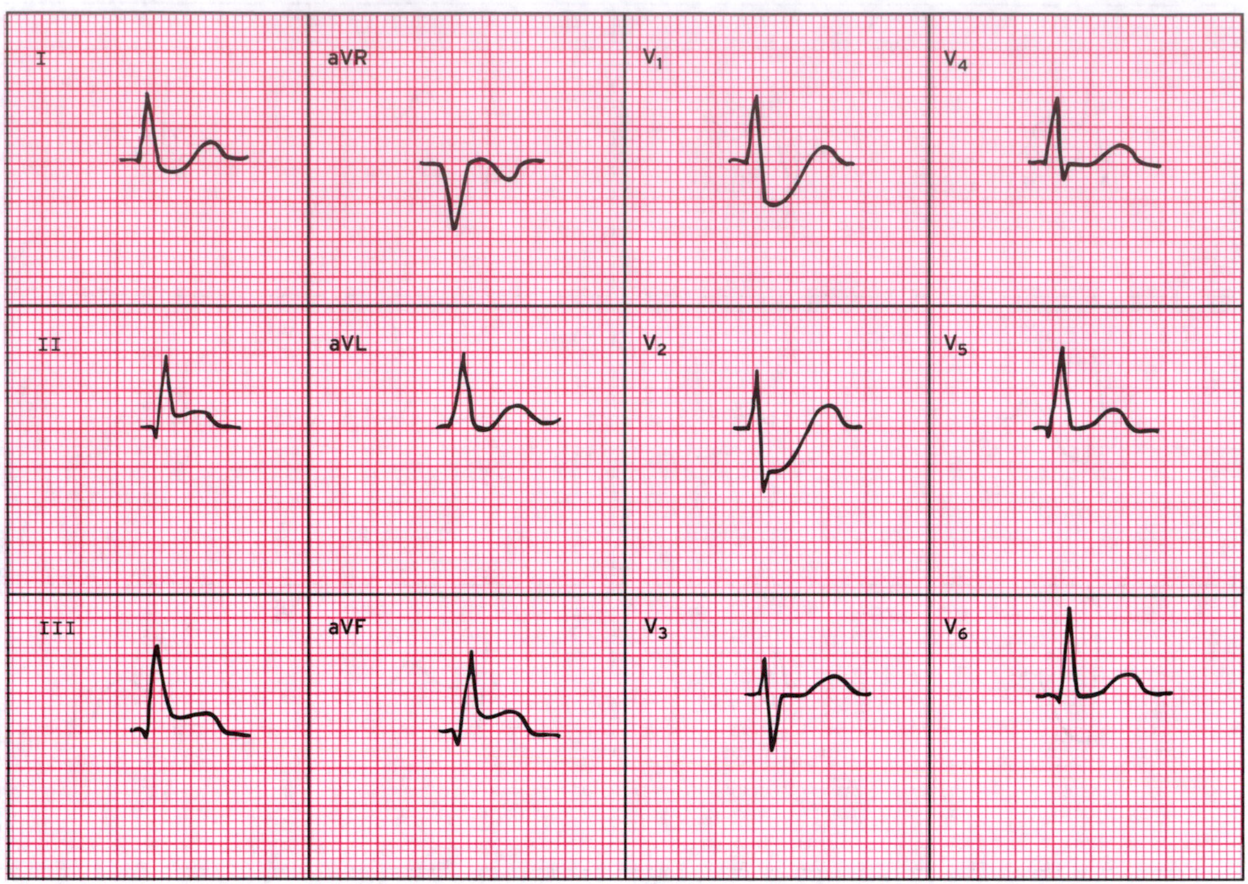

This is an **acute posterior wall MI**. Note the tall R wave in V_1 to V_2 along with ST segment depression and an upright T wave. Remember, a posterior MI is diagnosed by a mirror image of the normal indicative changes of an MI in V_1 to V_2. Note that there is an acute inferior MI as well.

An **age indeterminate posterior MI** would have more normal ST segments, a tall R wave, and an upright T wave.

The **old posterior MI** would have only the tall R wave remaining. The ST segments would be at baseline and the T wave would be inverted.

Extensive Anterior MI

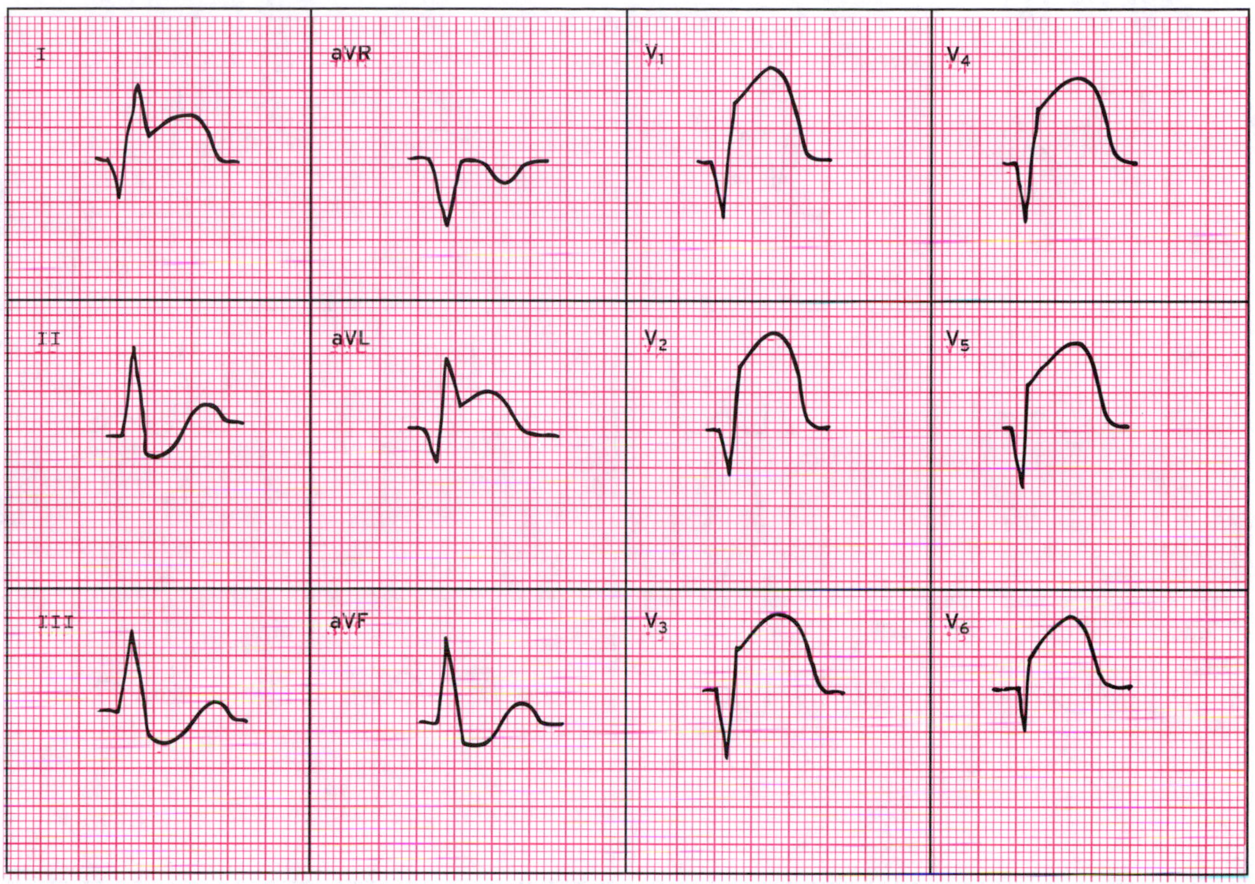

Here we have a huge MI, the **acute extensive anterior MI**. Note the significant Q waves and ST elevation in I, aVL, and V_1 to V_6 and the reciprocal ST depression in II, III, and aVF.

The **age indeterminate extensive anterior MI** would have more normal ST segments along with significant Q waves and T wave inversion.

The **old extensive anterior MI** would have baseline ST segments, significant Q waves, and upright T waves in I, aVL, and V_1 to V_6.

Anteroseptal MI

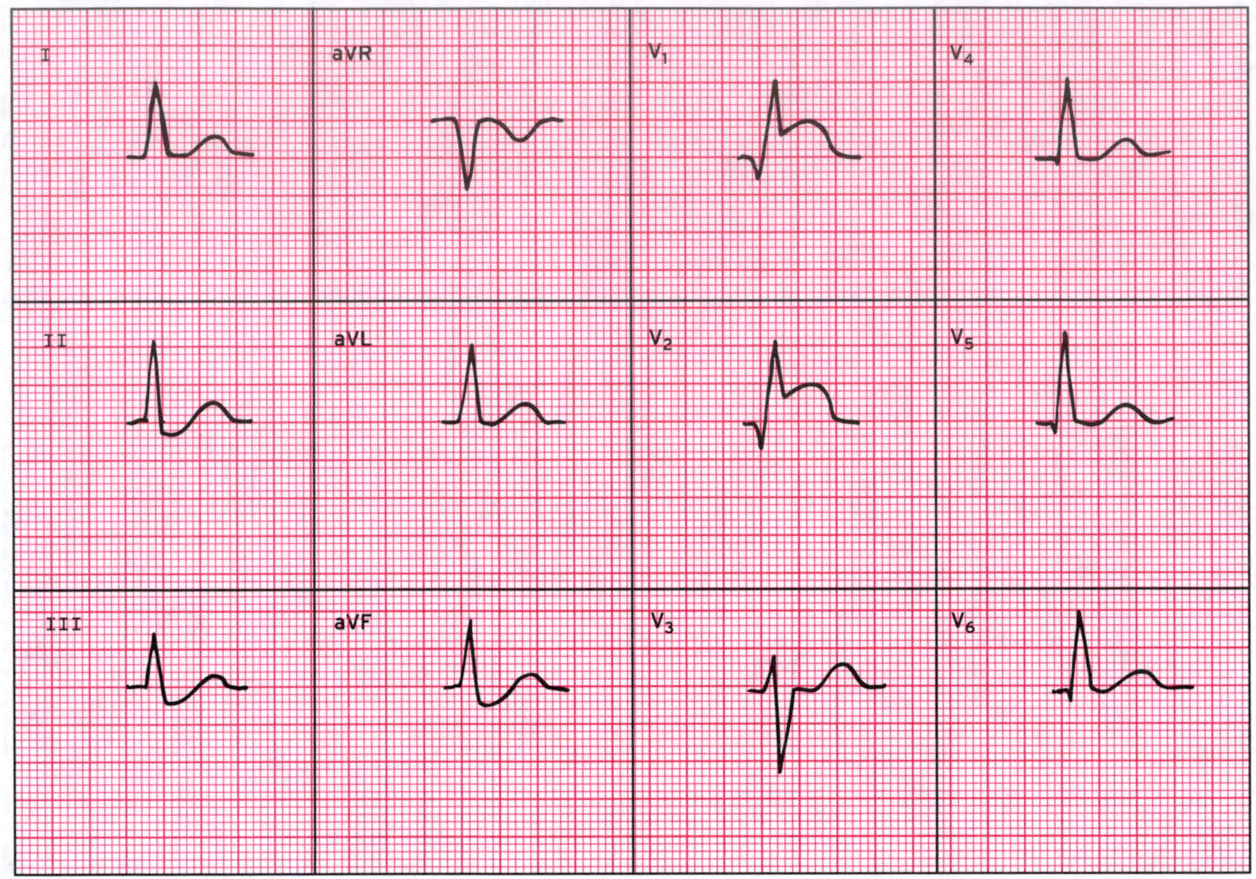

This is an **acute anteroseptal MI**. Note the ST elevation in leads V_1 to V_2. Recall V_1 is a septal lead and V_2 is an anterior lead. *The combination of V_1 plus any anterior lead results in an anteroseptal MI.*

An **age indeterminate anteroseptal MI** would have more normal ST segments, significant Q waves, and inverted T waves in V_1 to V_2.

The **old anteroseptal MI** would have only significant Q waves remaining in V_1 to V_2. The ST segments would be at baseline and the T waves would be upright.

Subendocardial MI

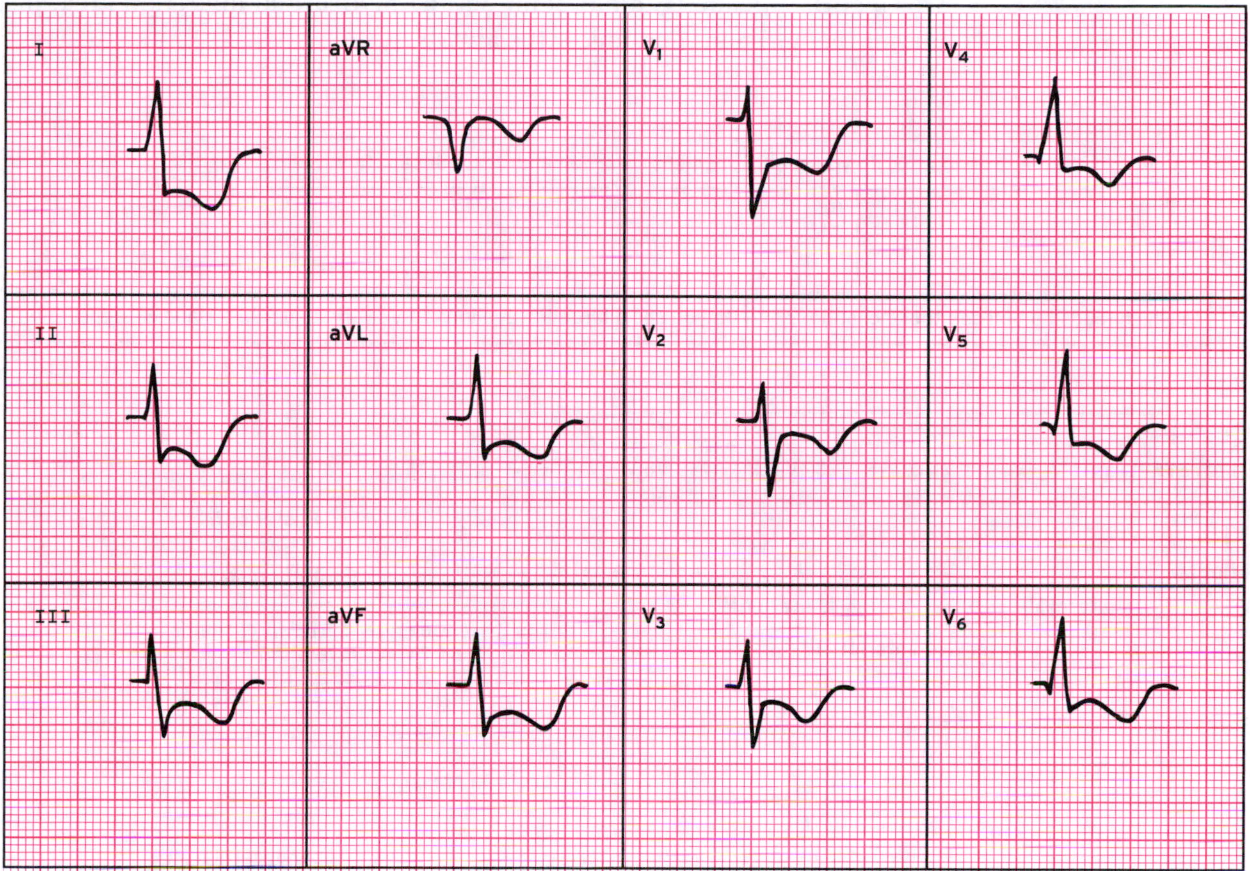

This is an **acute subendocardial MI**. It is one kind of non–Q wave MI. It is characterized by widespread ST depression and T wave inversions. Subendocardial infarctions are diagnosed only in the acute phase, as they do not cause significant Q waves, and their T waves are already inverted.

Myocardial Infarction Algorithm

This algorithm is designed to point out the myocardial infarction area. Just answer the questions and follow the arrows.

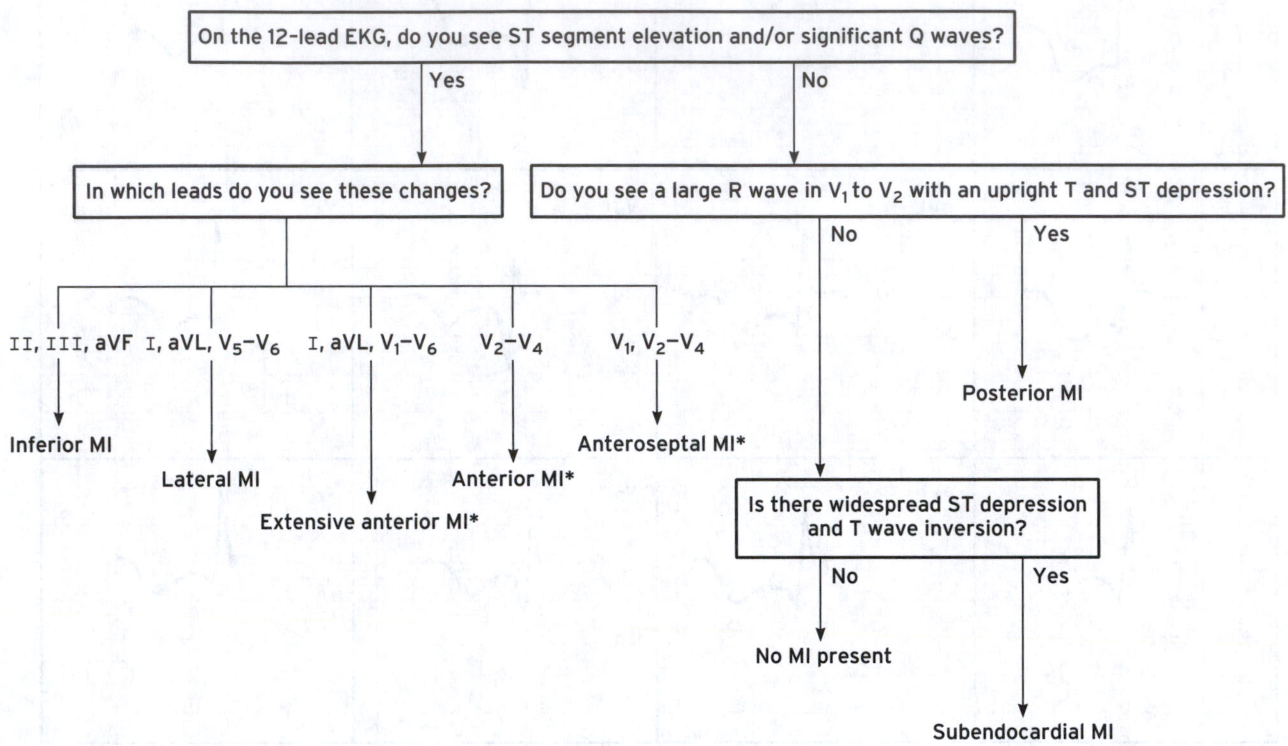

*If LBBB is present, these types of MIs cannot be diagnosed. The high take-off to the T wave of LBBB mimics the ST elevation of these kinds of MI.

How to Use the MI Algorithm

Refer to the EKG in Figure 14-12. Do you see any ST segment elevation or significant Q waves? Yes, there are significant Q waves, and also there is ST elevation.

In which leads do you see these changes? These are noted in V_1 to V_4. The arrow points to anteroseptal MI.

Right Ventricular Infarction

On occasion, an inferior MI will be accompanied by a right ventricular (RV) infarction. RV infarctions occur when the blockage to the right coronary artery system is so extensive that damage extends into the right ventricle. RV infarctions are not detectable by the routine 12-lead EKG, which looks at the left ventricle. To diagnose an RV infarction, two conditions must be met: First, there must be electrocardiographic evidence of an inferior wall MI on a standard 12-lead EKG. Second, a right-sided EKG must reveal ST elevation in V_3R and/or V_4R. This right-sided EKG is done only if an RV infarction is suspected (i.e., the patient exhibits symptoms, particularly hypotension, beyond what is expected with just an inferior MI).

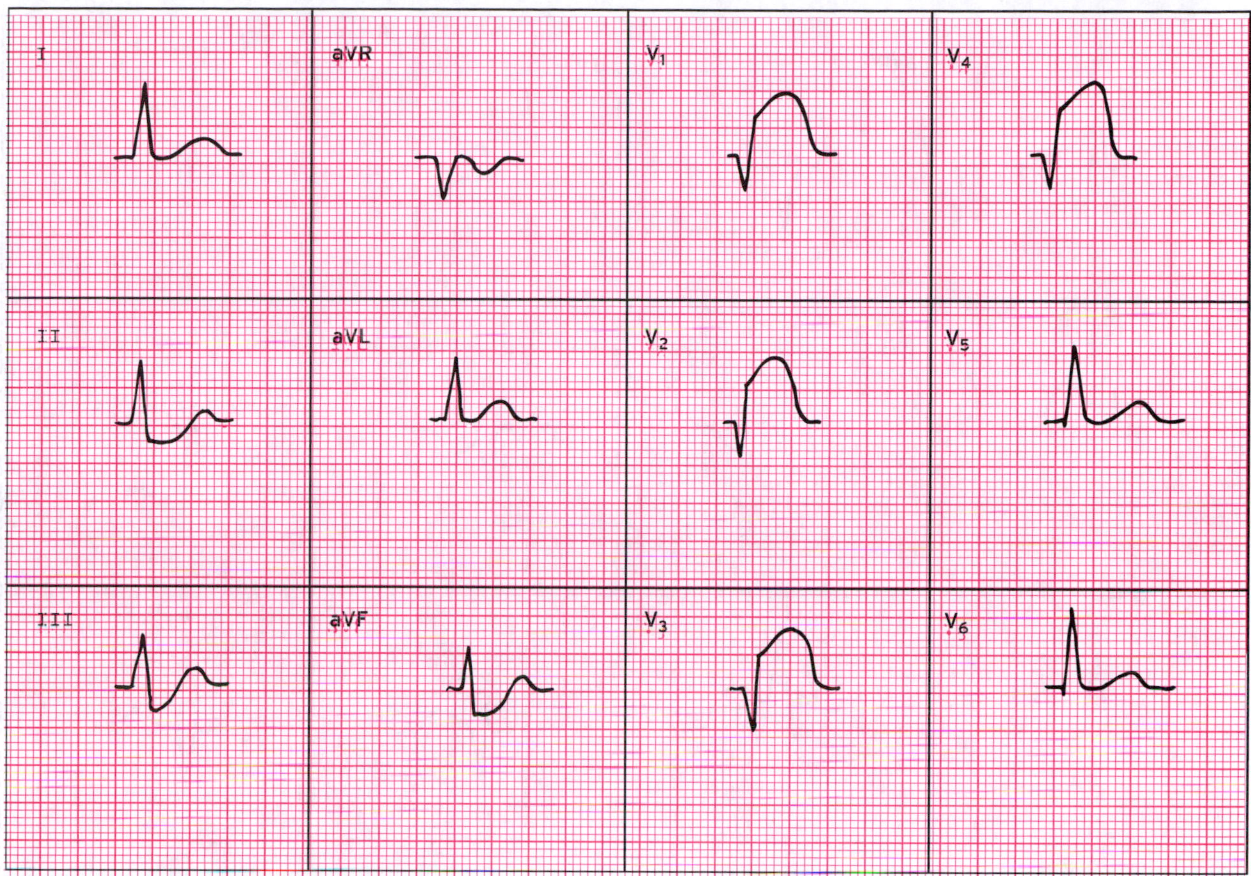

Figure 14-12 MI for algorithm.

A right-sided EKG is done with the limb leads in their normal places, but with the precordial leads placed on the right side of the chest instead of the left. See lead placement for a right-sided EKG in Figure 14-13.

Right Ventricular Infarction (Right-Sided EKG)

See Figure 14-14. On this right-sided EKG, note the ST elevation in leads V_3R to V_4R. This proves there is an RV infarction. You'll note also that there

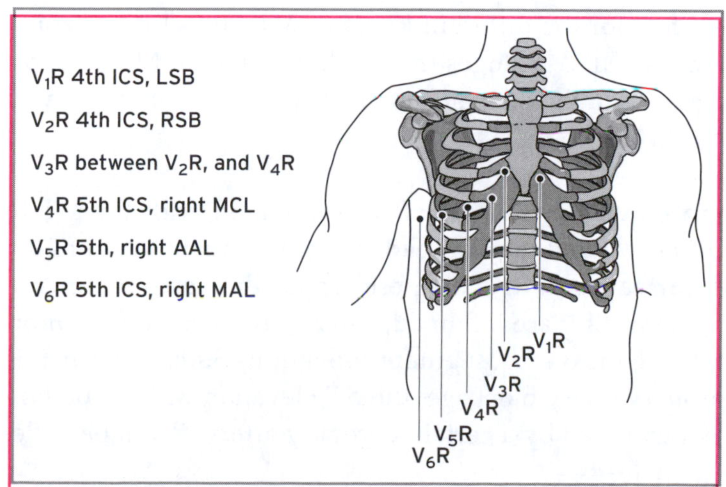

Figure 14-13 Lead placement for a right-sided EKG.

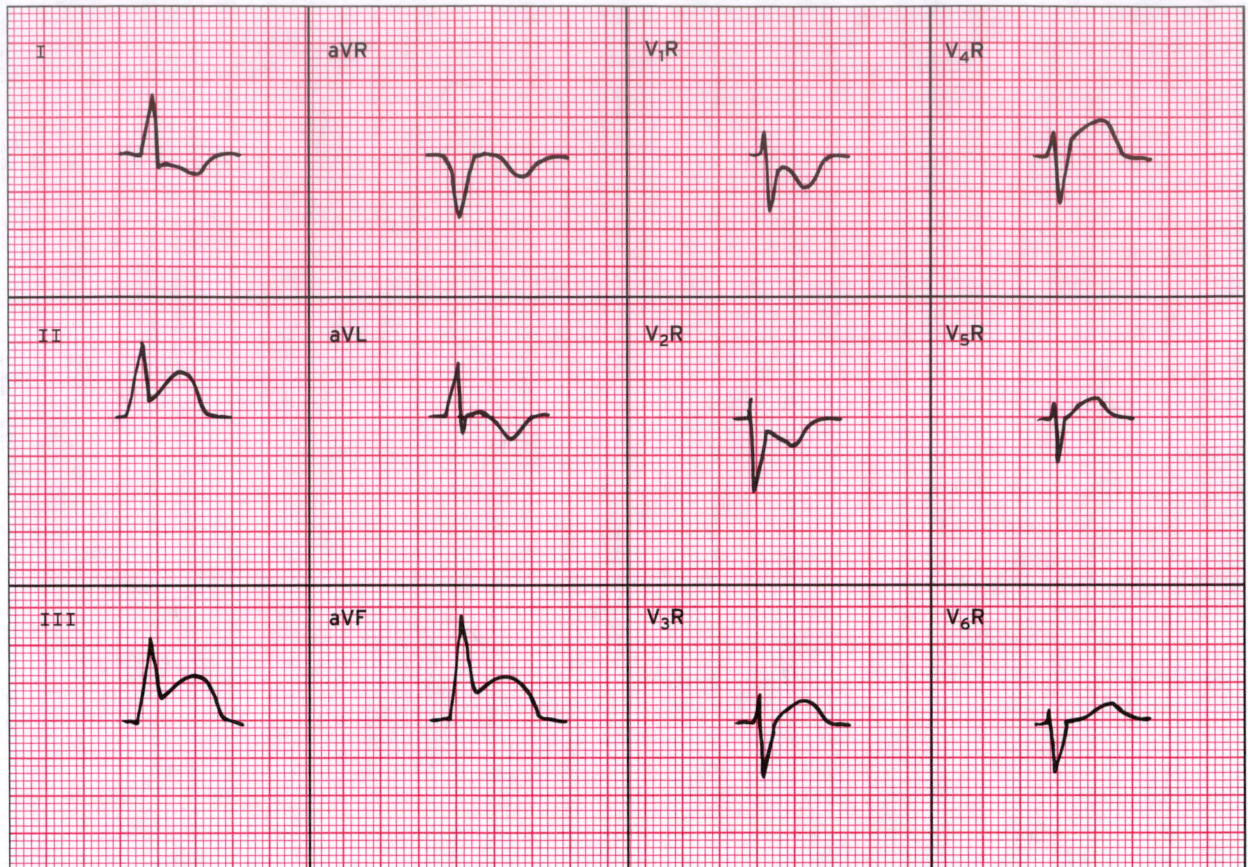

Figure 14-14 Right ventricular infarction (Right sided EKG).

is ST elevation in leads II, III, and aVF that indicate an inferior MI. Remember, the right-sided EKG leaves the limb leads in their normal place, but moves the precordial leads to the right side of the chest. So the inferior MI will still be obvious on the right-sided EKG.

Conditions That Can Mimic an MI

Now that you have a feel for the different kinds of MIs, let's look at some conditions that can cause EKG changes that look just like an MI. In most cases, the only difference is in the patient's medical symptoms and history.

Acute Pericarditis

Though ST segment elevation is most often associated with an MI in progress, there are times when it may instead imply an inflammation of the pericardium, called **pericarditis**. In acute pericarditis, the pericardium and the myocardium just beneath it are inflamed, causing repolarization abnormalities that present as concave ST segment elevation. Since pericarditis does not involve coronary artery blockage, the ST elevation will not be limited to leads overlying areas fed by a certain coronary artery–it will be widespread throughout many leads.

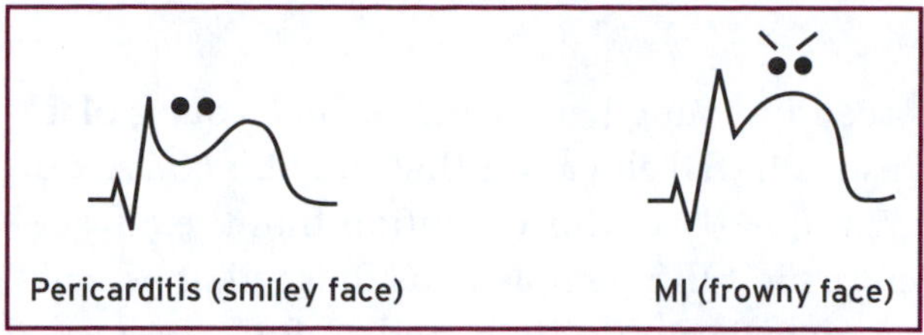

Figure 14-15 Smiley-face (concave) and frowny face (convex) ST elevations.

The ST elevation of pericarditis differs from that of an MI in that an MI usually produces *convex* ST elevation, whereas pericarditis produces *concave* elevation. These are often referred to as the *smiley-face* and *frowny-face* ST segments. The smiley face is concave ST elevation. The frowny face is convex. See Figure 14-15.

Like an MI, pericarditis also causes chest pain, and it is crucial to differentiate between the two, as treatment differs greatly. See Figure 14-16.

In Figure 14-16, note the widespread concave ST elevation in leads I, II, III, aVL, aVF, and V_1 to V_6. This is *not* typical of an MI because it is so widespread. Is it possible this is a huge MI instead of pericarditis? Sure. But based on the concave ST elevation scattered across many leads, it's more likely that it's pericarditis. Only by examining the patient would we know for sure.

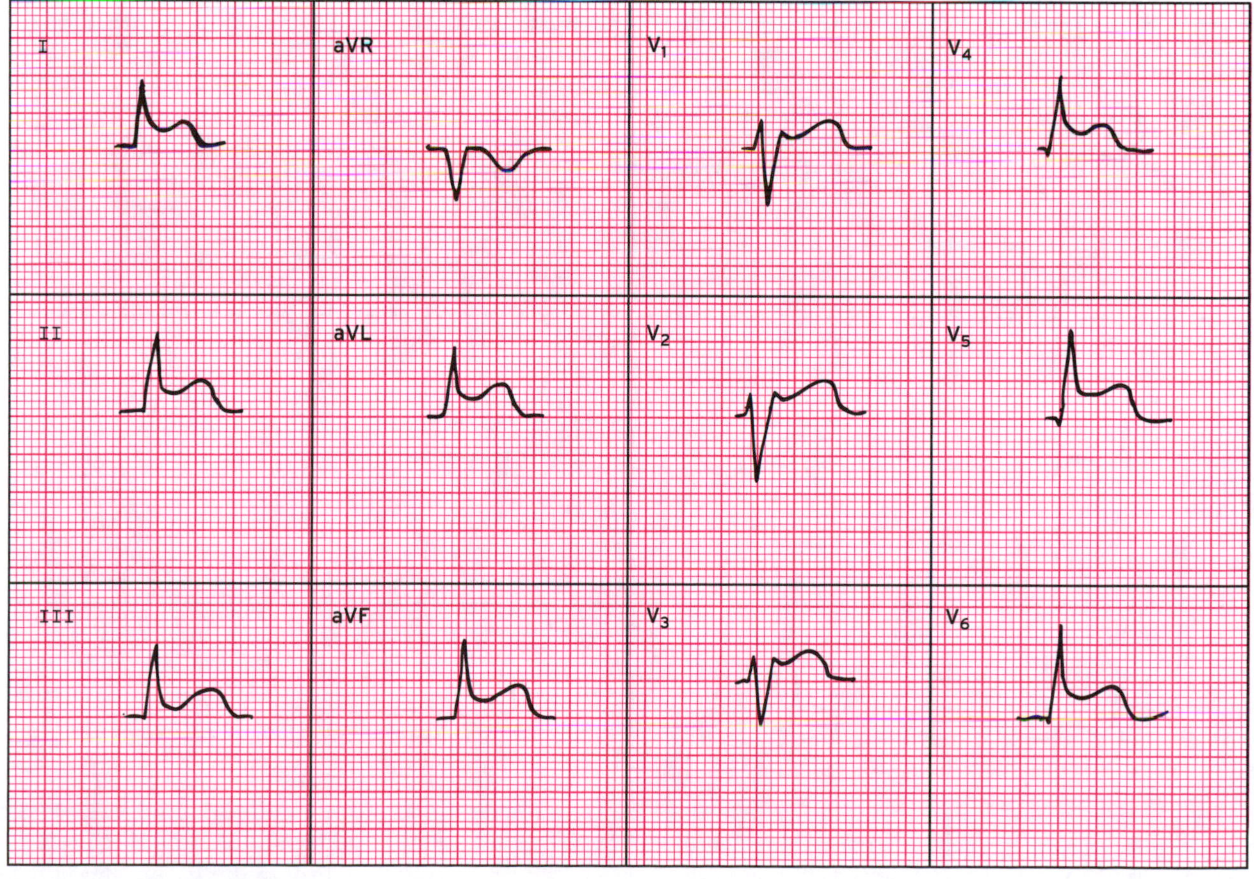

Figure 14-16 Pericarditis.

Early Repolarization

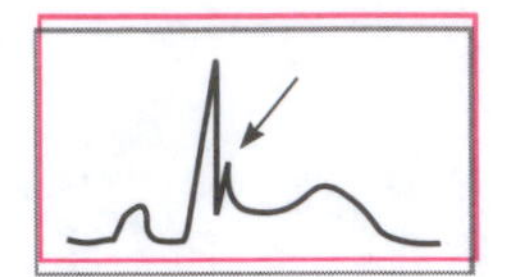

Figure 14-17 Fishhook of early repolarization.

A normal variant sometimes seen in young people, especially young black males, early repolarization results in ST elevation that may be convex or concave. Repolarization begins so early in this condition that the ST segment appears to start even before the QRS complex has finished, thus making it appear that the ST segment is mildly elevated. Often there is a "fishhook" at the end of some of the QRS complexes that makes recognition of early repolarization easier. Note the ST elevation and the fishhook (see arrow) in Figure 14-17.

It is not always possible to distinguish early repolarization from an MI based on only a single EKG. A series of EKGs would reveal the typical evolutionary changes if an MI is present, and they would remain unchanged if early repolarization is present. The ST segment elevations of early repolarization are most often evident in leads V_2 to V_4, though they may be more widespread. Of great help in differentiating early repolarization from an MI is the age and presentation of the patient. A 20-year-old black male with no cardiac complaints who has mild ST elevations probably has early repolarization. A 65-year-old male with chest pain and ST elevation is more likely to have an MI in progress. Only by examining the patient can the definitive diagnosis of early repolarization versus MI be made. But the EKG will give hints. See Figure 14-18.

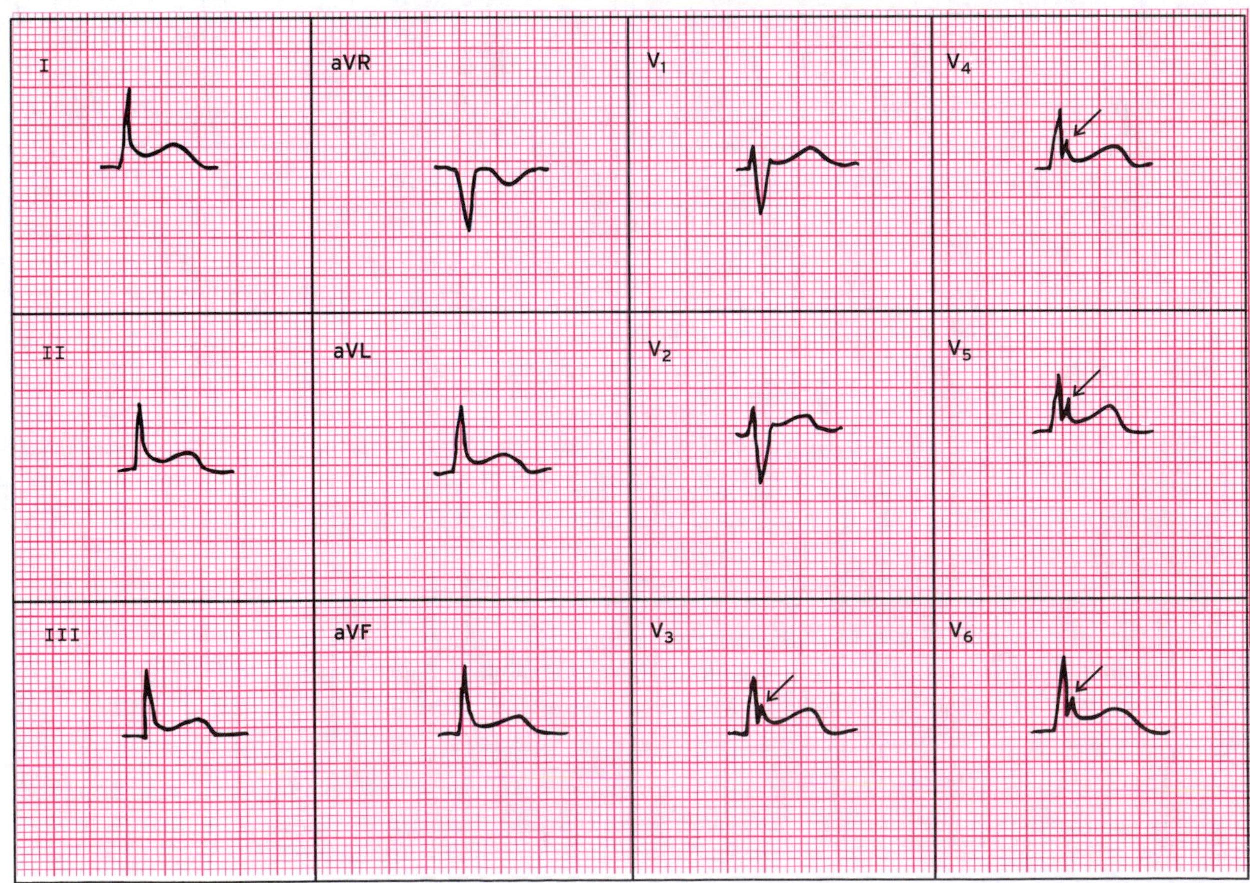

Figure 14-18 Early repolarization.

In Figure 14-18, note the mild ST segment elevation in almost all leads and the fishhook in V_3 to V_6 (see arrows). This is typical of early repolarization.

Now it's time for some practice. The EKGs that follow all represent standard left-sided EKGs. The first five EKGs are like the MI pictorials, consisting of only one beat in each lead box. The last five are genuine 12-lead EKGs. Use the infarction squares and/or the MI algorithm if you need help.

MI Practice

Tell which wall of the heart is affected and how old the MI is (if there is indeed an MI).

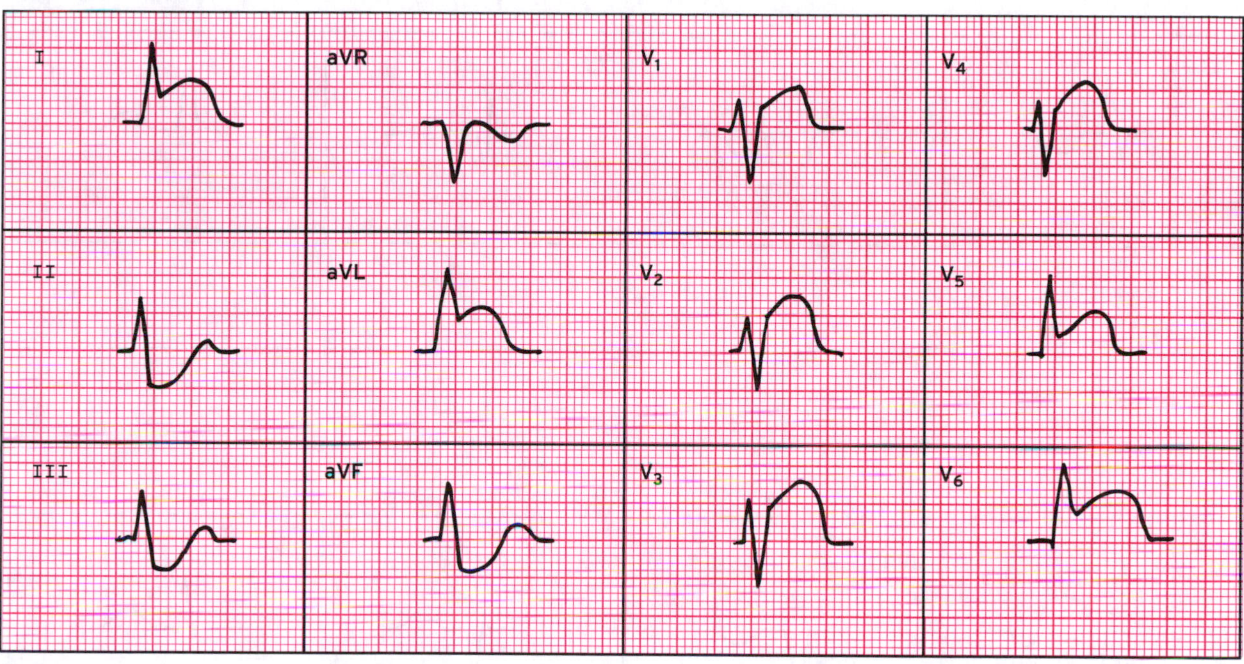

1. ______________________________

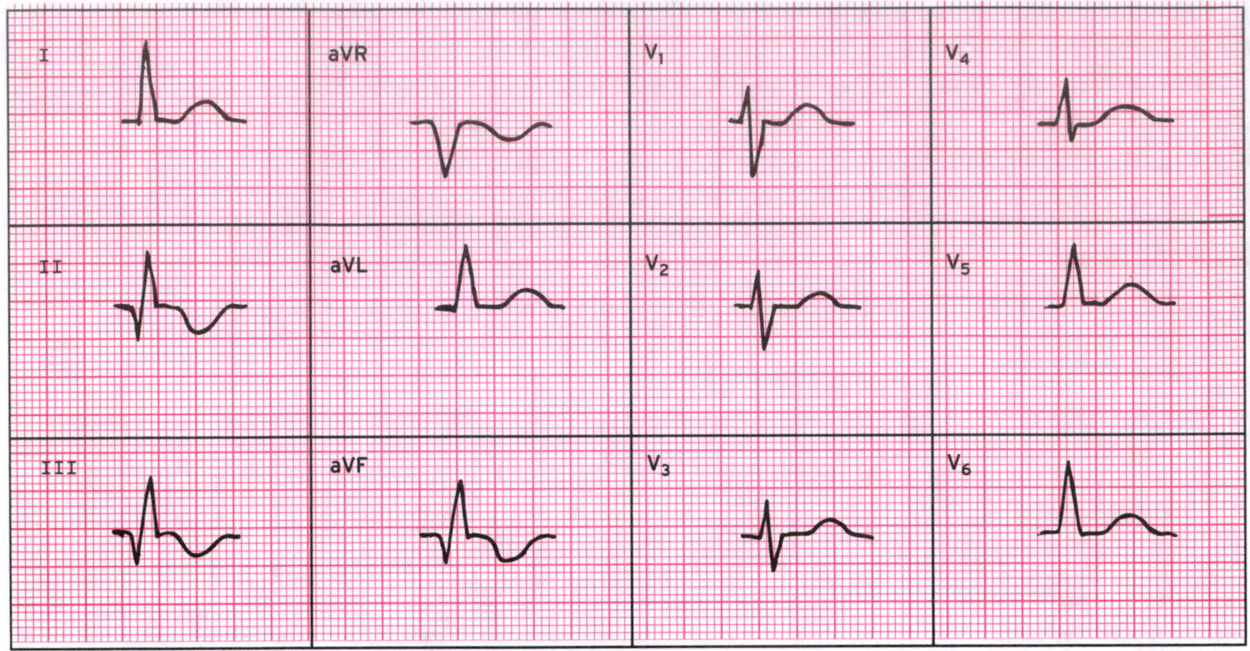
I
aVR
V_1
V_4
II
aVL
V_2
V_5
III
aVF
V_3
V_6

2. ____________________

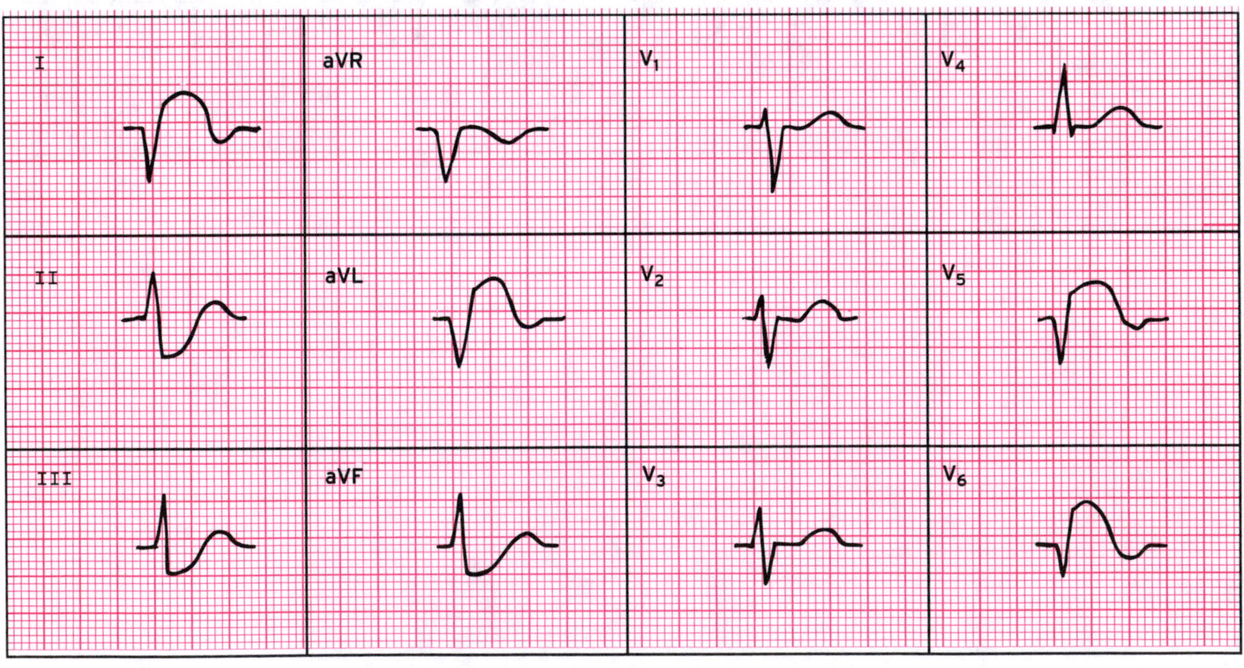
I
aVR
V_1
V_4
II
aVL
V_2
V_5
III
aVF
V_3
V_6

3. ____________________

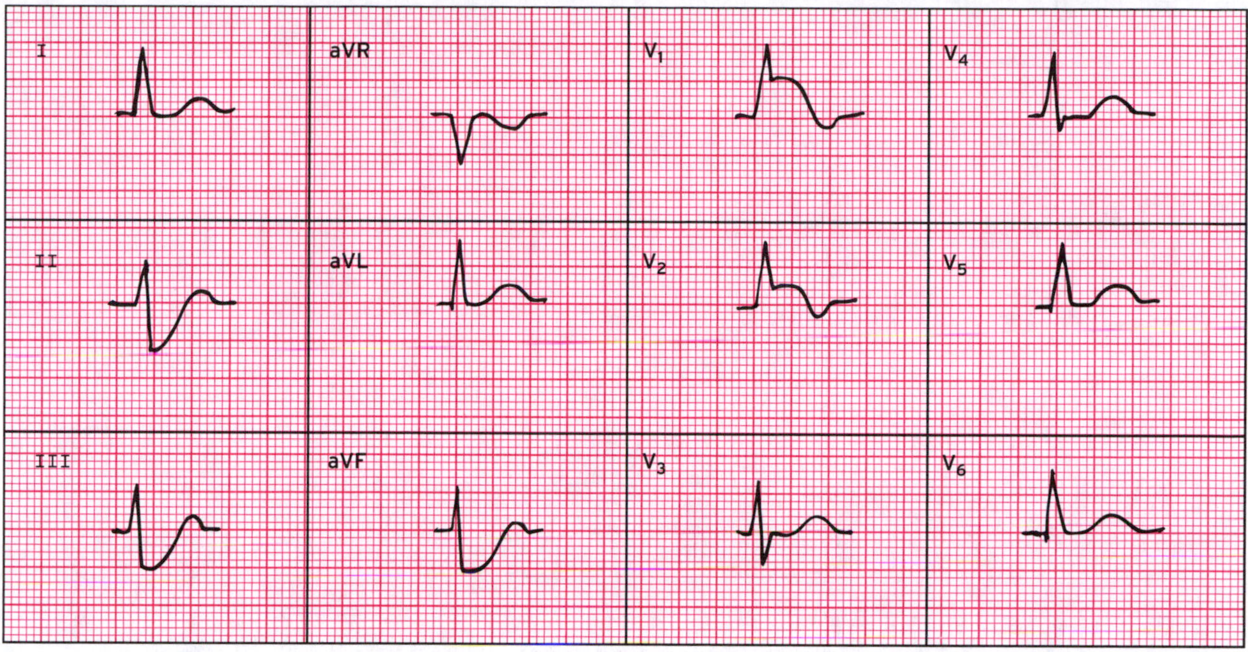
I
aVR
V1
V4
II
aVL
V2
V5
III
aVF
V3
V6

4. ______________________________

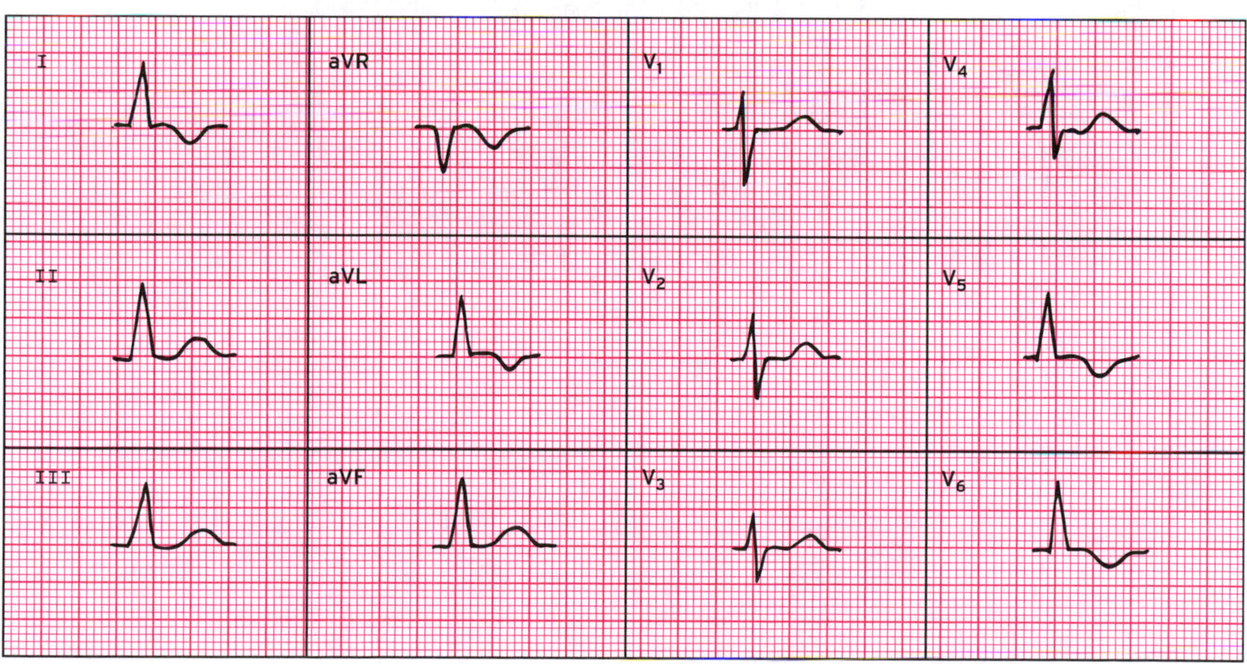
I
aVR
V1
V4
II
aVL
V2
V5
III
aVF
V3
V6

5. ______________________________

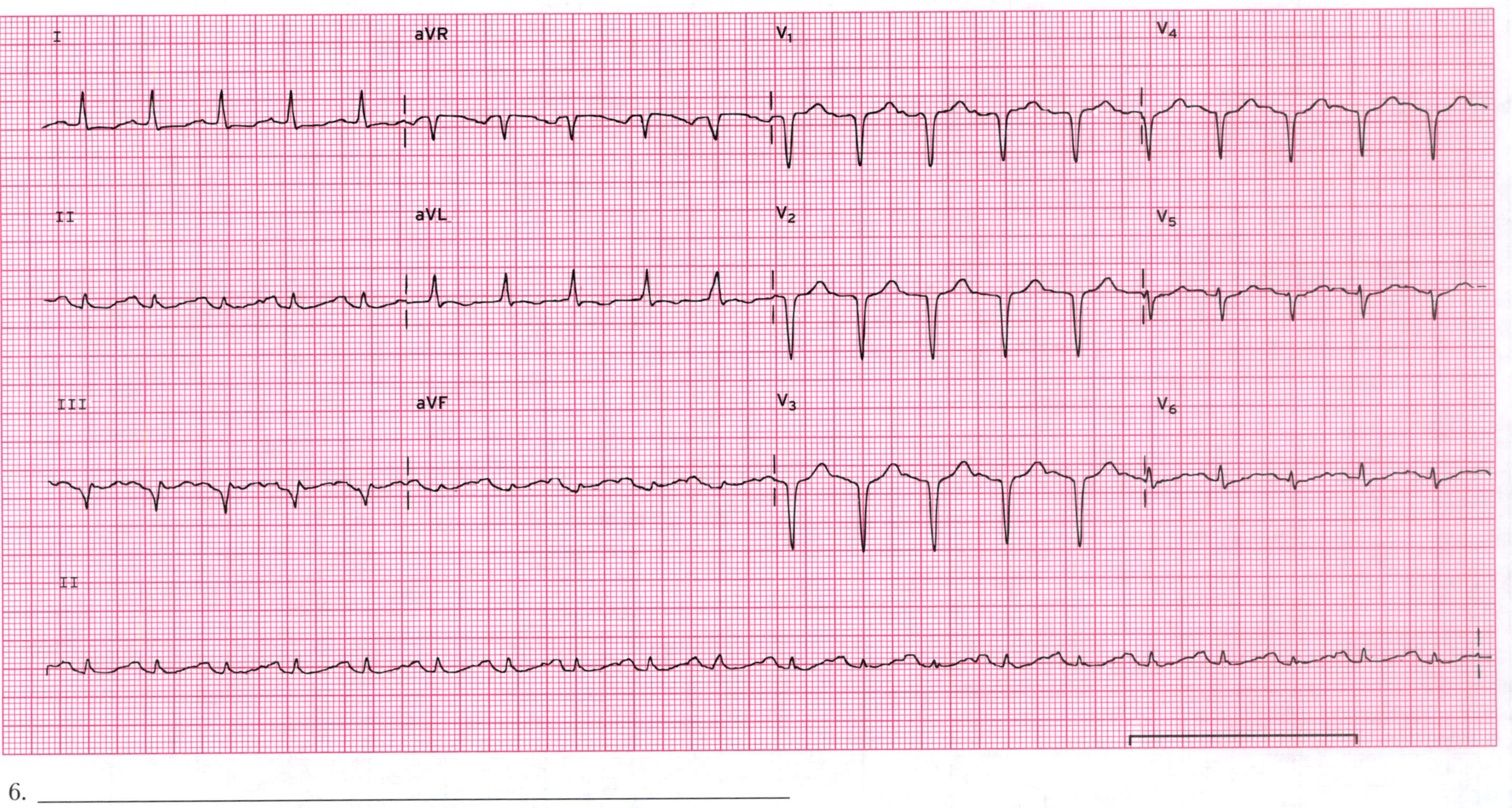

6. ______________________________

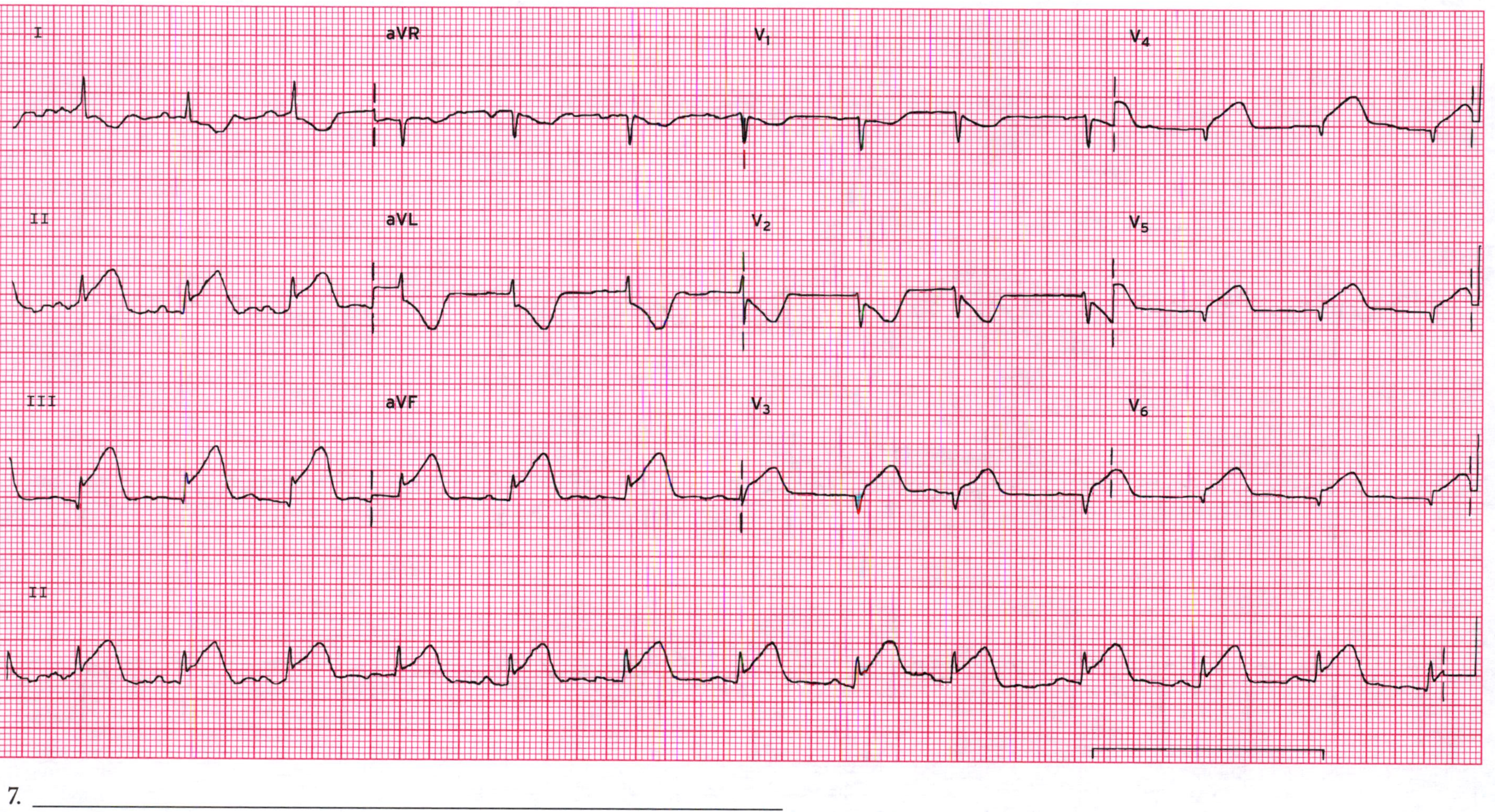

7. ______________________________

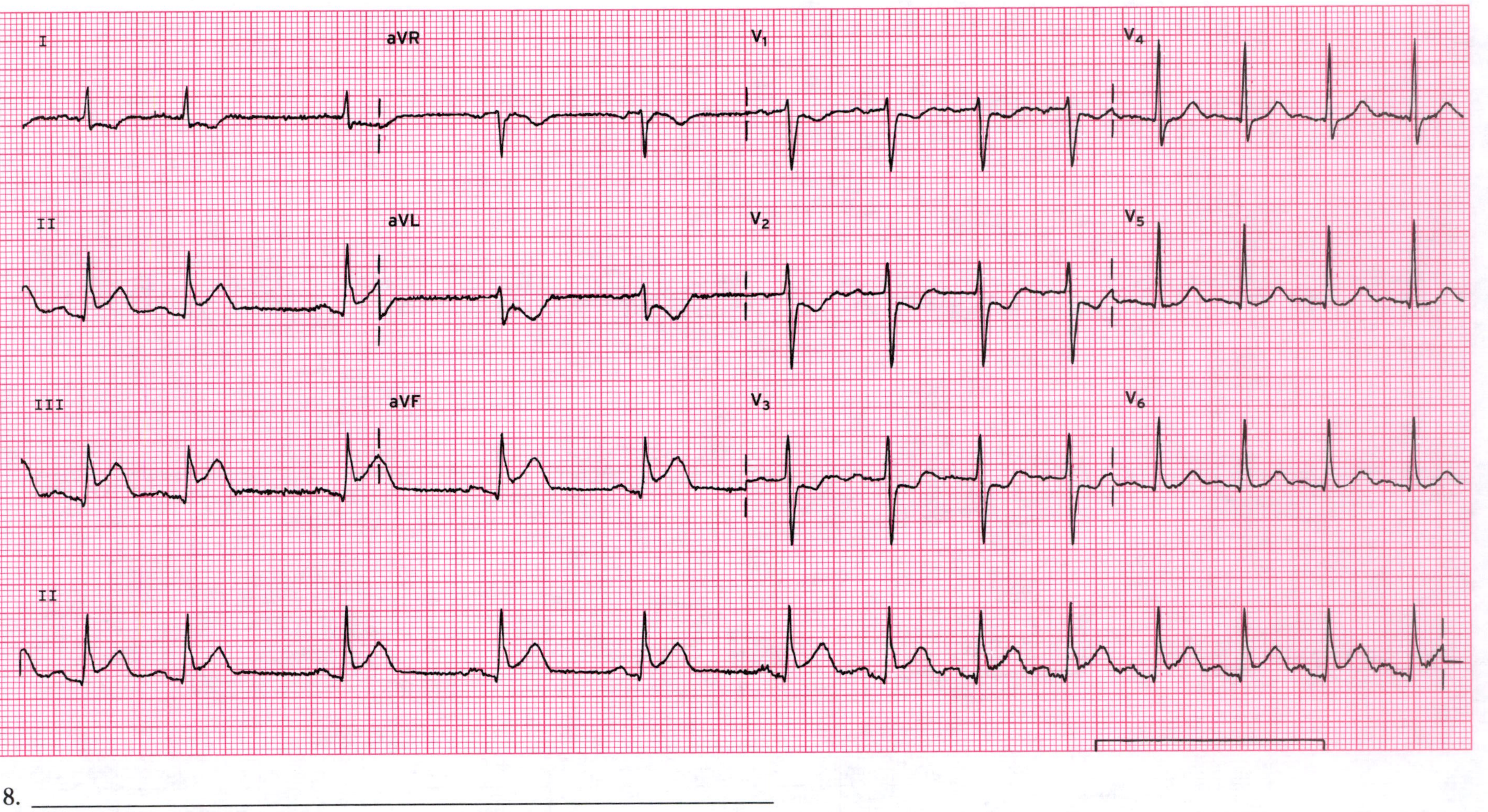

8. ______________________

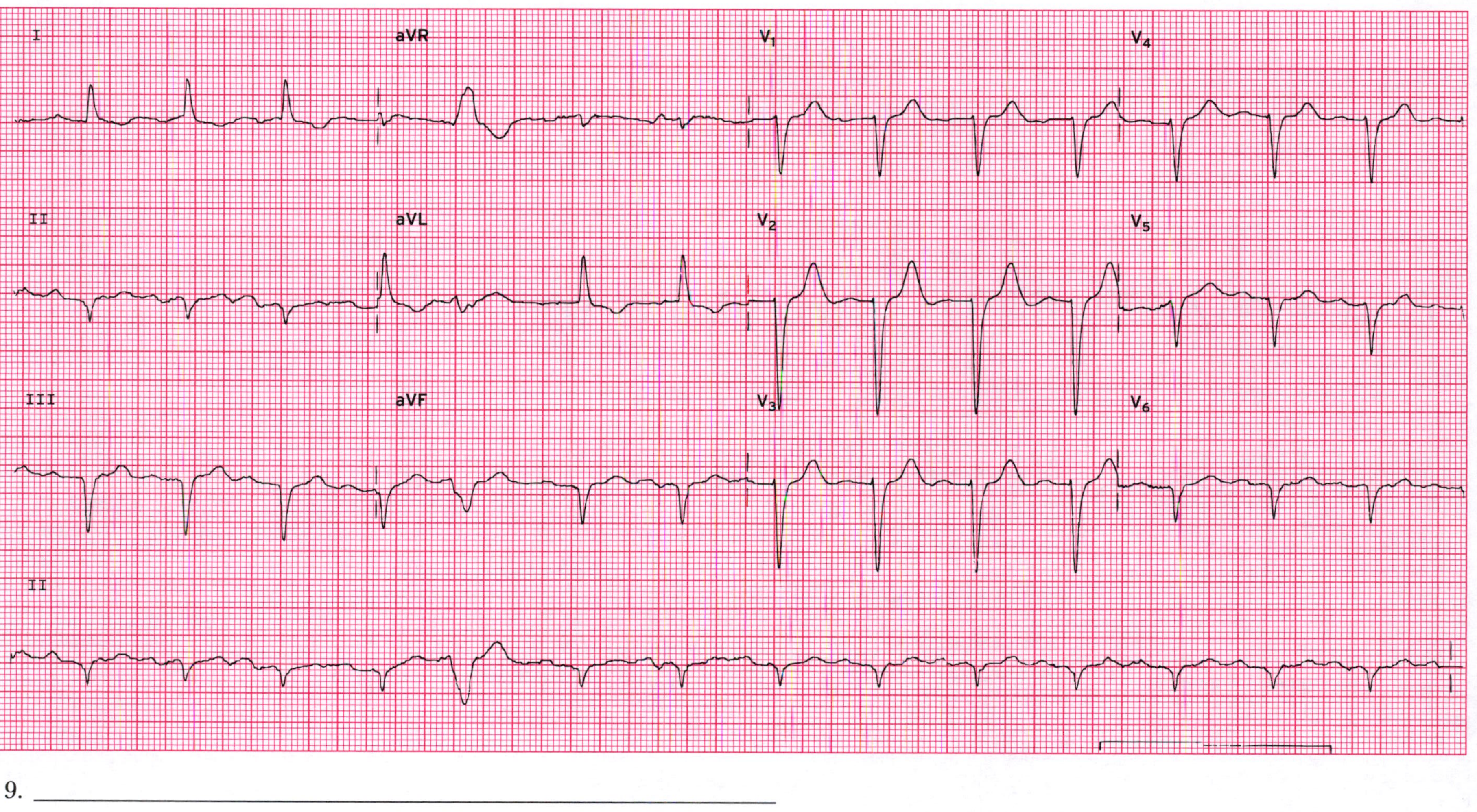

9. ______________________________

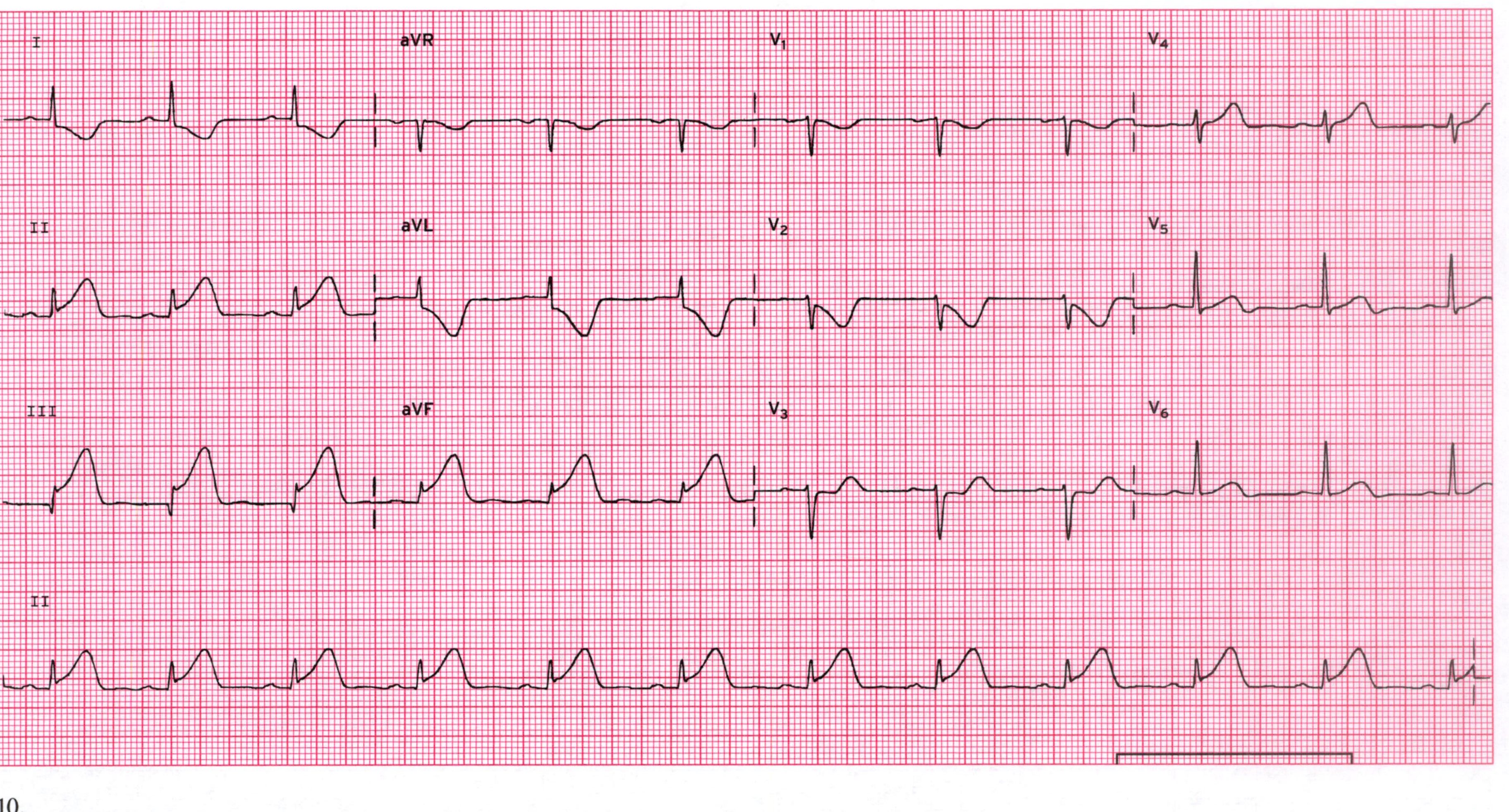

10. ______________________________

Answers to MI Practice

1. **Extensive anterior MI, acute**. Note the ST segment elevation in leads I, aVL, V_1 to V_6, along with reciprocal ST depression in II, III, and aVF. The T waves are upright.
2. **Inferior MI, age indeterminate**. Note the significant Q waves in II, III, and aVF, along with inverted T waves. The ST segment is at baseline.
3. **Lateral wall MI, acute**. Note the ST elevation, significant Q waves, and inverted T waves in I, aVL, and V_5 to V_6, along with reciprocal ST depression in II, III, and aVF.
4. **Anteroseptal MI, acute**. Note the ST elevation and inverted T in V_1 to V_2, along with reciprocal ST depression in II, III, and aVF.
5. **No MI. Lateral wall ischemia present**. Note the T wave inversion in I, aVL, and V_5 to V_6. Remember that T wave inversion represents ischemia. There is no ST elevation or depression and no significant Q waves.
6. **Anteroseptal and inferior MI, both old**. Note the significant Q waves in V_1 to V_4 (anterior and septal leads), along with essentially normal ST segments. The ST does slope upward a bit in V_1 to V_4, but it is not frankly elevated. There is also an old inferior MI. There are significant Q waves in III and aVF, but not in II. aVF is tiny, but you can see a Q wave there. That Q wave in aVF is significant because it is about half the size of the R wave–more than deep enough to meet the criteria. The T waves in the inferior leads are not inverted.
7. **Inferior and anterior-lateral MI, acute**. There is ST elevation in II, III, and aVF (inferior leads) and ST elevation and QS complexes in V_3 to V_6 (anterior and lateral leads). Leads V_1 and V_2 both have tiny R waves–those are not QS complexes there. It appears this patient started off with an anterior-lateral MI, which then extended into the inferior wall. The Q waves in V_3 to V_6 indicate that that infarct area is older than that in the inferior leads, where there are no significant Q waves.
8. **Inferior MI, acute**. There is ST elevation in II, III, and aVF, along with upright T waves and no significant Q waves as yet. Also note the reciprocal ST depression in I, aVL, and V_1 to V_3.
9. **Inferior-lateral MI, old**. There are significant Q waves in II, III, aVF (inferior leads), and V_6 (lateral lead) with upright T waves and baseline ST segments. Lead V_5 looks like it has a tiny R wave, not a Q wave. Also note the essentially nonexistent R wave progression in the precordial leads. This could imply an additional old anterior MI, or it could be caused by other factors.
10. **Inferior MI, acute**. Note the ST elevation in II, III, and aVF with reciprocal ST depression in I, aVL, and V_1 to V_3. There is a significant Q in III, but not yet in II or aVF.

Practice Quiz

1. List the three Is of infarction. ______________________________

____

____

2. State the differences between a Q wave MI and a non–Q wave MI. ____

____

3. Which coronary artery's occlusion results in an anterior wall MI? ______

____

4. Name the three normal indicative changes of an MI. ______________

____

5. Reciprocal changes are seen in which area of the heart? ____________

____

6. If there is ST elevation in leads II, III, and aVF, how old is the MI and in which wall of the heart?

____

____

7. If there is a significant Q wave in V_1 to V_3 with baseline ST segments and upright T waves, how old is the MI and in which wall of the heart?

____

____

8. If the transition zone of the precordial leads is in V_1 to V_2, what kind of rotation is the heart said to have? ______________________________

____

9. The kind of MI that can be diagnosed by inverting the EKG and looking at leads V_1 and V_2 from behind is the ______________________________

____

10. Which coronary artery supplies the lateral wall of the left ventricle?

____

Putting It All Together—Critical Thinking Exercises

These exercises may consist of diagrams to label, scenarios to analyze, brain-stumping questions to ponder, or other challenging exercises to boost your understanding of the chapter material.

1. Draw and label the evolution of EKG changes seen from immediately before the actual MI starts to an MI that is weeks, months, or years old.

2. If Mr. Milner, a 69-year old man with a history of chest pain, arrives in your ER with newly inverted T waves in leads II, III, and aVF, what do you suspect is happening?

____

3. If an hour later Mr. Milner is doubled over with crushing chest pain and his EKG now shows marked ST elevation in II, III, aVF and V_5-V_6, what is happening?

____

The following is a scenario which will provide you with information about a fictional patient and ask you to analyze the situation, answer questions, and decide on appropriate actions.

Mr. Jones is a 79-year old black male who arrives in the ER stating he'd had chest pain for about a half hour prior to arrival, but right now the pain is gone. See his EKG in Figure 14-19.

4. What do you see in leads II, III, and aVF that would be consistent with myocardial ischemia?

____

The ER physician orders lab work and the nurse keeps a close eye on Mr. Jones. Thirty minutes later Mr. Jones calls his nurse, complaining of crushing chest pain and shortness of breath. His blood pressure has dropped and his skin is ashen, cool, and clammy. The nurse calls for the physician and repeats an EKG. See Figure 14-20.

5. What is happening?

____

The physician orders medication for the pain and thrombolytic therapy (blood clot–dissolving medication) for the MI. Within 20 minutes Mr. Jones feels much better and his EKG is much improved. He is sent to the coronary care unit for a few days and sent home in a week.

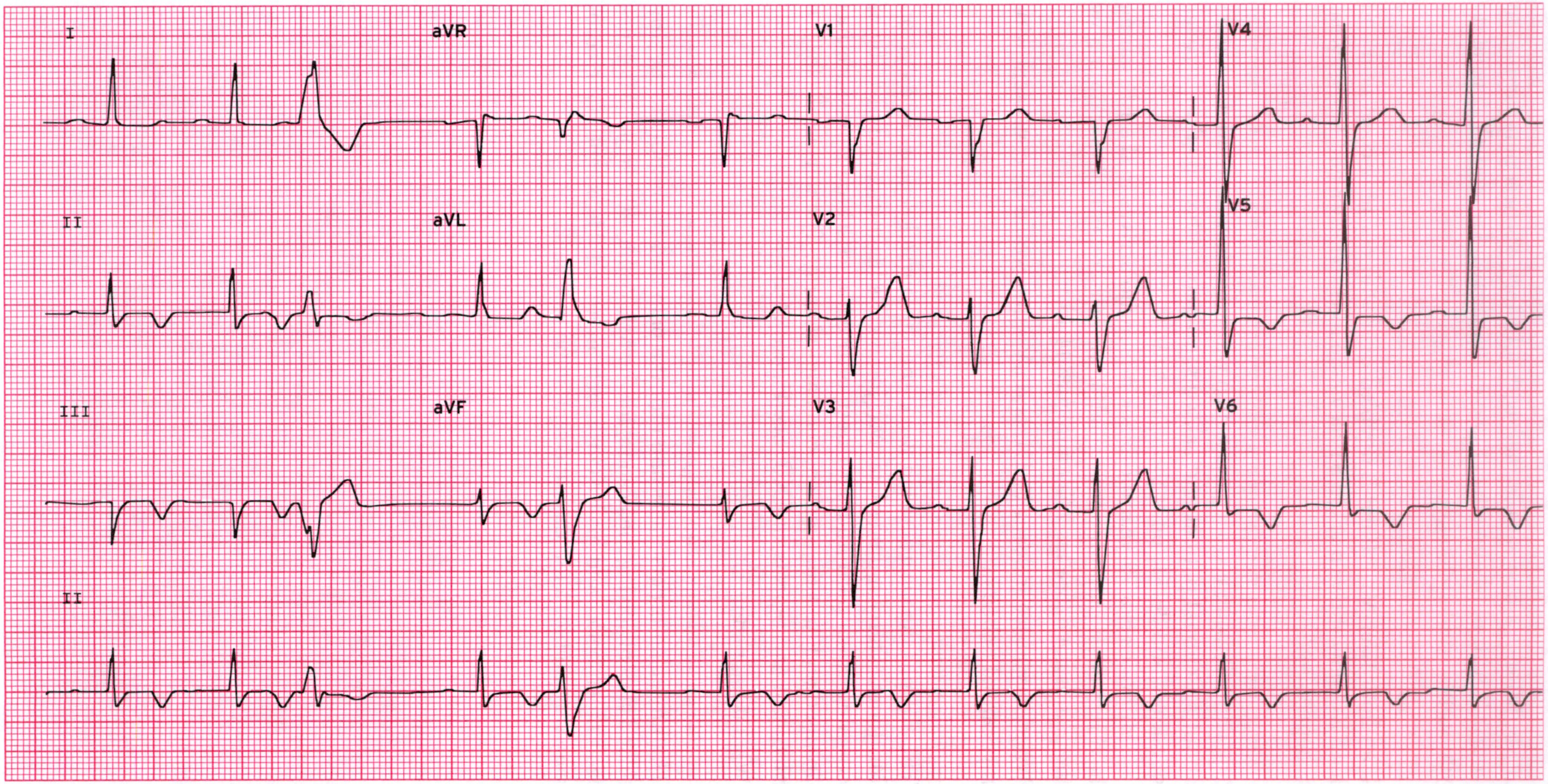

I
aVR
V1
V4
II
aVL
V2
V5
III
aVF
V3
V6
II

Figure 14-19 Mr. Jones's first EKG.

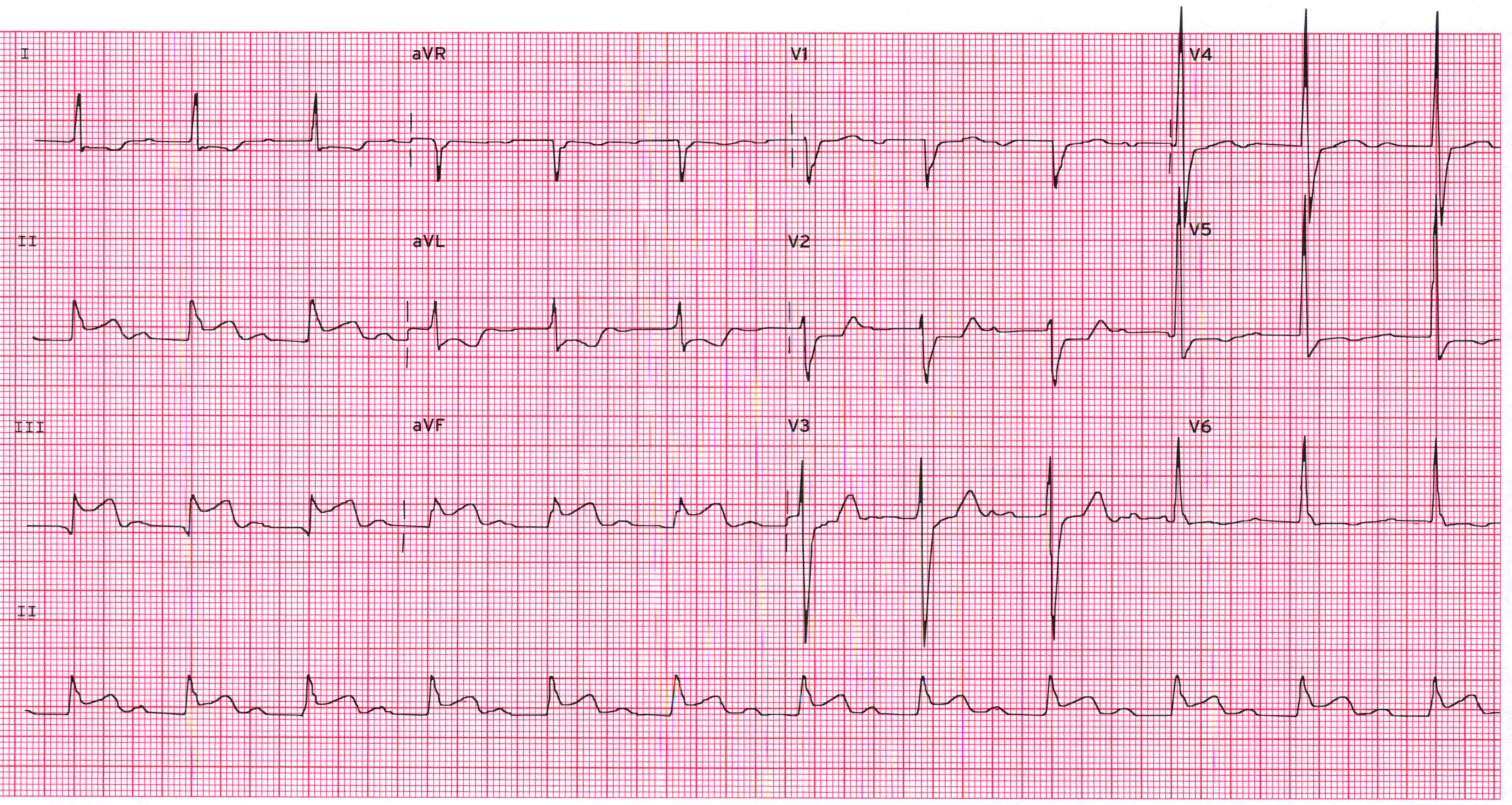

Figure 14-20 Mr Jones's second EKG.

CHAPTER **15**

Artificial Pacemakers

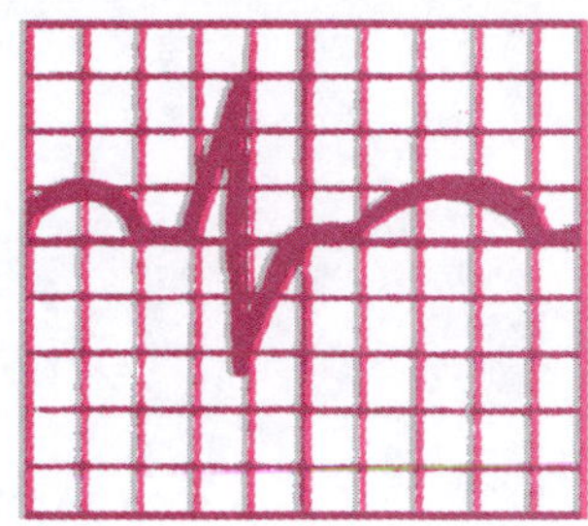

Chapter 15 Objectives

Upon completion of this chapter, the student will be able to:

- State the primary function of a pacemaker.
- Outline the indications for a pacemaker.
- Name the two components of a permanent pacemaker.
- Describe the types of temporary pacemakers.
- Define the terms ***firing, capture,*** and ***sensing.***
- State what each letter of the pacemaker code means.
- Identify pacemaker rhythms as being either VVI or DDD.
- Identify the different kinds of pacemaker malfunctions.

Introduction

The primary function of an artificial pacemaker is to prevent the heart rate from becoming too slow. Pacemakers provide an electrical stimulus when the heart is unable to generate its own or when its own is too slow to provide adequate cardiac output. You'll recall from chapter 10 that pacemakers can pace the atrium, the ventricle, or both.

Another use for pacemakers is overdrive suppression of tachydysrhythmias. Say the patient is in SVT with a heart rate of 180. If a pacemaker is in place, its rate can be set at a rate higher than the heart rate (set it at, say, 190 in this case). That puts the pacemaker in control of the heart. (Remember the fastest pacemaker, whether it be the normal conduction system or an artificial pacemaker, is the one in control.) Once the pacemaker is in control, the other rhythm is effectively knocked out of power. The pacemaker's rate is then slowly dialed back down to a rate low enough for the sinus to take back over.

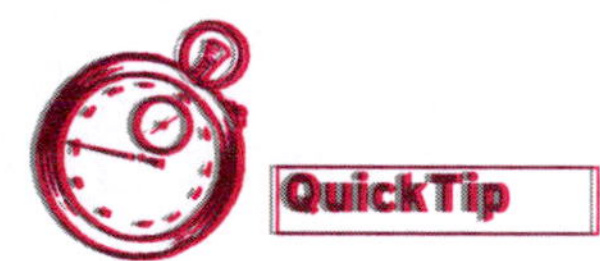

Pacemakers do not force the heart to beat. They simply send out an electrical signal, just as the heart's normal pacemakers do. If the heart is healthy enough, it should respond to that stimulus by depolarizing.

Indications

Indications for a pacemaker may include the following:

- Symptomatic sinus bradycardia
- Junctional rhythms
- Idioventricular rhythm
- Dying heart

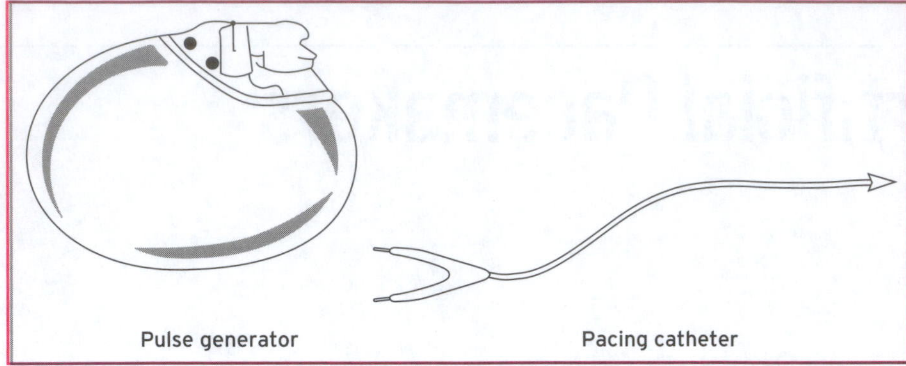

Figure 15-1 Pulse generator and pacing catheter of a permanent pacemaker.

- Asystole
- 2:1 AV block
- Type II second-degree AV block
- Third-degree AV block
- Overdrive suppression of tachydysrhythmias

Permanent versus Temporary Pacemakers

A **permanent pacemaker** has two components–a **pulse generator** (a battery pack), inserted surgically into a pocket made just under the right clavicle, and a **pacing catheter**, which is inserted via the subclavian vein into the superior vena cava and down into the right atrium or ventricle. Permanent pacemaker batteries are made of lithium and usually last between 5 and 15 years. See Figure 15-1.

Temporary pacemakers can be of various types, the two most common being the **transvenous**, in which a pacing catheter is inserted into a large vein and threaded into the right atrium and down into the right ventricle, and the **transcutaneous**, which involves large pacing electrodes attached to the chest and back that pace the heart through the chest wall. Both of these temporary pacer methods require a pulse generator at the patient's bedside. See Figures 15-2 and 15-3.

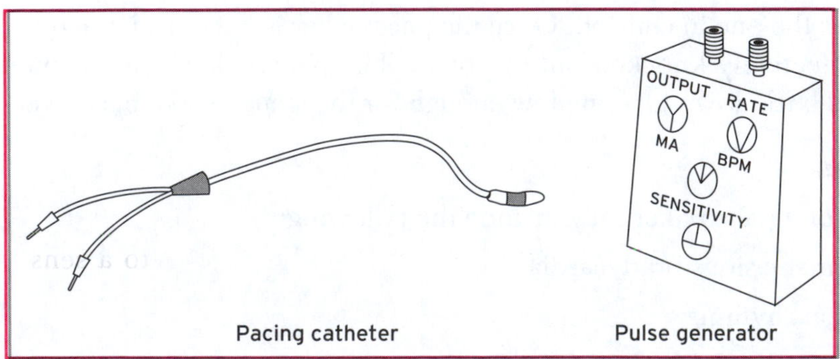

Figure 15-2 Transvenous pacemaker components.

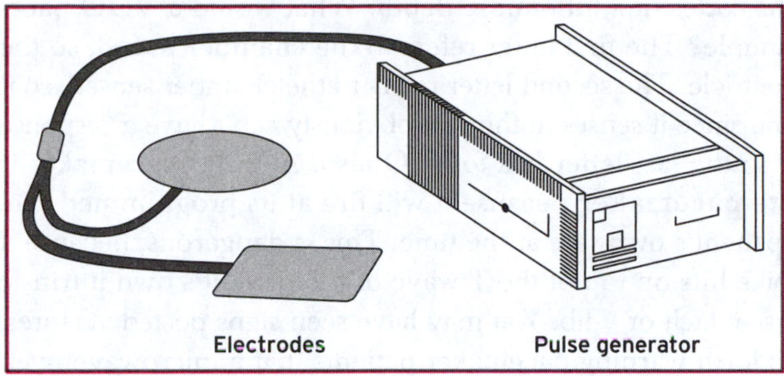

Figure 15-3 Transcutaneous pacemaker components.

Pacemaker Terminology

Firing refers to the pacemaker's generation of an electrical stimulus. It is noted on the EKG by the presence of a **pacemaker spike**.

Capture refers to the presence of a P wave or a QRS (or both) after the pacemaker spike. This indicates that the tissue in the chamber being paced has depolarized. The pacemaker is then said to have "captured" that chamber. Paced QRS complexes are wide and bizarre and resemble PVCs.

Sensing refers to the pacemaker's ability to recognize the patient's own intrinsic rhythm or beats in order to decide if it needs to fire. Most pacemakers function on a **demand mode**, meaning they fire only when needed (only on demand).

Three-Letter Pacemaker Code

Pacemakers are referred to by a three-letter code:

- The first letter refers to the chamber paced.

  V = ventricle

  A = atrium

  D = dual (atrium and ventricle)

  O = none

- The second letter refers to the *chamber sensed.*

  V = ventricle

  A = atrium

  D = dual (atrium and ventricle)

  O = none

- The third letter refers to the *response to sensed events.*

  I = inhibited (pacemaker watches and waits, does not pace until needed)

  T = triggered (pacemaker sends out a signal in response to a sensed event)

  D = dual (inhibited and triggered)

  O = none

Let's look at the codes in a little more depth. What would a VOO pacemaker do, for example? The first letter refers to the chamber paced, so the VOO paces the ventricle. The second letter refers to the chamber sensed, so it senses nothing. And since it senses nothing, it obviously can't have a response to sensed events, so the last letter has to be O also. A VOO pacemaker is called a **fixed-rate pacemaker** because it will fire at its programmed rate regardless of the patient's own rate at the time. This is dangerous, because if the pacemaker spike hits on top of the T wave of the patient's own intrinsic beats, it could cause v-tach or v-fib. You may have seen signs posted at stores, snack bars, and so forth warning pacemaker patients that a microwave oven was in use. Older pacemakers were poorly insulated and could be turned into fixed-rate pacemakers by microwaves. Newer pacemakers are well insulated and do not have that problem. VOO pacemakers are not used today.

VVI Pacemakers

The most common kinds of pacemakers in use today are the VVI and the DDD. The **VVI pacer**, also known as a **ventricular demand pacer**, was at one time the most commonly used permanent pacer. It's now in second place. The VVI pacer consists of a catheter with both pacing and sensing capabilities and is inserted into the right ventricle. See Figure 15-4.

The VVI pacemaker paces the ventricle, providing a spike and then a wide QRS complex. It senses the ventricle, so it looks for intrinsic QRS complexes to determine if it needs to fire. Let's say the patient is in a sinus rhythm with a heart rate of 80 and the pacemaker is set at a rate of 60. The sensor would "see" the patient's own QRS complexes and realize it does not need to fire. It will be inhibited. If the patient's heart rate falls to a rate below the pacemaker's preset heart rate, the pacer will see that the QRS complexes are not at a fast enough rate, so it will fire and pace the heart. As with your own conduction system, whichever is the fastest pacemaker is the one in control. Since the VVI pacer senses only intrinsic QRS complexes, it ignores the P waves. Therefore, *there will be no relationship between P waves and paced QRS complexes.*

VVI pacemakers provide two options:

- *Intrinsic beats only.* The pacemaker does not pace because it does not need to. The rhythm is fast enough, so the pacemaker is inhibited. There will be no pacemaker spikes.

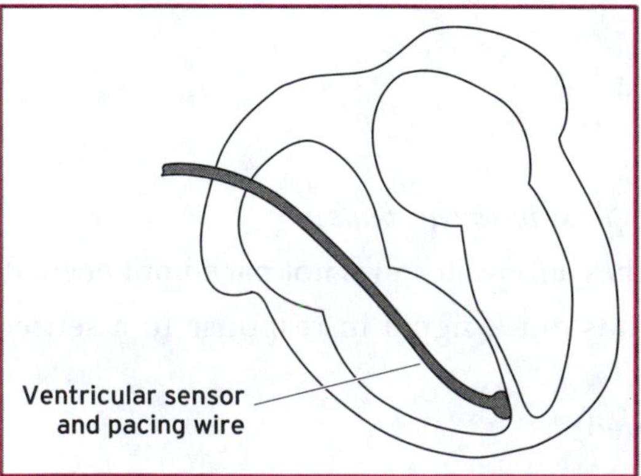

Figure 15-4 VVI pacemaker inserted into the right ventricle.

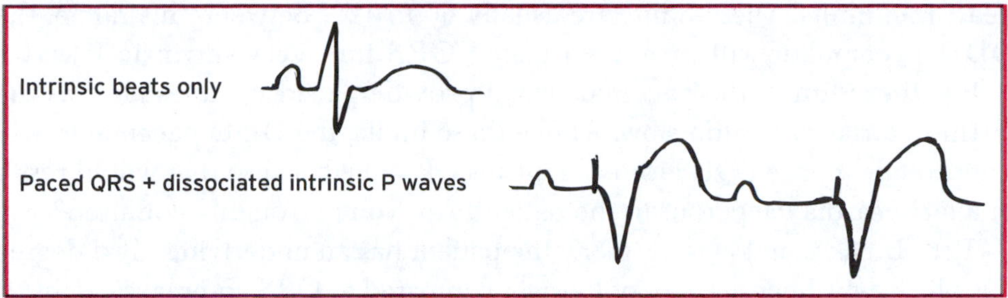

Figure 15-5 VVI pacemaker options.

- *Paced QRS, dissociated intrinsic P waves.* The pacemaker senses and paces only the ventricle. There will be pacemaker spikes preceding only the QRS complexes. Intrinsic P waves, if present, will be ignored by the pacemaker. See Figure 15-5.

DDD Pacemakers

The **DDD pacemaker** is the most modern and the most physiologic. It is known as an **AV universal pacemaker** and is now the most commonly inserted permanent pacemaker. It paces and senses both atrium and ventricle. See Figure 15-6.

The DDD pacemaker senses intrinsic atrial activity and takes advantage of the patient's own P waves. If the DDD pacemaker senses the patient's P waves within its preset rate, it will not need to give another P wave, so its atrial pacer will be inhibited. The ventricle, however, will then be triggered to give a QRS if the patient does not have his or her own QRS in the preset length of time after the P wave. *DDD pacemakers provide a constant relationship between P waves and QRS complexes.* If the pacemaker senses intrinsic P waves and QRS complexes within the appropriate time interval, it will be inhibited, and it will just watch and wait until it's needed. If there are no Ps or QRS complexes in the preset time interval, the pacemaker will pace both chambers, providing a paced P and a paced QRS. Basically, the DDD provides whatever the patient cannot do on his or her own.

DDD pacemakers are usually **rate-responsive**, meaning they will provide a paced QRS to follow the patient's intrinsic P waves between preset

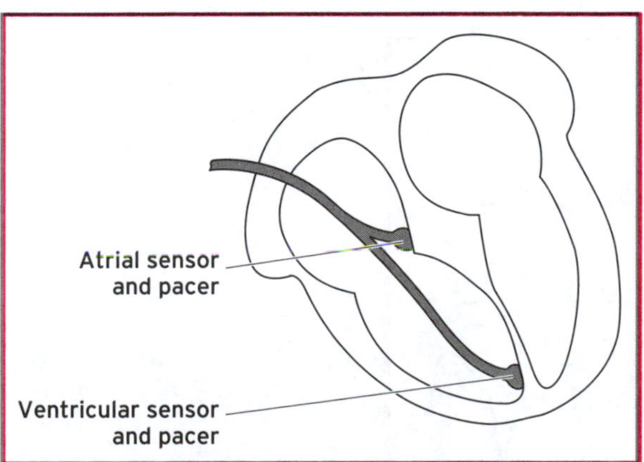

Figure 15-6 DDD pacemaker sensor and pacer wires in right atrium and ventricle.

heart rate limits. These limits are usually 60 to 125. Between this range, the DDD pacemaker will provide a paced QRS for every intrinsic P wave. Below these limits, the pacemaker will provide paced P waves also, as the intrinsic atrial rate is too slow. Above these limits, the DDD pacemaker will not provide a paced QRS for each intrinsic P wave because that would result in a tachycardia dangerous to the patient. Are you thoroughly confused?

Let's break that down a bit. Say the patient has an underlying third-degree AV block, which means a lot of P waves compared to QRS complexes, right? If the atrial rate is between 60 and 125, the DDD pacemaker will "track the P waves." The pacemaker will provide a paced QRS complex to follow each intrinsic P wave (assuming the patient does not have his or her own QRS at the right time after the P wave). It will not provide paced P waves, as it won't need to.

If the atrial rate drops below 60, the DDD pacemaker will provide paced P waves as well as QRS complexes as needed to keep the heart rate within the range of 60 to 125.

If the atrial rate exceeds 125, the DDD pacemaker will ignore some of those P waves and track others. Therefore, there may be paced QRS complexes after only every second or third intrinsic P wave, and so forth. Why does it do this? If the atrial rate is faster than 125, and the pacemaker provides a paced QRS after each P wave, the patient ends up with a heart rate of 125. That may be so fast that cardiac output drops. If the atrial rate exceeds the upper limit, the pacemaker senses the atrial rate and decides to obey only some, rather than all, of the intrinsic P waves.

DDD pacemakers provide four options:

- *Intrinsic beats only.* The pacemaker does not fire because it does not need to. The intrinsic rate is fast enough. There will be no pacemaker spikes.
- *Paced P wave, intrinsic QRS.* The pacemaker paces the atrium, providing a pacemaker spike and a paced P wave. Following this, the patient's own QRS occurs. There is therefore a spike only before the P wave.
- *Paced P wave, paced QRS.* The pacemaker paces both chambers, providing a spike before the P wave and a spike before the QRS.
- *Intrinsic P wave, paced QRS.* The patient has his or her own P waves, so the pacemaker tracks them and provides a paced QRS to follow. There is a pacemaker spike only before the QRS. See Figure 15-7.

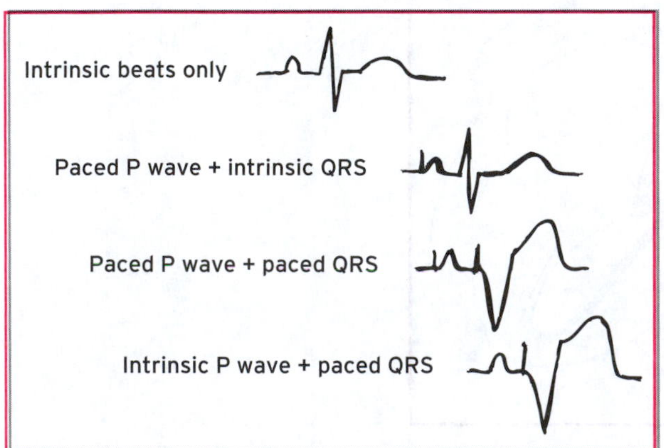

Figure 15-7 DDD pacemaker options.

DDD versus VVI Practice

On the following strips, tell whether the pacemaker is DDD or VVI (or undeterminable).

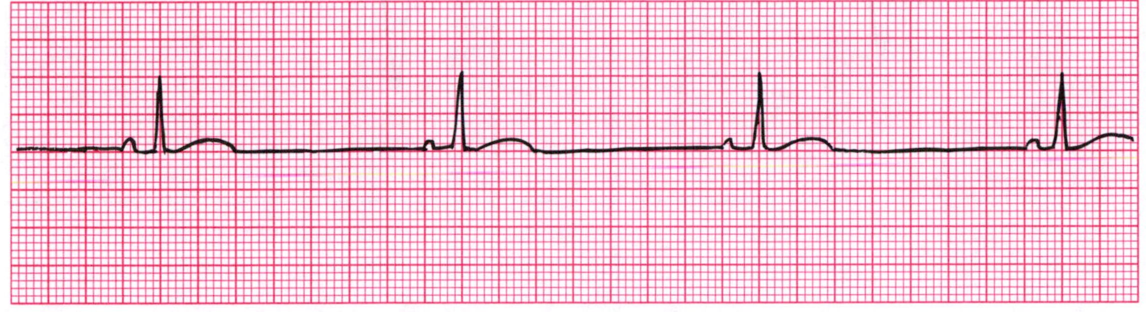

1. ______________________________

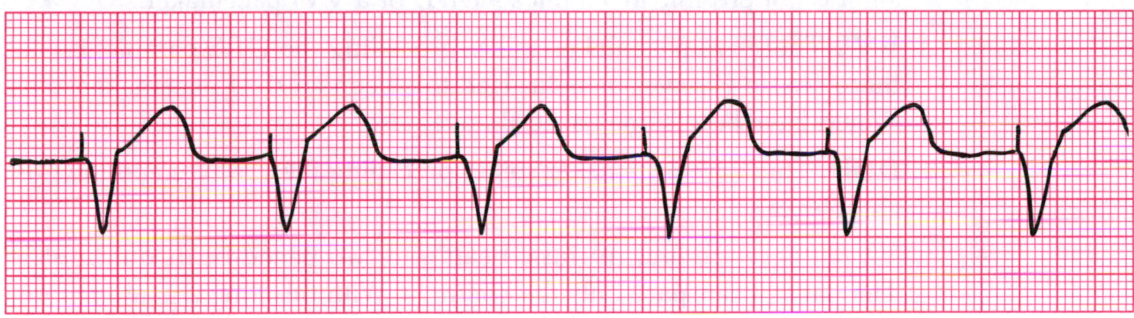

2. ______________________________

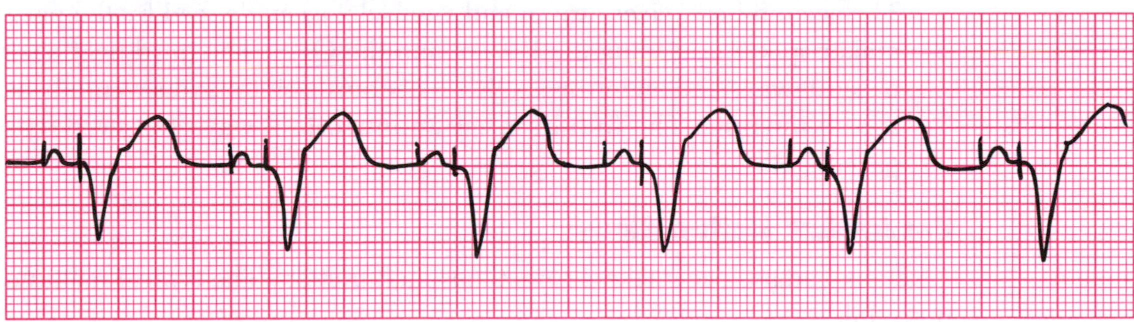

3. ______________________________

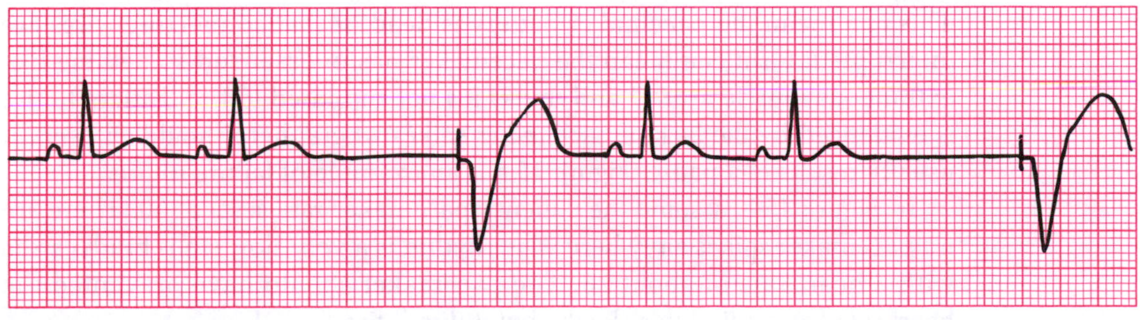

4. ______________________________

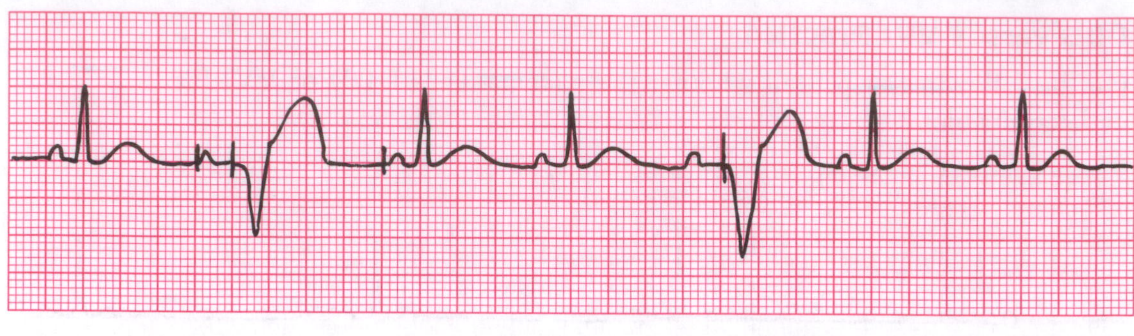

5. ______________________________

Answers to DDD versus VVI Practice

1. **Can't tell which kind of pacemaker.** Since there are no paced beats at all, it is not possible to tell if it's a DDD or a VVI pacemaker.
2. **VVI.** There are pacemaker spikes preceding the QRS complexes, and there are no P waves in sight. Had this been a DDD pacemaker, there should have been some paced P waves also.
3. **DDD.** There are pacemaker spikes preceding the P waves and the QRS complexes.
4. **VVI.** There are four intrinsic beats and two paced beats on the strip. The paced beats pace only the ventricle. With this long a pause before a paced beat kicks in, a DDD pacemaker would have provided a paced P wave as well.
5. **DDD.** This strip has a little of everything. The first beat is all intrinsic. The second beat paces atrium and ventricle, as evidenced by the pacemaker spikes preceding the P wave and the QRS. The third beat has a paced P wave and an intrinsic QRS. The fourth, sixth, and seventh beats are all intrinsic. The fifth beat has an intrinsic P wave followed by a paced QRS.

Pacemaker Malfunctions

Like any gadget, pacemakers sometimes malfunction. The typical malfunctions follow.

Failure to Fire

Here the pacemaker fails to send out its electrical stimulus when it should. This can mean the pacemaker battery is dead or that connecting wires are interrupted. Or it can mean the pacemaker has **oversensed** something like extraneous muscle artifact and thinks it's not supposed to fire. Failure to fire is evidenced by the lack of pacemaker spikes where there should've been. It usually results in a pause. Figure 15-8 is an example of failure to fire.

In Figure 15-8, assume the patient's pacemaker rate is set at 60. There are no pacemaker spikes anywhere. The rhythm is a very slow sinus bradycardia with a heart rate of about 28. The pacemaker should have prevented the heart rate from going this slowly, but it didn't fire.

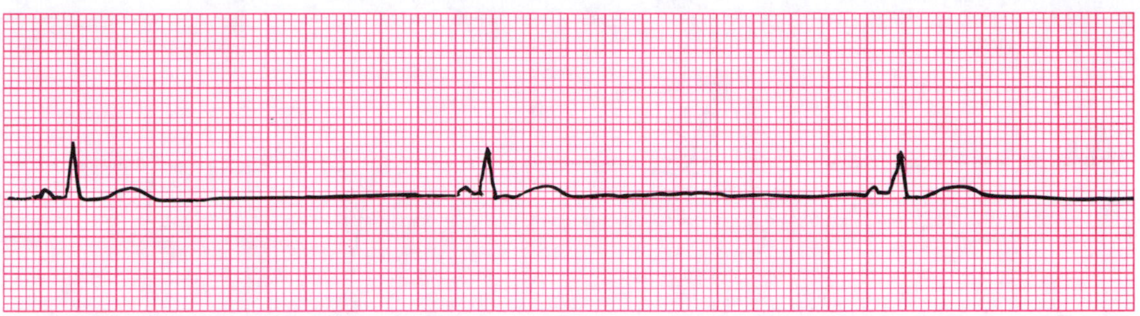

Figure 15-8 Failure to fire.

Loss of Capture

There is no P or QRS after the pacemaker spike in loss of capture. This is often simply a matter of turning up the pacemaker's voltage so that it sends out more "juice" to tell the heart what to do. Maybe the signal it sent out was too weak to get a response from the chamber. Another possibility is that the pacing catheter has lost contact with the wall of the chamber it's in and cannot cause depolarization. That could be corrected by a simple position change of the patient, or it could necessitate minor surgery to adjust the catheter placement. Loss of capture can also occur when the heart is too damaged to respond to the pacer's stimulus. See Figure 15-9 for an example of loss of capture.

In Figure 15-9 we have asystole with pacemaker spikes but no Ps or QRS complexes after the spikes. The pacemaker has fired, as evidenced by the spikes, but it has not captured the chamber it's in.

Undersensing

Here the pacemaker fires too soon after an intrinsic beat, often resulting in pacemaker spikes where there shouldn't have been, such as in a T wave, an ST segment, or right on top of another QRS. This happens when the pacemaker just doesn't see that other beat. The pacemaker's sensor needs adjusting. Another possibility is a fractured sensing wire or battery failure. In Figure 15-10, we have undersensing.

In Figure 15-10, note the spikes at times when the pacer should not have fired. How do you detect undersensing? Look at the distance between two consecutive pacemaker spikes. That's the normal **pacing interval,** which

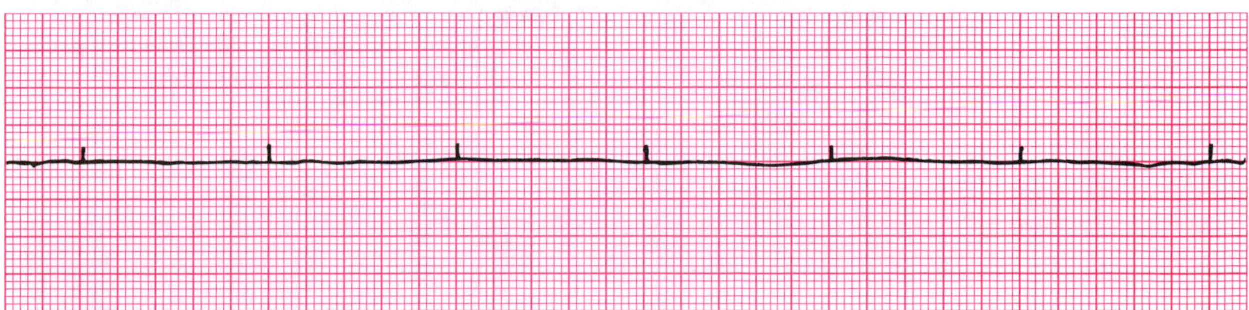

Figure 15-9 Loss of capture.

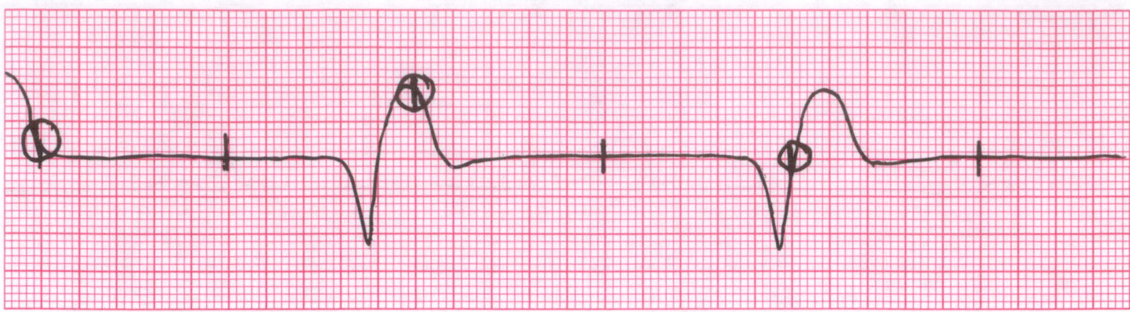

Figure 15-10 Undersensing.

will correspond to a certain paced heart rate. *There should be exactly that same distance between the patient's own intrinsic beats and the next paced beat.* If the distance is less than that, there is undersensing. In Figure 15-10, the circled pacemaker spikes indicate undersensing.

But this strip also shows another malfunction. Do you know what it is? Look it over carefully before continuing.

There is loss of capture in addition to the undersensing. All the uncircled spikes plus the first circled one did not result in a P or QRS complex at a time when they should have. The second and third circled ones would not be considered loss of capture even though they also don't result in a P or QRS. Why? Remember the refractory periods? From the beginning of the QRS to the upstroke of the T wave is the absolute refractory period. A spike that occurs during that time cannot possibly capture. That's not a pacemaker malfunction, it's just physiology.

For a summary of pacemaker malfunctions, see Table 15-1.

Table 15-1 Pacemaker Malfunctions Summary

PACEMAKER MALFUNCTIONS	EKG EVIDENCE
Failure to fire	Lack of pacemaker spikes where there should have been. Usually results in a pause.
Loss of capture	Pacemaker spikes not followed by P waves or QRS complexes.
Undersensing	Paced beats or spikes too close to previous beats. Often results in spikes inside T waves, ST segments, or QRS complexes.

Pacemaker Malfunctions Practice

On the strips that follow, indicate the pacer malfunction(s), if any.

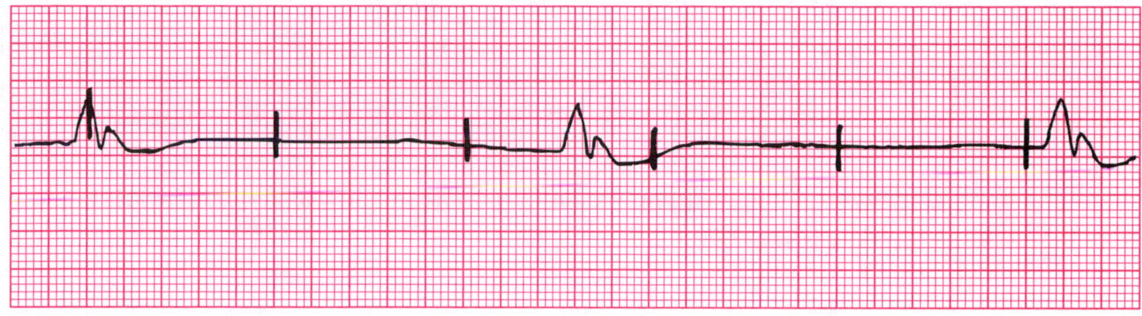

Situation: This patient passed out at home. The paramedics found him with a barely palpable, very slow pulse. His VVI pacemaker is set at 60.

1. ______________________________

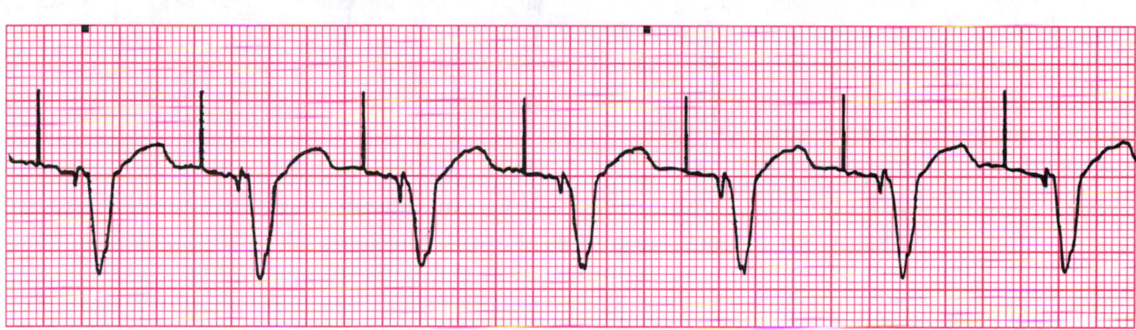

Situation: This patient had a DDD pacemaker inserted three years ago and now appears in the ER complaining of sudden onset of dizziness and syncope. The pacemaker rate is set at 68.

2. ______________________________

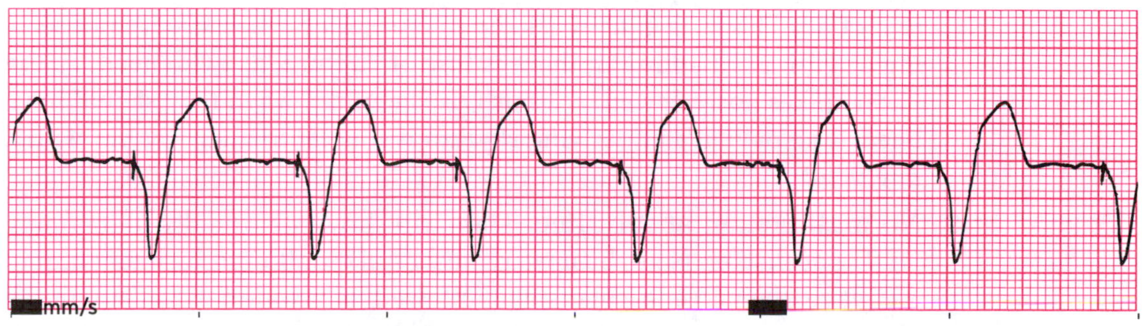

Situation: This patient has a DDD pacemaker set at 72. She's seen in her doctor's office for a routine checkup. She feels fine.

3. ______________________________

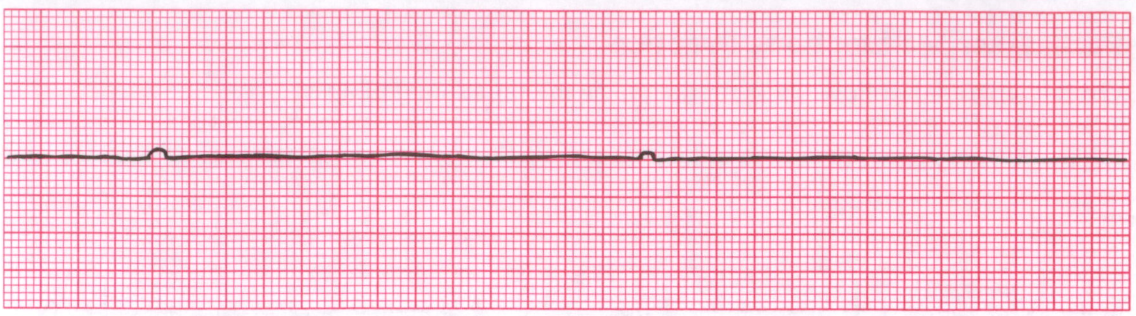

Situation: This patient is seen in the ER in cardiac arrest. His DDD pacemaker is set at 70.

4. ______________________________

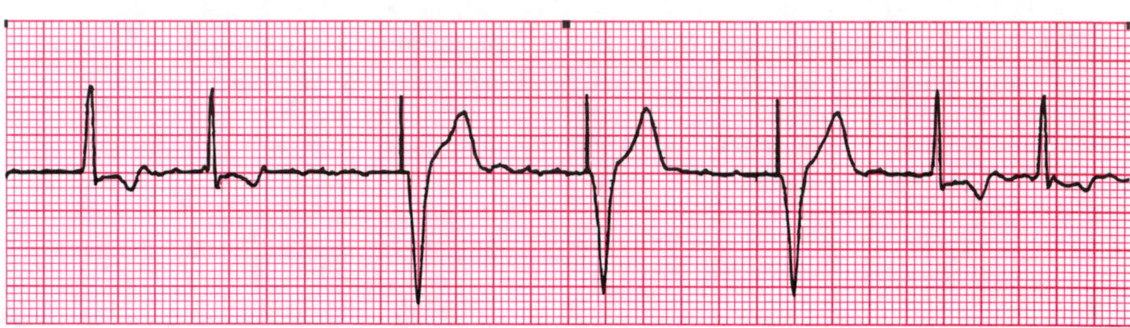

Situation: This patient had a VVI pacemaker inserted recently because of slow atrial fibrillation. It's set at 60. She feels fine.

5. ______________________________

Answers to Pacemaker Malfunctions Practice

1. **Undersensing and loss of capture.** We have pacer spikes in inappropriate places, such as inside the first QRS complex. It is clear this pacer is not sensing the QRS complexes, since it does nothing in response to those intrinsic complexes. The pacer should have been inhibited by the patient's intrinsic QRS complexes. Also note the spikes are regular at a rate of 60. This is essentially a fixed-rate pacer now because it's not sensing anything. In addition, there is loss of capture, as evidenced by the pacer spikes not followed by Ps or QRSs at times when they should have been. The patient's underlying rhythm is idioventricular rhythm with a rate of 23.
2. **No malfunction at this time.** This strip shows a normally functioning DDD pacemaker. Note the upward atrial spikes followed by a tiny blip of a P wave, then a ventricular spike followed by a wide QRS. Though the pacemaker seems fine right now, it could be that it malfunctions intermittently, causing the symptoms, so the patient will still need close observation. It is also possible that the patient's dizziness and syncope were caused by something totally unrelated to the pacemaker.
3. **No malfunction noted.** This strip shows a normally functioning DDD pacemaker. See the very small intrinsic P waves preceding each QRS?

The pacemaker senses them and tracks them, providing the paced QRS to follow those Ps since the patient does not have her own QRS complexes in the programmed time.

4. **Failure to fire.** There are two intrinsic P waves on this strip. The pacemaker should have sensed them and provided a paced QRS to follow them. In addition, it should have paced the atrium and then the ventricle, as necessary, at its programmed rate of 70. It didn't. There's not a pacemaker spike in sight.
5. **No malfunction noted.** The pacemaker rate is set at 60, and it fires at 60 when the atrial fibrillation slows down. Note the pacing interval from spike to spike on the three paced beats. Now look at the interval between the second QRS and the paced beat that follows. It's exactly the same interval. The pacemaker is therefore sensing the underlying rhythm, and it's firing and capturing appropriately.

Practice Quiz

1. List five indications for an artificial pacemaker. ____________________
2. The first letter of the pacemaker code refers to ____________________
3. The second letter of the pacemaker code refers to ____________________
4. The third letter of the pacemaker code refers to ____________________
5. Name the malfunction of a pacemaker that has no P wave or QRS after the pacemaker spike. ____________________
6. The pacemaker's ability to recognize the patient's own intrinsic rhythm in order to decide if it needs to fire is called ____________________
7. The pacemaker's generation of an electrical impulse is called ____________________
8. A DDD pacemaker paces which chamber(s)? ____________________

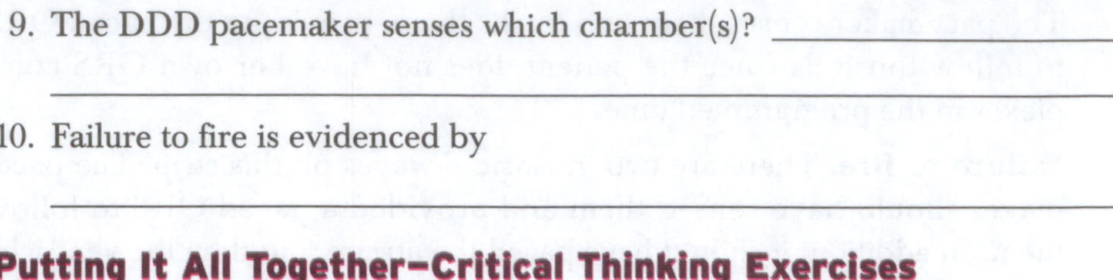

9. The DDD pacemaker senses which chamber(s)? ______________________

10. Failure to fire is evidenced by ______________________

Putting It All Together—Critical Thinking Exercises

These exercises may consist of diagrams to label, scenarios to analyze, brain-stumping questions to ponder, or other challenging exercises to boost your understanding of the chapter material.

The following scenario will provide you with information about a fictional patient and ask you to analyze the situation, answer questions, and decide on appropriate actions.

Mr. Johnson had a temporary transvenous VVI pacemaker inserted yesterday because of slow atrial fibrillation It's set at a rate of 60. This morning he calls you to his room complaining of feeling faint. His blood pressure has dropped and his rhythm is as seen on the strip below. See Figure 15-11.

1. What is this rhythm and heart rate? ______________________
2. What is the pacemaker doing? ______________________
3. Describe how to utilize the pacemaker to abolish this rhythm. ______________________

Within a few minutes Mr. Johnson's rhythm has changed. See below in Figure 15-12. His blood pressure remains low and he still feels faint.

4. What is this rhythm and heart rate? ______________________
5. What is the pacemaker doing? ______________________
6. Is there a pacer malfunction? Explain. ______________________
7. What corrective measures can help remedy the pacer malfunction? ______________________

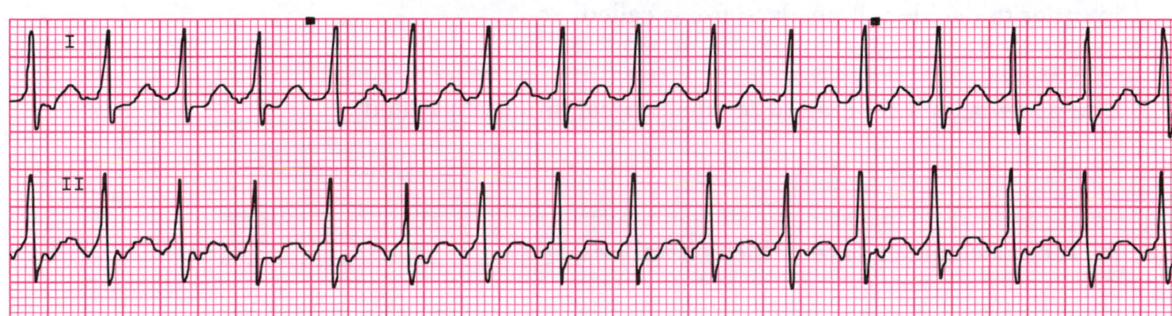

Figure 15-11 Mr. Johnson's first rhythm strip.

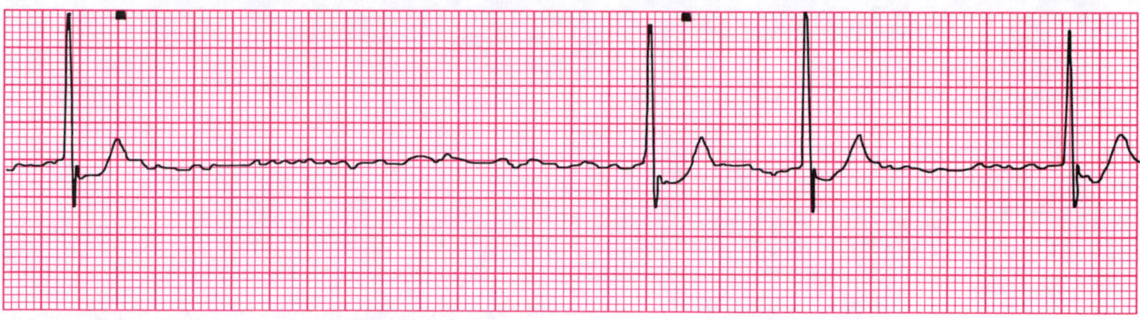

Figure 15-12 Mr. Johnson's second strip.

8. Explain the physiologic reason that he had low blood pressure and a feeling of faintness with both rhythms seen on his rhythm strips.

 ____

 ____

After corrective measures, the pacemaker now works properly and Mr. Johnson is in paced rhythm with a good blood pressure. He feels much better.

CHAPTER **16**

12-Lead EKG Practice

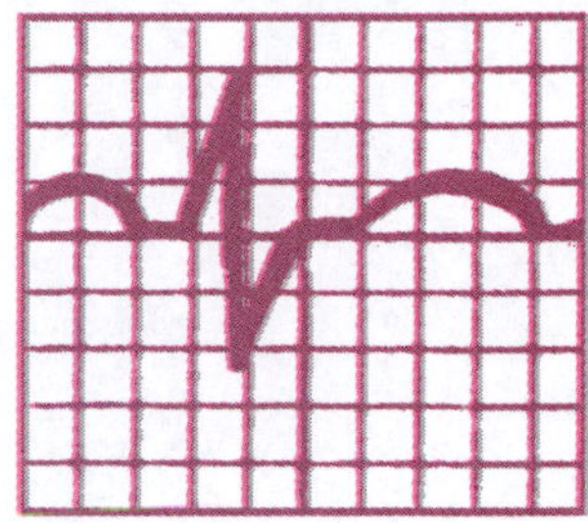

Chapter 16 Objectives

Upon completion of this chapter, the student will be able to:

- Practice the six steps in analyzing EKGs.
- Using this method, correctly interpret a variety of 12-lead EKGs.

Introduction

This chapter pulls together everything you've learned so far about rhythm and 12-lead EKG interpretation. First, you will find a comprehensive summary of what to look for on every EKG, then a checklist. Refer to these when evaluating the 12-lead EKGs that follow.

There are 20 EKGs to interpret in this chapter. Take your time and be methodical. Don't hesitate to go back and review portions of this text if you find that you're a little weak in certain areas. Practice does indeed make perfect.

Now let's get down to work.

12-Lead EKG Interpretation in a Nutshell

You've seen all the criteria for 12-lead EKG interpretation. Let's put it all in condensed form. Look for the following on every 12-lead EKG:

The Basics	Rhythm, Rate, Intervals (PR, QRS, QT)
Axis quadrant	Normal, LAD, RAD, or indeterminate?
BBB	RBBB = RSR' in V_1, QRS ≥ 0.12 s LBBB = QS or RS in V_1, QRS ≥ 0.12 s
Hypertrophy	RVH = R ≥ S in V_1, inverted T, RAD LVH = S in V_1 + R in V_5 or V_6 ≥ 35
Miscellaneous effects	Digitalis effect = Sagging ST segments, prolonged PR interval Hyperkalemia = Tall, pointy, narrow T waves Severe hyperkalemia = Wide QRS complex Hypokalemia = Prominent U waves, flattened T waves Hypercalcemia = Shortened ST segment causing short QT interval Hypocalcemia = Prolonged ST segment causing prolonged QT
Infarction	Anterior MI = ST elevation and/or significant Q in V_2 to V_4 Inferior MI = ST elevation and/or significant Q in II, III, aVF Lateral MI = ST elevation and/or significant Q in I, aVL, V_5 to V_6 Septal MI = ST elevation and/or significant Q in V_1 Extensive anterior (extensive anterior-lateral) = ST elevation and/or significant Q in I, aVL, V_1 to V_6 Posterior MI = Large R + upright T in V_1 to V_2; may also have ST depression Subendocardial = Widespread ST depression and T wave inversion in many leads Ischemia = Inverted T waves in any lead, as long as not BBB-related

12-Lead EKG Interpretation Checklist

The Basics

- Rhythm ______________________________
- Rate ________________________________
- Intervals: PR ________ QRS ________ QT ________

Axis

Circle one:

- Normal
- Abnormal (what quadrant?) ____________________________

Bundle Branch Blocks

Circle if present:

- RBBB
- LBBB

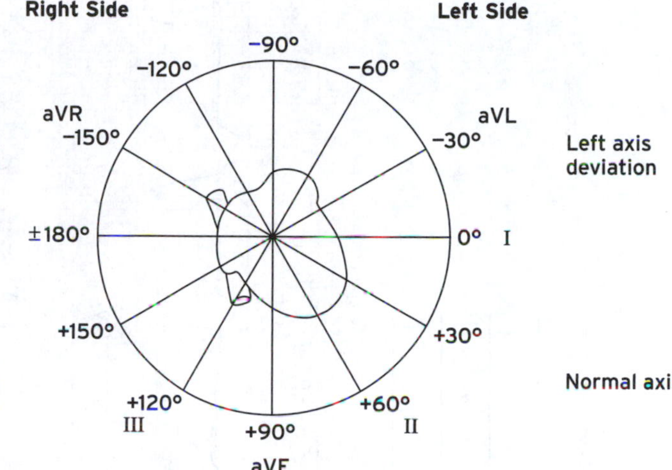

Hypertrophy

Circle if present:

- RVH
- LVH

Infarction/Ischemia

What leads? ____________

Miscellaneous Effects

Circle if present:

- Digitalis effect
- Hyperkalemia
- Severe hyperkalemia
- Hypokalemia
- Hypercalcemia
- Hypocalcemia

Practice EKGs

1. Rhythm and rate ________ PR ________ QRS ________ QT ________

   Axis ______________________ BBB ______________________

   Hypertrophy ______________________________________

   Miscellaneous effects ______________________________

   Infarction ____

I aVR V_1 V_4

II aVL V_2 V_5

III aVF V_3 V_6

II

2. Rhythm and rate ________ PR ________ QRS ________ QT ___________

Axis ___________________________ BBB ______________________________

Hypertrophy ____

Miscellaneous effects ____

Infarction ____

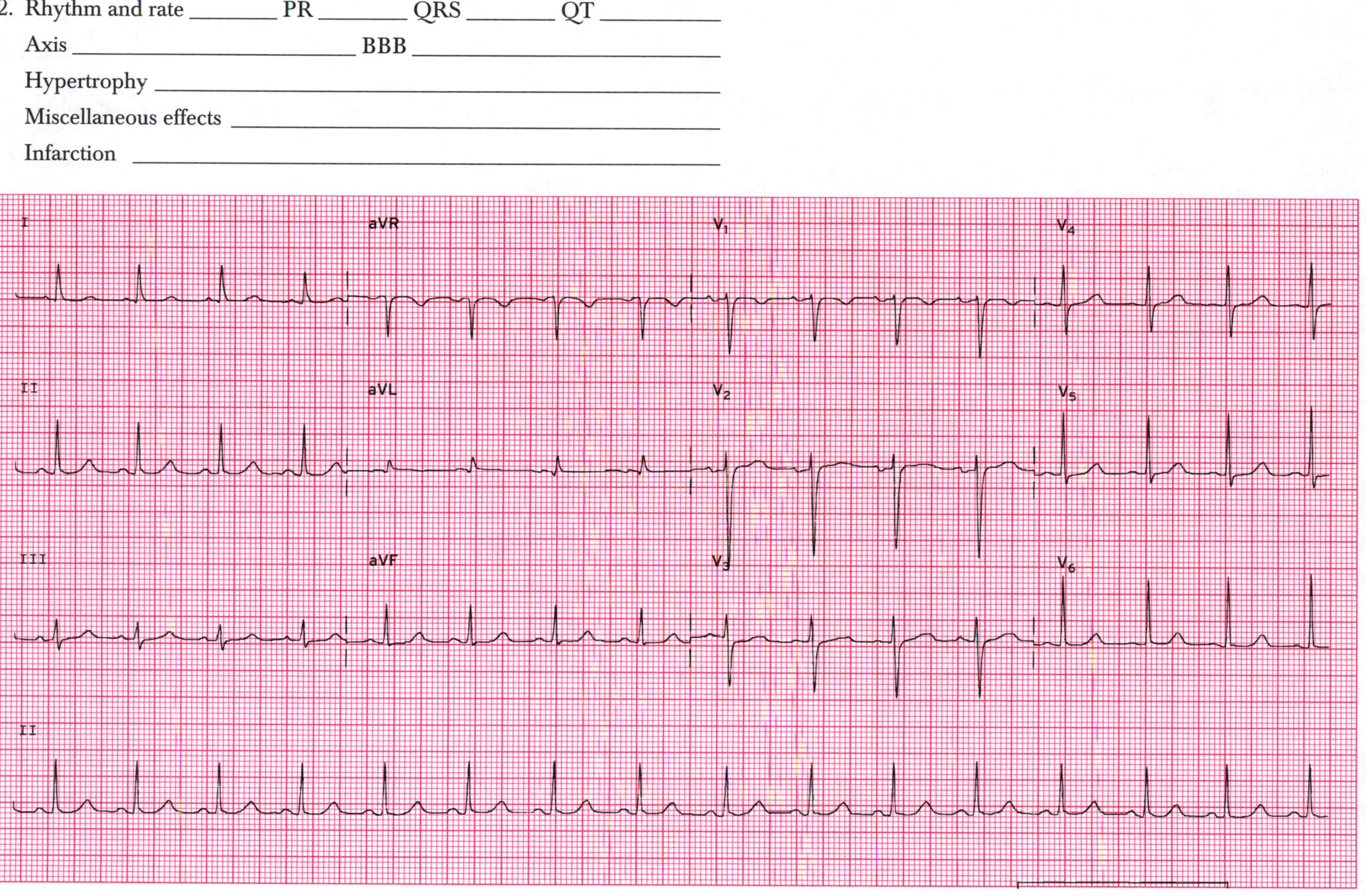

3. Rhythm and rate ________ PR ________ QRS ________ QT ___________

Axis __________________________ BBB ____________________________

Hypertrophy ____

Miscellaneous effects ____

Infarction ____

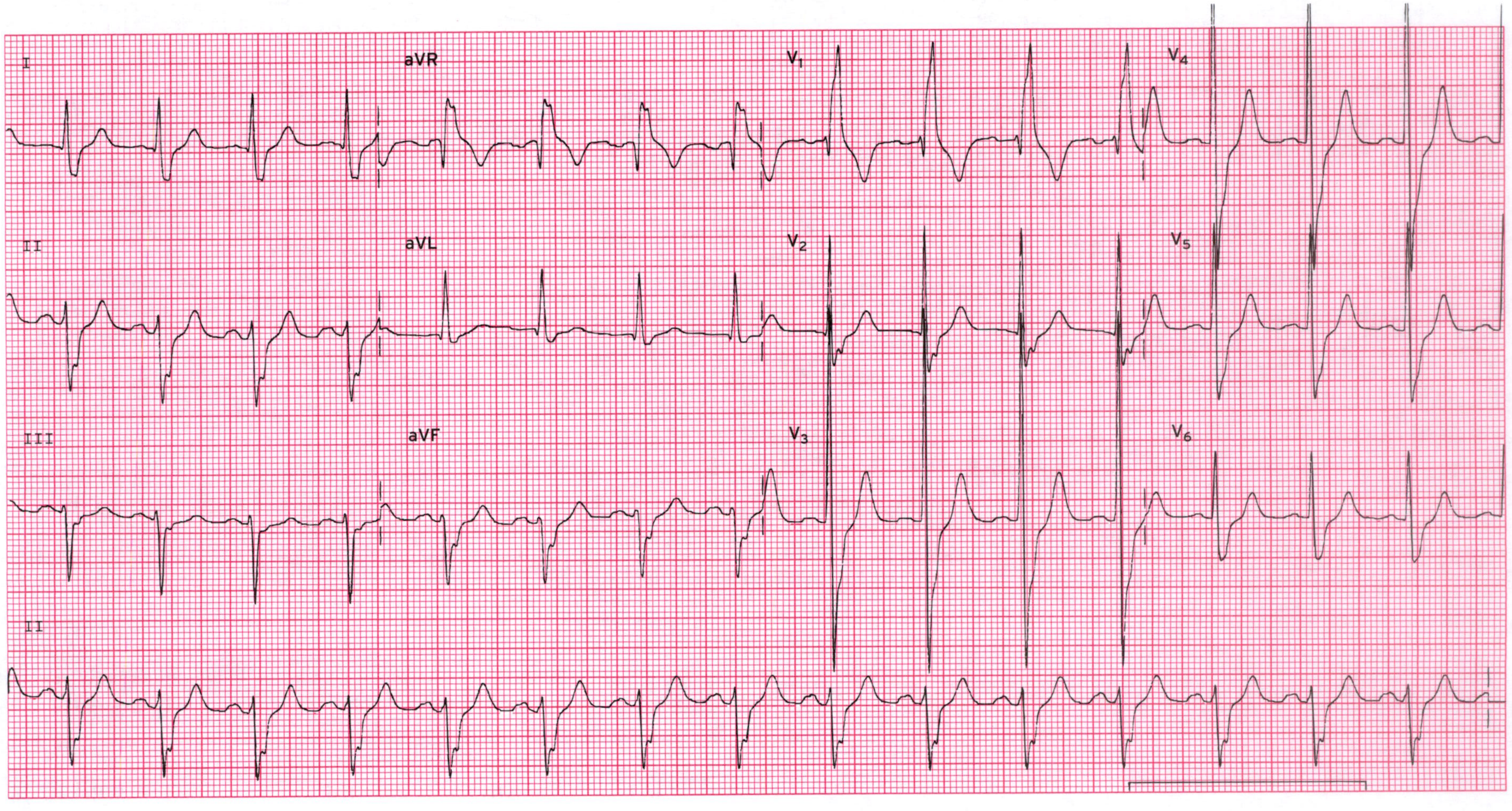

4. Rhythm and rate ________ PR ________ QRS ________ QT ___________

Axis __________________________ BBB __________________________

Hypertrophy ____

Miscellaneous effects ____

Infarction ____

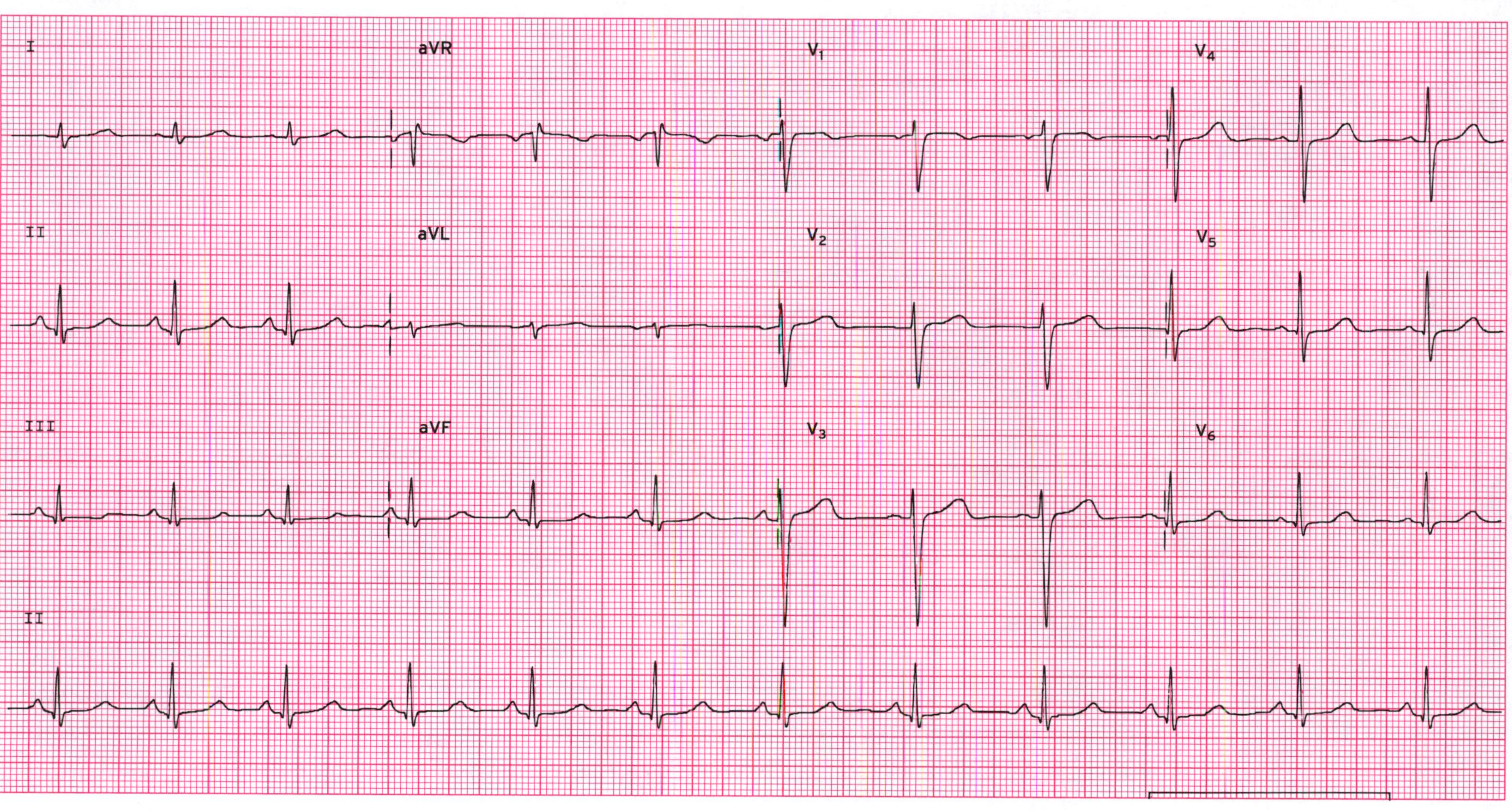

5. Rhythm and rate ________ PR ________ QRS ________ QT ________

Axis ________________ BBB ________________

Hypertrophy ________________________________

Miscellaneous effects ________________________________

Infarction ________________________________

6. Rhythm and rate ________ PR ________ QRS ________ QT ___________

Axis __________________________ BB ______________________________

Hypertrophy ____

Miscellaneous effects ____

Infarction ____

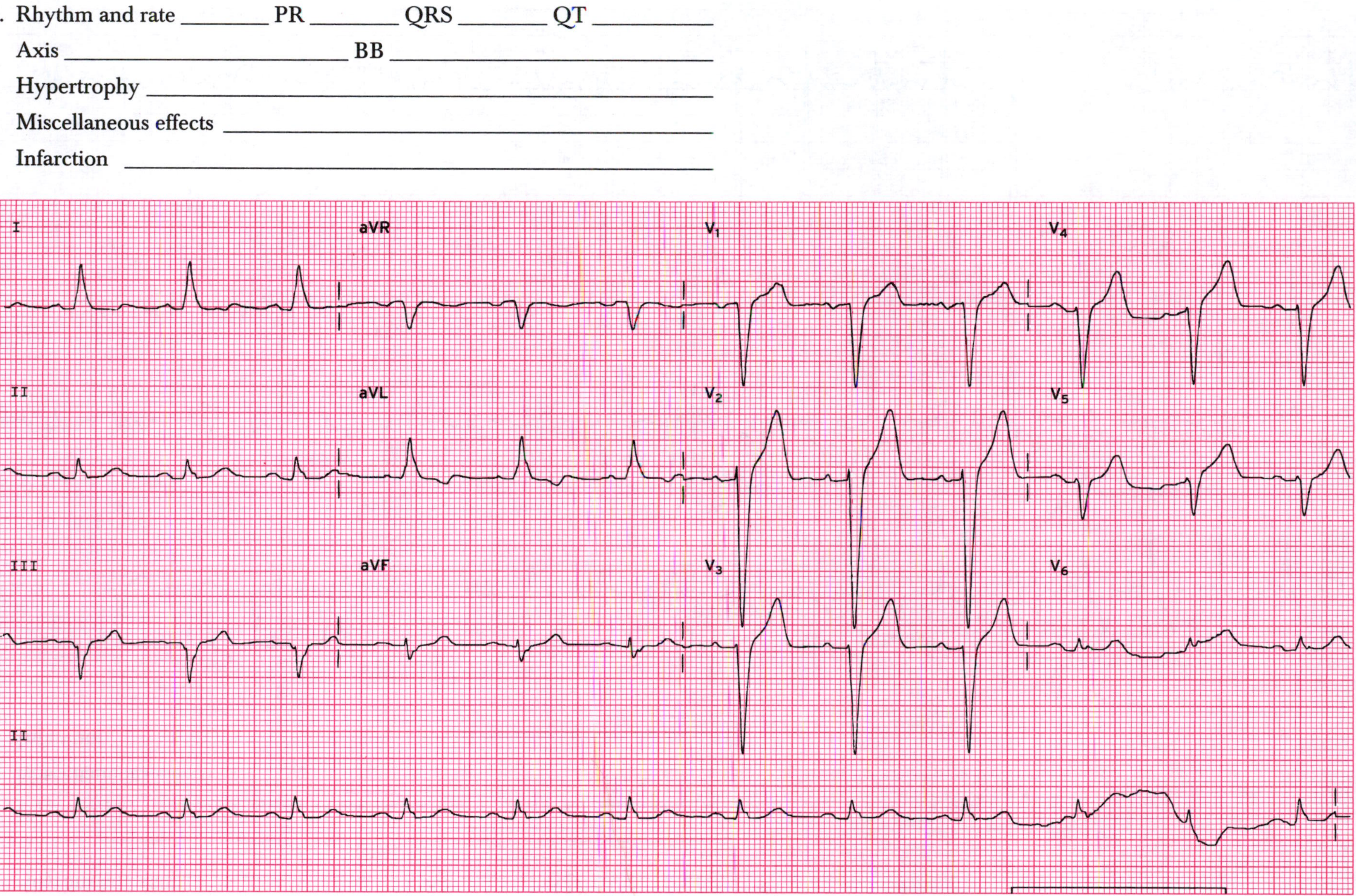

7. Rhythm and rate _______ PR _______ QRS _______ QT _________

Axis _________________________ BBB ___________________________

Hypertrophy ____

Miscellaneous effects ____

Infarction ____

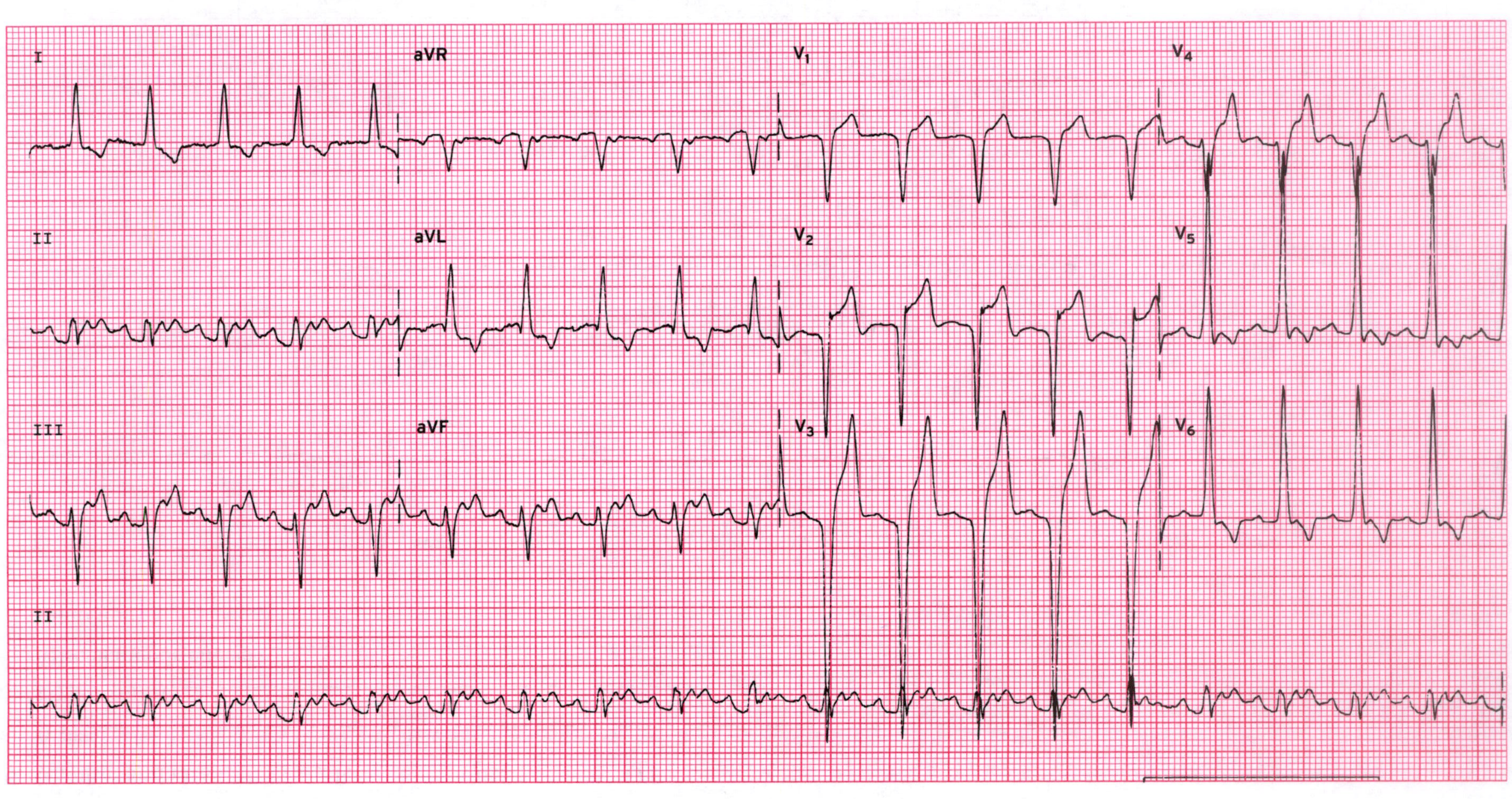

8. Rhythm and rate ________ PR ________ QRS ________ QT ___________

Axis ___________________________ BBB _____________________________

Hypertrophy ____

Miscellaneous effects ____

Infarction ____

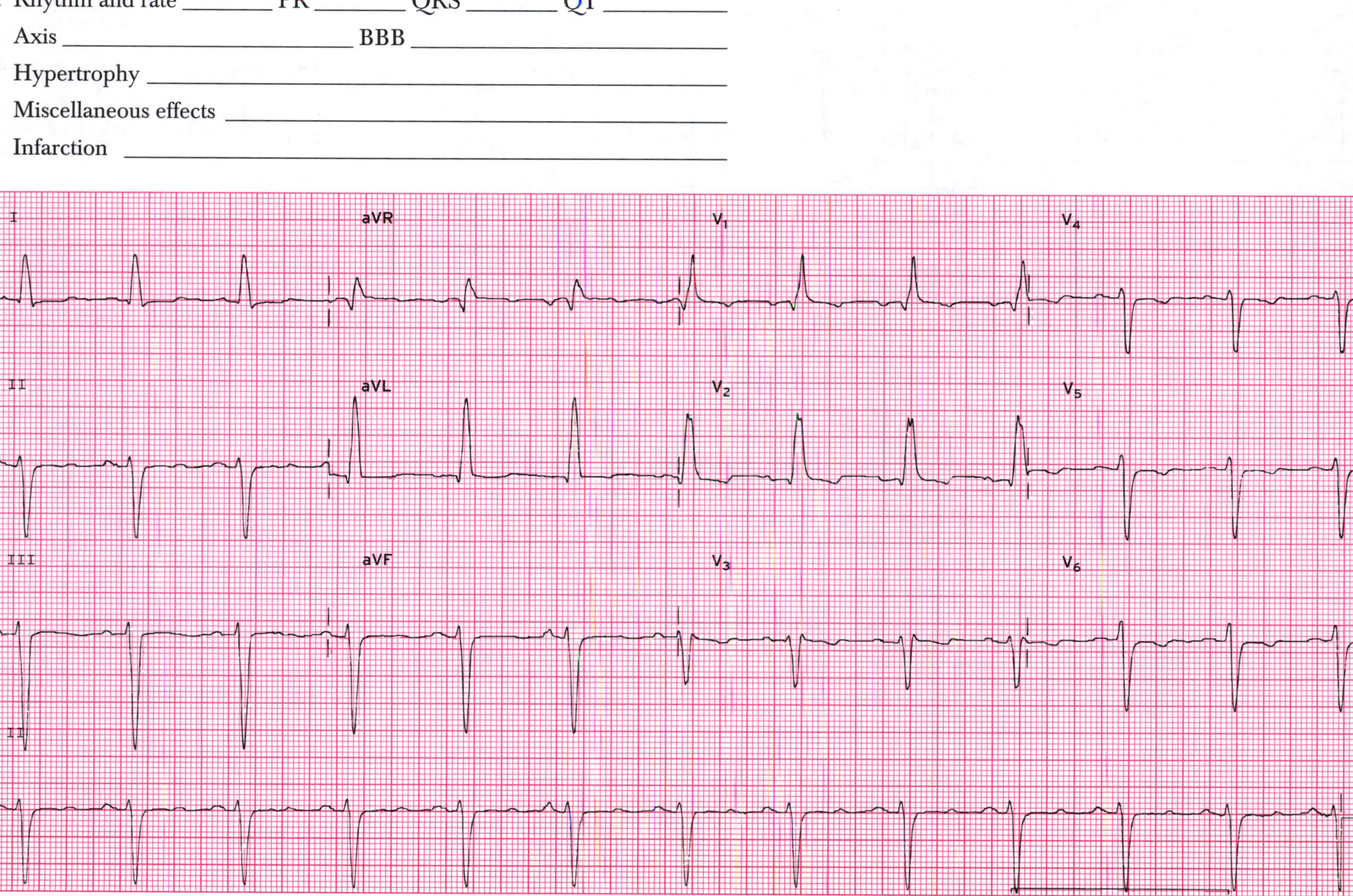

9. Rhythm and rate ________ PR ________ QRS ________ QT ___________
   Axis ___________________________ BBB ______________________________
   Hypertrophy ____
   Miscellaneous effects ____
   Infarction ____

I aVR V_1 V_4

II aVL V_2 V_5

III aVF V_3 V_6

II

10. Rhythm and rate ________ PR ________ QRS ________ QT ________

Axis ________________ BBB ________________

Hypertrophy ________________________________

Miscellaneous effects ________________________________

Infarction ________________________________

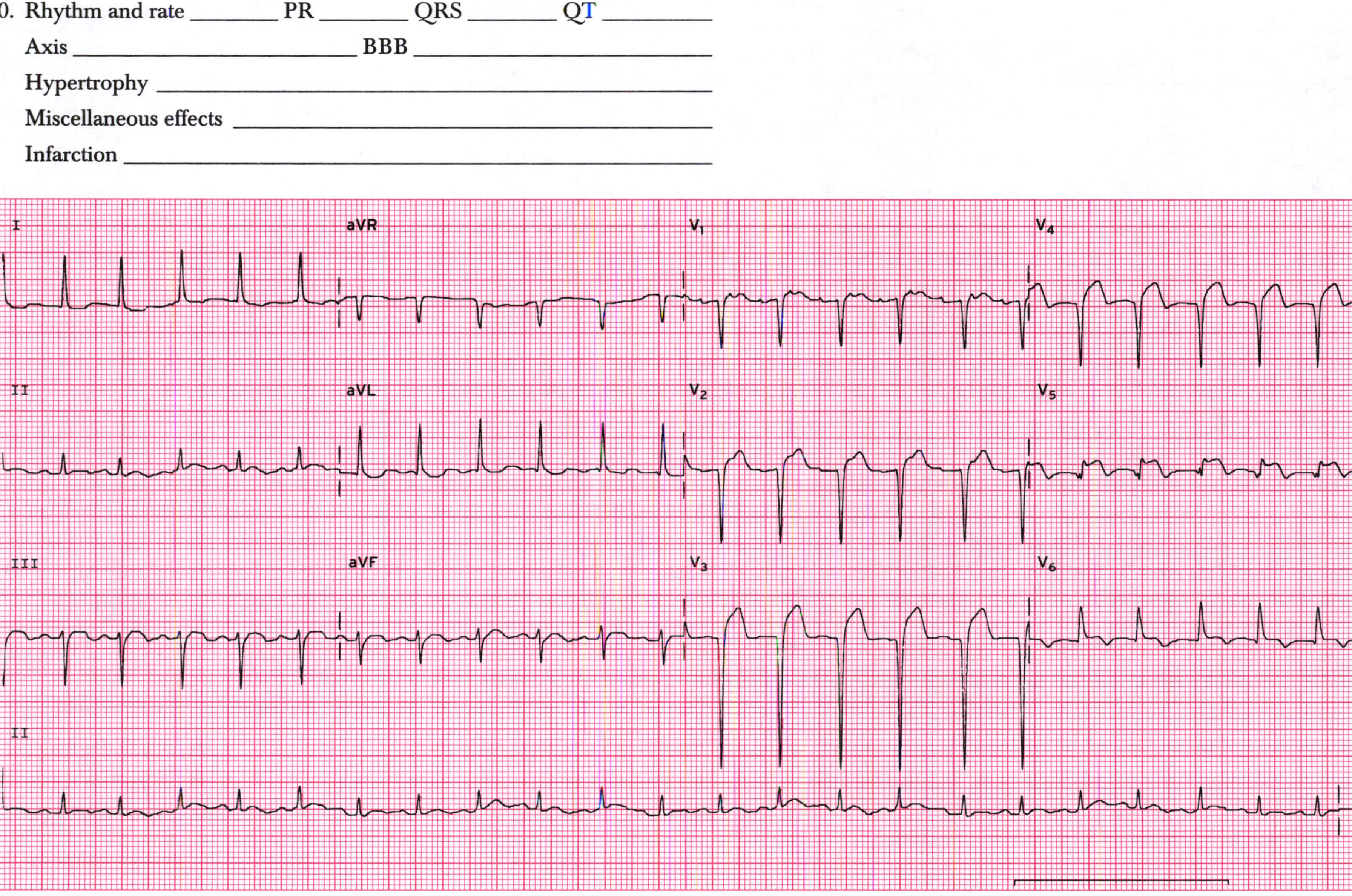

11. Rhythm and rate ________ PR ________ QRS ________ QT ________

Axis ________________________ BBB ________________________

Hypertrophy ____

Miscellaneous effects ______________________________________

Infarction ____

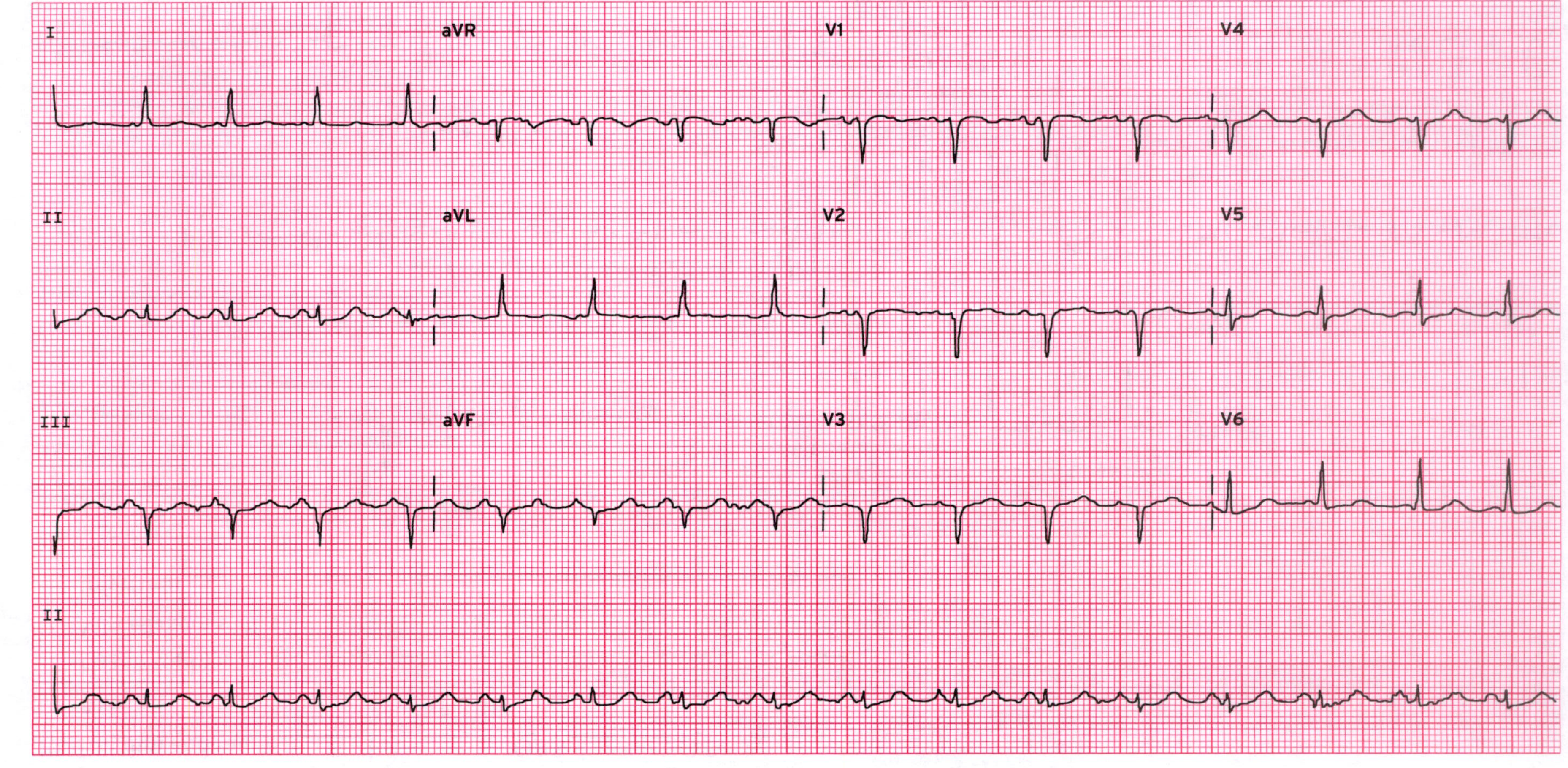

12. Rhythm and rate ________ PR ________ QRS ________ QT __________

Axis __________________________ BBB ___________________________

Hypertrophy ____

Miscellaneous effects ____

Infarction ____

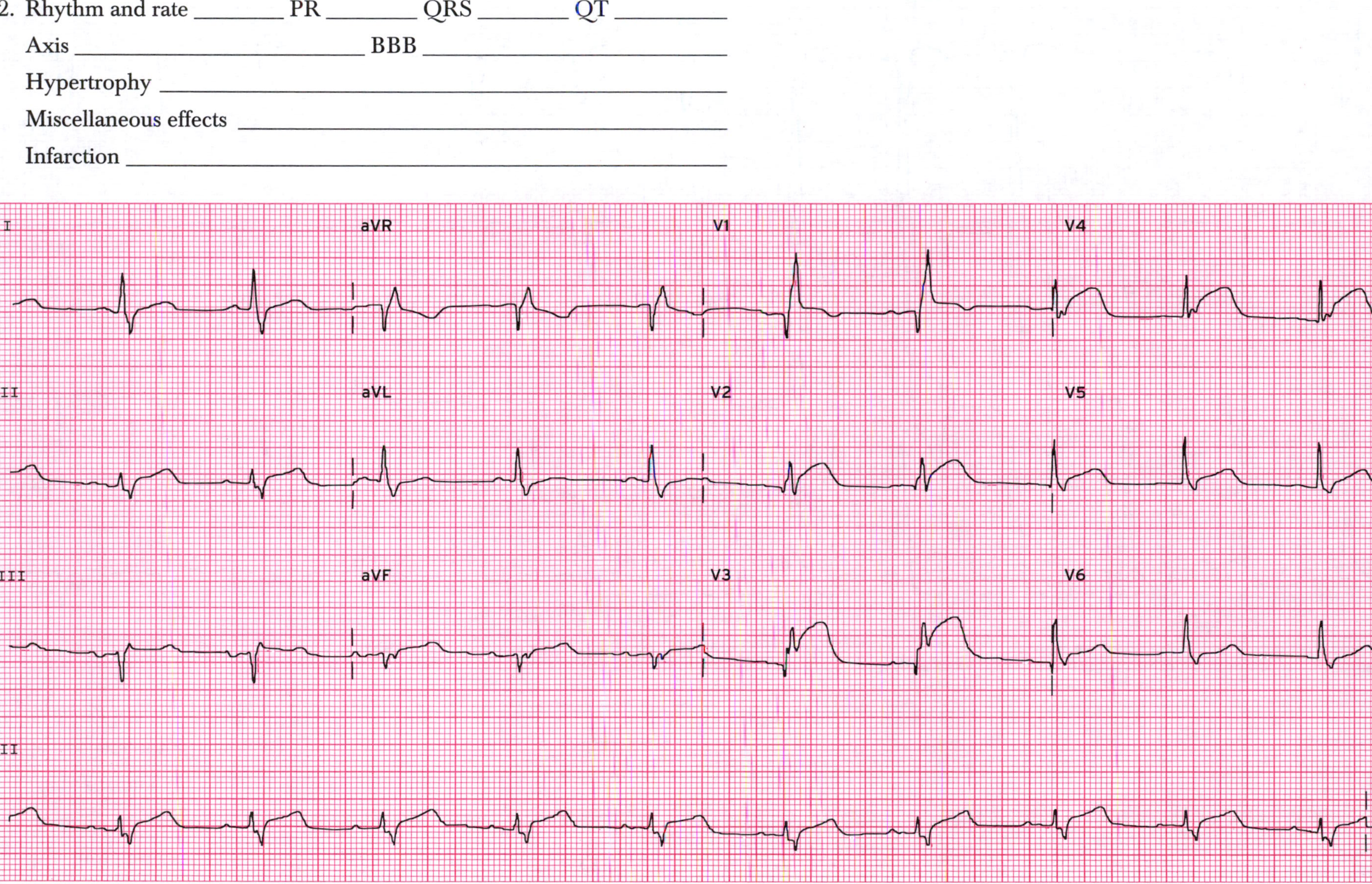

13. Rhythm and rate ________ PR ________ QRS ________ QT __________

Axis __________________________ BBB ___________________________

Hypertrophy ____

Miscellaneous effects ____

Infarction ____

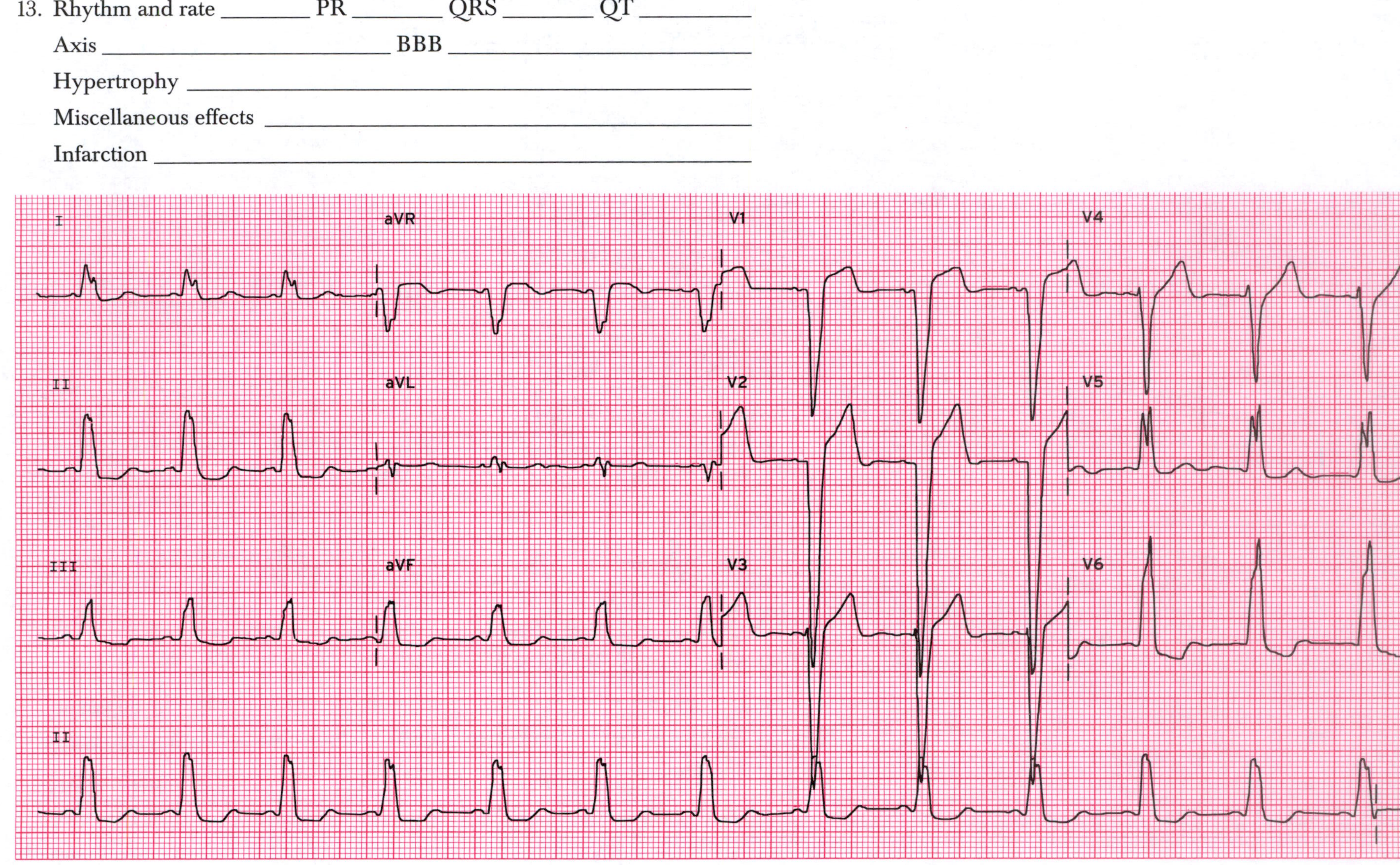

14. Rhythm and rate _______ PR _______ QRS _______ QT _________

Axis _________________________ BBB ___________________________

Hypertrophy ____

Miscellaneous effects ____

Infarction ____

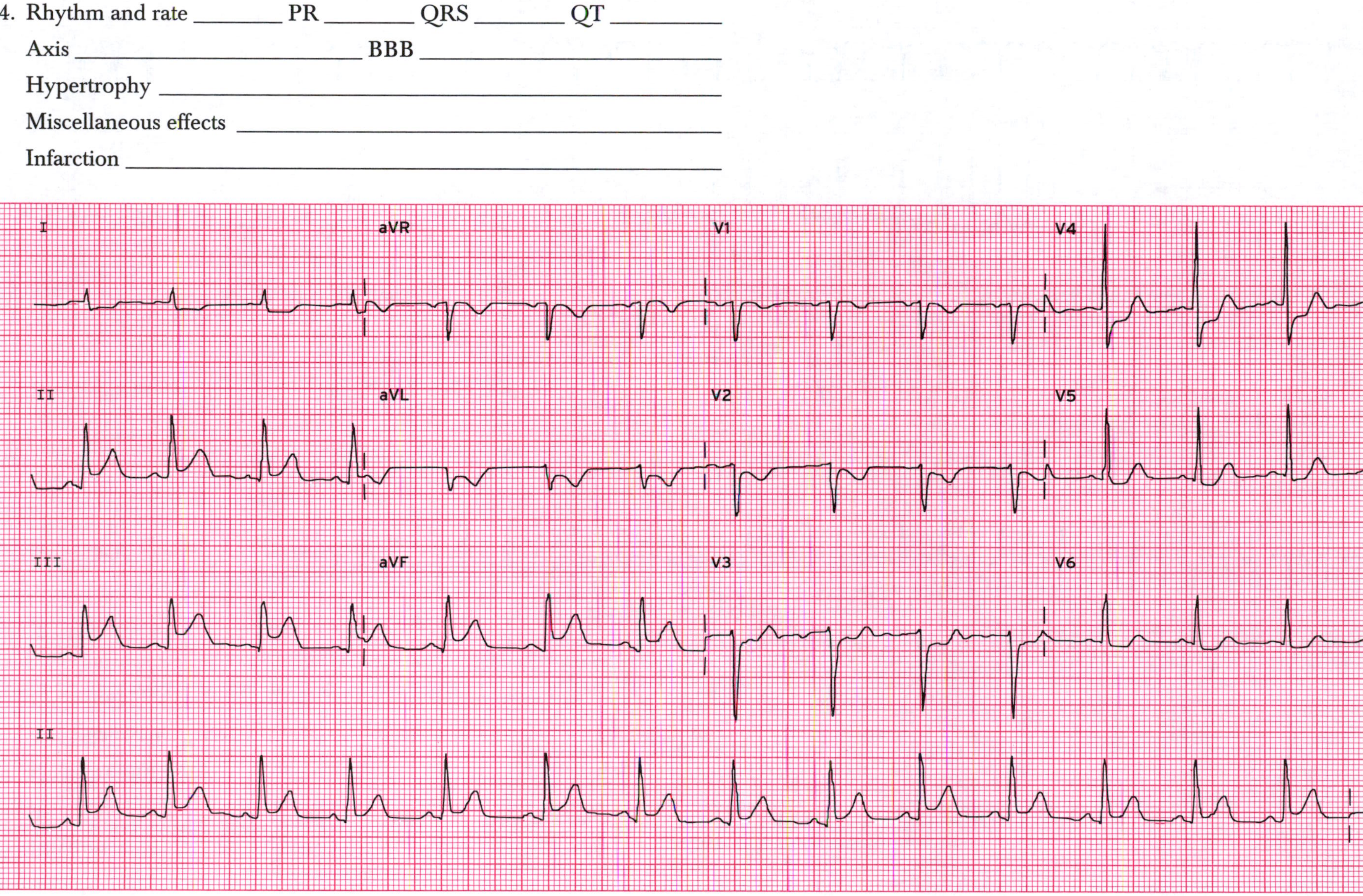

15. Rhythm and rate ________ PR ________ QRS ________ QT ________

Axis ____________________ BBB ____________________

Hypertrophy ____

Miscellaneous effects ____

Infarction ____

I aVR V1 V4

II aVL V2 V5

III aVF V3 V6

II

16. Rhythm and rate _______ PR _______ QRS _______ QT _________

Axis ________________________ BBB ________________________

Hypertrophy ____

Miscellaneous effects______________________________________

Infarction ____

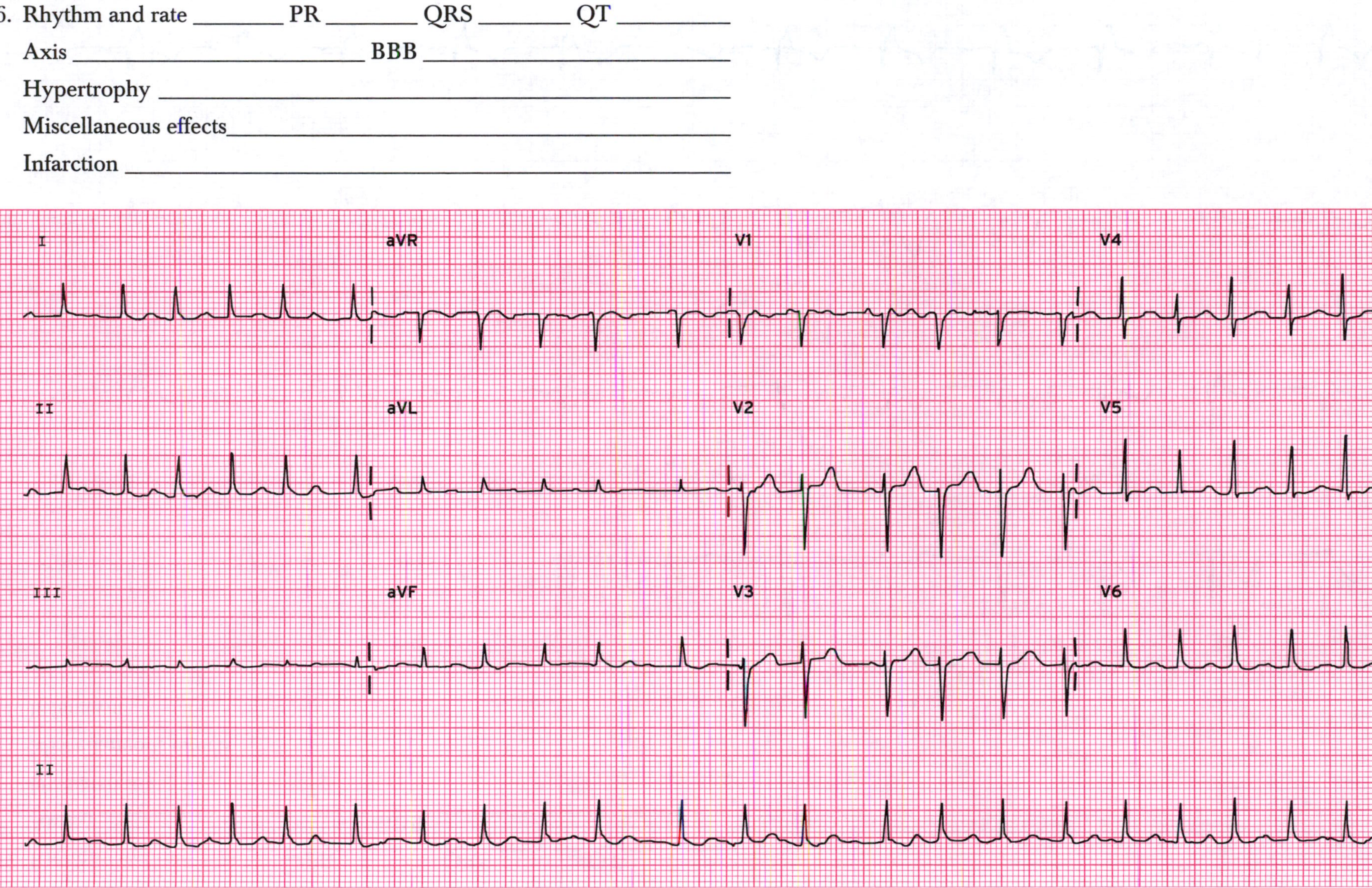

17. Rhythm and rate ________ PR________ QRS_______ QT_________

Axis __________________________ BBB__________________________

Hypertrophy ____

Miscellaneous effects ____

Infarction ____

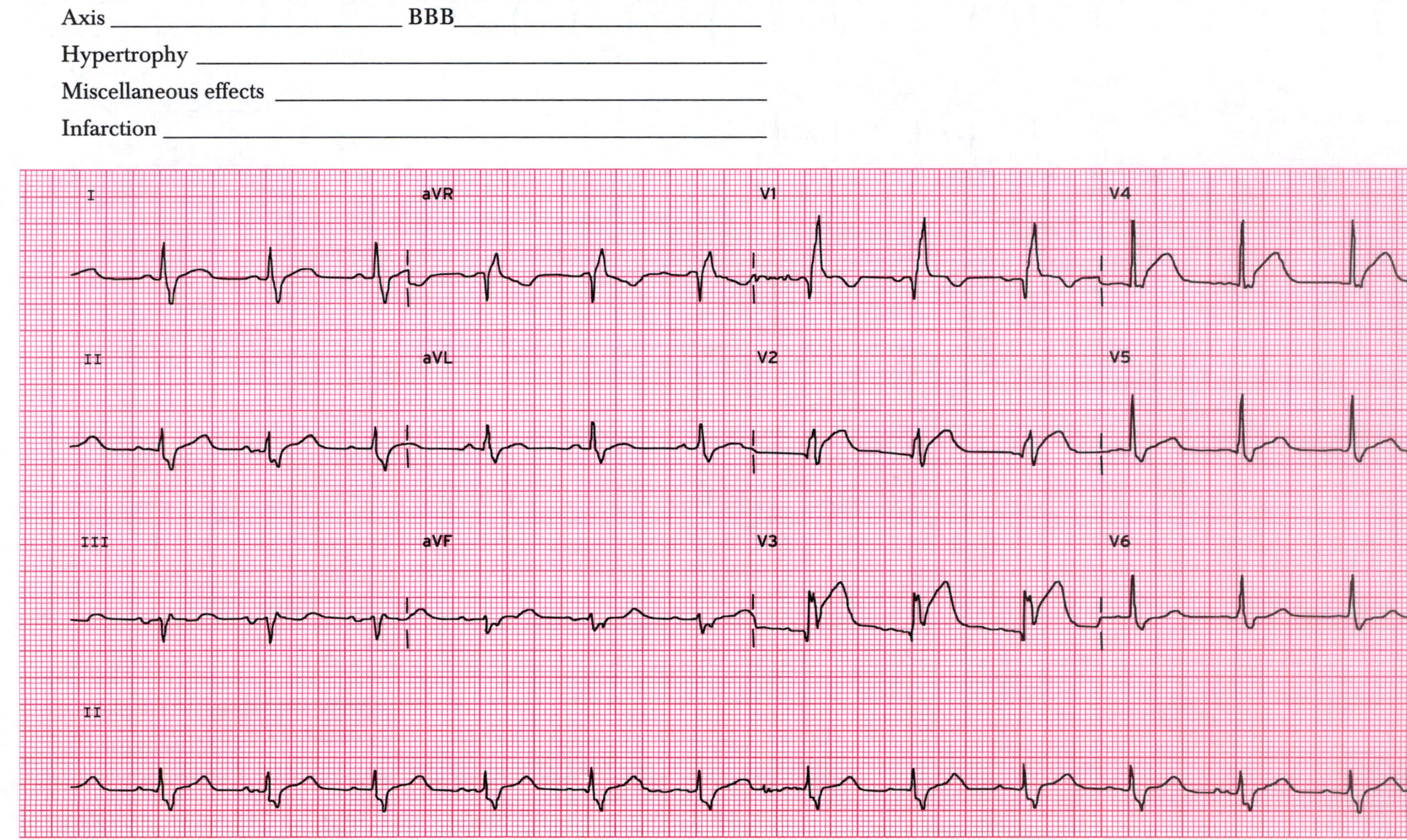

18. Rhythm and rate ________ PR________ QRS_______ QT_________

Axis ___________________________ BBB____________________________

Hypertrophy ____

Miscellaneous effects ______________________________________

Infarction ____

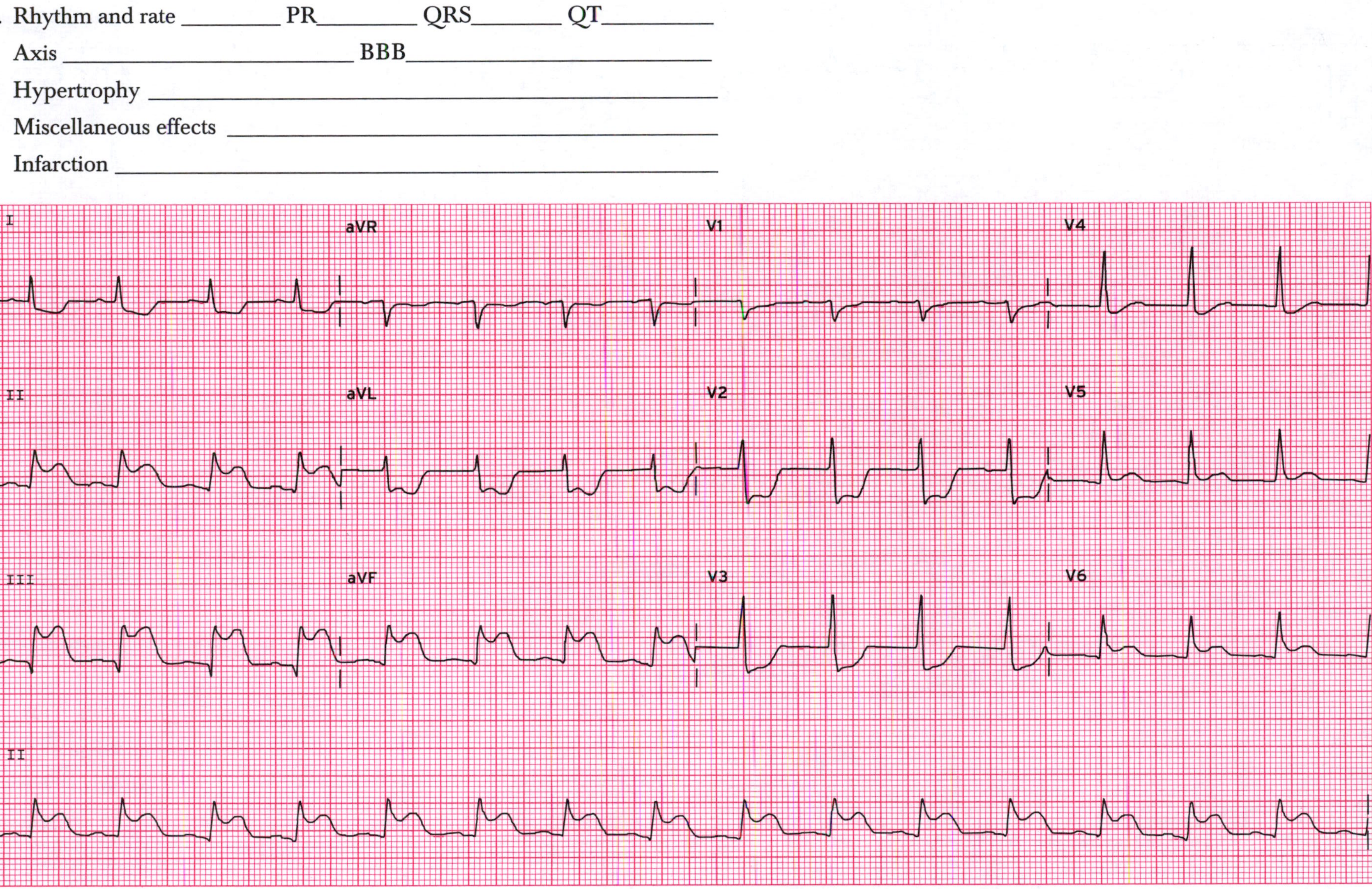

19. Rhythm and rate ________ PR________ QRS_______ QT_________

Axis _________________________ BBB__________________________

Hypertrophy ____

Miscellaneous effects ____

Infarction ____

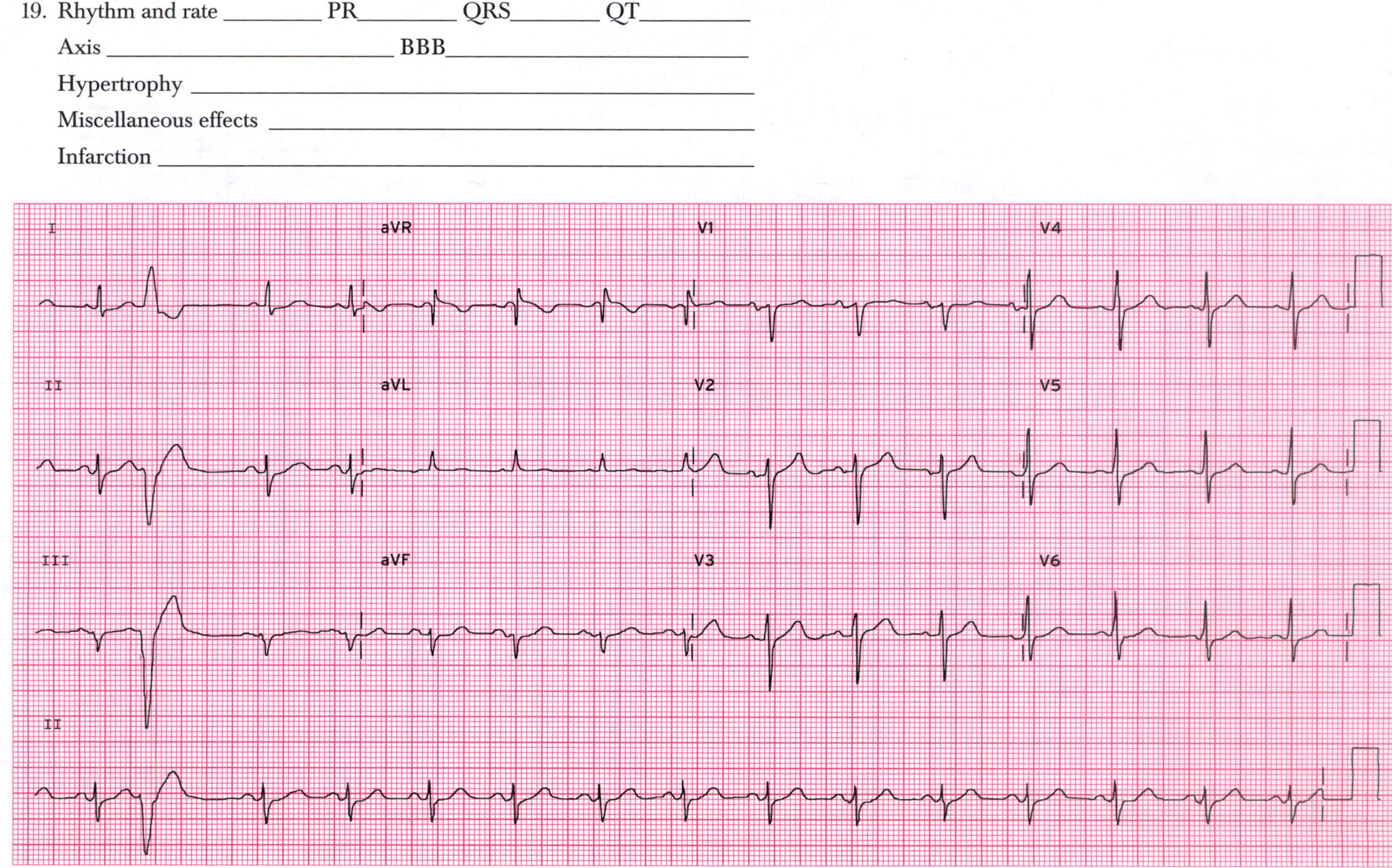

20. Rhythm and rate ________ PR________ QRS_______ QT_________

Axis ___________________________ BBB_____________________________

Hypertrophy ____

Miscellaneous effects ____

Infarction ____

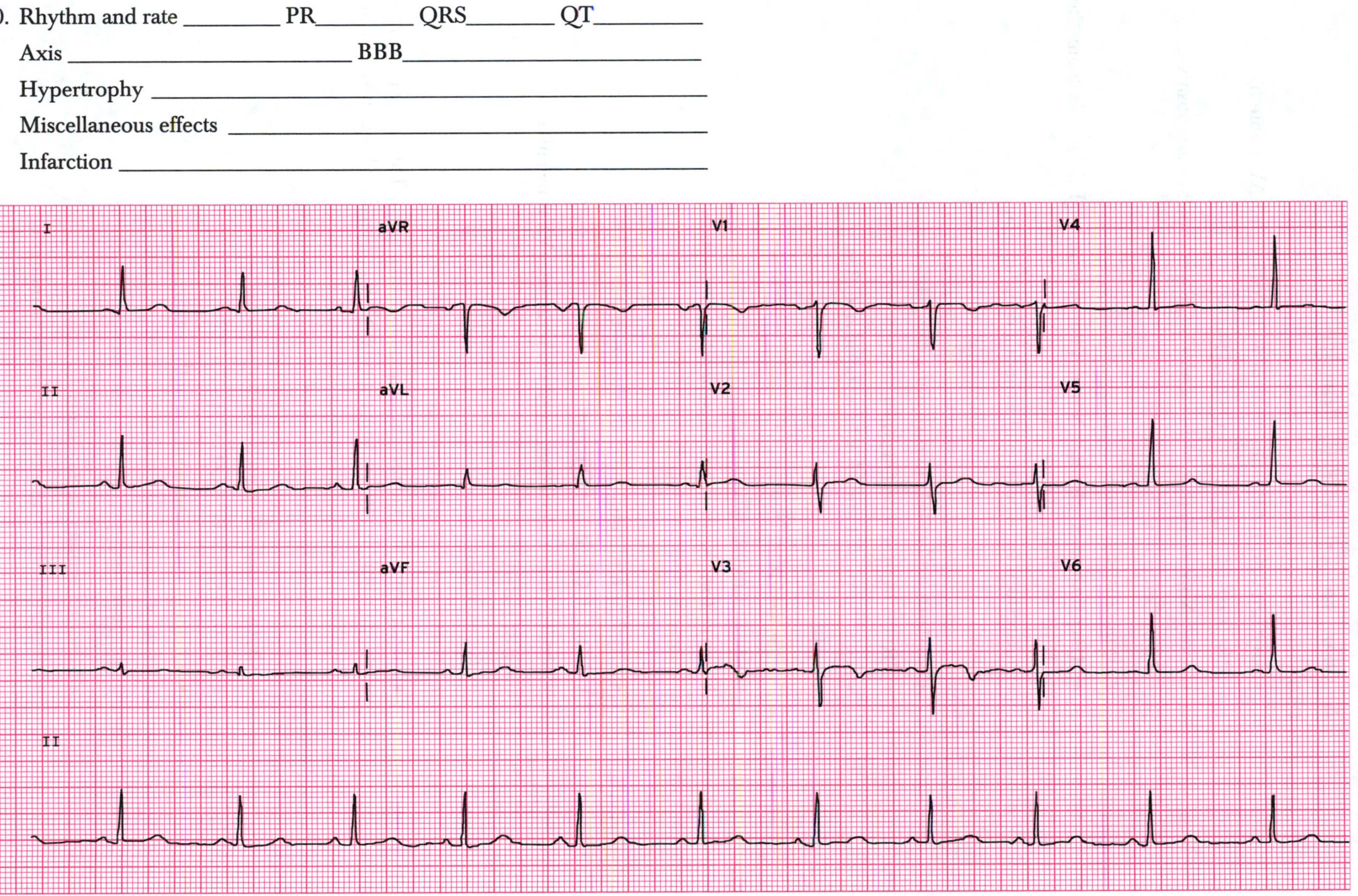

Answers to 12-Lead EKG Practice

EKG 1

- **Rhythm and rate:** Sinus rhythm with first-degree AVB, rate 62.
- **PR:** 0.20–0.24 **QRS:** 0.16 **QT:** 0.44–0.48
- **Axis:** Normal. Both lead I and aVF's QRS complexes are positive.
- **BBB:** Left bundle branch block.
- **Hypertrophy:** None.
- **Miscellaneous effects:** None. The widened QRS here is from the LBBB, not from hyperkalemia
- **Infarction:** No evidence of ischemia or infarction.

EKG 2

- **Rhythm and rate:** Sinus rhythm, rate 94.
- **PR:** 0.12 **QRS:** 0.06 **QT:** 0.34.
- **Axis:** Normal. I and aVF have positive QRSs.
- **BBB:** None.
- **Hypertrophy:** None.
- **Miscellaneous effects:** None.
- **Infarction:** No evidence of ischemia or infarction.

EKG 3

- **Rhythm and rate:** Sinus rhythm, rate 94.
- **PR:** 0.16 **QRS:** 0.14 **QT:** 0.40.
- **Axis:** Left axis deviation. Lead I is positive, aVF is negative.
- **BBB:** RBBB.
- **Hypertrophy:** None.
- **Miscellaneous effects:** None.
- **Infarction:** No evidence of ischemia or infarction. There is ST depression in many leads, but this is probably bundle-related rather than true ischemia.

EKG 4

- **Rhythm and rate:** Sinus rhythm, rate 68.
- **PR:** 0.16 **QRS:** 0.08 **QT:** 0.40
- **Axis:** Normal. I and aVF are both positive.
- **BBB:** None.
- **Hypertrophy:** None.
- **Miscellaneous effects:** None.
- **Infarction:** No evidence of ischemia or infarction.

EKG 5

- **Rhythm and rate:** Sinus tachycardia, rate 150.
- **PR:** 0.14 **QRS:** 0.06 **QT:** 0.24
- **Axis:** Normal
- **BBB:** None.
- **Hypertrophy:** None. In fact, the voltage is pretty low throughout most leads.
- **Miscellaneous** effects: None.
- **Infarction:** No evidence of ischemia or infarction. Those are not Q waves in V_1 to V_2, in case you thought it was an anteroseptal MI. There's a small R wave there.

EKG 6

- **Rhythm and rate:** Sinus rhythm, rate 71.
- **PR:** 0.20 **QRS:** 0.12 **QT:** 0.40
- **Axis:** Left axis deviation. Lead I is positive and aVF is negative.
- **BBB:** LBBB
- **Hypertrophy:** None
- **Miscellaneous effects:** None.
- **Infarction:** No evidence of ischemia or infarction.

EKG 7

- **Rhythm and rate:** Atrial flutter with 2:1 conduction? Atrial rate 250, ventricular rate 115.
- **PR:** 0.16 **QRS:** 0.10 **QT:** 0.28
- **Axis:** Left axis deviation. Lead I is positive and aVF is negative.
- **BBB:** No BBB. QRS too narow for a BBB.
- **Hypertrophy:** LVH by voltage criteria.
- **Miscellaneous effects:** No miscellaneous effects. The incredibly tall, pointy T wave in V_3 is related to the huge QRS voltage in that lead.
- **Infarction:** Anterior and inferior wall MI. Note the ST segment elevation in II, III, aVF, and V_1 to V_4. There are already significant Q waves in V_1 to V_3. This is a massive MI.

EKG 8

- **Rhythm and rate:** Sinus rhythm, rate 75.
- **PR:** 0.18 **QRS:** 0.13 **QT:** 0.42
- **Axis:** Left axis deviation. Lead I is positive, aVF is negative.
- **BBB:** RBBB.
- **Hypertrophy:** LVH. See how tall the R wave is in aVL? It's taller than 11 mm, so it meets the criteria for LVH.

- **Miscellaneous effects:** None.
- **Infarction:** Probable old anteroseptal MI, as there is a loss of the normal small R wave in V_1 to V_2.

EKG 9

- **Rhythm and rate:** Sinus rhythm, rate 65.
- **PR:** 0.18 **QRS:** 0.06 **QT:** 0.36
- **Axis:** Nornal. Lead I and aVF are both positive.
- **BBB:** None.
- **Hypertrophy:** None, but very close to meeting voltage criteria for LVH.
- **Miscellaneous effects:** None.
- **Infarction:** Probable early repolarization. Note the very slight concave ST elevation in II, III, aVF, and V_3 to V_5. It would help to know the age of this patient and the symptoms (if any) to identify this with a higher probability of accuracy.

EKG 10

- **Rhythm and rate:** Atrial flutter with 2:1 conduction. No way, you say? Look at V_1. See the spike in the ST segment? That's a flutter wave. There's another one before the QRS. Atrial rate is about 250, ventricular rate is 125.
- **PR:** Not applicable **QRS:** 0.06 **QT:** 0.24
- **Axis:** Left axis deviation. Lead I is positive and aVF is negative.
- **BBB:** None.
- **Hypertrophy:** None. In fact, the voltage is rather low in the frontal leads.
- **Miscellaneous effects:** None.
- **Infarction:** Acute anterior-lateral MI. Note the ST elevation in V_1 to V_6. There are significant Q waves in V_1 to V_5. There is also *very slight* ST coving in III and aVF, so there may also be an inferior MI starting up.

EKG 11

- **Rhythm and rate:** Sinus tachycardia, rate 101.
- **PR:** 0.12 **QRS:** 0.06 **QT:** 0.32
- **Axis:** Left axis deviation. Lead I is positive and aVF is negative.
- **BBB:** None.
- **Hypertrophy:** None
- **Miscellaneous effects:** None.
- **Infarction:** Old inferior MI and old anterior MI. Note the significant Q waves in leads III and aVF and also in V_2–V_3.

EKG 12

- **Rhythm and rate:** Sinus rhythm, rate 60.
- **PR:** 0.20 **QRS:** 0.14 **QT:** 0.46
- **Axis:** Left axis deviation. Lead I is positive and aVF is negative.
- **BBB:** RBBB. There is a QR configuration in V_1.
- **Hypertrophy:** None
- **Miscellaneous effects:** None.
- **Infarction:** Acute anterior-lateral MI. Note the ST elevation in V_1 to V_5. There are significant Q waves in V_1 to V_3.

EKG 13

- **Rhythm and rate:** Sinus rhythm, rate 75.
- **PR:** 0.12 **QRS:** 0.14 **QT:** 0.42
- **Axis:** Normal.
- **BBB:** LBBB. Note the **HUGE** QS wave in V_1.
- **Hypertrophy:** None.
- **Miscellaneous effects:** None.
- **Infarction:** None.

EKG 14

- **Rhythm and rate:** Sinus rhythm, rate 83.
- **PR:** 0.14 **QRS:** 0.08 **QT:** 0.34.
- **Axis:** Normal.
- **BBB:** None.
- **Hypertrophy:** None.
- **Miscellaneous effects:** None.
- **Infarction:** Acute inferior MI. Note the ST elevation in II, III, and aVF along with reciprocal ST depression in I, aVL, and $V_{2–6}$.

EKG 15

- **Rhythm and rate:** Atrial fibrillation with uncontrolled ventricular response.
- **PR:** Not applicable **QRS:** 0.04 **QT:** 0.16.
- **Axis:** Normal.
- **BBB:** None.
- **Hypertrophy:** None. In fact, the voltage is rather low in the frontal leads.
- **Miscellaneous effects:** Digitalis effect? ST segments look a bit scooped in leads II and V_6. This may be simply from the rapid heart rate, however.
- **Infarction:** None.

EKG 16

- **Rhythm and rate:** Atrial fibrillation.
- **PR:** Not applicable **QRS:** 0.06 **QT:** 0.28
- **Axis:** Normal.
- **BBB:** None.
- **Hypertrophy:** None. In fact, the voltage is rather low in the frontal leads.
- **Miscellaneous effects:** None.
- **Infarction:** None.

EKG 17

- **Rhythm and rate:** Sinus rhythm, rate 75.
- **PR:** 0.16 **QRS:** 0.14 **QT:** 0.40.
- **Axis:** Left axis deviation. Lead I is slightly more positive than negative and aVF is slightly more negative than positive.
- **BBB:** RBBB.
- **Hypertrophy:** None.
- **Miscellaneous effects:** None.
- **Infarction:** Acute anterior MI. Note the ST elevation in V_{2-4}.

EKG 18

- **Rhythm and rate:** Sinus rhythm, rate 94.
- **PR:** 0.16 **QRS:** 0.10 **QT:** 0.36
- **Axis:** Normal. AVF's QRS has a little blip downward, then is positive.
- **BBB:** None.
- **Hypertrophy:** None.
- **Miscellaneous effects:** None.
- **Infarction:** Acute inferior-lateral MI. Note the ST elevation in II, III, aVF and V_{5-6}.

EKG 19

- **Rhythm and rate:** Sinus rhythm, rate 88, with one PVC.
- **PR:** 0.12 **QRS:** 0.08 **QT:** 0.32
- **Axis:** Left axis deviation. Lead I is positive and aVF is negative.
- **BBB:** None.
- **Hypertrophy:** None. In fact, the voltage is rather low in the frontal leads.
- **Miscellaneous effects:** None.
- **Infarction:** None.

EKG 20

- **Rhythm and rate:** Sinus rhythm, rate 65.
- **PR:** 0.16 **QRS:** 0.06 **QT:** 0.36.
- **Axis:** Normal.
- **BBB:** None.
- **Hypertrophy:** None
- **Miscellaneous effects:** None.
- **Infarction:** None.

CHAPTER **17**

Cardiac Medications and Electrical Therapy

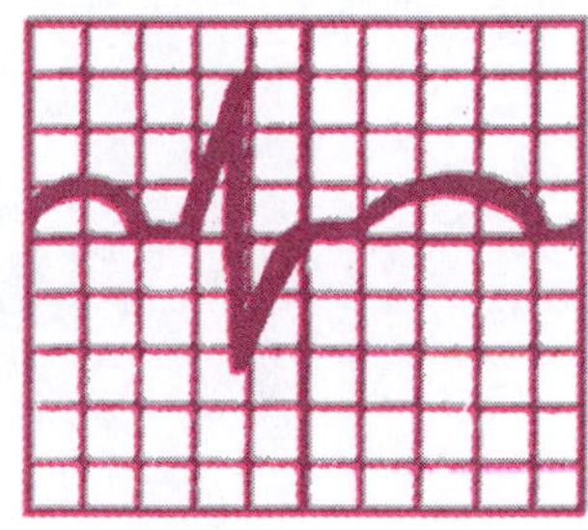

Chapter 17 Objectives

Upon completion of this chapter, the student will be able to:

- Describe the effect of each class of antiarrhythmic medication on the action potential.
- Give examples of each class of antiarrhythmic medication.
- Describe the effects of digitalis and adenosine on the heart rate.
- Name the emergency medications and describe the mode of action of each.
- Describe the danger of giving supplemental oxygen to patients with chronic lung disease.

Cardiac Medications

Cardiac medications are used to treat dysrhythmias or abnormalities in cardiac function. Let's look at the various classifications of medications.

Antiarrhythmics

These medications are used to treat and/or prevent dysrhythmias. They all affect the action potential. See Figure 17-1 for the effects of each class on the action potential. There are four classes of antiarrhythmic medications. Let's look at the four classes.

Class I: Sodium Channel Blockers

Class I medications block the influx of sodium ions into the cardiac cell during depolarization. This results in decreased excitability of the cardiac cell and decreased myocardial contractility. Class I antiarrhythmic medications affect phase 0 of the action potential. There are three categories of class I antiarrhythmics:

- **Class Ia.** These medications include *quinidine* and *procainamide*, and they cause prolonged QT interval as well as decreased cardiac contractility. They can also cause hypotension. Quinidine is especially notorious for causing wide T waves. Most class Ia antiarrhythmics can be used to treat supraventricular as well as ventricular arrhythmias. Quinidine is usually given orally. In rare instances it may be given intravenously. Procainamide can be given orally or intravenously.

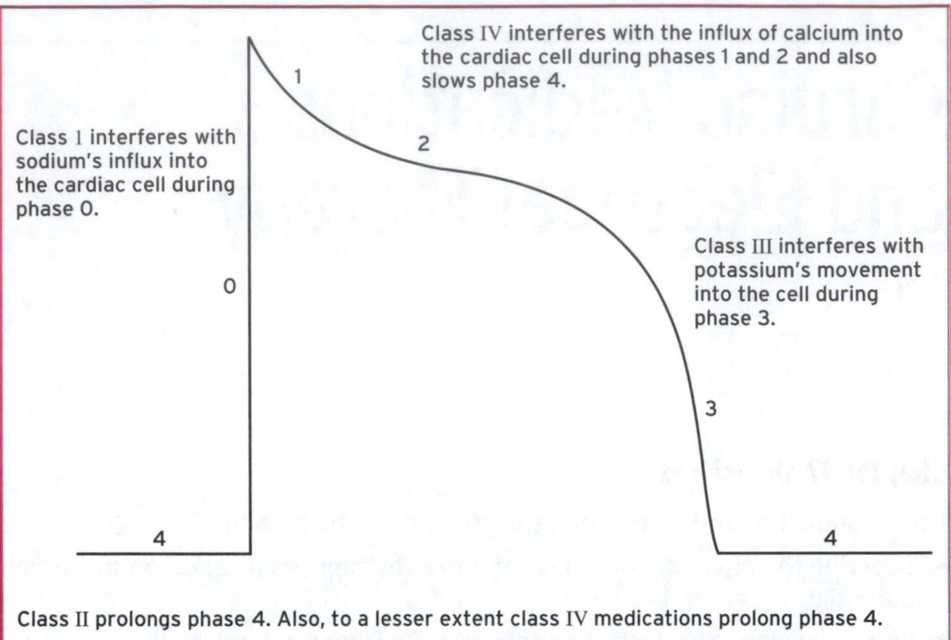

Figure 17-1 Effects of each class of antiarrhythmic medications on the action potential.

- **Class Ib.** These medications include *lidocaine* and *tocainide,* both of which have a local anesthetic effect. They are used for treatment of ventricular arrhythmias only. They suppress the ventricles' irritability and raise the fibrillatory threshold, making it less likely the ventricles will fibrillate. Class Ib medications have minimal, if any, effect on conductivity. Lidocaine is given intravenously. Tocainide is given orally.
- **Class Ic.** These medications slow impulse conduction and are useful in treating SVT and ventricular arrhythmias. Unfortunately, they are also very prone to causing arrhythmias and are therefore used only in life-threatening situations. These medications include *flecainide* and *propafenone,* both of which are given orally.

Class II: Beta-Blockers

Beta-blockers slow the heart rate by blocking the sympathetic nervous system's beta receptors. There are two kinds of beta receptors: *Beta-1 receptors* increase heart rate, conductivity, and contractility. *Beta-2 receptors* relax smooth muscle in arteries and bronchi. Blocking these receptors decreases or blocks these actions. Beta-blockers decrease the automaticity of the sinus node, slow AV conduction, and slow the process of depolarization. They are used to treat supraventricular tachyarrhythmias. They depress phase 4 of the action potential. Beta-blockers include medications such as *propranolol* and *atenolol.* Propranolol can be given orally or intravenously. Atenolol is given orally. Beta-blockers should be used with caution in patients with asthma or heart failure, as the effects could be life threatening.

Class III: Potassium Channel Blockers

These medications interfere with the movement of potassium ions into the cardiac cell during phase 3 of the action potential. They therefore can prolong the PR, QRS, and QT intervals. Class III medications can be used to treat supraventricular and/or ventricular arrhythmias. Medications include *amiodarone,* which is used to treat ventricular and supraventricular tachyarrhythmias, and *ibutilide,* used for supraventricular tachyarrhythmias. Amiodarone can be given orally or intravenously. Ibutilide is given intravenously.

Class IV: Calcium Channel Blockers

These medications interfere with the influx of calcium into the cardiac cell during phases 1 and 2 of the action potential and also slow phase 4 of the action potential. Thus, AV conduction is prolonged and contractility decreased. The PR interval will prolong and the heart rate will slow. Calcium blockers are used for supraventricular arrhythmias. Medications include *verapamil* and *diltiazem,* both of which can be given orally or intravenously.

There are other antiarrhythmic medications that do not fall into any of the four classes. These include but are not limited to *adenosine,* which is used to treat SVT, and *digitalis,* classified as a cardiac glycoside, which is used to treat heart failure and supraventricular arrhythmias.

Let's summarize the antiarrhythmic medications. See Table 17-1.

Table 17-1 Antiarrhythmic Medications Summary

CLASS	KNOWN AS	MODE OF ACTION	EXAMPLES	KIND OF DYSRHYTHMIAS TREATED
I	Sodium channel blockers	Block sodium's influx into the cardiac cell, decrease myocardial excitability and contractility	*Ia.* Quinidine, procainamide *Ib.* Lidocaine, tocainide *Ic.* Flecainide, propafenone	*Ia.* Supraventricular and ventricular *Ib.* Ventricular only *Ic.* Supraventricular and ventricular
II	Beta-blockers	Block the sympathetic nervous system's beta receptors, slow the heart rate	Propranolol , atenolol	Supraventricular
III	Potassium channel blockers	Decrease potassium's movement into the cardiac cell, prolong PR, QRS, and QT intervals	Amiodarone, bretylium, ibutilide	Ventricular *or* supraventricular
IV	Calcium channel blockers	Decrease calcium's influx into the cardiac cell, slow AV, conduction,decrease contractility	Verapamil, diltiazem	Supraventricular

Emergency Cardiac Medications

These medications are used during cardiac arrest or in situations in which the patient's condition is rapidly deteriorating because of a dysrhythmia.

- **Atropine.** Atropine is used to increase the heart rate during asystole or bradycardias. It reverses any vagal influence that could slow or stop the heart. It is usually given intravenously, but in situations in which there is no IV line in place, it can be given via the **endotracheal tube,** a breathing tube inserted into the trachea by way of the nose or mouth.
- **Epinephrine.** Epinephrine causes vasoconstriction (narrowing of the arteries), thus increasing the blood pressure, and beta receptor stimulation, thus restoring the heartbeat in cardiac arrest. It is given intravenously (or endotracheally if an IV line is not in place) and is used for asystole, v-fib, pulseless v-tach, pulseless electrical activity, and profound bradycardias.
- **Amiodarone.** A class III antiarrhythmic, Amiodarone has become the first-line medication for treatment of ventricular fibrillation and pulseless ventricular tachycardia. Additionally, it can be used to treat supraventriular arrhythmias as well. It is given intravenously during an emergency and can later be given by mouth to prevent dysrhythmia recurrences.
- **Adenosine.** Adenosine is used in emergency situations to convert supraventricular tachycardias back to sinus, or to slow the heart rate to a more tolerable level if conversion is not possible. It is given intravenously in emergency situations and can have the unnerving side effect of causing transient asystole of six or seven seconds before the rhythm coverts to sinus. Adenosine cannot be given endotracheally.
- **Sodium bicarbonate.** This medication combats the acidity of the blood caused by lactic acid buildup in a cardiac arrest situation. Lactic acid builds up in an anaerobic (oxygen-deprived) environment. Cardiac arrest produces just such an environment. Combating this acidity can help convert dyshythmias back to normal in a cardiac arrest.
- **Isoproterenol (Isuprel).** Isuprel was once a first-line drug used to treat cardiac arrest and bradycardias. It has fallen out of favor in recent years because it causes a monumental increase in the heart's oxygen consumption and can extend the size of an MI. Nowadays, it is used only as a last resort to treat symptomatic bradycardias that are resistant to atropine and epinephrine. It is turned off once a pacemaker can be utilized. Isuprel is given by continuous intravenous infusion. It cannot be given endotracheally.
- **Oxygen.** Though most people do not think of oxygen as a medication, when it is used to treat disease or a medical condition it is indeed a medication. And, like any medication, oxygen has its benefits and its risks. Oxygen is used in emergency situations to provide the tissues with the oxygen they are lacking. This alone can help convert dysrhythmias back to normal. Oxygen can be given by mask, nasal cannula (small prongs in the nose), endotracheal tube, and **tracheostomy** (surgically inserting a tube through the neck into the trachea).

Table 17-2 Emergency Medications Summary

MEDICATION	MODE OF ACTION	INDICATION
Atropine	Increases heart rate	Bradycardias, asystole
Epinephrine	Stimulates contractility, increases heart rate and BP	Cardiac arrest, bradycardias
Amiodarone	Helps convert rapid ventricular and supraventricular dysrhythmias back to sinus	Rapid ventricular dysrhythmias, PVCs, supraventricular dysrhythmias
Adenosine	Decreases heart rate	Supraventricular tachycardias
Sodium bicarbonate	Decreases blood's acidity	Cardiac arrest with acidosis
Isoproterenol	Increases heart rate	Bradycardias resistant to atropine and epinephrine
Oxygen	Increases tissue oxygenation	Symptomatic dysrhythmias, cardiac arrest

Let's summarize the emergency medications. See Table 17-2.

Electrical Therapy

Electrical therapy involves shocking the heart out of a dangerous or unstable rhythm into a more acceptable one, preferably sinus. There are two kinds of electrical therapy–cardioversion and defibrillation.

Cardioversion

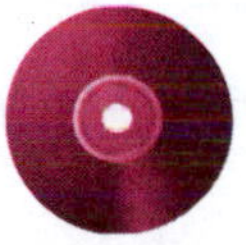

The word **cardioversion** means changing the heart (see CD-ROM for a video on the topic of cardioversion). Electrical cardioversion is usually performed to convert supraventricular tachycardias back to sinus, but it can also be used for ventricular tachycardia, provided the patient has a pulse. (Pulseless V-tach requires defibrillation, not cardioversion). The goal here is to interrupt an abnormal electrical circuit within the heart that is allowing a dysrhythmia to continue. Electrical cardioversion is performed using a defibrillator that can be set to "synchronous" mode. *Synchronizing is what differentiates cardioversion from defibrillation.* Once the synchronizer button is activated on the defibrillator, the machine delays delivery of the shock until it has synchronized with the patient's QRS complexes. The shock must be delivered at a critical point in the cardiac cycle. **If a shock is delivered at the wrong point in the cardiac cycle, it can put the patient into ventricular fibrillation**–not a good thing if the patient was just in SVT. Perhaps the most critical thing to know about cardioversion is **when not to use it**: Do not try to cardiovert v-fib–this rhythm requires defibrillation. **Turn the synchronizer button off when defibrillating or the shock will not be delivered!**

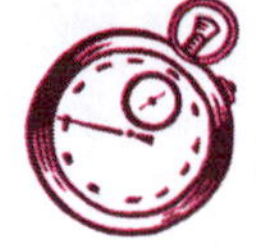

QuickTip

If the rhythm is **v-fib** you must **defib**!

Defibrillation

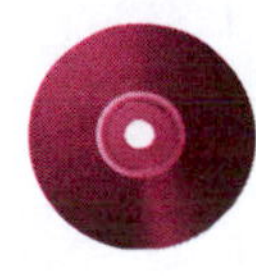

Defibrillation differs from cardioversion in that the shock is delivered immediately upon pressing the button (see CD-ROM for a video on the topic of defibrillation). There is no synchronizing in defibrillation. And the electrical current delivered tends to be much larger, causing the entire myocardium to depolarize at once. This interrupts the abnormal rhythm and causes a brief asystole, after which the hope is that the heart's normal automaticity will allow it to restart with normal conduction. **Defibrillation is the treatment for ventricular fibrillation and pulseless ventricular tachycardia.** There are several kinds of defibrillators: the monitor/defibrillator used in hospitals, AICDs (automated internal cardioverter-defibrillator), and AEDs (automated external defibrillator). Let's look at each of those:

- The ***monitor/defibrillator*** *is a combination of a cardiac monitor with a three- or five- lead cable plus a cardioverter-defibrillator.* It is attached to the patient, then health care personnel analyze the rhythm and activate the buttons to either cardiovert or defibrillate the patient. It requires knowledge of rhythms and their appropriate treatment by the user.
- The ***AICD*** *is an implanted device that is programmed to analyze abnormal rhythms and deliver a small internal electrical shock to abort an abnormal rhythm such as V-tach or V-fib.* It is completely contained within the body. The AICD also has a pacemaker that allows it to pace the heart if the shock causes asystole.
- The ***AED*** *is a defibrillator that is meant for use by the lay public.* It can be found in airports, shopping malls, and on airplanes. It is extremely simple to use. The device is attached to the patient and automatically analyzes the rhythm and tells the rescuer what to do (as in "push the button to defibrillate" or to check for a pulse). It requires no knowledge by the rescuer. The machine, once plugged in, tells the rescuer step by step what to do next.

Cardiac medications and electrical therapy are being constantly updated and improved. Keeping up with these advances is critical in caring for your patients.

Practice Quiz

1. Digitalis is classified as what kind of medication? ________________
2. Class I antiarrhythmic medications have what effect on the action potential?
   ____
   ____
3. What effect does atropine have on the heart rate? ________________
4. What effect does vasoconstriction have on the blood pressure? ________
   ____
5. True or false: An AED is meant for use by lay people.
6. What effect do class III antiarrhythmic medications have on the action potential? ________________________________
   ____
7. True or false: Defibrillation involves a small electrical shock synchronized with the cardiac cyle.
8. True or false: Epinephrine is classified as a cardiac glycoside.

9. How does cardioversion differ from defibrillation? ____________

____

10. Isoproterenol is used nowadays in treating what problem? ____________

____

Putting It All Together—Critical Thinking Exercises

These exercises may consist of diagrams to label, scenarios to analyze, brain-stumping questions to ponder, or other exercises to help boost your understanding of the chapter material.

For the following "shockable" rhythms, state whether the rhythm should be cardioverted or defibrillated:

1. Atrial fibrillation. ____________
2. Ventricular tachycardia with a pulse. ____________
3. Ventricular fibrillation. ____________
4. Ventricular tachycardia without a pulse. ____________
5. SVT. ____________

Diagnostic Electrocardiography

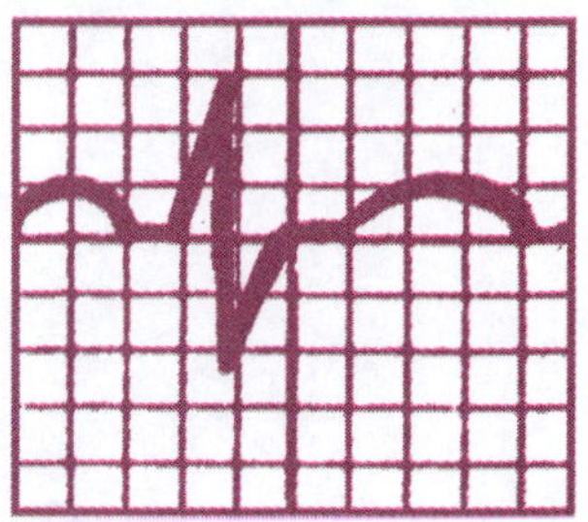

Chapter 18 Objectives

Upon completion of this chapter, the student will be able to:

- Define *stress testing.*
- State the goal of stress testing.
- Define *MET.*
- Describe the indications for stress testing.
- Describe the relative and absolute contraindications to stress testing.
- State how to calculate target heart rate.
- Describe how a stress test is done.
- Describe how a pharmacologic stress test is done.
- Name the three most commonly used protocols for treadmill exercise testing.
- Describe the reasons to terminate the test.
- Describe normal signs and symptoms during the stress test.
- Describe the normal EKG changes that occur during stress testing.
- Describe the EKG changes that indicate a positive stress test.
- Explain Bayes's theorem as it relates to the reliability of stress testing.
- Define *specificity* and *sensitivity.*
- Describe the indications for Holter monitoring.
- State the contraindications to Holter monitoring.
- Describe the artifact associated with Holter monitoring.
- Explain why an event monitor might be superior to a Holter monitor for some patients.
- State what a positive Holter or event monitor is.

Introduction

Diagnostic electrocardiography involves an EKG done to rule out disease. It can involve a resting EKG, a stress test, or ambulatory monitoring such as Holter monitoring. We've talked about resting EKGs in depth. Let's look at the other two now.

Stress Testing

Stress testing is a diagnostic procedure done to determine the likelihood of coronary artery disease (CAD). The heart is stressed by physical exertion, usually on a bicycle or a treadmill, or by administration of medication that causes increased heart rate and thus stresses the heart. The patient's symptoms and EKG during the stress test give vital information regarding the **patency** (openness) of his or her coronary arteries.

Goal of Stress Testing

The goal of stress testing, whether exercise or pharmacologic, is to increase the heart rate to a maximal level that increases myocardial oxygen demand and to evaluate the EKG and subjective responses of the patient. Decreased flow through narrowed coronary arteries will usually become evident as the test progresses. In other words, are there EKG changes that signal ischemia or infarction? Does the patient experience chest pain or arrhythmias with this stress? The test is concluded when the patient's symptoms (chest pain, fatigue, or ST segment changes) preclude continuing, or, for submaximal tests, when a target heart rate is reached.

Indications for Stress Testing

Stress testing is usually done to search for coronary artery disease in a patient having suspicious symptoms. But there are other indications as well. Here are a few:

- **Post-CABG or postangioplasty evaluation.** The patient has had bypass surgery or a balloon procedure to open up blocked coronary arteries. The stress test is a way to determine if those procedures have improved coronary flow.
- **Diagnosis or treatment of exercise-induced arrhythmias.** Some patients have arrhythmias only on exertion. The stress test is a safe way to induce those arrhythmias in a controlled environment so they can be identified and treated.
- **Follow-up to cardiac rehab.** The post-MI patient has gradually worked up to more normal exercise levels. The stress test helps determine if his or her heart is tolerating this increased exertion.
- **Family history of heart disease.** The individual with a family history of heart disease and two or more of the recognized heart disease risk factors is advised to have a stress test at age 40 and periodically thereafter. If coronary artery disease is detected, treatment can begin early.

Absolute Contraindications

Who is *not* a candidate for stress testing under any circumstances? For people with the following conditions, the risks of the test greatly outweigh the potential benefits. Testing these people could have serious or fatal consequences.

- **Acute MI.** The heart is too unstable to tolerate exertion. Stress testing could cause the infarct area to extend.

- **Unstable angina or angina at rest.** Patients who have angina at rest will not tolerate stress. It could cause them to infarct.
- **Uncontrolled ventricular rhythms.** The rhythm could deteriorate to v-fib.
- **Severe aortic stenosis.** Due to a very narrowed aortic valve opening, cardiac output is low, and stressing these patients could cause them to pass out or suffer cardiac arrest.
- **Dissecting aneurysm.** This is a ballooning out of the wall of an artery. Stress causes an increase in blood pressure, which could cause the aneurysm to blow.
- **Heart block greater than first degree.** These patients cannot get their heart rate up to the target level, and they may already have decreased cardiac output that exertion would worsen.

Relative Contraindications

Some individuals can have a stress test *only* if the benefits outweigh the risks. In other words, it must be determined that the information to be gained from the stress test is so valuable that it outweighs the risks involved to individuals with the following conditions:

- **Uncontrolled rapid supraventricular rhythms.** With the heart rate already fast prior to the stress test, it won't take much to make the cardiac output fall.
- **Frequent PVCs.** It's possible that ventricular tachycardia or fibrillation could result, so it's important to determine if the information the stress test will provide is worth the risk.
- **Uncontrolled hypertension.** The person with this condition has either not received treatment for hypertension or has not taken the prescribed medication, and his or her BP is extremely high. Stress testing this person could result in stroke.
- **Mild or moderate aortic stenosis.** The cardiac output could drop.

Preparation Techniques

The single most important piece of equipment in performing a stress test is a 12-lead EKG machine that has the capability to run continuously for a period of time. The electrode patches should adhere securely to the skin, and they may be taped if necessary. Female patients are advised to wear a bra in order to decrease artifact. To prevent nausea, patients are advised not to eat a large meal for at least four hours prior to the test. They should wear comfortable, loose clothing and walking shoes or other appropriate footwear. They should take their routine medications as usual unless specifically instructed not to by the physician. Certain medications, such as beta-blockers and calcium channel blockers, may be held for a period of time before the test, as they prevent the heart rate from reaching target levels. Also, nitrates might be held, as they could prevent symptoms of coronary artery disease, such as chest pain, and could thus result in a false-negative test.

How is it Done?

Before all stress tests, a resting EKG is done. A history is obtained, with special emphasis on a description of any symptoms the patient has been having that prompted the test (chest pain, shortness of breath, etc.). Baseline vital signs (heart rate, blood pressure, respiratory rate) are checked with the patient lying down and standing. An EKG will be done with the patient standing up **hyperventilating** (breathing very rapidly). ST segment and T wave changes can be caused by hyperventilation, and during the stress test it's important to know if any ST-T changes are from ischemia or simply from hyperventilating.

For the **exercise test**, the patient then exercises on a treadmill or bicycle, or uses a special arm bicycle called an *arm ergometer,* while a continuous EKG is run. A nurse or technician checks the patient's blood pressure at frequent intervals and inquires about any symptoms the patient may be developing. The stress test is continued until at least 85% of the target heart rate is achieved or the patient develops EKG changes or symptoms that require termination of the test. *The target heart rate is 220 minus the patient's age.* A 60-year-old patient would thus have a target heart rate of 220 − 60 = 160. For the test to be valid for interpretation, a heart rate of 85% of 160, or 136, would be required. For a **submaximal test** following an MI, the test is concluded when 70% of the target heart rate is achieved, assuming the patient is asymptomatic. If myocardial perfusion is to be studied, radioisotopes such as **thallium-201** can be injected during the last minute of exercise and then special x-rays done. Thallium follows potassium ions into the heart and diffuses into the tissues. Poor myocardial uptake of the thallium produces a "cold spot" on the X-ray (compared to the "hot spots" from adequate thallium uptake) and indicates impaired myocardial blood flow in the artery supplying that area. Multiple gated acquisition (MUGA) scans can also be done after the exercise test to check myocardial perfusion. MUGA scans are nuclear scans that use an injected radioisotope to point out areas of poor myocardial blood flow.

The **pharmacologic stress test** does not involve exercise. This kind of testing is appropriate for individuals with physical limitations that preclude exercise, such as amputations, or for the elderly who could not do enough exercise to reach the target heart rate. For this test, an IV line is started, and the patient is given an intravenous dose of medication that causes the heart rate to climb to the target level. This increased heart rate stresses the heart and should provide the same symptoms and EKG changes as an exercise test. As with the exercise test, a continuous EKG is run, vital signs are checked, and symptoms are assessed. After at least 85% of the target heart rate is achieved, the test is concluded. The most common medications used in pharmacologic stress tests are *cardiolyte, dobutamine, dipyridamole,* and *adenosine.*

Exercise Protocols

There are three main protocols used in treadmill exercise stress tests. Speed and incline of the treadmill, as well as the frequency of the changes in the protocol's stages, are determined by the protocol used. The intensity of

Table 18-1 Bruce Protocol Stages

STAGE	SPEED	INCLINE
I	1.7 mph	10°
II	2.5 mph	12°
III	3.4 mph	14°
IV	4.2 mph	16°
V	5.0 mph	18°
VI	5.5 mph	20°
VII	6.0 mph	22°

exercise is measured in metabolic equivalents (**METs**), which are reflections of oxygen consumption. One MET is the oxygen consumption of a person sitting down resting. Most average adults can reach a MET level of 13 with exertion. Those with coronary artery disease (CAD) may have symptoms of ischemia at very low MET levels, such as four METs. Sometimes a **double product** is calculated in order to determine the level of exercise achieved. Double product is calculated as the heart rate times the systolic blood pressure (HR × SBP = DP). A double product greater than 25,000 indicates that an acceptable level of exercise has been achieved during stress testing. Let's look at the different protocols.

- **Bruce.** This is the most commonly used protocol, used for maximal testing. The treadmill's speed and incline are increased every 3 minutes up to a total of 21 minutes. Let's look at the stages of the Bruce protocol. See Table 18-1.

  As you can see in Table 18-1, the speed starts out at a comfortable walking pace at a low incline, then every 3 minutes accelerates until by stage VII the patient is running uphill at a 22° incline. An advantage of the Bruce protocol is the relatively short duration needed to produce maximal effort in the patient. On the downside, this protocol can be very demanding and may be too ambitious for the sedentary individual.
- **Modified Bruce.** Many institutions have modified the Bruce protocol so that the initial work is less strenuous, and the stages change in smaller increments. This is appropriate for patients who might not tolerate the standard Bruce protocol.
- **Naughton.** This is a slower-moving submaximal test in which the settings are changed every two minutes. Though the settings change more quickly than in the Bruce protocol, they are more gradual and allow the individual to adjust more easily. The Naughton protocol is used most often for testing post-MI patients just before or shortly after hospital discharge.

Termination of the Test

The stress test should be immediately stopped if any of the following occur:

- *ST segment elevation.* This indicates severe transmural myocardial ischemia and injury. The sudden development of ST segment elevation is an ominous sign. Continuing the test could result in irreversible cardiac damage.

- *Ventricular tachycardia.* Cardiac arrest could result if the test is not stopped.
- *Chest pain, especially if accompanied by ST segment depression or elevation.* Mild chest pain unaccompanied by ST segment changes may not be indicative of significant coronary artery disease. More severe chest pain, especially that accompanied by ST segment changes, is more reflective of significant disease.
- *Drop in blood pressure or failure of the BP to rise with exercise.* The blood pressure usually rises in response to exercise. Failure of the blood pressure to rise with exercise indicates poor cardiac reserve. A drop in BP can indicate pump failure.
- *Bradycardia, especially the development of AV blocks.* The heart rate should increase with exertion. If it slows down, it is a sign of poor cardiac reserve. The development of AV blocks, especially type II second-degree AV block and third-degree AV block, could signal ischemia to the AV node or bundle branches, which are supplied by the right coronary artery and the LAD, respectively. Continuing the test could prove dangerous to the patient.
- *Patient indicates inability to continue due to fatigue, shortness of breath, or dizziness.* Trust the patient who says he or she feels too bad to continue.
- *Patient requests to stop.* Again, listen to the patient. But inquire about the symptoms that prompt the patient to want to stop the test. There may be an occasional unmotivated patient who requests to stop the test before achieving target levels. In this case the physician might gently encourage the patient to continue, since the test that is stopped at too early a stage will be inadequate at ruling out CAD.
- *ST depression greater than 3 mm.* This is a strongly positive stress test. Continuing the test could cause the patient to infarct.
- *Elevation of the systolic blood pressure above 240 mmHg or the diastolic blood pressure above 120 mmHg.* This is controversial. Though some experts say that blood pressure that rises too high during exercise puts the patient at risk for stroke, others downplay this risk.
- *Patient becomes very pale and diaphoretic (cold and clammy).* These are signs of decreased cardiac output. The patient is not tolerating the test.

Test Interpretation

The following EKG changes are normal on the stress test:

- **Shortened PR interval.** AV conduction and heart rate usually accelerate with exertion.
- **Tall P waves.** This is often a result of increased lung capacity.
- **Lower-voltage QRS complexes.** This may be due to increased volume of air in the lungs muffling the cardiac impulse as it heads toward the skin.
- **Increased heart rate (shorter R-R intervals).** The ability of the heart rate to increase with exercise is known as the **chronotropic reserve.** Heart rate that does not increase with stress is **chronotropic incompetence.**

Normal Signs and Symptoms

The following patient signs and symptoms are normal during a stress test:

- *Decreased systemic vascular resistance due to vasodilation.* Exercise causes blood vessels to dilate, lowering the resistance to the outflow of blood from the heart and increasing cardiac output.
- *Increased respiratory rate.* Exercise causes increased oxygen demand, so the respiratory rate increases to allow more oxygen intake.
- *Sweating.*
- *Fatigue.*
- *Muscle cramping in calves or sides.* This is a common phenomenon in exercise and does not imply poor myocardial function.
- *Increased blood pressure.* The ability of the blood pressure to rise with exercise is known as **inotropic reserve.** Blood pressure that does not rise with exercise can imply **inotropic incompetence.**
- *J point depression.* The J point is the point at which the QRS joins the ST segment. J point depression means the ST segment takes off before the QRS complex has gotten back up to the baseline. Note the J point in Figure 18-1. It is below the baseline. This is J point depression.

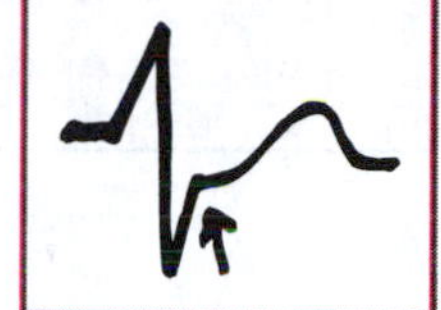

Figure 18-1 J point depression.

Positive Stress Test

The following indicate a positive (abnormal) stress test:

- *ST segment depression greater than or equal to 1.0 to 1.5 mm that does not return to the baseline within 0.08 s (two little blocks) after the J point.* ST depression can be of three different types: upsloping, horizontal, and downsloping. In terms of cardiac implications, upsloping is the least indicative of coronary artery disease, horizontal is intermediate, and downsloping is the most indicative of CAD. See Figure 18-2.

Let's compare ST segments on a preexercise resting EKG and a stress test EKG. See Figures 18-3 and 18-4. Ignore the QRS width on these examples. In Figure 18-3, note the normal ST segments and the relatively slow heart rate. Now see Figure 18-4 for the stress test EKG. Note the normal increase in heart rate along with significant downsloping ST segment depressions in leads II, III, and a VF. This is a positive stress test.

- *U wave inversion or new appearance of U waves.* Though a much less common phenomenon than ST segment changes, U wave inversion–or indeed the sudden appearance of U waves during the exercise test–is

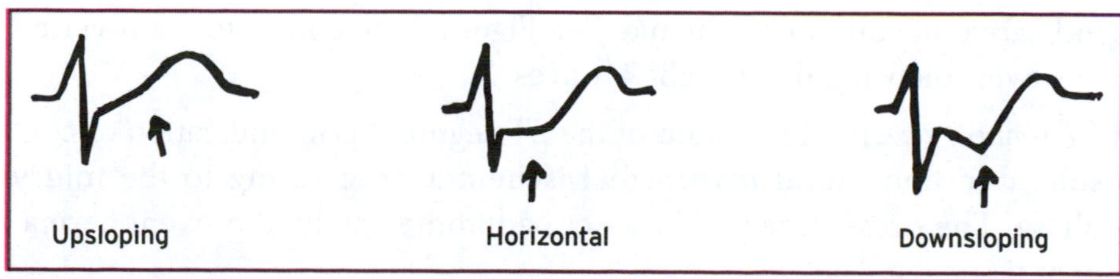

Figure 18-2 Types of ST segment depression.

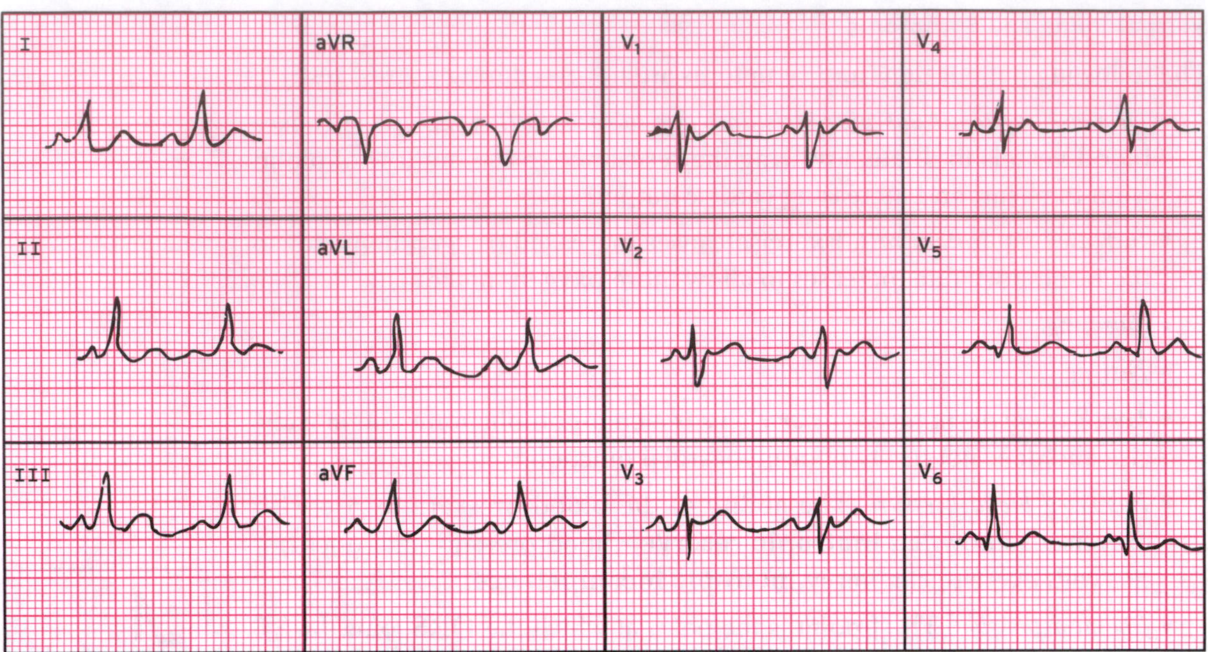

Figure 18-3 Preexercise resting EKG.

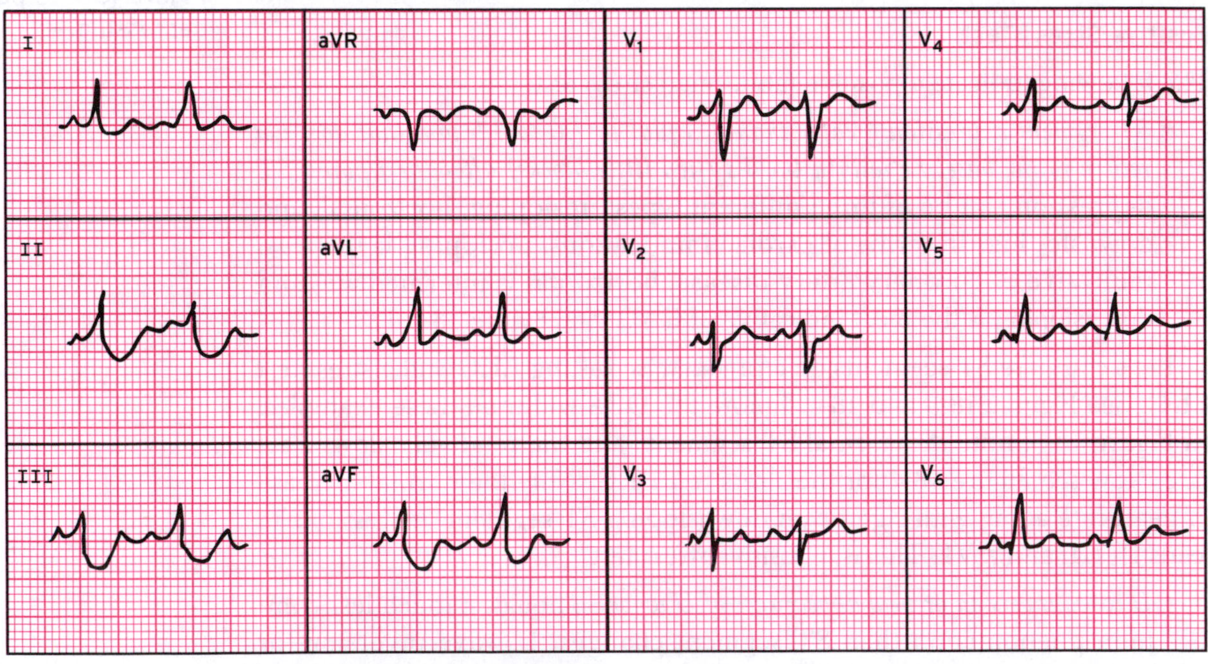

Figure 18-4 Stress test EKG.

indicative of coronary ischemia. See Figure 18-5, and note the inverted U waves following the upright T waves.

- *ST segment elevation.* Elevation of the ST segment is an indication of considerable transmural myocardial ischemia progressing to the injury phase. The stress test should be stopped immediately to prevent permanent tissue damage.

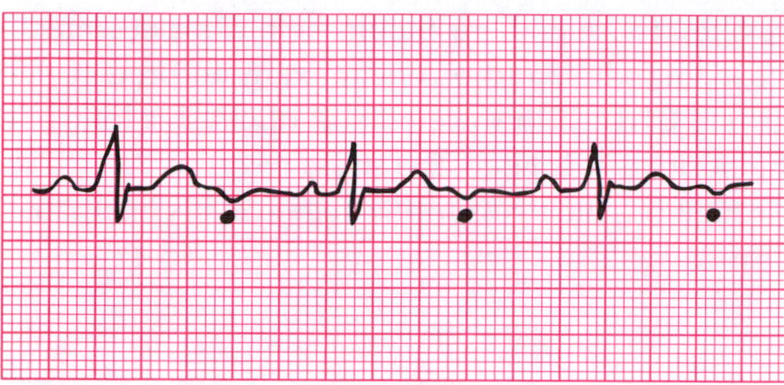

Figure 18-5 Inverted U waves.

Reliability of Stress Tests

How reliable are stress tests in diagnosing coronary artery disease? Like any medical testing, the stress test is not infallible. There can be false positives and false negatives. The validity of stress test results can be absolutely determined only by **angiogram**, a procedure in which dye is injected into the coronary arteries to determine if there is indeed coronary artery disease. For the stress EKG to show any diagnostic changes that indicate CAD, the coronary artery in question must be at least 75% narrowed. And conditions other than CAD can result in a positive test. To better understand the reliability of the test results, it is necessary to understand the terms *sensitivity* and *specificity*.

Sensitivity refers to the percentage of patients who have a positive stress test and CAD as proven by angiogram. In other words, is the stress test sensitive enough to pick up those individuals who truly have coronary artery disease?

Specificity refers to the percentage of patients who have negative (normal) stress tests and normal coronary arteries as proven by angiogram. Is the stress test specific enough to exclude individuals who do not have CAD?

Thus the term *positive* refers to the test's sensitivity and *negative* refers to its specificity.

If the stress test and angiogram results differ–if one is positive and the other is negative, for example–**the stress test result will be considered false. If stress test and angiogram agree, the stress test result is true.** The stress test result will then tell you positive or negative. If stress test is negative and angiogram is positive, for example, the stress test result is said to be false (because stress test and angiogram results differ) negative (because the stress test was negative).

Categories of Stress Tests

Stress test results fall in four categories:

- *True positive.* The stress test is positive (indicating coronary artery disease) and the angiogram is also positive, confirming CAD.
- *False positive.* The stress test is positive for CAD, but the angiogram is negative, revealing normal coronary arteries.
- *True negative.* The stress test and angiogram are both negative for CAD.
- *False negative.* The stress test is negative, but the angiogram is positive for CAD.

Bayes's theorem suggests that the true predictive value of any test is not just in the accuracy (sensitivity and specificity) of the test itself, but also in the patient's probability of disease, as determined before the test was done. In other words, before the stress test is done, there should be a risk assessment, based on the patient's history, heredity, and physical exam, to predict the likelihood of that patient having CAD. If this pretest risk of CAD is low, but his stress test turns out to be positive, it is likely the stress test result is a false positive. If the pretest risk is high but the stress test is negative, it's likely that the stress test is a false-negative.

After the Stress Test

What happens after the stress test? If the stress test is positive, the patient will likely be either treated with medications or scheduled for an angiogram for further diagnostic evaluation. If the test is negative, there may be no treatment indicated.

Stress Test Assessment Practice

Let's look at a few EKGs from stress tests. On the first five, **assess the EKG and decide if the test should continue or be terminated.** Assume that each person's rhythm was sinus rhythm with a heart rate of 70 and the EKG was otherwise completely normal at the start of the stress test. Assume this EKG was done 3 minutes into the Bruce protocol.

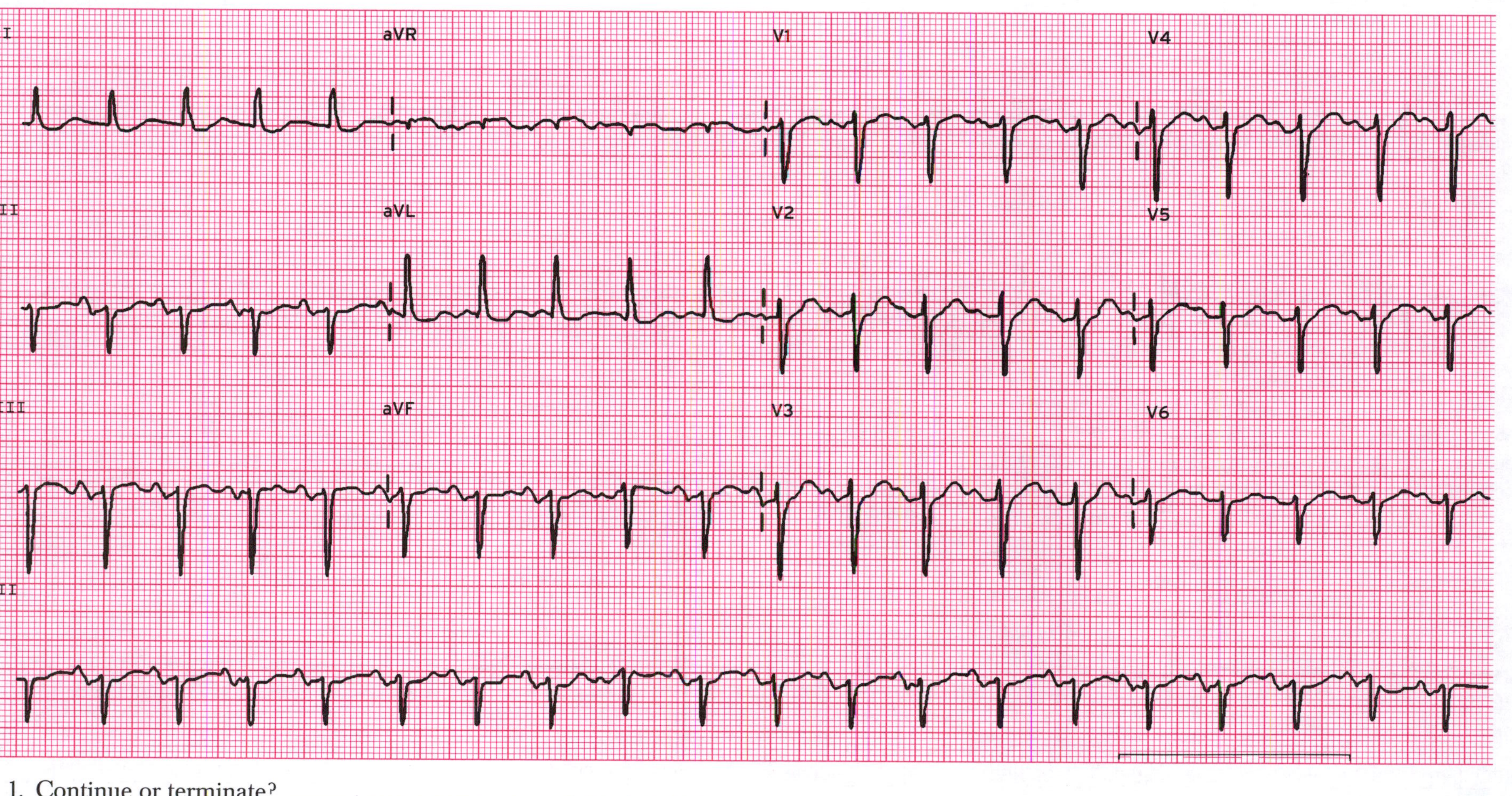

1. Continue or terminate? ______________________

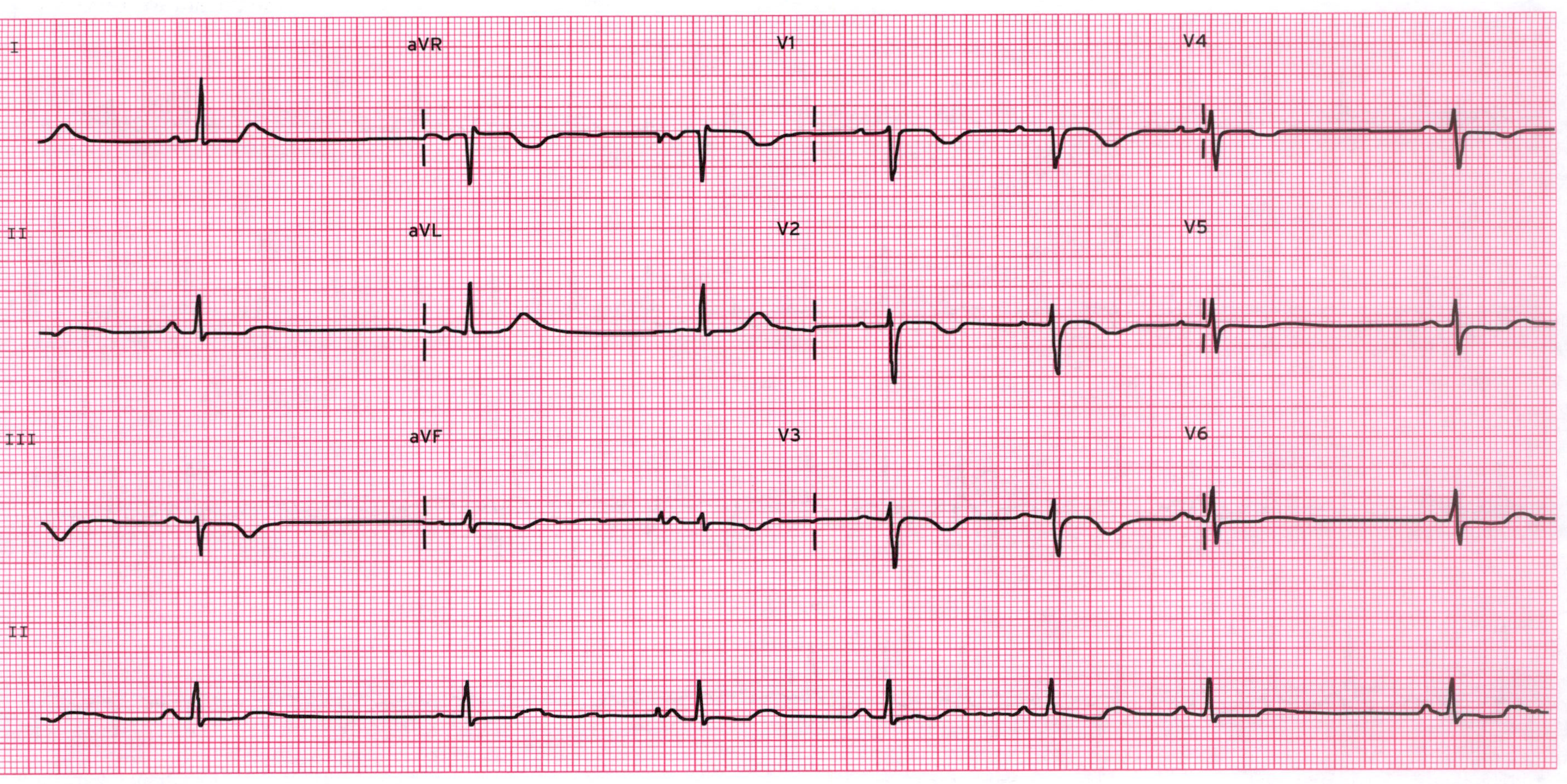

2. Continue or terminate?______________________________

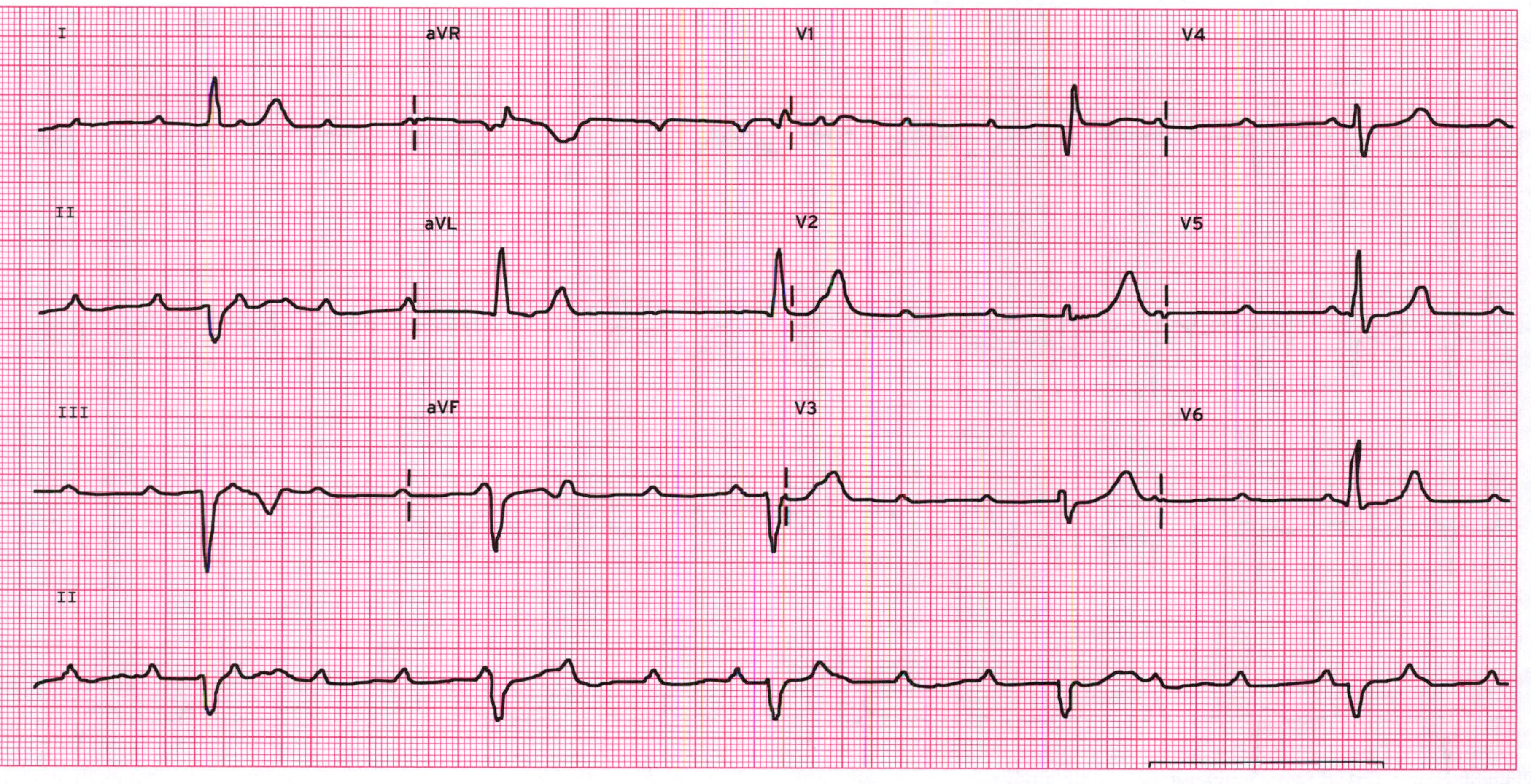

3. Continue or terminate? ______________________________

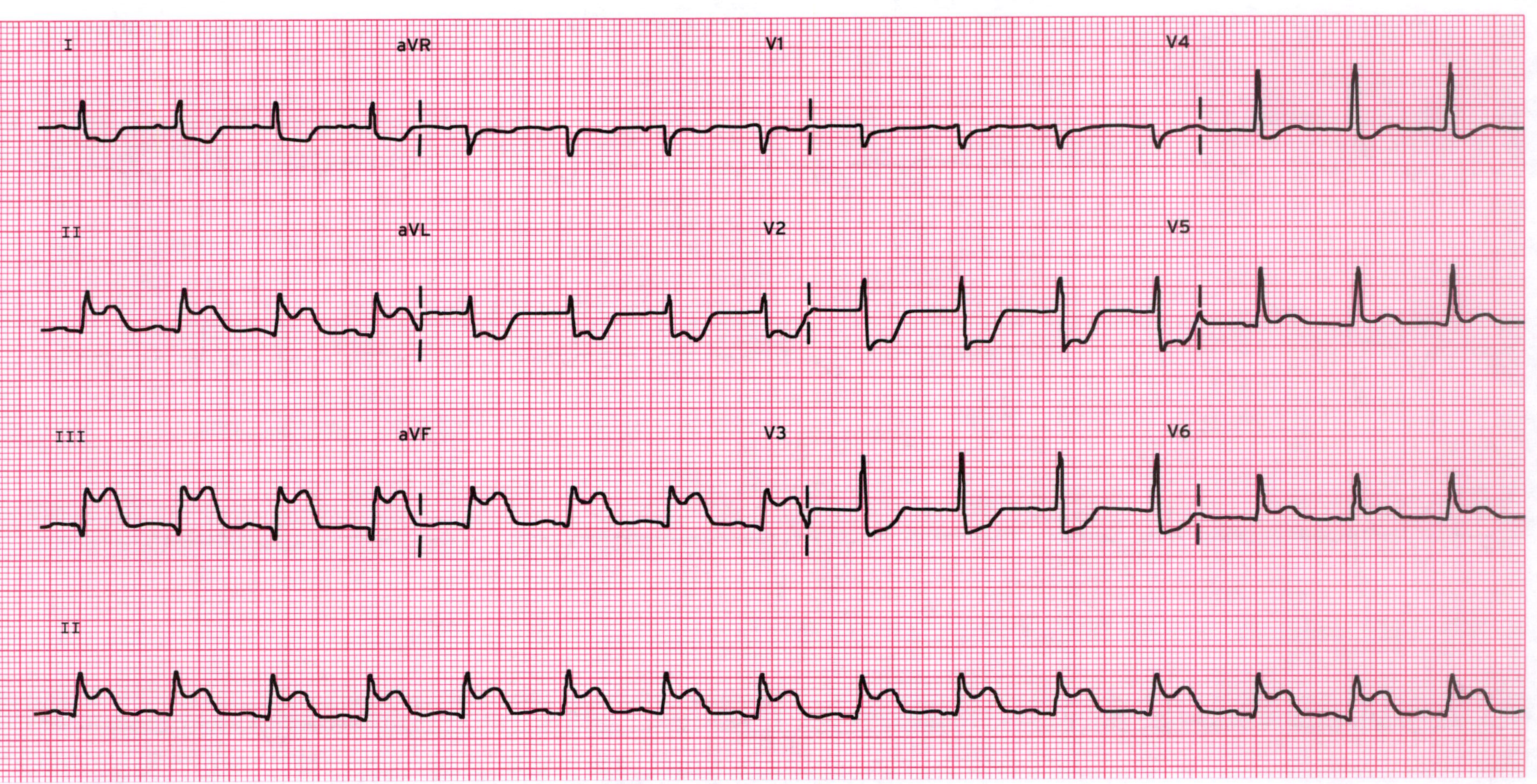

4. Continue or terminate? ______________

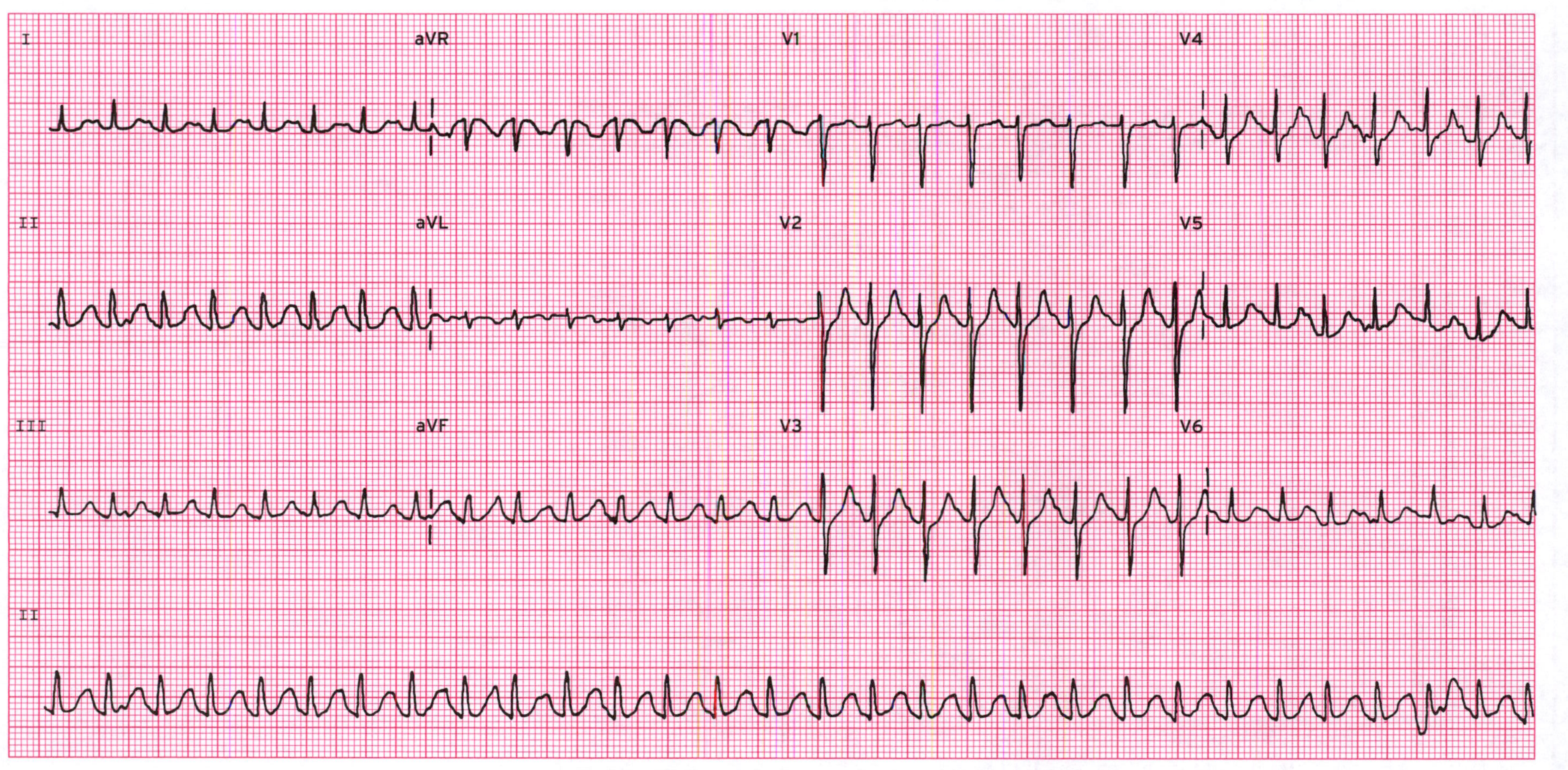

5. Continue or terminate? ______________________

On these final five, assume all patients have had a negative angiogram. Assess the EKG and determine if the stess test is positive or negative for CAD, and **state whether the stress test is true positive, false positive, true negative, or false negative.** Again, assume all pretest EKGs were normal.

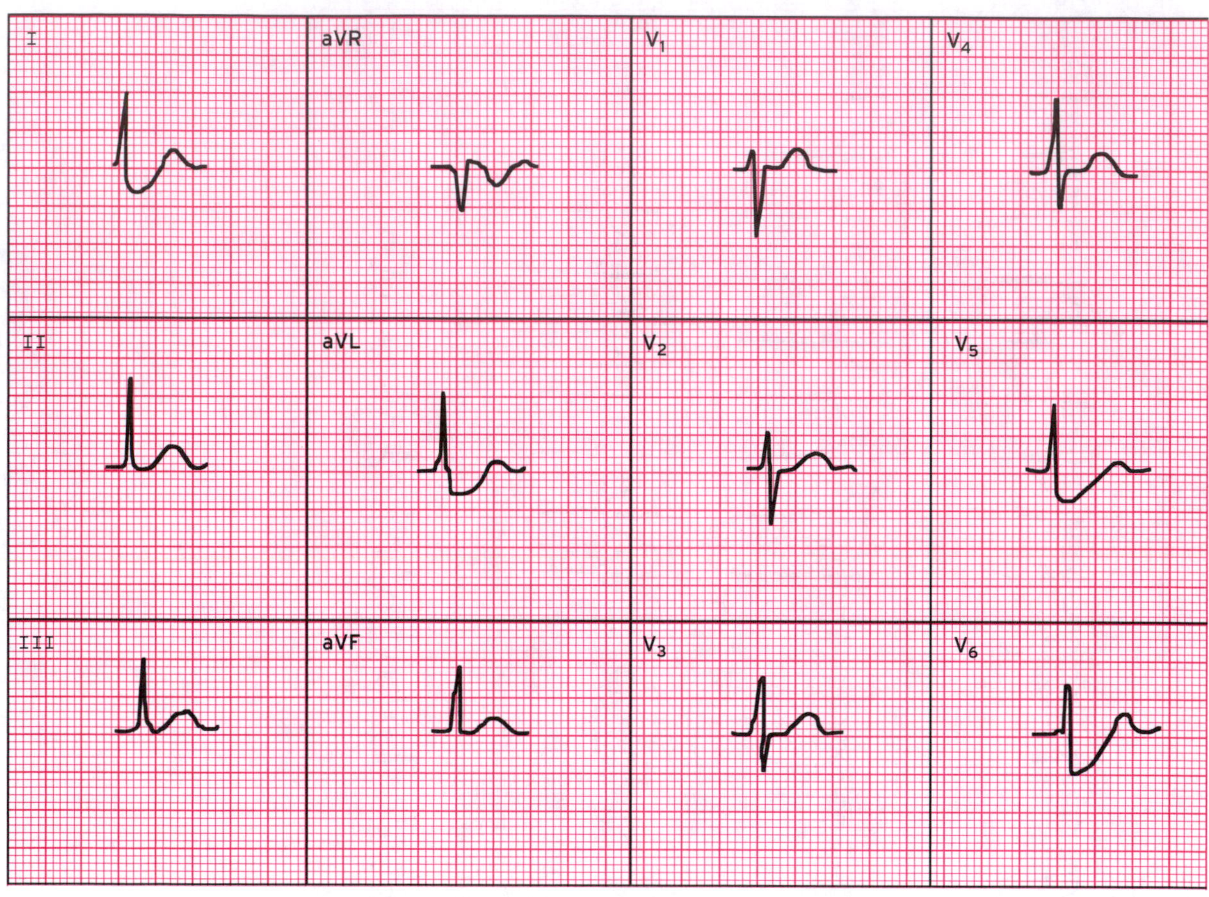

6. If the angiogram is negative, this stress test result is ________________

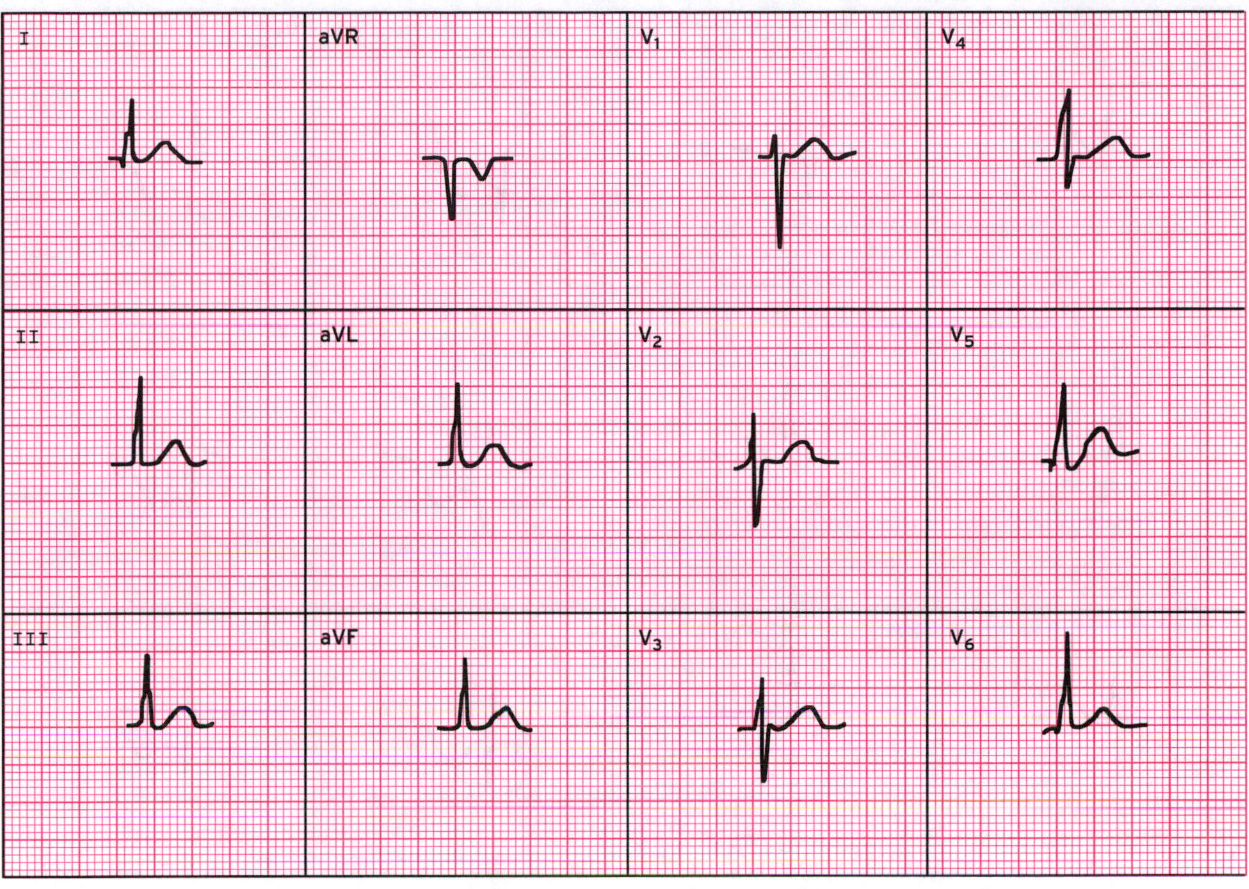

7. If the angiogram is positive, this stress test result is ____________________

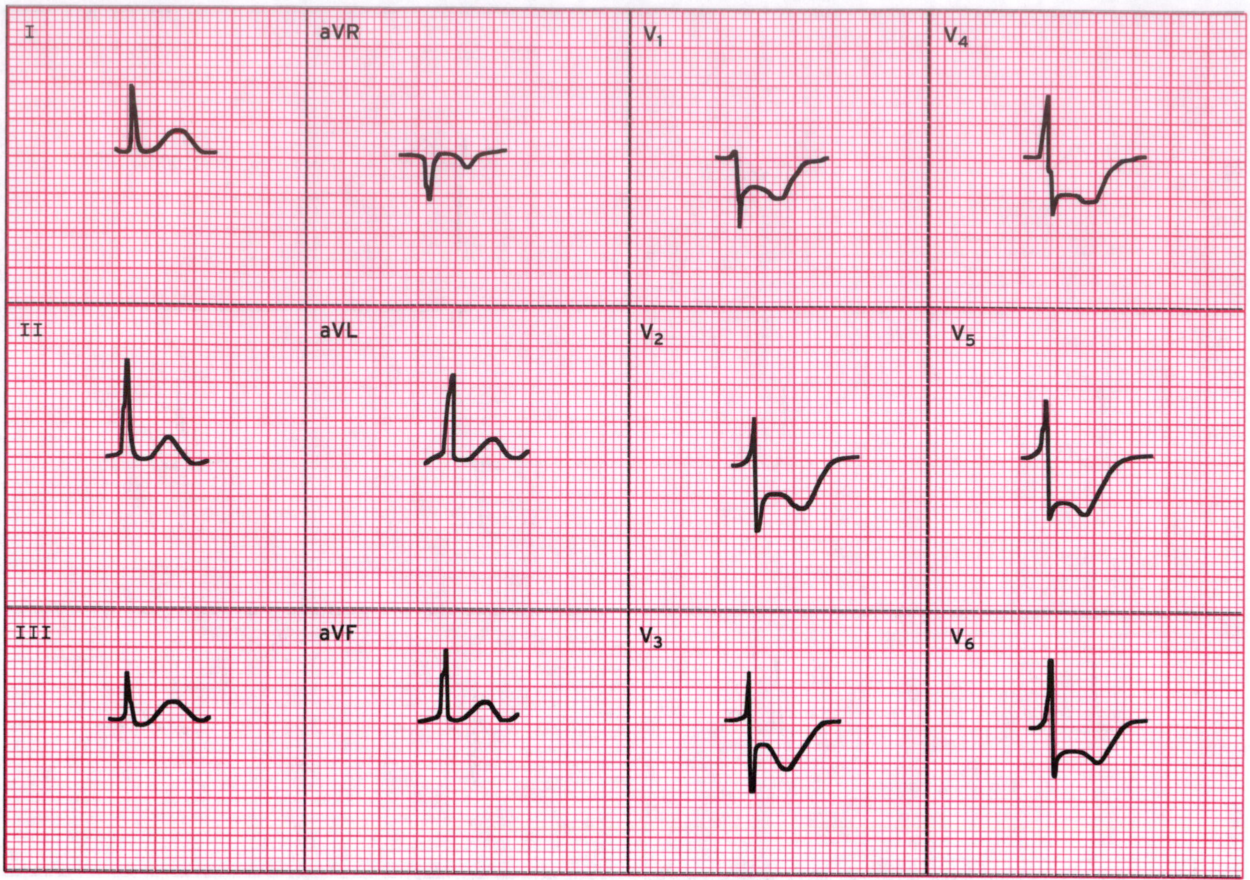

8. If the angiogram is negative, this stress test result is ___________________

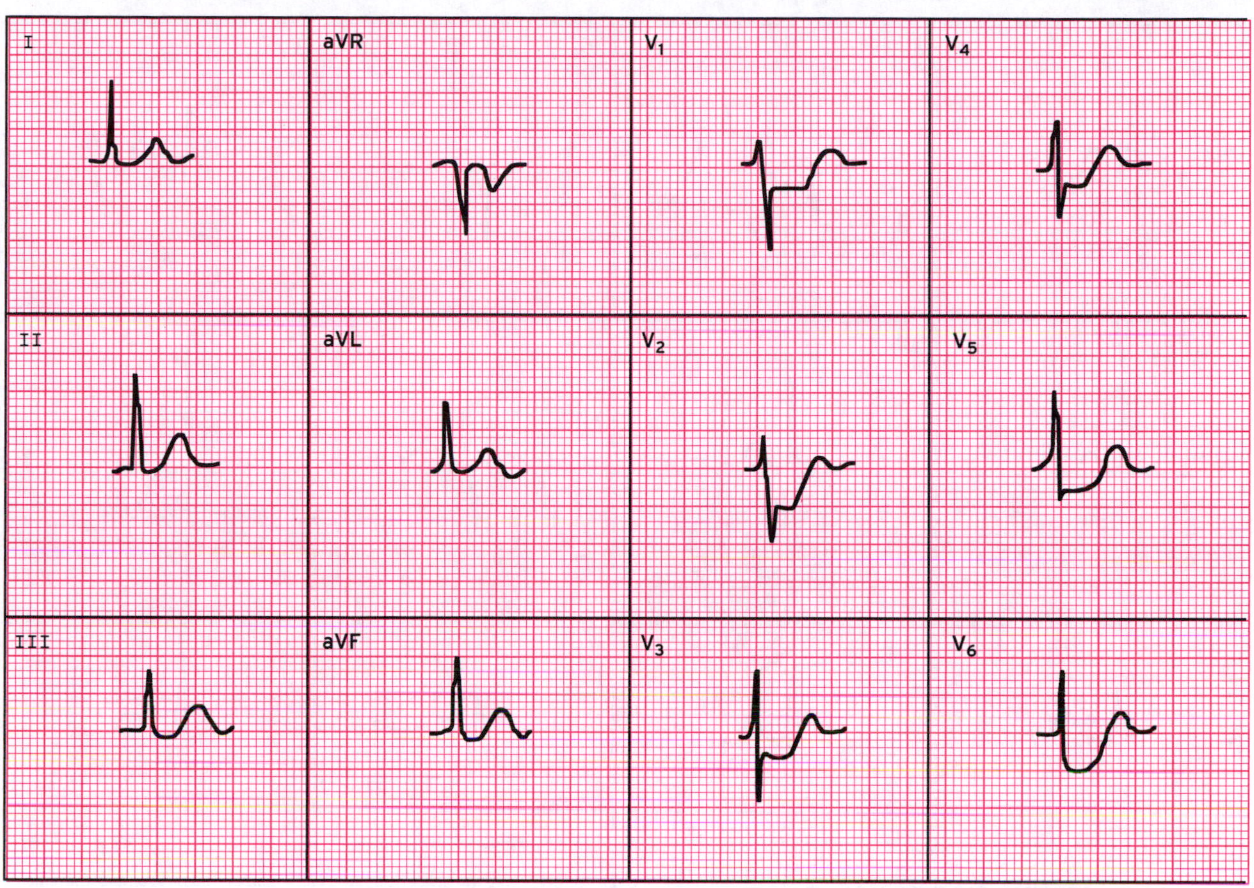

9. If the angiogram is positive, this stress test result is ________________

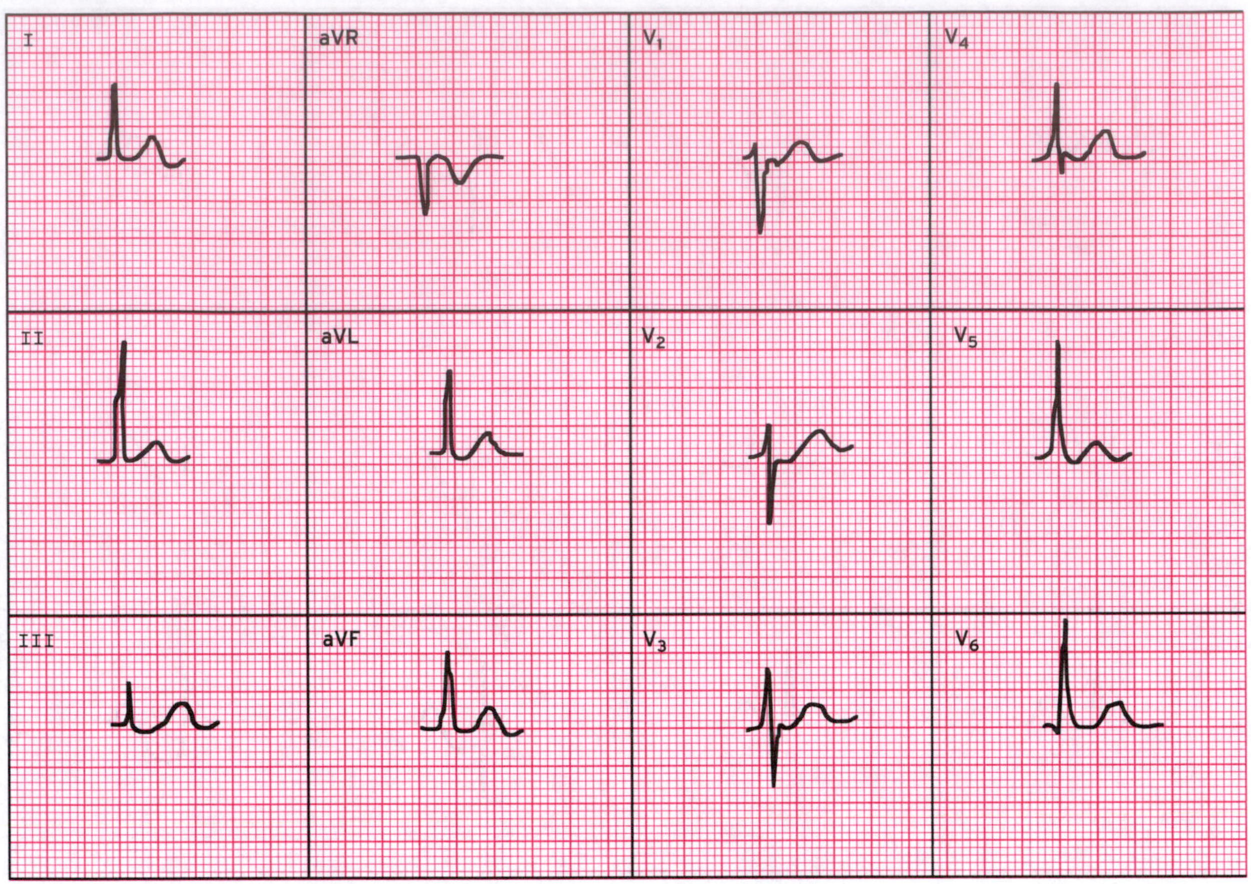

10. If the angiogram is negative, this stress test result is ________________

Stress Test Assessment Practice Answers

1. **Continue.** The EKG shows sinus tachycardia, which is expected. There are no ST segment changes that warrant stopping the test.
2. **Terminate.** The heart rate before the test was 70 and now varies from about 33 to 58. Note the P wave shapes vary also. The heart rate during a stress test should increase, not decrease. This decreased heart rate could signal decreased cardiac reserve.
3. **Terminate.** This is third degree AV block, an ominous development during a stress test. The heart rate should speed up during the test.
4. **Terminate.** There is marked ST segment elevation in leads II, III,and aVF and V_5–V_6. This is an indication of an MI in progress. Note the reciprocal ST depression in I, aVL, and V_2–V_4.
5. **Continue.** Sinus tachycardia is expected during a stress test. As long as the patient is tolerating the rhythm, the test may continue.
6. **False positive.** The stress test is positive for CAD–note the >1.5 mm ST segment depression in I, aVL, V_5–V_6. But the angiogram is negative, and that's the gold standard for diagnosing CAD. The stress test result is therefore a false positive.

7. **False negative.** The stress test is negative–no ST depression–but the angiogram is positive.
8. **False positive.** The stress test is positive–striking ST depression in V_1–V_6–but the angiogram is negative.
9. **True positive.** Both stress test and angiogram are positive. Note the ST depression in V_1–V_6.
10. **True negative.** Both stress test and angiogram are negative.

Holter Monitoring

Holter monitoring is an ambulatory EKG done to rule out intermittent arrhythmias or cardiac ischemia that might otherwise be missed on a routine EKG. The Holter monitor consists of electrodes and a small, battery-powered tape recorder onto which the rhythm is recorded in two leads. The device is small enough to be worn in a pocket or on a strap over the shoulder. It may be done as an inpatient or outpatient, though most often it is done on an outpatient basis.

Indications

- *Syncope or near-syncopal episodes.* Fainting spells could be caused by arrhythmias, which could be evident on Holter monitoring.
- *Intermittent chest pain or shortness of breath.* These could be signs of myocardial ischemia, which could be detected with a Holter monitor.
- *Suspicion of arrhythmias.* The patient who complains of palpitations, dizzy spells, or skipped beats may have arrhythmias that the Holter monitor would demonstrate.
- *Determine the effectiveness of treatment for arrhythmias.* Holter monitoring can reveal if the rhythm being treated is still occurring and can demonstrate if a newly implanted pacemaker is functioning properly.

Contraindications

- *Terminal disease state.* This is controversial. On the one hand, if a patient is terminally ill, the information obtained using the monitor would be of no long-term benefit to the patient. On the other hand, treating any newly discovered arrhythmias or ischemia might help reduce or prevent symptoms and could improve the quality of the remainder of the patient's life.
- *Severe symptoms.* Patients with severe symptoms would more appropriately be monitored in the hospital than at home.

Preparation Techniques

The patient is attached to five electrodes, which are put on the trunk instead of the arms and legs in order to prevent muscle artifact. Male patients with considerable chest hair might need the electrode sites to be shaved in order for the electrode patches to adhere properly. Female patients should have chest leads positioned beneath, not on top of, the breast. The skin is prepped prior to attaching the electrodes. This skin prep involves abrading the thin outer layer of skin so the electrodes adhere to the skin without losing contact. The electrodes are then taped to the skin to prevent dislodgment, since they will be on for 24 hours or longer. Typically, at least two leads are simultaneously recorded–either leads V_1 and V_5 or leads V_1 and II.

After being attached to the Holter monitor, the patient is given instructions, including not to remove the electrodes and not to take a bath or shower during the time the Holter is in progress, as this could cause the electrodes to become dislodged. A careful sponge bath is OK. The patient is otherwise instructed to go about normal daily activities. This includes work, hobbies, sex, and so on. The patient should not curtail activities just because the Holter is in progress. The whole purpose of the Holter monitor is to catch abnormalities that show up in the course of daily activities. Curtailing those activities defeats the purpose.

The patient is advised to document any symptoms experienced while the Holter is in progress in a small diary provided for that purpose. By pressing the marker button on the Holter monitor, the patient marks the point in the EKG at which he or she feels symptoms so that this part of the EKG can be more closely examined for changes that could cause the symptoms. For example, if at four o'clock P.M. the patient feels very dizzy, and the Holter reveals a short run of v-tach at that time, the arrhythmia would explain the dizziness. Treatment could then be started to prevent further ventricular arrhythmias. After the prescribed duration of Holter monitoring, the patient returns the Holter to the hospital or physician's office, whereupon it is entered into a computer and scanned for abnormalities.

Artifact Associated with Holter Monitoring

Several types of artifact can be seen on Holter monitoring. See Figure 18-6.

- *Loose electrode.* Sometimes an electrode will loosen or fall off, creating artifact that can resemble v-tach, v-fib, or asystole. The other monitored lead should prove this artifact to indeed be artifact and not the true rhythm.
- *Scratching artifact.* The patient scratches at the electrode sites, causing artifact that can resemble atrial flutter or ventricular tachycardia. Remember "toothbrush tachycardia"? Scratching artifact can look just like that. This type of artifact is also usually obvious in the other monitored lead. Scratching is common, as the electrode adhesive can cause skin irritation.
- *Incomplete erasure of a previously used Holter tape.* In this type of artifact, an incompletely erased Holter tape is reused, resulting in the new rhythm being recorded over the incompletely erased old one. This can make deciphering the rhythm difficult, as there will be extra P waves, QRS complexes, or T waves from the other rhythm superimposed onto this rhythm. In Figure 18-6, the arrows indicate leftover P waves and QRS complexes that were not erased.
- *Slowing of the tape during recording.* Sometimes the battery or recorder motor fails, causing the tape to slow while recording. When played back at

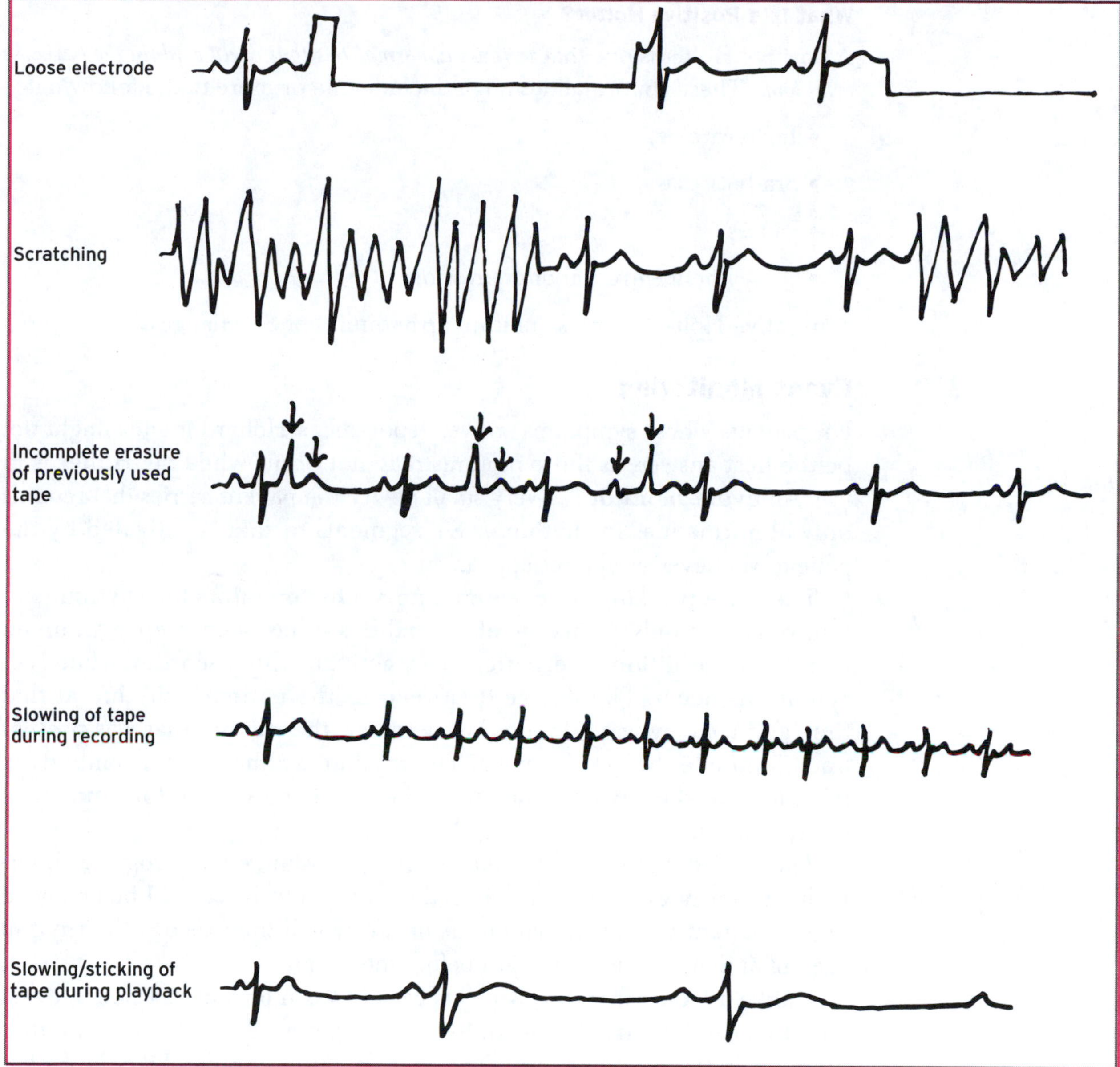

Figure 18-6 Types of artifact seen on Holter monitoring.

normal speed, the rhythm will look very fast. The abnormally shortened P, QRS, and T waves and intervals will be clues to the true cause of the apparent tachycardia.

- *Slowing or sticking of the tape during playback.* If the tape sticks while being played back, the rhythm will look abnormally slow. The abnormally prolonged P, QRS, and T waves and intervals will be clues to the true cause of this apparent bradycardia.

Using modern digital recorders rather than the older tape recorders can prevent the artifact problems commonly associated with tape recorder malfunctions.

What Is a Positive Holter?

A positive Holter is one that reveals *abnormalities that could explain the patient's symptoms*. These abnormalities might include one or more of the following:

- Tachycardias
- Bradycardias
- Pauses
- ST segment elevation or depression

A negative Holter has no significant arrhythmias or ST changes.

Event Monitoring

For patients whose symptoms are very sporadic, a Holter monitor might not be the best answer, as the symptoms may not occur while the Holter is in use. An **event monitor** is a very small device the patient carries that records only abnormalities in rhythm or ST segments or that is activated by the patient whenever symptoms appear.

There are two kinds of event monitors. One monitors the rhythm continuously, but only prints out abnormalities it has been preprogrammed to find. In addition, the patient can activate this recorder whenever symptoms occur. The device then records the patient's rhythm at that time and also, by way of a built-in memory, the rhythm that was present up to 5 minutes before the event. The rhythm can then be transmitted via telephone or the device turned in to the physician's office for immediate interpretation.

The second type of event monitor is not programmed to recognize abnormalities, nor does it monitor the rhythm continuously. It must be activated by the patient whenever symptoms occur. It will then record the rhythm present at that time as well as just before the event.

Unlike a Holter monitor, which is usually worn for only 24 hours, event monitors can be carried or worn for extended periods of time and are thus more likely to pick up abnormalities that are only sporadic. Like the Holter monitor, the event monitor is said to be *negative* if arrhythmias or ST-T changes are not found.

Practice Quiz

1. The type of monitor that is worn for 24 hours to uncover any arrhythmias or ST segment changes that might be causing the patient's symptoms is the ______________________________
2. List three indications for stress testing. ____________________
3. What does Bayes's theorem have to say about the validity of test results?

   ____
4. Is ST segment elevation of 5 mm indicative of a positive stress test or a negative stress test? ____________________

5. True or false: Patients on medications such as beta-blockers and nitrates might be advised to avoid taking these medications for a period of time before the stress test. ________________

6. Target heart rate is ________________

7. Event monitoring differs from Holter monitoring in what ways? ________________

8. The most commonly used protocol for treadmill stress testing is the ________________

9. The protocol used most often for post-MI patients just before or following hospital discharge is the ________________

10. What is a MET? ________________

Putting It All Together—Critical Thinking Exercises

These exercises may consist of diagrams to label, scenarios to analyze, brainstumping questions to ponder, or other challenging exercises to boost your knowledge of the chapter material.

The following scenario will provide you with information about a fictional patient and ask you to analyze the situation, answer questions, and decide on appropriate actions.

Mr. Cameron, a 46-year old male, is having a stress test required by his new insurance company. He is 5 feet 9 inches tall and weighs 325 pounds. He smokes two packs of cigarettes daily. Aside from an occasional twinge in his chest when he mows the lawn (the only exercise he gets), he has had no chest pain. Blood pressure is 160/90 (high), respiratory rate is 22 (slightly fast). The plan is to do a maximal test using the Bruce protocol.

You explain the stress test procedure and attach Mr. Cameron to the EKG. His resting EKG is below in Figure 18-7.

1. Do you see anything in this EKG that is of concern? ________________

   You start the Bruce protocol and all is going well, though Mr. Cameron does seem to be getting winded (slightly short of breath) quickly.

2. What in his history tells you this is nothing to be surprised about? ________________

   By stage two of the Bruce protocol Mr. Cameron's heart rate is 148 and his PR intervals have shortened.

3. Should the test continue or be terminated at this point? ________________

   The test continues and at seven minutes into the test Mr. Cameron complains of fatigue and dizziness. Blood pressure is now 82/64 and his skin is cool and clammy. He looks pale but denies chest pain. You continue the test and two minutes later he loses consciousness. Mr. Cameron's rhythm is seen below in Figure 18-8.

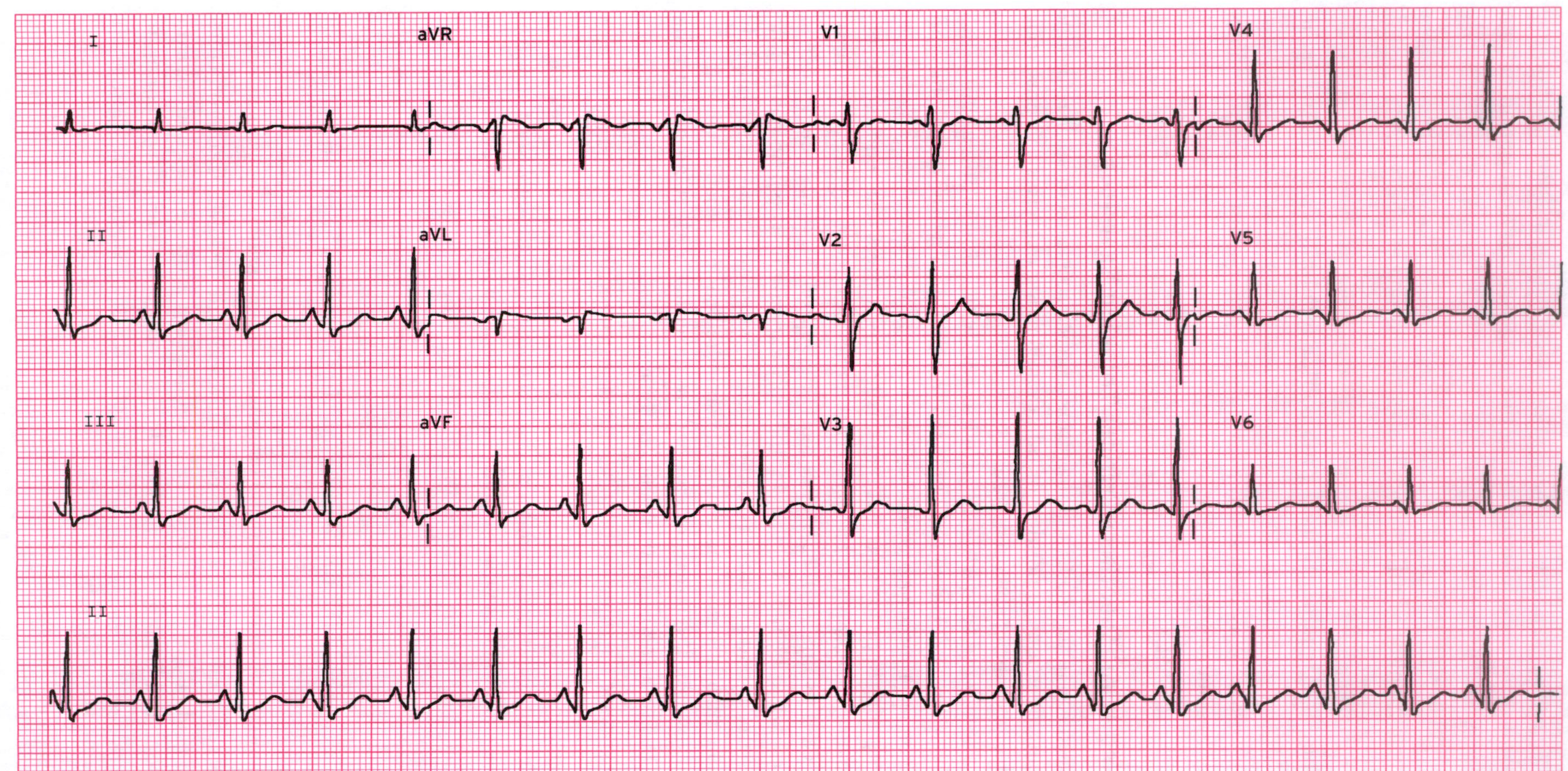

Figure 18-7 Mr. Cameron's resting EKG.

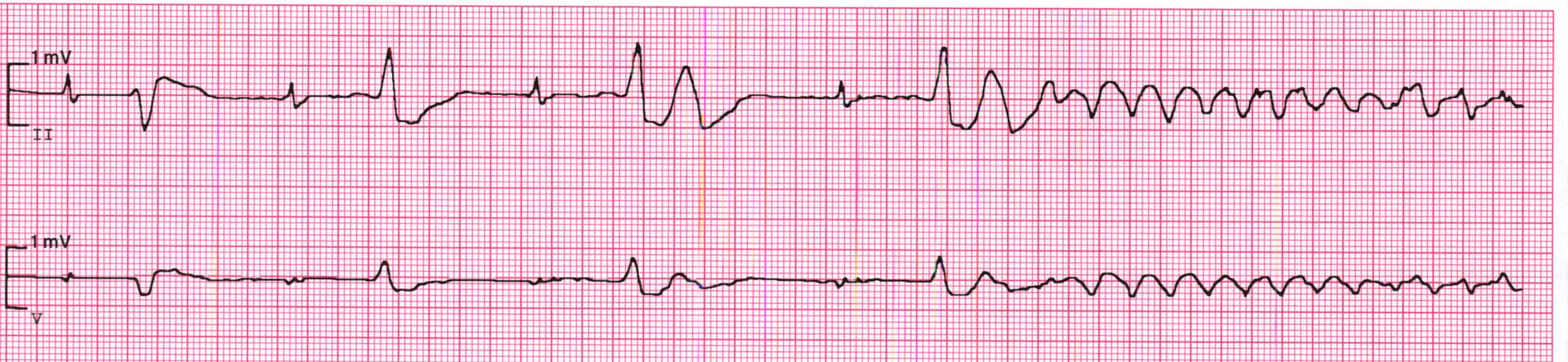

Figure 18-8 Mr. Cameron's rhythm when he loses consciousness.

4. What is this rhythm? ________________________
5. What is the appropriate course of action? ________________
6. After appropriate treatment, Mr. Cameron is sent to the coronary care unit. Looking back on the test, what should you have done differently?

   ____

   ____

CHAPTER **19**

Putting It All Together: Critical Thinking Scenarios

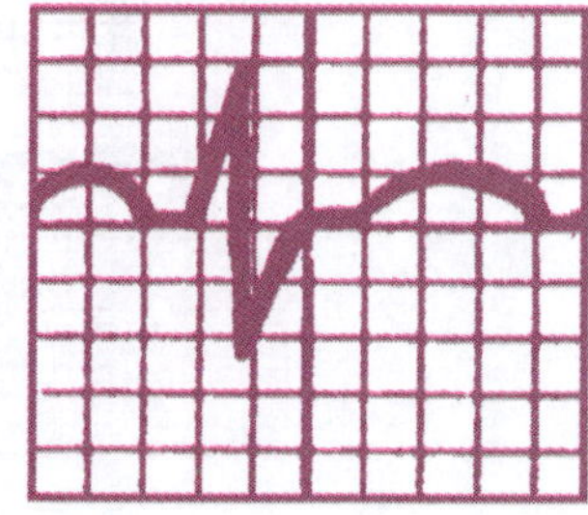

Chapter 19 Objectives

Upon completion of this chapter, the student will be able to:

- Correlate certain rhythms and 12-lead EKGs with their treatment.
- Display critical thinking skills.

Introduction

Throughout the previous chapters you've been working with practice skills and critical thinking exercises to boost your understanding of the chapter material. It's time now to put everything you've learned together in a big way. In the following scenarios you will use every skill you've learned. You will analyze rhythms and 12-lead EKGs and decide on a course of action. What's going on? Why is it happening? What was done about it in the scenario? What **should have** been done? Is there an MI? What's the rhythm? What medication is indicated? This is the pinnacle of the learning experience–not just mindlessly memorizing material, but using it in a practical way. Let's get started.

Scenario A: Mr. Johnson

Mr. Johnson, age 52, was admitted to the hospital's telemetry floor complaining of mild chest discomfort that lasted 2 hours and was unrelieved by antacids. His parents both had a history of heart disease, so Mr. Johnson was afraid he might be having a heart attack. His initial EKG in the emergency department was completely normal, and his pain was relieved with one sublingual nitroglycerin tablet. Medical history included a two-pack-a-day cigarette habit, as well as major surgery the previous week to remove a small colon cancer. Mr. Johnson had been asleep in his room for about an hour when the nurse observed the strip shown in Figure 19-1 on his cardiac monitor.

1. What do you see of concern on the rhythm strip in Figure 19-1? _______

   ____

   The nurse went to check on Mr. Johnson and found him just awakening and complaining of a dull ache in his chest. Per unit protocol, the nurse did a 12-lead EKG, shown in Figure 19-2.

2. What conclusion do you draw from the EKG in Figure 19-2? _________

   ____

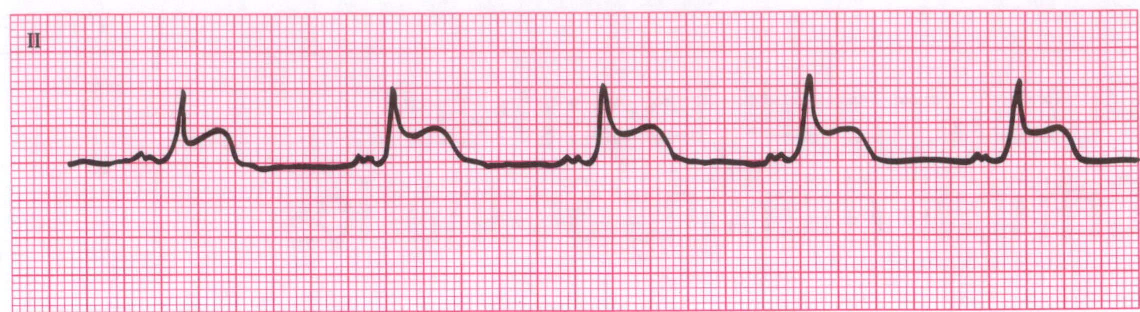

Figure 19-1 Mr. Johnson's rhythm.

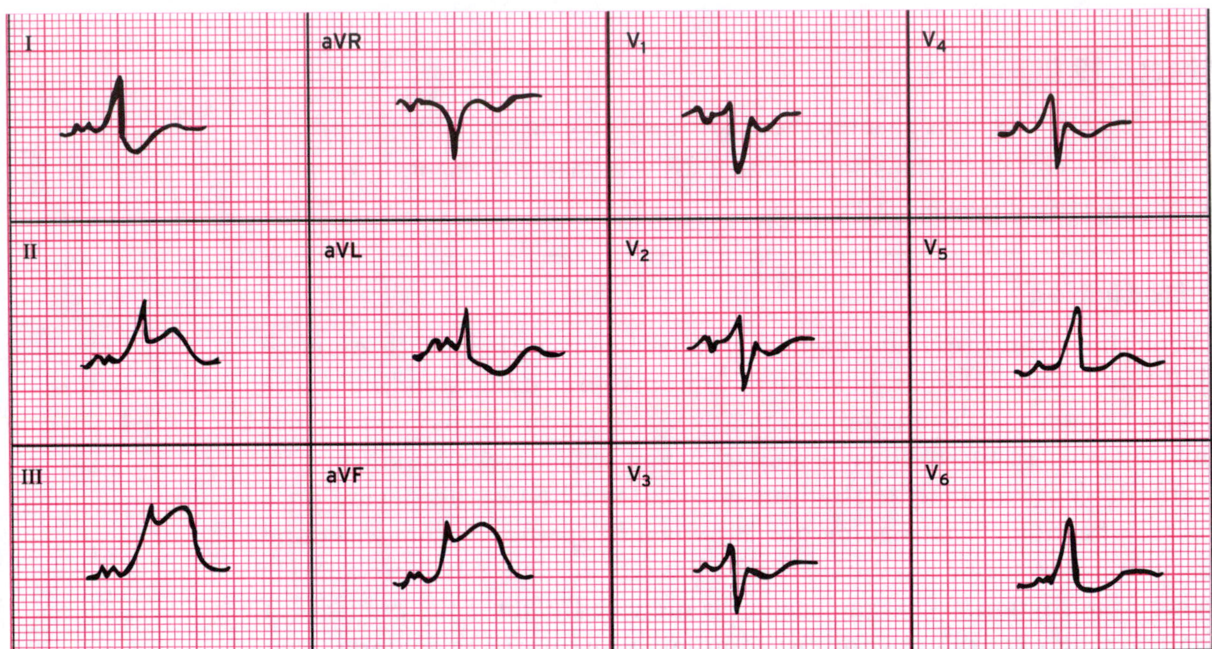

Figure 19-2 Mr. Johnson's 12-lead EKG done during chest pain.

3. Mr. Johnson was moved to the coronary care unit and was started on a nitroglycerin infusion and a heparin infusion. For what purpose were these infusions started? ____

4. Mr. Johnson was also started on oxygen by nasal prongs. What beneficial effect would the oxygen be expected to have? ____________________

5. The physician considered starting thrombolytic therapy, but due to Mr. Johnson's recent surgery decided he was not a candidate for thrombolytics. What is the mode of action of thrombolytic medications? ______

6. What is the danger of giving thrombolytics to someone who had recent surgery? ____

Shortly after arrival in CCU, Mr. Johnson called his nurse and told her he felt "funny." He denied pain but stated he felt "full in the head." The nurse noticed the rhythm in Figure 19-3 on the monitor in Mr. Johnson's room.

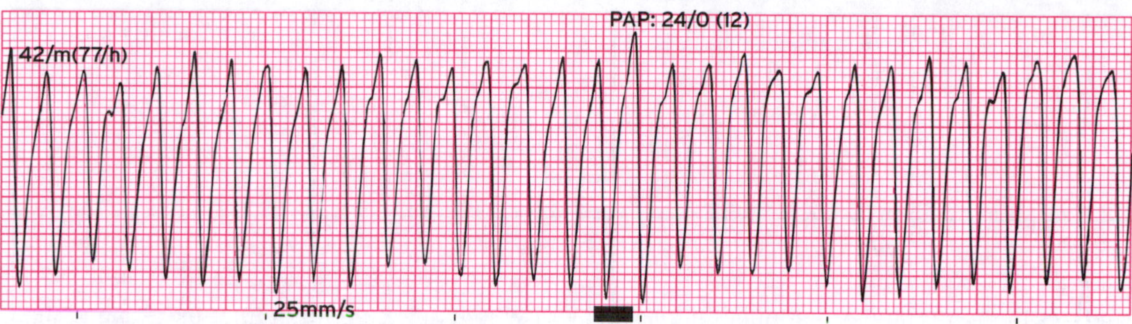

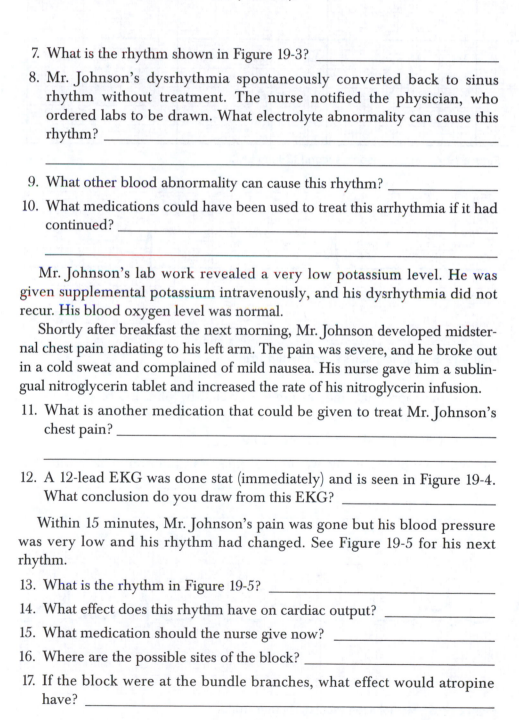

Figure 19-3 Mr. Johnson's second rhythm strip.

7. What is the rhythm shown in Figure 19-3? ____________________
8. Mr. Johnson's dysrhythmia spontaneously converted back to sinus rhythm without treatment. The nurse notified the physician, who ordered labs to be drawn. What electrolyte abnormality can cause this rhythm? ____________________
9. What other blood abnormality can cause this rhythm? ____________________
10. What medications could have been used to treat this arrhythmia if it had continued? ____________________

Mr. Johnson's lab work revealed a very low potassium level. He was given supplemental potassium intravenously, and his dysrhythmia did not recur. His blood oxygen level was normal.

Shortly after breakfast the next morning, Mr. Johnson developed midsternal chest pain radiating to his left arm. The pain was severe, and he broke out in a cold sweat and complained of mild nausea. His nurse gave him a sublingual nitroglycerin tablet and increased the rate of his nitroglycerin infusion.

11. What is another medication that could be given to treat Mr. Johnson's chest pain? ____________________
12. A 12-lead EKG was done stat (immediately) and is seen in Figure 19-4. What conclusion do you draw from this EKG? ____________________

Within 15 minutes, Mr. Johnson's pain was gone but his blood pressure was very low and his rhythm had changed. See Figure 19-5 for his next rhythm.

13. What is the rhythm in Figure 19-5? ____________________
14. What effect does this rhythm have on cardiac output? ____________________
15. What medication should the nurse give now? ____________________
16. Where are the possible sites of the block? ____________________
17. If the block were at the bundle branches, what effect would atropine have? ____________________

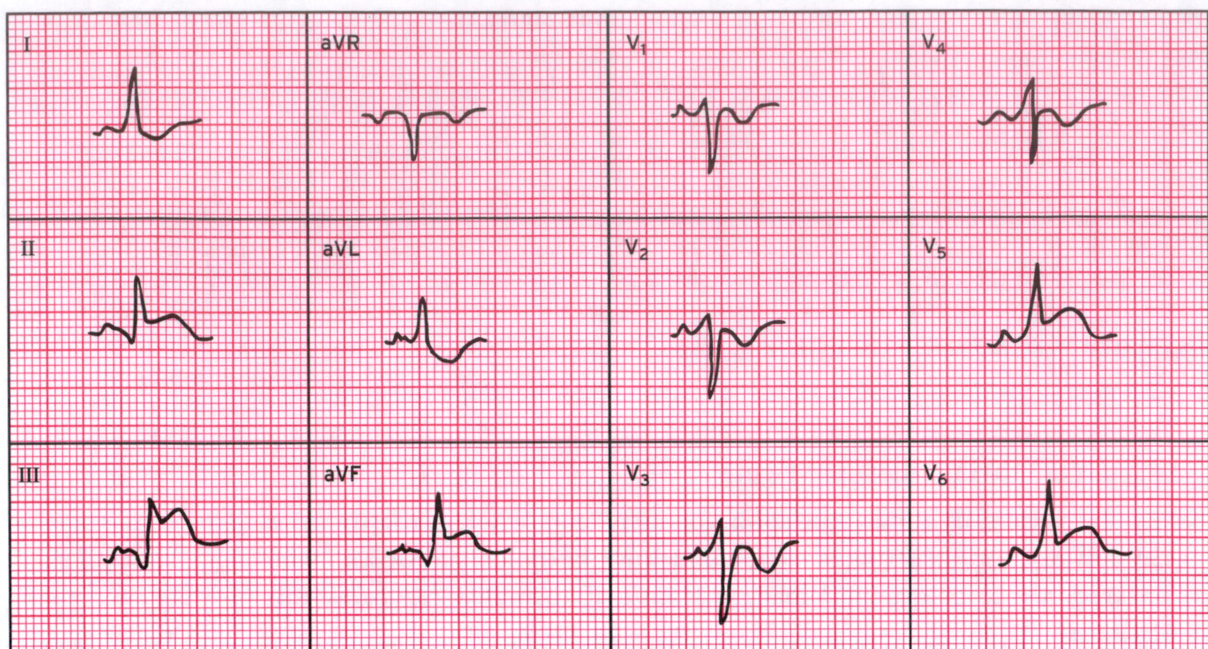

Figure 19-4 Mr. Johnson's second 12-lead EKG.

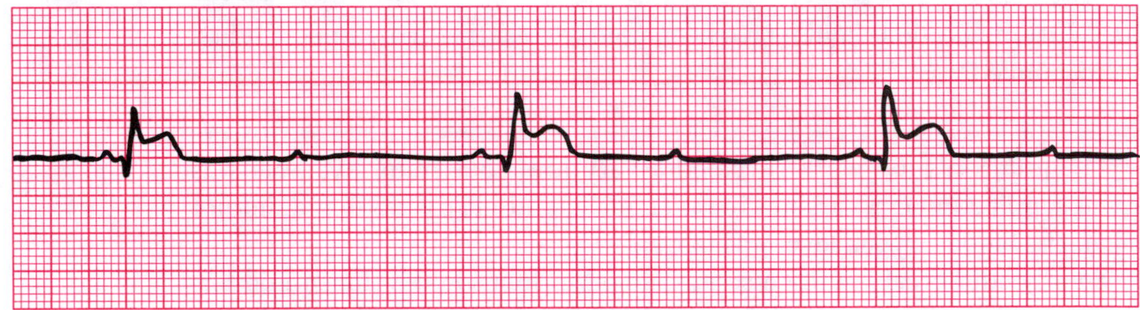

Figure 19-5 Mr. Johnson's third rhythm strip.

After the appropriate medication was given, Mr. Johnson's blood pressure returned to normal, and his rhythm was as seen in Figure 19-6.

18. What rhythm is shown in Figure 19-6? ______________________

19. What symptoms, if any, would you expect Mr. Johnson to have with this rhythm? ______________________

____

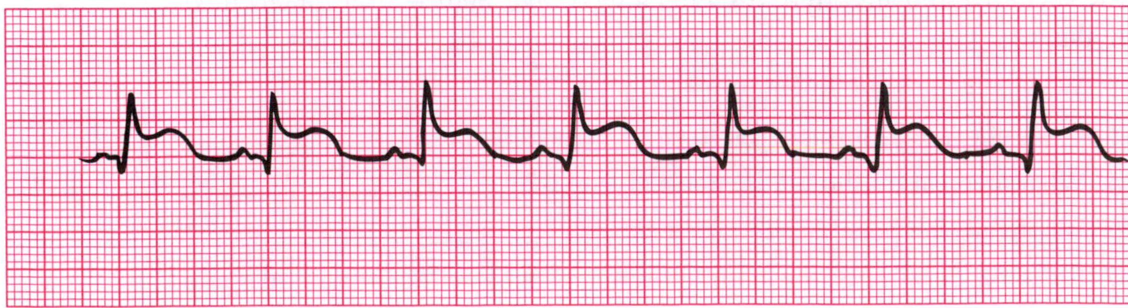

Figure 19-6 Mr. Johnson's fourth rhythm strip.

Mr. Johnson's cardiologist was concerned about the implications of the most recent EKG and his dysrhythmias. He took Mr. Johnson to the cardiac catheterization lab to do an angiogram. It revealed significant blockage in two of his coronary arteries.

20. Based on the two EKGs in Figures 19-2 and 19-4, which two coronary arteries do you suspect were blocked? ______________________

Balloon angioplasty was attempted but was unsuccessful, so Mr. Johnson was taken to the operating room to have bypass surgery. He did well and was home in a week.

Scenario B: Ms. Capitano

Ms. Capitano was a 23-year-old woman who presented to the ER with complaints of fatigue and dizziness. She had a negative medical history and did not smoke. Aside from birth control pills, she took no medication and denied illegal drug use. She did drink five or six soft drinks daily and had two to three cups of coffee every morning. Cardiac monitor revealed the rhythm seen in Figure 19-7.

1. What is the rhythm shown in Figure 19-7? ______________________
2. What is the likely cause of this rhythm in Ms. Capitano's case? ________ ______________________
3. The physician ordered adenosine to be given intravenously. The rhythm strip shown in Figure 19-8 was the result. What happened?___________ ______________________

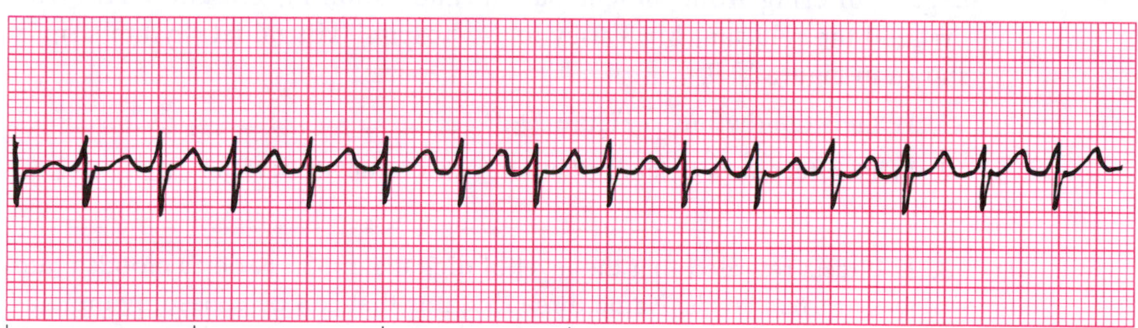

Figure 19-7 Ms. Capitano's initial rhythm in the ER.

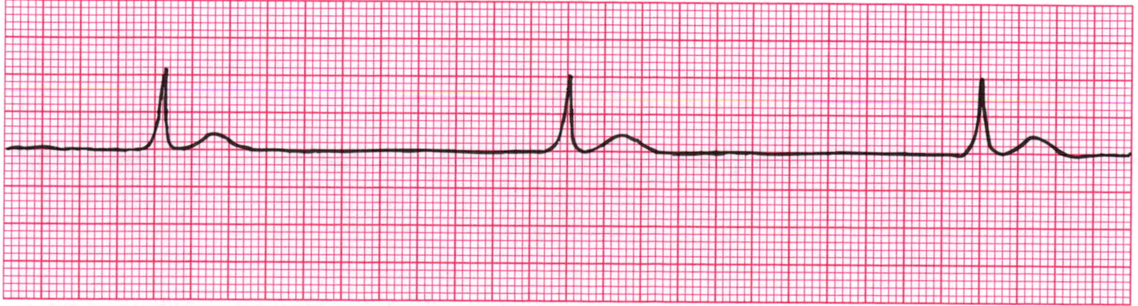

Figure 19-8 Ms. Capitano's rhythm after adenosine administration.

After a few seconds of the slow heart rate, Ms. Capitano's heart rate sped back up–to the 250s this time–and she stated that she felt as though she were going to pass out. Her blood pressure, which had been 110/60, dropped to 68/50, and she was now very pale and drenched in a cold sweat.

4. What effect was the tachycardia having on her cardiac output? ________

____

Ms. Capitano's condition had worsened–she was now in shock. The ER physician elected to perform synchronized electrical cardioversion. After a low-voltage shock, Ms. Capitano's rhythm converted to sinus rhythm with a heart rate in the 90s and her blood pressure improved. Soon her color was back to normal and her skin was dry. She was admitted to the coronary care unit for close observation and was started on calcium channel blockers to prevent recurrences of her tachycardia. The physician advised her to curtail her caffeine intake. After a day in CCU, Ms. Capitano was transferred to the telemetry floor. She was sent home a day later, doing well.

Scenario C: Mr. Farley

A few years ago, Mr. Farley was diagnosed with chronic atrial fibrillation and was started on digitalis. He'd done well, with a heart rate running in the 70s and 80s since then. For the last few days, however, Mr. Farley had felt lousy–nothing specific, just "not right," as he would later describe it. He didn't think it was important enough to bother his physician, though his wife had fussed at him to do so. Believing his problem to be related to his atrial fibrillation, Mr. Farley doubled up on his digitalis dose. If one pill a day was good, two a day had to be better, he reasoned. After five days of this, he began suffering from violent nausea and vomiting episodes. His wife dragged the reluctant Mr. Farley to the hospital. His initial rhythm strip is shown in Figure 19-9.

1. What is the rhythm in Figure 19-9? ________________
2. What effect does atrial fibrillation have on the atrial kick? ________

   ____

3. Lab tests revealed that the level of digitalis in Mr. Farley's bloodstream was at toxic levels. Name three rhythms that can be caused by digitalis toxicity. ________________

   ____

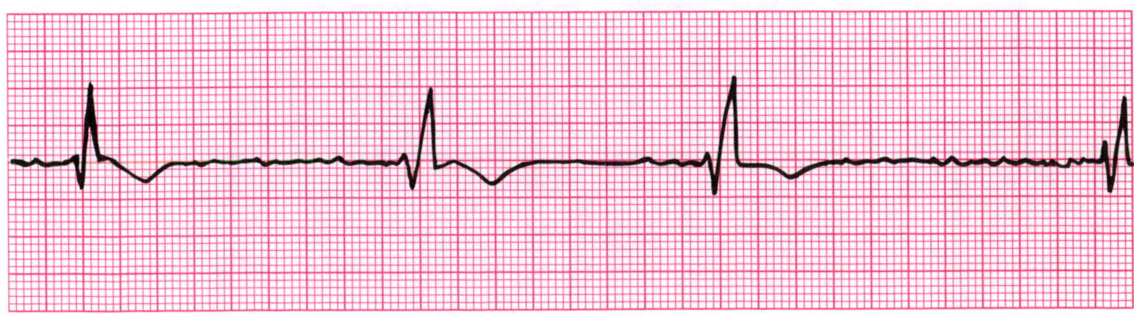

Figure 19-9 Mr. Farley's initial rhythm strip.

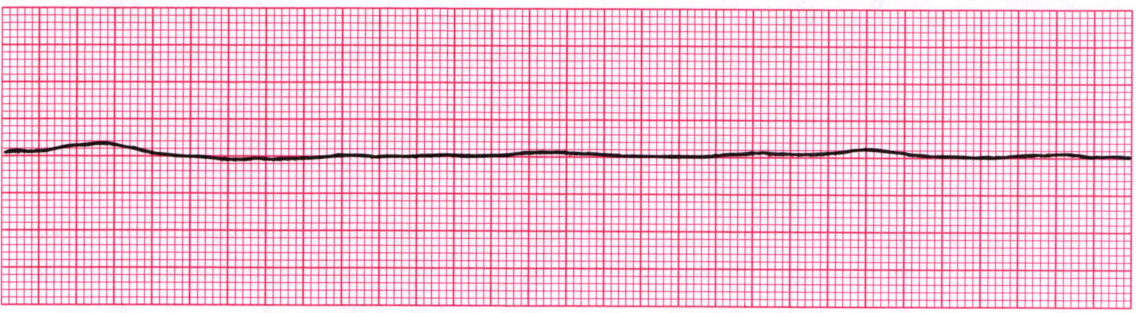

Figure 19-10 Mr. Farley's second rhythm strip.

The physician contemplated sending Mr. Farley to the CCU, but since his blood pressure was good and he looked OK, he was sent to the telemetry floor instead. His nausea was treated with medication and he was taken off digitalis. Three hours after arriving on the telemetry floor, Mr. Farley passed out in the bathroom. His wife ran to get the nurse just as the nurses, having seen his rhythm on the monitor, were running toward his room. His new rhythm is shown in Figure 19-10.

4. What is the rhythm in Figure 19-10? ____________________
5. The emergency team was called and CPR was initiated. What two medications would be appropriate to give at this time? ____________________
6. After successful resuscitation, Mr. Farley was transferred to the CCU, where a temporary pacemaker was inserted. What beneficial effect would the pacemaker have? ____________________
7. A few hours after the pacemaker was inserted, the nurse noticed evidence of loss of capture on the monitor. On the monitor strip in Figure 19-11, what would tell her there was loss of capture? ____________________
8. What can be done to restore capture? ____________________

Capture was restored, and Mr. Johnson rested well for the next few hours. Suddenly, he went into v-tach with a heart rate of 200. The nurses could tell

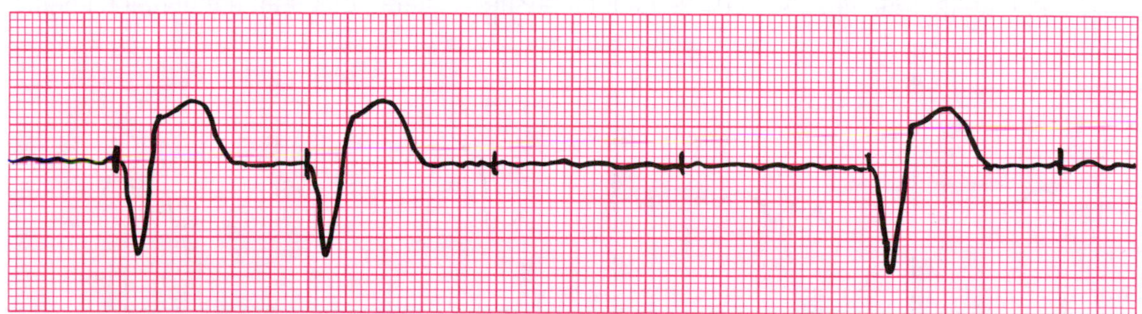

Figure 19-11 Mr. Farley's third rhythm strip.

the v-tach was originating in the left ventricle, so they knew it was not induced by irritation from the pacemaker wire in the right ventricle.

9. With a pacemaker in place, what can be done to terminate the tachycardia? ____

10. With the v-tach now resolved, Mr. Farley was started on an amiodarone infusion to prevent a recurrence of the v-tach. What is amiodarone's effect on the ventricle? ____

11. The rest of Mr. Farley's hospital stay was uneventful. Since his problem began with his inappropriate self-dosing of digitalis, what would you tell Mr. Farley regarding his digitalis dose in the future? ____________

Scenario D: Mr. Lew

Age 78, Mr. Lew had outlived his wife and most of their friends. He had never been in the hospital and had not seen his physician in seven years. By all accounts, he was unusually healthy for his age. He was not alarmed by the occasional tightness in his chest–and in fact took it as a sign that he was out of shape and needed to exercise more. One summer day, while mowing the lawn, the chest tightness came back, but this time it was much more intense, and Mr. Lew became concerned. He called his son to take him to the hospital. On the way, Mr. Lew passed out in the car and slumped over onto his son, causing an accident. Ambulances rushed the duo to the closest ER. Stephen, the son, was treated for a fractured arm and was discharged in a cast. Though not injured in the accident, Mr. Lew was in much worse shape. See his EKG in Figure 19-12.

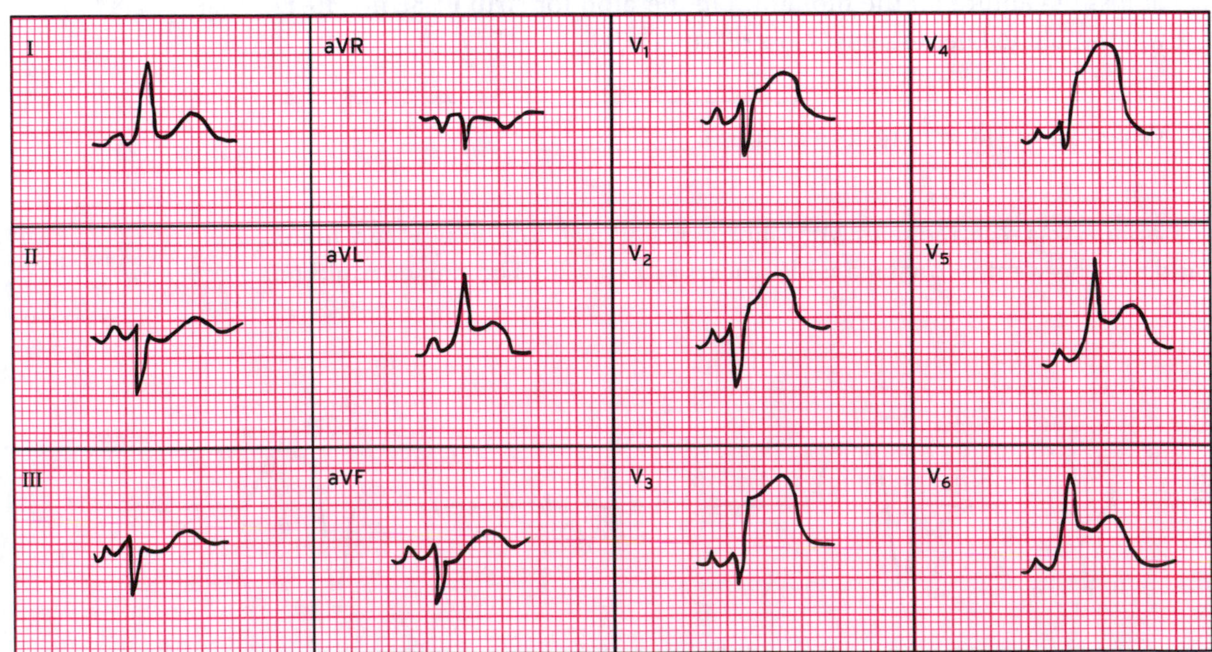

Figure 19-12 Mr. Lew's initial 12-lead EKG.

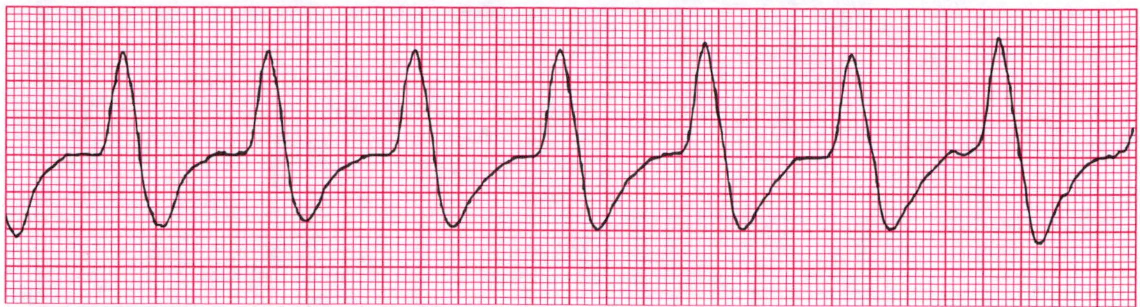

Figure 19-13 Mr. Lew's rhythm strip after thrombolytic therapy.

1. What conclusion do you draw from the EKG in Figure 19-12? ________
____

Mr. Lew's condition was precarious. His blood pressure was low and he was in danger of cardiac arrest. Thrombolytic therapy was started, and within one hour Mr. Lew's blood pressure had improved. Soon he was in the rhythm shown in Figure 19-13.

2. What is the rhythm in Figure 19-13? ____________________
3. What, if any, treatment does this rhythm require in this case? ________
____
4. What was the likely cause of this rhythm? ________________

This rhythm converted back to sinus rhythm within 30 minutes. Mr. Lew's condition improved over the next hour, and he was transferred to the coronary care unit, where he stabilized.

When Stephen came by to see his dad the next day, Mr. Lew whispered to him that he was having mild chest pain again, but that it wasn't bad enough to bother the nurses. Stephen, however, alerted the nurse, who did an EKG while the pain was in progress. See the EKG in Figure 19-14.

5. What conclusion do you draw from the EKG in Figure 19-14? ________
____

Mr. Lew's nitroglycerin and heparin infusions, which had been started in the ER, were adjusted and Mr. Lew was taken for an emergency angiogram. An occlusion of the left main coronary artery was noted, along with blockage in another coronary artery.

6. Based on the two EKGs in Figures 19-12 and 19-14, which other coronary artery is involved? ____________________
7. What is the cause of the ST segment depression noted on Mr. Lew's first EKG? ____________________
____

Mr. Lew was taken to the operating room for emergency bypass surgery. Following cardiac arrest in the operating room, he returned to the CCU in critical condition. Before the surgical nurses had gotten back to the OR after having brought Mr. Lew to CCU, they heard the emergency page on the loudspeaker. Mr. Lew was cardiac arresting again. They rushed back to

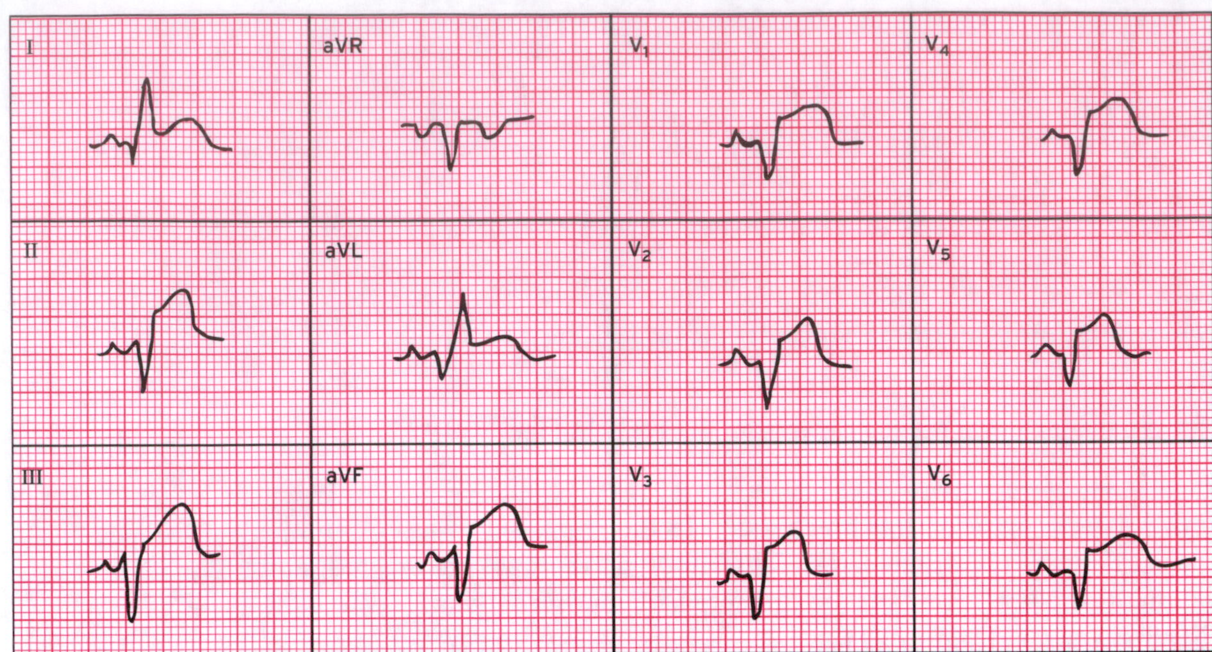

Figure 19-14 Mr. Lew's EKG done during chest pain.

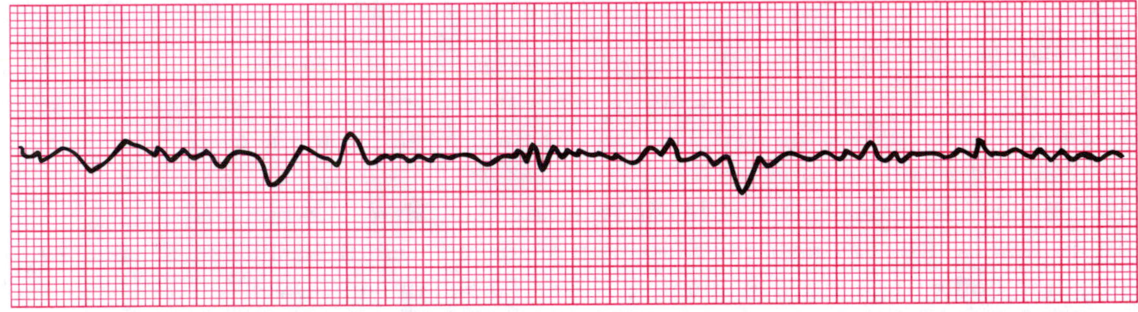

Figure 19-15 Mr. Lew's rhythm during cardiac arrest.

CCU to help. The cardiac surgeon had opened the chest sutures and was doing manual chest compressions by squeezing Mr. Lew's heart in his hands. Mr. Lew's rhythm strip is shown in Figure 19-15.

8. What is the rhythm in Figure 19-15? ______________________

Internal defibrillator paddles were inserted into the open chest cavity and placed on either side of Mr. Lew's heart. A small volt was discharged, and Mr. Lew's rhythm changed to the one shown in Figure 19-16.

9. What is the rhythm in Figure 19-16? ______________________

CPR was started again, and the staff administered various medications as well as temporary pacing–all to no avail. Mr. Lew did not make it.

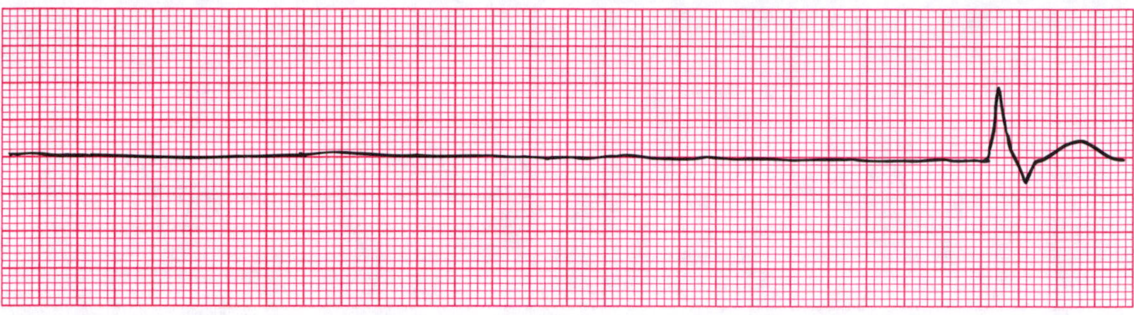

Figure 19-16 Mr. Lew's rhythm after defibrillation.

Scenario E: Mrs. Epstein

Mrs. Epstein had had her pacemaker implanted four years ago because of third-degree AV block. She'd been doing well until this morning, when she began to feel dizzy. She took her pulse as she'd been taught to do and found it to be 38. Her rate-responsive DDD pacemaker was set at a rate of 60 to 125. At the physician's office, the cardiologist found that the pacemaker needed a new battery. Because her heart rate was now in the 60s, he felt the battery change could wait until the next morning. He sent Mrs. Epstein to the hospital, where she was admitted to the telemetry floor.

A few hours after arrival, Mrs. Epstein complained again of dizziness, this time much worse. Her rhythm is shown in Figure 19-17.

1. What is the rhythm in Figure 19-17? ______________________________
2. What is her pacemaker doing? ______________________________
3. What is the likely cause of this problem? ______________________________

The nurse, following hospital protocol, gave atropine, and Mrs. Epstein's heart rate climbed to the 60s.

After notifying the cardiologist of the situation, the nurse rushed Mrs. Epstein to the cardiac catheterization lab, where an emergency pacemaker battery change was done. After her return to the telemetry floor, the nurse noted her rhythm as shown in Figure 19-18.

4. What is the rhythm in Figure 19-18? ______________________________
5. Is the pacemaker functioning properly? If not, what is the problem?

____

____

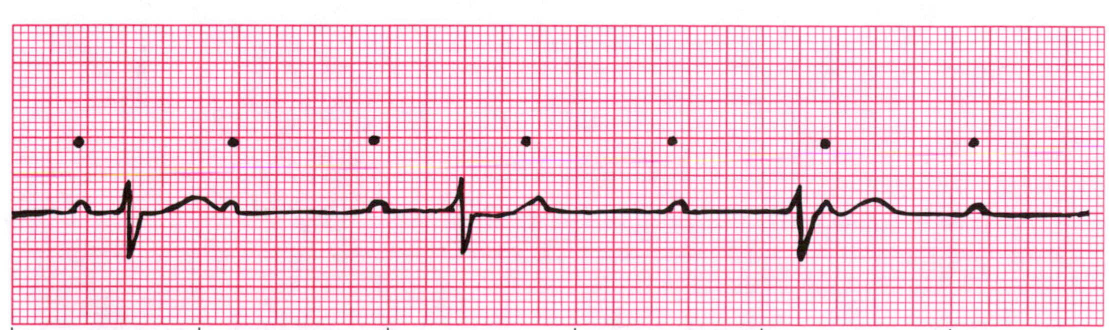

Figure 19-17 Mrs. Epstein's rhythm during a dizzy spell in the hospital.

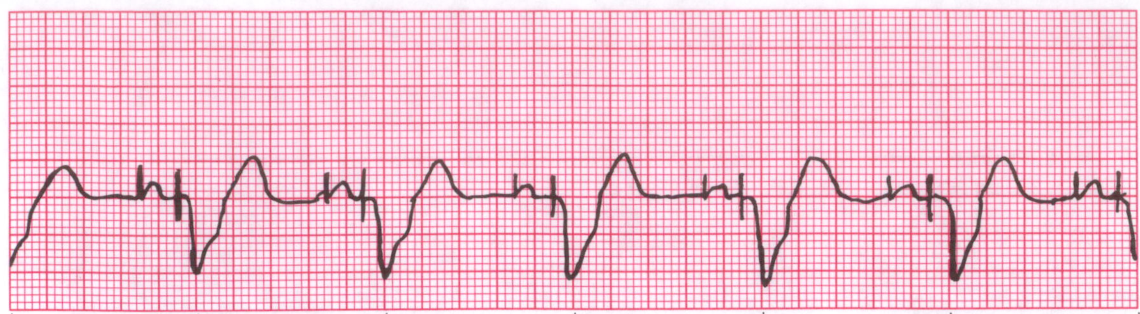

Figure 19-18 Mrs. Epstein's rhythm on return from her pacemaker battery change.

Mrs. Epstein was discharged the following day in good condition.

Scenario F: Mr. Calico

Mr. Calico, age 76, was taking a walk when he developed chest heaviness. He went inside and told his wife he was going to lie down on the sofa for a while. She grew concerned an hour later when she called his name and he didn't answer. Mrs. Calico called 911 and the paramedics arrived to find Mr. Calico in the rhythm seen in Figure 19-19.

1. What is this rhythm?____________________________________
2. What symptoms would you expect to see in Mr. Calico?________________ ____
3. Mr. Calico was unconscious and had no pulse and no breathing. What should the paramedics do to resuscitate Mr. Calico? ________________

After appropriate initial treatment, Mr. Calico's pulse returned and he began to awaken. The paramedics ran another rhythm strip. See Figure 19-20.

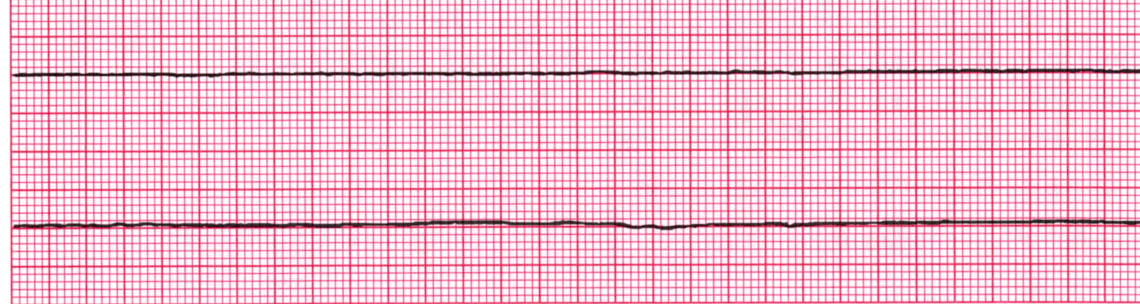

Figure 19-19 Mr. Calico's initial rhythm.

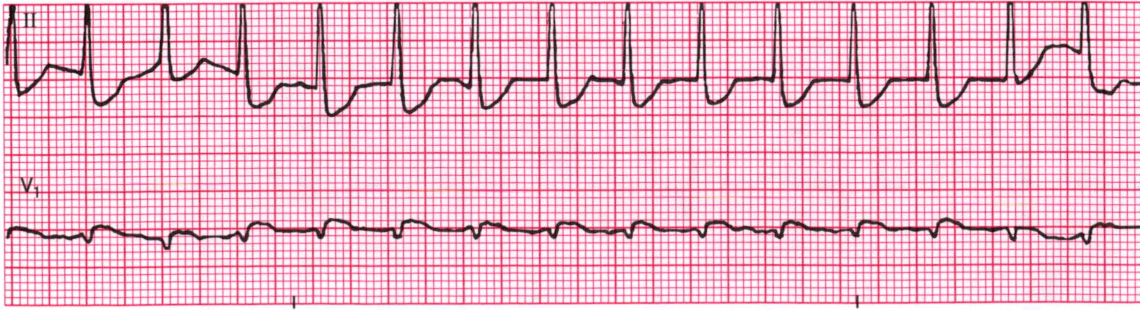

Figure 19-20 Mr. Calico's rhythm after initial treatment.

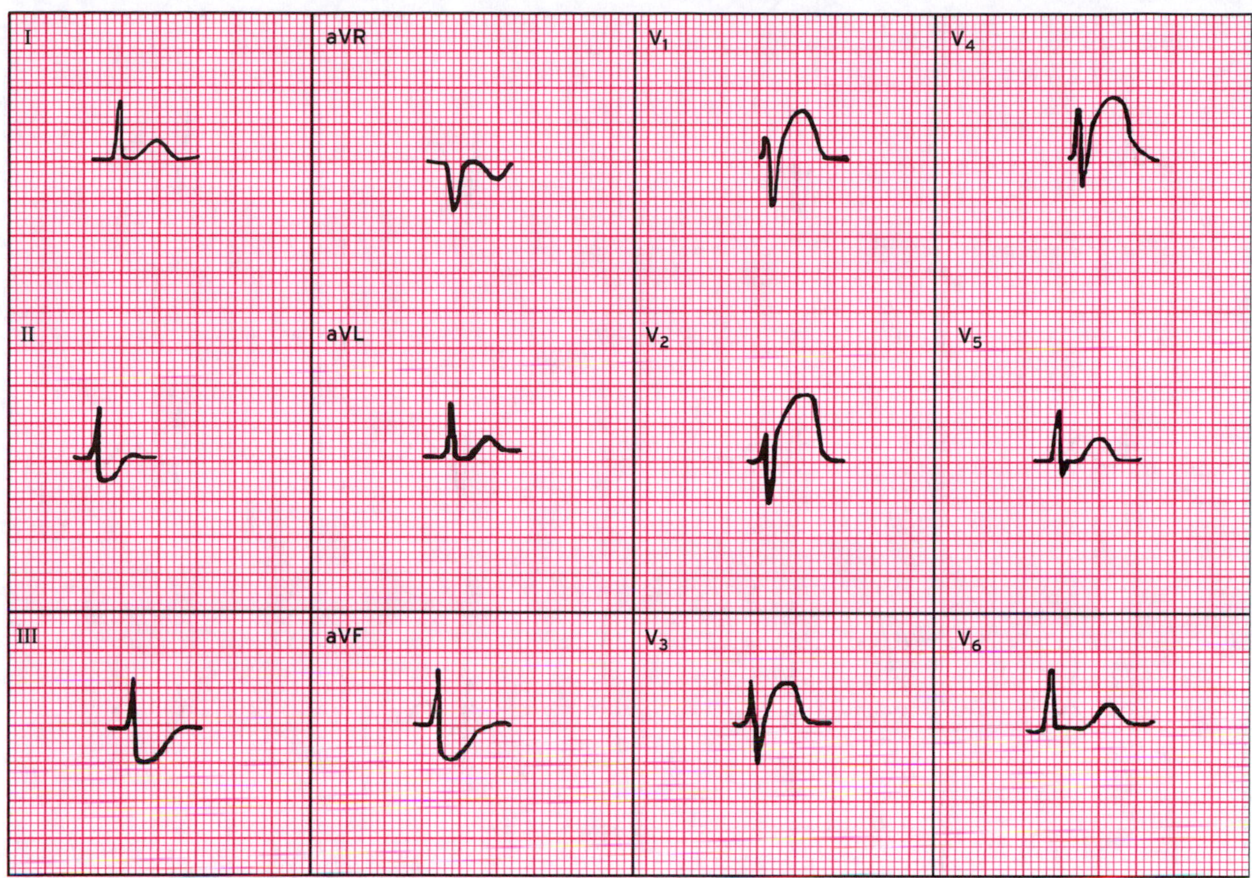

Figure 19-21 Mr. Calico's initial 12-lead EKG.

4. What is this rhythm? ________________________

Paramedics rushed Mr. Calico to the nearest hospital, where a 12-lead EKG was done. His 12-lead EKG is seen in Figure 19-21.

5. What conclusion do you draw from this EKG? ________________
6. Thrombolytic medication was started and the EKG was repeated. See Figure 19-22. What has changed since the last EKG?______________

____
7. Mr. Calico went into ventricular fibrillation a few minutes later. The nurse prepared to cardiovert the rhythm, but when he depressed the buttons to deliver the shock, nothing happened. Why and what corrective action is needed for this problem?____________________

____

After correctly defibrillating Mr. Calico, the ER staff sent him to the CCU, where he spent a week recovering. He went home and did well with no further problems.

Scenario G: Mrs. Taylor

Mrs. Taylor hated dialysis (a method of removing waste from the bloodstream when the kidneys are unable to do so). Being attached to a machine

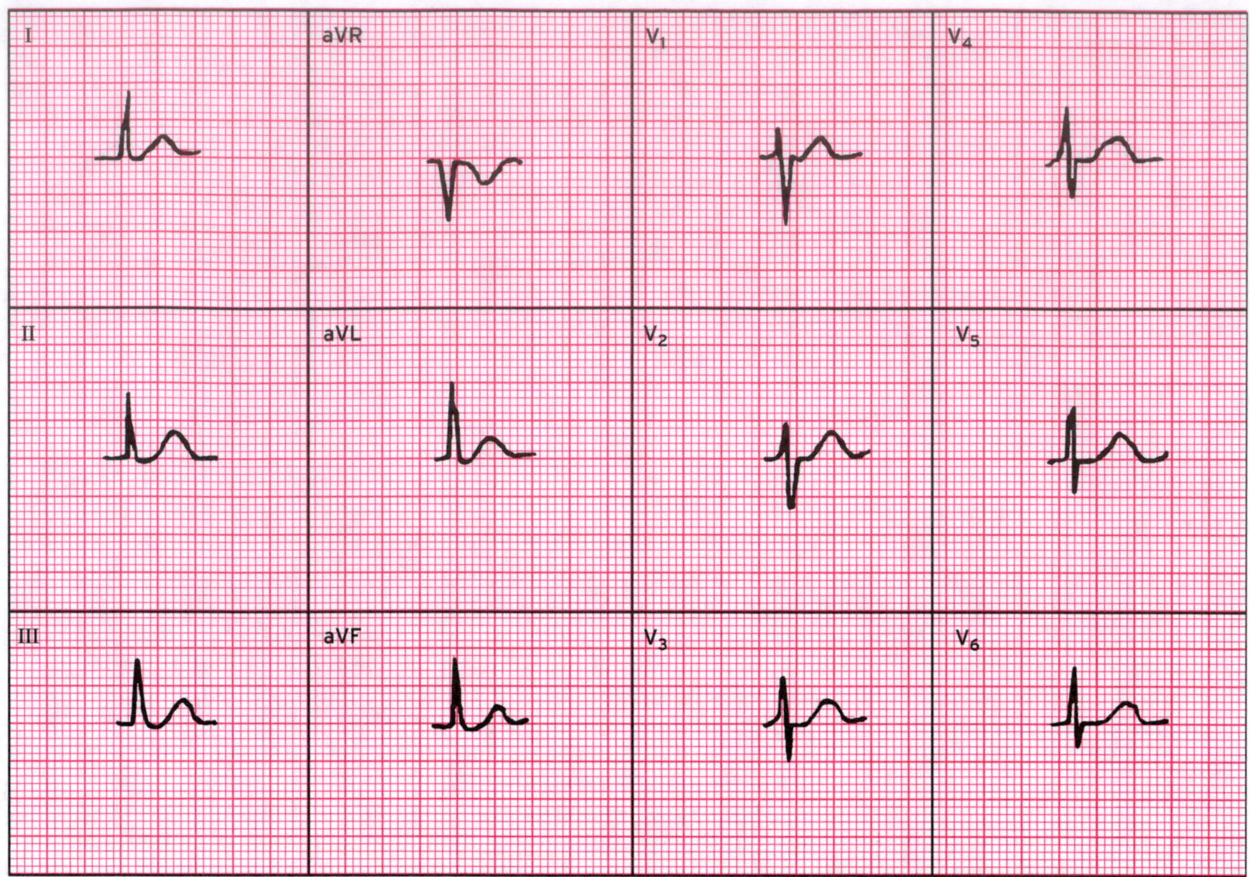

Figure 19-22 Mr. Calico's EKG after thrombolytic medication.

for three days a week, four hours each time, was, in her words, "not my idea of living." Age 45, she'd been in kidney failure for 15 years, and had required dialysis for most of that time. Because of other health problems (diabetes, heart disease, asthma), she was not a candidate for a kidney transplant. At her local hospital, Mrs. Taylor was notorious for coming in critically ill after having skipped two or three dialysis treatments. She'd be admitted to the intensive care unit, treated, and released a week or so later, with a warning not to skip dialysis any more. But a few months later she'd be back again.

Tonight Mrs. Taylor comes in yet again. Her potassium level, which should be 5.0 at the most, is 8.9, dangerously high. Her EKG is below. See Figure 19-23.

1. In chapter 13 you learned that elevated potassium levels can cause two main effects on the EKG. What are they and which one or ones do you see on this EKG?______________________________________

____

Almost immediately after arrival in the ER, Mrs. Taylor loses consciousness and suffers cardiac arrest. The nurse records the following rhythm strip as she begins CPR. See Figure 19-24.

2. What is this rhythm?____

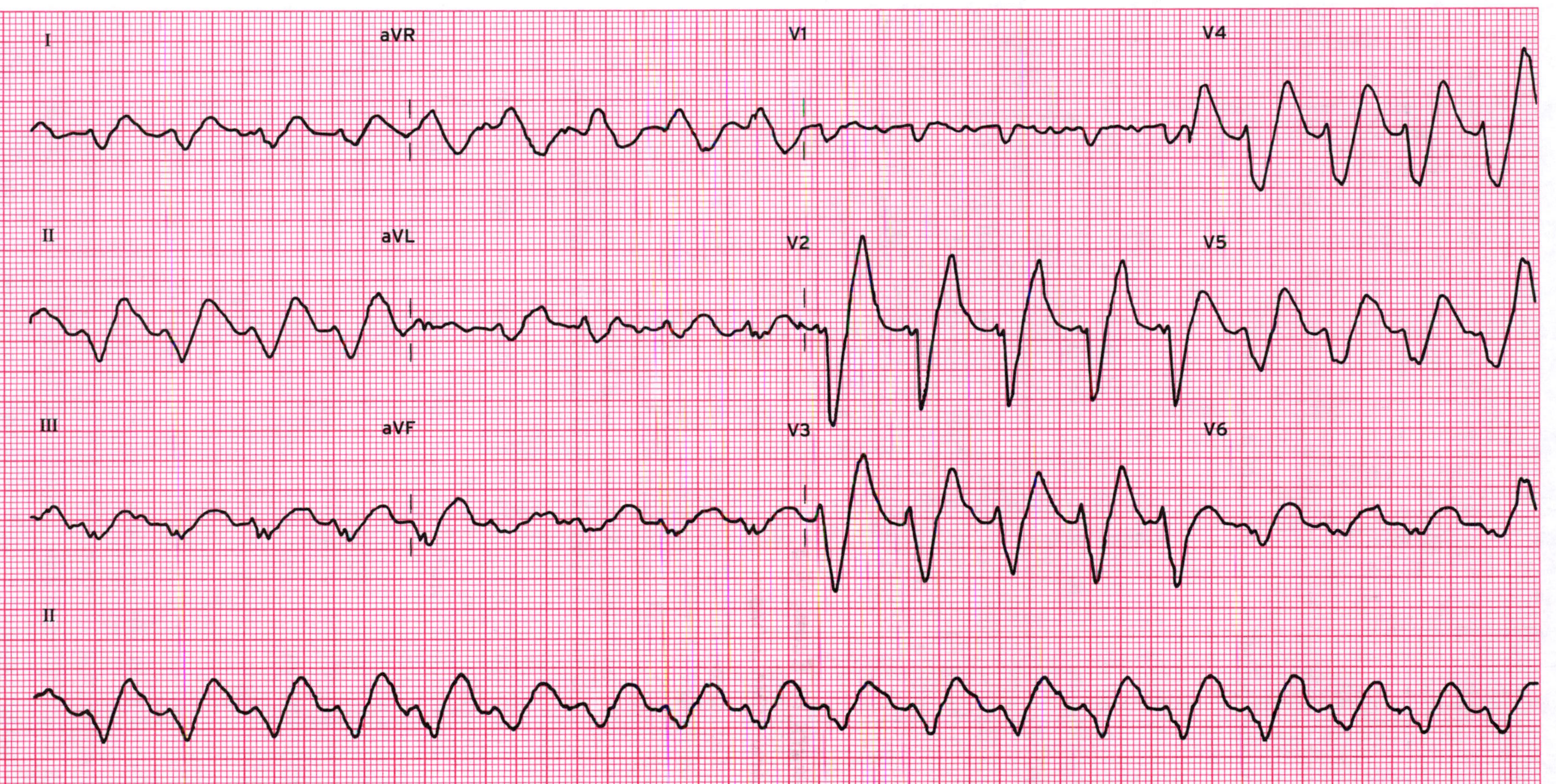

Figure 19-23 Mrs. Taylor's first EKG.

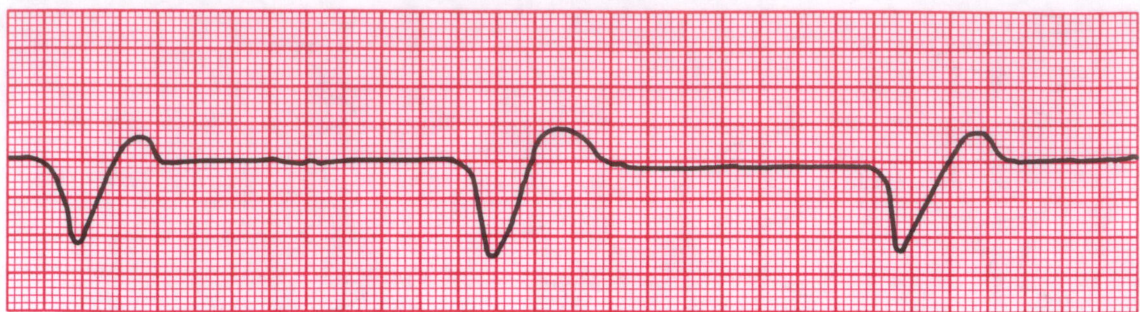

Figure 19-24 Rhythm strip during cardiac arrest.

The physician orders calcium to be given intravenously. Calcium is a potassium antagonist that decreases the potassium level in the bloodstream. After giving the calcium, the nurse runs the following EKG. See Figure 19-25.

3. What change do you see in the QRS complex? ____________________

Mrs. Taylor's pulse and breathing have resumed after the calcium. She is sent to the intensive care unit, where she is dialyzed. Four days later, she is well enough to go home. Once again she is warned that the next time she skips dialysis, it could be fatal. She smiles at the nurses and says, "I know, I know."

Answers to Scenarios

Scenario A: Mr. Johnson

1. Of concern is the ST segment elevation in lead II on this strip. The sinus bradycardia is not a concern, especially since Mr. Johnson had been asleep, but the ST elevation is worrisome.
2. Mr. Johnson is having an inferior wall MI, as evidenced by the ST elevation in leads II, III, and aVF and by the reciprocal ST depression in the anterior leads.
3. Nitroglycerin dilates coronary arteries and thus increases the flow to the tissues. Heparin is an anticoagulant that will prevent clots from forming in the coronary arteries. It will not, however, dissolve any that may already be there.
4. The oxygen will improve tissue concentration of oxygen and can help prevent arrhythmias and decrease the heart's workload.
5. Thrombolytic medications dissolve blood clots.
6. The danger of giving thrombolytics to someone who had recent surgery is that severe bleeding may occur at the surgical site.
7. The rhythm is ventricular tachycardia. Heart rate is about 300.
8. Potassium deficit (hypokalemia) can cause v-tach.
9. Hypoxia is another blood abnormality that can cause v-tach.
10. Procainamide and amiodarone could be used to abolish the v-tach.
11. Morphine is another medication that can be used to treat chest pain.

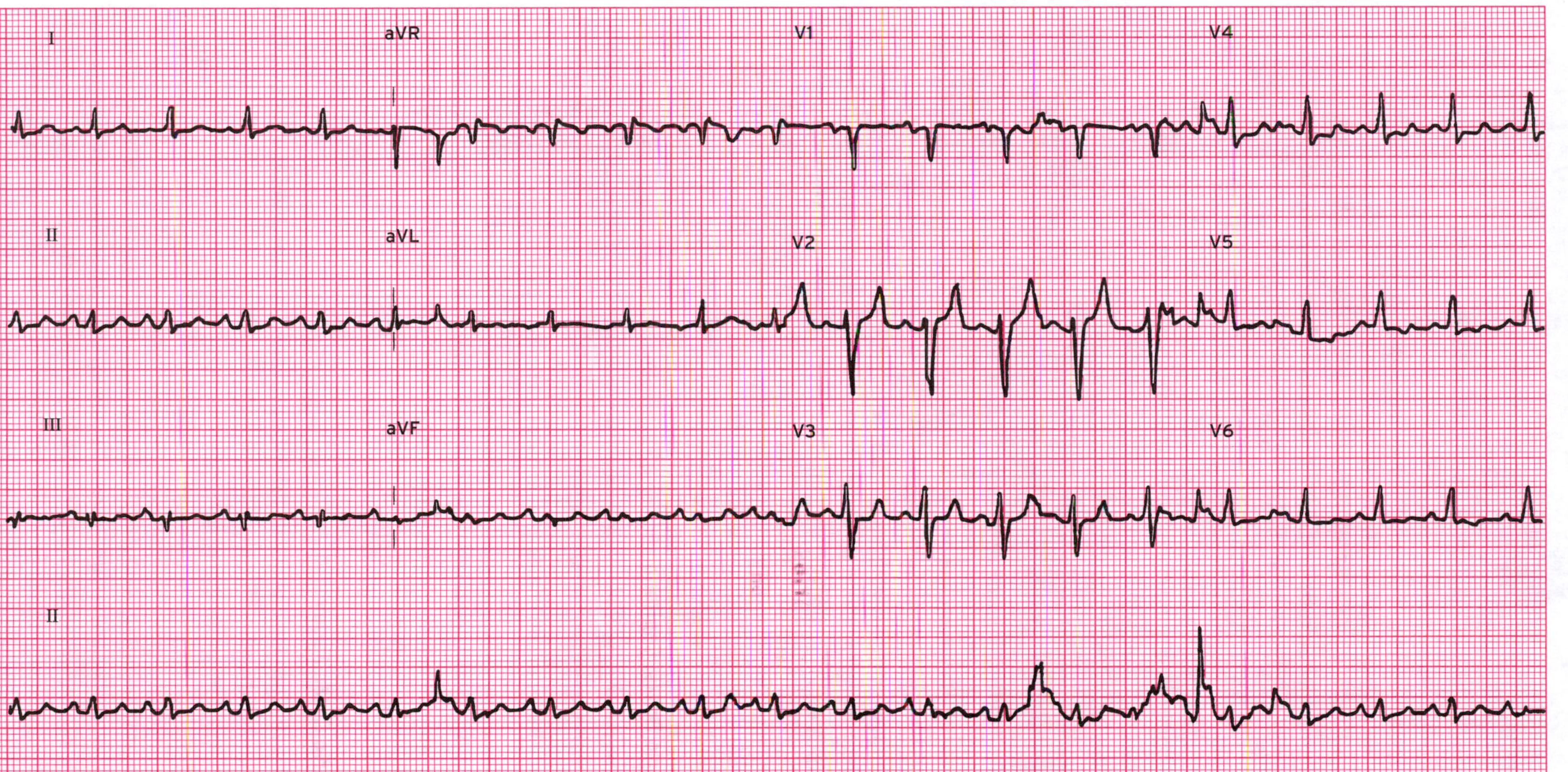

Figure 19-25 EKG after calcium.

12. The MI is extending into the lateral wall now, as evidenced by the new ST elevation in leads V_5 to V_6.
13. This rhythm is 2:1 AV block. There are two P waves to every QRS on this strip.
14. This rhythm can cause the cardiac output to drop.
15. The nurse should now give atropine to speed up the heart rate.
16. The block could be at the AV node or the bundle branches.
17. If the block were at the bundle branches, atropine may have no effect on the heart rate, or it could make things worse by speeding up the sinus rate and increasing the block ratio. Atropine speeds up the rate of the sinus node and increases AV conduction, causing the impulses to come more rapidly. The impulses blast through the AV node only to arrive at the still-blocked bundle branches (atropine has no effect on the bundle branches). Epinephrine and/or pacing would be indicated for a block at the bundle branches.
18. This rhythm is sinus rhythm.
19. Mr. Johnson should have no symptoms from this rhythm. He should in fact feel much better now that his heart rate is more normal.
20. The two coronary arteries blocked were probably the right coronary artery, which supplies the inferior wall of the left ventricle, and the circumflex, which supplies the lateral wall. It is also possible that Mr. Johnson is left-dominant, with a circumflex coronary artery that is very prominent and supplies not only the lateral wall, but the inferior wall as well. (Review chapter 2 for a refresher on the coronary arteries.)

Scenario B: Ms. Capitano

1. The rhythm is SVT. The heart rate is about 150, the rhythm is regular, and P waves are not discernible.
2. The likely cause of this rhythm in this case is caffeine overdose.
3. The heart rate slowed dramatically to a junctional bradycardia. This is not unusual after adenosine administration. In fact, sometimes the heart completely stops for a few seconds before the sinus node kicks back in.
4. The tachycardia is dropping her cardiac output to dangerously low levels.

Scenario C: Mr. Farley

1. The rhythm is slow atrial fibrillation. Note the wavy, undulating baseline and the absence of P waves.
2. In atrial fibrillation, there is no atrial kick at all, thus causing a drop in cardiac output of about 15% to 30%.
3. Digitalis toxicity can cause almost any arrhythmia, such as junctional tachycardia; atrial tachycardia; sinus arrests, sinus blocks; all degrees of AV blocks; and slow junctional and ventricular rhythms.
4. The rhythm is asystole.

5. Atropine and epinephrine would be appropriate to give, as they both work to speed up the heart rate. Epinephrine also helps restore pumping function in cardiac arrest.
6. A pacemaker would prevent Mr. Farley's heart rate from going too slow.
7. Loss of capture is evidenced by the pacemaker spikes not followed by a QRS complex.
8. Capture might be restored by repositioning Mr. Farley in bed or by increasing the voltage sent out by the pacemaker.
9. A pacemaker provides the possibility of overdriving the tachycardia. The pacemaker rate is dialed up to a rate exceeding the patient's heart rate. The pacemaker then assumes control of (usurps) the underlying rhythm. The pacemaker can then be slowly turned down, allowing the sinus node to assume control.
10. Amiodarone decreases the irritability of the ventricle and makes it less responsive to ventricular impulses.
11. Mr. Farley should be instructed to follow his physician's prescription, not to add or subtract doses on his own. If he feels bad, he should contact his physician or go to the hospital ER.

Scenario D: Mr. Lew

1. This EKG reveals that Mr. Lew has suffered an extensive anterior MI, as evidenced by the ST elevation in I, aVL, and all the precordial leads, along with reciprocal ST depression in the inferior leads.
2. This rhythm is accelerated idioventricular rhythm.
3. It usually requires no treatment. AIVR is a common rhythm after thrombolytic therapy and is believed to be a sign of reperfusion of the tissue that was in jeopardy.
4. The probable cause of this rhythm is reperfusion.
5. Mr. Lew has now extended his MI into the inferior wall, as evidenced by the new ST elevation in II, III, and aVF. This is a catastrophic development.
6. The right coronary artery is also blocked. (It is possible also that Mr. Lew is left-dominant, with his inferior wall supplied by the circumflex coronary artery. In that case, occlusion of the left main coronary artery would also disrupt flow to the inferior wall.)
7. The ST depression in the first EKG was reciprocal changes.
8. The rhythm is ventricular fibrillation.
9. The rhythm is agonal rhythm (dying heart).

Scenario E: Mrs. Epstein

1. The rhythm is third-degree AV block. Note that the P-P intervals are regular and the R-R intervals are also regular, but at a different rate. The PR intervals vary.

2. Her pacemaker is doing nothing. There are no pacemaker spikes anywhere.
3. The likely cause of this is a dead pacemaker battery.
4. The rhythm is dual-chamber pacing. Note the pacemaker spikes preceding the P waves and QRS complexes.
5. The pacemaker is functioning properly.

Scenario F: Mr. Calico

1. The rhythm is asystole. There is a flat line–no P waves, QRS complexes, or T waves.
2. He would have no pulse, no breathing, no movement. His skin would be cool and ashen or cyanotic in color.
3. Treatment would include immediate CPR and administration of intravenous atropine and perhaps epinephrine. Other medications or infusions could be added if these initial medications are ineffective in restoring the rhythm.
4. The rhythm is SVT, heart rate 150. This is a typical reaction to atropine and/or epinephrine–the heart rate speeds up dramatically.
5. There is an anteroseptal MI. Note the ST elevation in V1-4, with reciprocal ST depression in II, III, and aVF.
6. The ST segment has returned to normal, indicating the MI has been aborted.
7. The problem was the nurse tried to **cardiovert** vfib. Cardioversion requires that the electrical shock to the heart be synchronized with the QRS complex. In vfib there are no QRS complexes with which to to synchronize, so the shock is never delivered. The nurse must change the machine setting to **defibrillate** (take it off synchronous mode) and try again.

Scenario G: Mrs. Taylor

1. Hyperkalemia, you'll recall, is elevated blood potassium level. It can cause tall pointy T waves, typically at levels up of about 6 to 7, and wide QRS complexes at levels of about 8 or higher.
2. The rhythm is idioventricular rhythm, rate about 28. Note the slow heart ate and the wide QRS complexes.
3. The QRS complex has narrowed.

APPENDIX

Answers to Practice Quizzes and Critical Thinking Exercise Questions

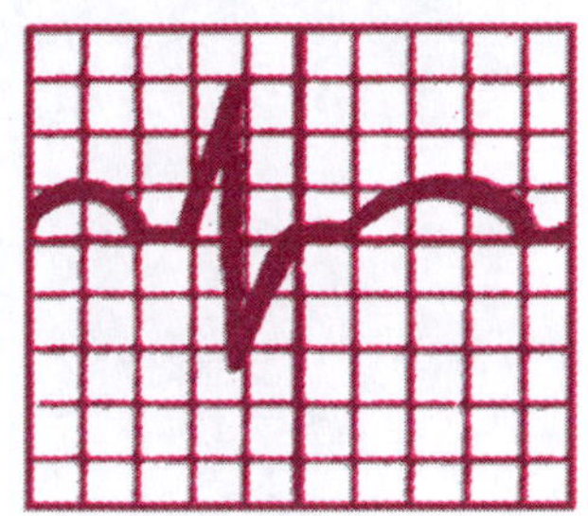

Chapter One

Practice Quiz

1. The function of the heart is to **pump enough blood to meet the body's metabolic needs.**
2. The four layers of the heart are the **endocardium, myocardium, epicardium,** and **pericardium.**
3. The four chambers of the heart are the **right atrium, left atrium, right ventricle,** and **left ventricle.**
4. The four heart valves are the **tricuspid, mitral, pulmonic,** and **aortic valves.**
5. The purpose of the heart valves is to **prevent backflow of blood.**
6. The five great vessels are the **aorta, pulmonary artery, pulmonary veins, superior vena cava,** and **inferior vena cava.**
7. The phases of diastole are **rapid filling, diastasis, and atrial kick.**
8. The phases of systole are **isovolumetric contraction, ventricular ejection, protodiastole, and iovolumetric relaxation.**
9. Once the atria have delivered their blood to the ventricles, the ventricles depolarize and a **QRS complex** is written on the EKG.
10. The three main coronary arteries are the **left anterior descending, the right coronary artery, and the circumflex.**

Critical Thinking Exercises

1.

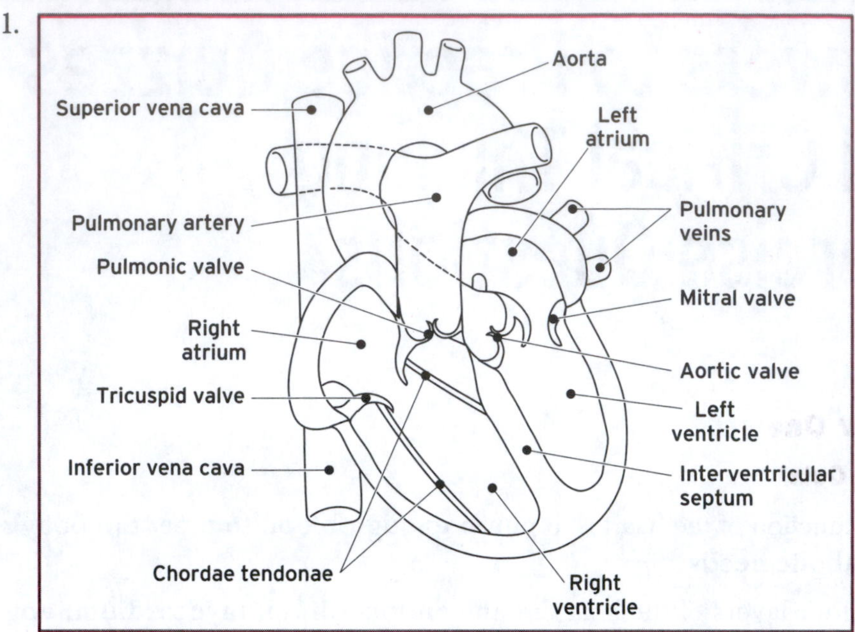

2. Here are the following structures numbered 1–14 in order of blood flow through the heart:

_____1_____superior and inferior vena cava

_____3_____tricuspid valve

_____10_____mitral valve

_____12_____aortic valve

_____5_____pulmonic valve

_____14_____body

_____13_____aorta

_____6_____pulmonary artery

_____7_____lungs

_____8_____pulmonary veins

_____2_____right atrium

_____9_____left atrium

_____4_____right ventricle

_____11_____left ventricle

3. If the chordae tendonae of the tricuspid and mitral valves “snapped” loose, the valves would lose their ability to remain closed during systole, allowing blood to flow backward into the atria.

Chapter Two

Practice Quiz

1. Cardiac cells at rest are electrically **negative.**
2. Depolarization and repolarization are **electrical events.**
3. Phase 4. **The cardiac cell is at rest.**

   Phase 0. **Depolarization occurs when sodium rushes into the cell.**

   Phase 1. **Early repolarization. Calcium is released.**

   Phase 2. **The plateau phase of early repolarization. Calcium is released.**

   Phase 3. **Rapid repolarization. Sodium rushes out of the cell.**
4. The P wave represents **atrial depolarization.**

   The QRS complex represents **ventricular depolarization.**

   The T wave represents **ventricular repolarization.**
5. **No impulse can result in depolarization during the absolute refractory period.**
6. The four characteristics of heart cells are **automaticity, conductivity, excitability, and contractility.**
7. The inherent rates of the pacemaker cells are: **sinus node-60 to 100, AV junction-40 to 60, ventricle-20 to 40.**
8. The structures of the cardiac conduction pathway are: **sinus node, interatrial tracts, atrium, internodal tracts, AV node, bundle of His, bundle branches, Purkinje fibers, and ventricle.**
9. **Escape occurs when the prevailing pacemaker slows or fails and a lower pacemaker takes over as the pacemaker at a slower rate than before.**
10. **Usurpation occurs when a lower pacemaker becomes "hyper" and fires at an accelerated rate, stealing control away from the predominant pacemaker and providing a faster heart rate than before.**

Critical Thinking Exercises

1. If the sinus node is firing at a rate of 65 and the AV junction kicks in at a rate of 70, **the AV junction will usurp the sinus node and become the heart's pacemaker.** The sinus node would be inhibited and would stop firing out impulses as long as the AV junction is faster. Remember, the fastest pacemaker at any given time is the one in control.
2. If your patient's PR interval last night was 0.16 seconds and this morning it is 0.22, **the AV node is becoming incapable of transmitting impulses at its normal rate, causing the PR interval to prolong.**
3. The heart's pumping ability can fail but its electrical conduction ability remain **intact if there is a heart attack or other condition that damages**

the myocardium but leaves the conduction system unaffected. The conduction system would send out its impulses as usual, but the damaged myocardium would be unable to respond by pumping.

4. 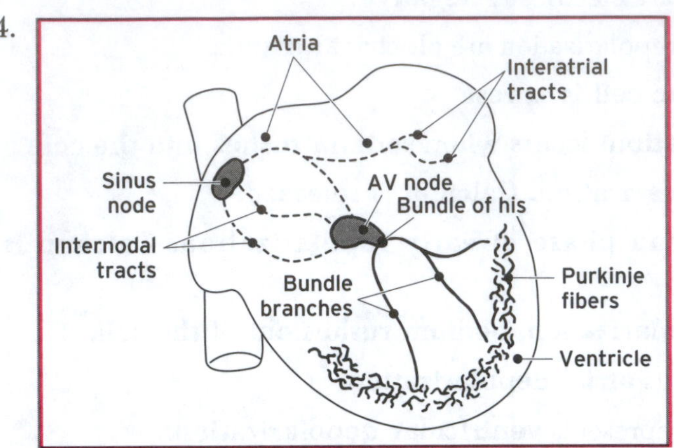

Chapter Three

Practice Quiz

1. **Willem Einthoven won the Nobel Prize for inventing the EKG machine.**
2. The three bipolar leads are **leads I, II,** and **III. Lead I connects the right and left arms. Lead II connects the right arm and left foot. Lead III connects the left arm and left foot.**
3. The three augmented leads are as follows:

   aVR **Positive pole is on the right arm.**

   aVL **Positive pole is on the left arm.**

   aVF **Positive pole is on the left foot.**
4. The six leads composing the hexiaxial diagram are **leads I, II, III, aVR, aVL,** and **aVF.**
5. The precordial leads see the heart from the **horizontal plane.**
6. The precordial leads and their locations are as follows:

   V_1 **4th ICS, RSB**

   V_2 **4th ICS, LSB**

   V_3 **Between V_2 and V_4**

   V_4 **5th ICS, MCL**

   V_5 **5th ICS, AAL**

   V_6 **5th ICS, MAL**
7. The two leads most commonly used for continuous monitoring are **leads II** and **V_1.**
8. An impulse traveling toward a positive electrode writes a **positive** complex on the EKG.

9. aVR should have a **negative** QRS complex.
10. The QRS complexes in the precordial leads start out primarily **negative.**

Critical Thinking Exercises

1. If Lead I + Lead III do not equal Lead II it could imply that **the electrodes were placed on the incorrect limbs.**
2. If the QRS complex in lead III is isoelectric, **the heart's current is traveling perpendicular to that lead.**
3. If your patient has a heart rhythm in which the current starts in the left ventricle and travels upward toward the sinus node, the frontal leads would look like the following: **Lead I's QRS would be negative, Lead II would be negative, lead III would be negative, aVR would be positive, aVL would be negative, and aVF would be negative.** You'll note this is the exact opposite of how the frontal leads normally look. This is because the current would be traveling away from all the positive electrodes except aVR's. Recall that aVR's positive electrode sits on the right arm and would be watching this current come straight toward it, resulting in a positive QRS in aVR.

Chapter Four

Practice Quiz

1. The function of the EKG machine is to print out a representation of the electrical signals generated by the heart.
2. Normal chart speed for running a 12-lead EKG is 25 millimeters per second.
3. The sensitivity control **adjusts the height of the waves and complexes.**
4. When 1 millivolt of electricity is thrown into the EKG machine's system, the stylus should be deflected **10 millimeters.**
5. Macroshock **is a high-voltage electrical shock that results from inadequate grounding of electrical equipment.**
6. Microshock is **a lower voltage shock that involves a conduit directly into the patient, such as a pacemaker.**
7. The first anatomic landmark to look for when placing electrodes is the **clavicle on the patient's right side.**
8. The four kinds of artifact are **somatic tremors, baseline sway, 60-cycle interference,** and **broken recording.**
9. If there is artifact in I, aVR, and II, troubleshooting efforts should be directed toward the **right arm.**
10. Three ways to determine if a rhythm is real or artifact are any three of the following: **Observe the rhythm in another lead such as V_1. Check to see if the rhythm meets the normal criteria. Check the monitor wires and patches. See if the patient has any muscle tremors that could cause artifact. Check the patient's vital signs for evidence of decreased cardiac output.**

Critical Thinking Exercises

1. If your patient, who is on telemetry monitoring, is noted to have two electrodes that have fallen off–the right arm and left foot, **you would expect to see artifact in any leads that use either or both of those limbs: Lead I, lead II, lead III, aVR, and aVF.**
2. You would know that your patient is having artifact and not a life-threatening arrhythmia by **assessing the patient for signs of decreased cardiac output, checking the rhythm in another lead, checking the electrode patches and wires to see if any are loose or detached, and assessing for any muscle tremors or twitches that could mimic artifact.**

Chapter Five

Practice Quiz

1. The three methods for calculating heart rate are the **6-second strip method,** the **little block method,** and the **memory method.**
2. The least accurate method of calculating heart rate is the **6-second strip method.**
3. When using the little block method, count the number of little blocks between QRS complexes and divide into **1,500.**
4. The memory method is **300–150–100–75–60–50–43–37–33–30.**
5. With regular rhythms interrupted by premature beats, the heart rate is calculated by **ignoring the premature beat and calculating the heart rate on an uninterrupted portion of the strip.**
6. The three types of regularity are **regular, regular but interrupted,** and **irregular.**
7. A rhythm with R-R intervals that vary throughout the strip is an **irregular** rhythm.
8. A rhythm that is regular except for premature beats or pauses is a **regular but interrupted** rhythm.
9. A rhythm in which the R-R intervals vary by only one or two little blocks is a **regular** rhythm.
10. R-R interval is defined as **the distance between two consecutive QRS complexes.**

Critical Thinking Exercises

1. A rhythm whose R-R intervals are 23, 24, 23, 23, 12, 24, 23, 24, 23, 23 would be considered **regular but interrupted (by a premature beat). The heart rate would be 65 (1500 divided by 23).** On a rhythm that's regular-but-interrupted by a premature beat, ignore the premature beat (the R-R interval of 12) and the short pause that normally follows it (R-R of 24) and just find an uninterrupted part of the strip. Most R-R intervals are 23, so calculate the heart rate based on this.
2. A rhythm with R-R intervals of 12, 17, 22, 45, 10, and 18 would be considered **irregular. Heart rate would be mean rate of 60 and a range of**

33 to 150. How did we come up with the mean rate? To get the first R-R of 12 requires two QRS complexes. Then each R-R is one more QRS for a total of six on the strip. So the mean rate is 60. Then for the heart rate range, find the two QRS complexes the farthest apart (R-R of 45) and the two closest together (R-R of 10) and divide each set into 1500. Slowest heart rate is 33, fastest is 150.

3. A rhythm with R-R intervals of 22, 23, 22, 22, 23, 22, 22, 22 would be considered **regular. Heart rate is 68 (R-R of 22 divided into 1500).**

Chapter Six

Practice Quiz

1. A heart rate that is greater than 100 is said to be a **tachycardia.**
2. A heart rate less than 60 is a **bradycardia.**
3. **False.** A sudden drop in heart rate from a tachycardia of 125 to a normal heart rate of 65 is indeed cause for concern, as it may cause the cardiac output (the amount of blood pumped out by the heart each minute) to drop. This could cause the patient to have symptoms such as low blood pressure, dizziness, cold clammy skin, or other problems.
4. Dysrhythmia means **abnormal heart rhythm.**
5. The five steps to rhythm interpretation are
   - **Evaluate the QRS complexes.**
   - **Assess rhythm regularity.**
   - **Calculate the heart rate.**
   - **Assess P waves.**
   - **Assess PR interval and QRS intervals.**

Chapter Seven

Practice Quiz

1. **False.** Most rhythms from the sinus node are regular rhythms.
2. The only difference between sinus rhythm, sinus bradycardia, and sinus tachycardia is the **heart rate.**
3. Sinus arrhythmia is typically caused by the **breathing pattern.**
4. A sinus exit block differs from a sinus arrest in that **in a sinus exit block, the pause is a multiple of the previous R-R intervals. In sinus arrest, the pause is *not* a multiple.**
5. **False.** Atropine is inappropriate for sinus tachycardia, as it would speed up the already-fast heart rate even more.
6. An individual with a fever of 103°F would be expected to be in **sinus tachycardia.**
7. A regular rhythm from the sinus node with heart rate of 155 is called **sinus tachycardia.**
8. **True.** That is the most basic criterion for sinus rhythms.

9. **Atropine causes the heart rate to increase.**
10. **False.** Atropine is indicated for sinus bradycardia with symptoms. Remember, athletes very often have sinus bradycardia and tolerate it very well.

Critical Thinking Exercises

1. The rhythm is **sinus rhythm.** Note the matching upright P waves and the heart rate between 60-100.
2. The rhythm is **sinus tachycardia,** rate 115.
3. The change in heart rate is most likely caused by **Mr Cavernum's increasing temperature.** Recall that the heart rate speeds up about ten beats per minute for every one degree increase in temp. Since his temp has climbed just over two degrees, his heart rate has increased by about 20 beats per minute.
4. **Acetaminophen or ibuprofen** is the medication Mr. Cavernum needs. It will lower his body temperature and that will decrease his heart rate. Atropine is indicated for bradycardias, not tachycardias. Beta-blockers would indeed lower the heart rate, but since it is likely the heart rate is related to the fever, acetaminophen or ibuprofen is the best choice.
5. The rhythm **is sinus arrhythmia.** Note the irregularity. The first two QRS complexes are 37 little blocks apart. The last two are 41 blocks apart–enough to say this rhythm is irregular and is therefore sinus arrhythmia.
6. As long as Mr. Cavernum is tolerating the rhythm without ill effects, **he requires no treatment.** If he did show signs of decreased cardiac output, however, he'd probably need atropine to speed up his heart rate. Though his heart rate is slow (between 37–40), it is not necessarily in need of treatment.
7. **Past history of sleep apnea** is a possible cause of sinus arrhythmia.

Chapter Eight

Practice Quiz

1. The complication of atrial fibrillation that can be prevented by the use of anticoagulants is **blood clots.**
2. The rhythm that is the same as wandering atrial pacemaker except for the heart rate is **multifocal atrial tachycardia.**
3. The rhythm that produces V-shaped waves between QRS complexes is **atrial flutter.**
4. Atrial rhythms take **the normal conduction pathway to the ventricles after depolarizing the atria.**
5. All rhythms that originate in a pacemaker other than the sinus node are called **ectopic rhythms.**
6. Treatment for atrial fibrillation is dependent **on its duration–specifically whether or not the atrial fib has lasted longer than 48 hours.**

7. **False.** Some PACs are nonconducted.
8. The classic cause of multifocal atrial tachycardia is **chronic lung disease.**
9. The test than can determine the presence of atrial blood clots in an emergency is **transesophageal echocardiogram.**

Critical Thinking Exercises

1. The rhythm is **atrial fibrillation.** Heart rate varies from a **low of 71 to a high of 166. Mean rate is 110.** Note the rhythm is very irregular with a wavy baseline and no P waves between QRS complexes.
2. Mr. Baldo is relatively asymptomatic, with stable vital signs. He does feel intermittent palpitations but this is not unusual. **This is NOT an emergency.**
3. **Coumadin (or Heparin),** an anticoagulant, is not needed in this situation, since the duration of atrial fib is less than 48 hours.
4. Appropriate treatment could include **beta-blockers, calcium channel blockers, amiodarone, or digitalis. Electrical cardioversion** could also be performed, but this is usually reserved for emergencies or for patients in whom medications have not been successful.
5. This rhythm strip catches Mr. Baldo converting from **atrial fib to sinus rhythm.**
6. The rhythm on discharge is **sinus rhythm.**

Chapter Nine

Practice Quiz

1. The three possible locations for the P waves in junctional rhythms are **before the QRS complex, after the QRS complex,** and **hidden inside the QRS complex.**
2. The P wave is inverted in junctional rhythms because **the impulse travels in a backward direction to reach the atria.**
3. A junctional rhythm with a heart rate greater than 100 is **junctional tachycardia.**
4. **False.** PJCs do not imply that a lethal arrhythmia is imminent.
5. A junctional rhythm with a heart rate less than 40 is **junctional bradycardia.**
6. Treatment for junctional bradycardia would consist of **atropine if the patient is symptomatic, consideration of starting oxygen, discontinuing or decreasing the dosage of any medications that could slow the heart rate down, and consideration of a pacemaker.**
7. PJCs cause the regularity to be **regular but interrupted.**
8. Junctional bradycardia is usually the result of **escape.**
9. Junctional tachycardia is best called SVT if the P waves are **hidden inside the QRS.**
10. Junctional tachycardia is the result of **usurpation.**

Critical Thinking Exercises

1. The medication used to speed up the heart rate is **atropine.** That's what Mrs. Dubos would have been given.
2. The rhythm is **junctional bradycardia with a heart rate of 37.**
3. **The ER nurse was incorrect** in her assertion that the rhythm was sinus bradycardia. Recall all rhythms from the sinus node have matching upright P waves. Since this rhythm has no P waves at all it cannot be sinus. Additionally, the heart rate is slower than the ER nurse reported.
4. The treatment in the ER would have been **atropine,** which would have been appropriate for any slow rhythm that produced symptoms. So even though the nurse identified the rhythm incorrectly, the treatment was still correct.
5. Mrs. Dubos **complained of chest pain and shortness of breath, both of which imply decreased cardiac output.** If the heart rate is too slow, the myocardium is deprived of oxygen and chest pain can result. Shortness of breath is a result of the slow heart rate's inability to transport adequate oxygen throughout the body. The low blood pressure, rapid respiratory rate, and the dazed and confused demeanor are also signs of decreased cardiac output.

Chapter Ten

Practice Quiz

1. The three main causes of PVCs are **heart disease, hypokalemia,** and **hypoxia.**
2. The rhythm that has no QRS complexes, but instead has a wavy, static-looking baseline is **ventricular fibrillation.**
3. Appropriate treatment for PVCs interrupting a sinus bradycardia with a heart rate of 32 would be **atropine** or **epinephrine** to increase the heart rate. Do not give lidocaine!
4. Torsades de pointes is a French term meaning **twisting of the points.**
5. Asystole differs from P wave asystole in that **asystole is flat-line** and **P wave asystole still has P waves.**
6. For a patient with a ventricular rhythm with a heart rate of 39 and no pulse, the treatment would be **CPR, epinephrine, atropine, oxygen, dopamine.**
7. **False.** Asystole is *not* treated with electric shock to the heart. Electric shock's goal is to recoordinate the heart's electrical activity. In asystole, there is no electrical activity to coordinate.
8. The treatment of choice for ventricular fibrillation is **defibrillation.**
9. **True.** Pacemakers can pace the atrium, the ventricle, or both.
10. **False.** Lidocaine should *not* be used to treat agonal rhythm. The lidocaine would suppress the only pacemaker this person has left–the ventricle–and would likely be fatal. Try atropine or epinephrine instead to speed up the heart rate.

Critical Thinking Exercises

1. The rhythm is **sinus rhythm with PVCs in trigeminy and quadrigeminy.**
2. **No, this rhythm does not require emergency treatment.** The patient is stable.
3. Three causes of PVCs **are hypoxia, hypokalemia, and MI.**
4. **This is ventricular fibrillation.**
5. **Yes, this is an emergency.** Patients in v-fib have no pulse and no breathing.
6. **Mr. Winston needs immediate defibrillation. Medications such as lidocaine, amiodarone and procainamide can make defibrillation more successful, but will not convert this lethal rhythm back to normal on their own.**

Chapter Eleven

Practice Quiz

1. The two typical locations for the block in AV blocks are the **AV node** and the **bundle branches.**
2. **False.** First-degree AV block causes no symptoms and does not require pacemaker insertion.
3. Wenckebach is another name for **type I second-degree AV block.**
4. AV dissociation is a hallmark of **third-degree AV block.**
5. **False.** Atropine has no effect on blocks at the bundle branches.
6. The AV block that provides merely a prolonged PR interval is **first-degree AV block.**
7. Atropine's mode of action is **to speed up the sinus node's rate of firing and to accelerate conduction through the AV node.**
8. The most dangerous type of AV block is **third-degree AV block.**
9. The least dangerous type of AV block is **first-degree AV block.**
10. **False.** First-degree AV blocks do not require atropine or epinephrine.

Critical Thinking Exercises

1. The rhythm is **sinus rhythm with first-degree AV block** (PR interval 0.24), heart rate 68.
2. **No, this is not an emergency.** First degree AV block does not cause symptoms, and the underlying rhythm is sinus, which is normal.
3. The rhythm has changed to **sinus rhythm with type I second degree AV block (Wenckebach).**
4. Both **digoxin and beta-blockers** can cause decreased conduction through the AV node, resulting in AV blocks. Insulin is not a likely cause of this rhythm.
5. Treatment should include **withholding digoxin until her level returns to normal, teaching her not to take extra medication without approval from her physician, and perhaps giving atropine if her**

heart rate slows enough to cause her symptoms. The "funny" spell in the physician's office could have reflected a slower heart rate, which might have been missed by the time the second rhythm strip was obtained. Atropine should be close by in case Ms. Watson needs it.

Chapter Thirteen

Practice Quiz

1. If the QRS complex in leads I and aVF are both negative, **the axis is in the indeterminate axis quadrant.**
2. **False.** Right bundle branch block can be a normal variant, seen in normal hearts.
3. Sagging ST segments are associated with **digitalis effect.**
4. **False.** Tall pointy T waves are typical of hyperkalemia, not RBBB.
5. Three causes of axis deviations are any three of the following: **normal variant, advanced pregnancy or obesity, myocardial infarction, hypertrophy, dysrhythmias, chronic lung disease and pulmonary embolism.**
6. The voltage criteria for LVH is: **If the S wave in V_1 added to the R wave in V_5 or V_6 (whichever is taller) is greater than or equal to 35, there is LVH.**
7. **False.** RVH is not always associated with an inverted T wave.
8. Hypertrophy is **excessive growth of tissue.**
9. Hypokalemia **causes the T wave to flatten.**
10. In a BBB, the **QRS interval must be at least 0.12 seconds.**

Critical Thinking Exercises

1. If both bundle branches became blocked simultaneously and no lower pacemaker took over, the rhythm would initially be **P-wave asystole, then eventually asystole.** The sinus node, unaffected by the BBB, would continue sending out its impulses as usual for awhile. This would provide the P waves. There would be no QRS complexes following these P waves because the bundle branch blocks would prevent the sinus impulses from reaching the ventricles. Thus the rhythm is initially P-wave asystole. Eventually the sinus node would slow down and stop, as it becomes more and more compromised by the lack of blood flow. Thus the P waves would stop. This would be asystole. Remember, if there are no QRS complexes there is no pulse and no blood flow. The sinus node, like all heart tissues, requires blood flow to function. Thus the sinus node would eventually fail because of a lack of perfusion.

2.

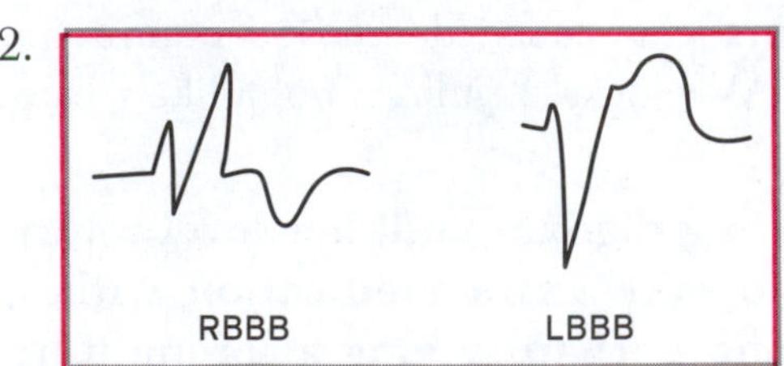

3. What happened is **she delivered the baby and her axis, which had been deviated to the left because of advanced pregnancy, is now back to normal.**

Chapter Fourteen

Practice Quiz

1. The three Is of infarction are **ischemia, injury,** and **infarction.**
2. **A Q wave MI causes ST elevation, T wave inversion, and significant Q waves to develop on the EKG. The non-Q wave MI does not cause development of significant Q waves.**
3. Occlusion of the **left anterior descending coronary artery** causes anterior MI.
4. The normal indicative changes of an MI are **ST elevation, significant Q waves,** and **T wave inversions.**
5. Reciprocal changes are seen **in the area electrically opposite the damaged area.**
6. If there is ST elevation in II, III, and aVF, **the MI is acute inferior.**
7. If there is a significant Q wave in V_1 to V_3 with baseline ST segments and upright T waves, **the MI is an old anteroseptal MI.**
8. If the transition zone is in V_1 to V_2, **there is counterclockwise rotation of the heart.**
9. The kind of MI that can be diagnosed by inverting (turning over) the EKG and looking at leads V_1 and V_2 from behind is the **posterior MI.**
10. The **circumflex coronary artery** supplies the lateral wall of the left ventricle.

Critical Thinking Exercises

1.

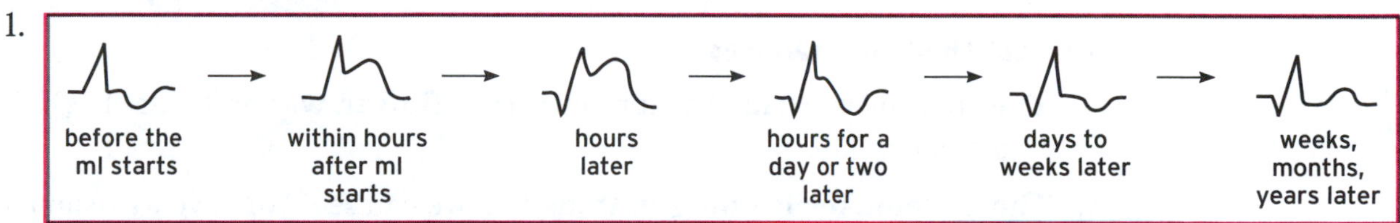

2. If Mr. Milner, a 69-year old man with a history of chest pain, arrives in your ER with newly inverted T waves in leads II, III, and aVF, it is likely **he has new ischemia in the inferior wall of the left ventricle.**
3. If an hour later Mr. Milner is doubled over with crushing chest pain and his EKG now shows marked ST elevation in II, III, aVF and V_{5-6}, **he is now injuring the inferior and lateral wall of the left ventricle.** This is an acute MI in progress which is reversible if he receives thrombolytic medications. If the MI in progress is untreated, myocardial tissue will die and significant Q waves will develop in the inferior and lateral leads on his EKG.

4. Mr. Jones's EKG shows inverted T waves in II, III, and aVF–changes consistent with ischemia.
5. He is now having an MI. Leads II, III, and aVF show ST segment elevations and upright T waves. Notice that the T waves, which were inverted on the first EKG showing ischemia, now become upright once myocardial injury begins.

Chapter Fifteen

Practice Quiz

1. Five indications for an artificial pacemaker would include any of the following: **symptomatic sinus bradycardia, junctional rhythms, idioventricular rhythm, dying heart, asystole, 2:1 AV block, type II second-degree AV block, third-degree AV block, sick sinus syndrome,** and **overdrive suppression of tachyarrhythmias.**
2. The first letter of the pacemaker code refers to the **chamber paced.**
3. The second letter of the pacemaker code refers to the **chamber sensed.**
4. The third letter of the pacemaker code refers to the **pacemaker's response to sensed events.**
5. A pacemaker that has no P wave or QRS after the pacemaker spike has **failure to capture.**
6. The pacemaker's ability to recognize the patient's own intrinsic rhythm in order to decide if it needs to fire is called **sensing.**
7. The pacemaker's generation of an electrical impulse is called **firing.**
8. A DDD pacemaker paces **dual chambers–atrium and ventricle.**
9. The DDD pacemaker senses **dual chambers–atrium and ventricle.**
10. Failure to fire is evidenced by the **lack of pacemaker spikes where there should have been.**

Critical Thinking Exercises

1. The rhythm **is atrial flutter with two flutter waves to each QRS.** Heart rate is 150.
2. **The pacemaker is doing nothing** that we can see. We have to assume it is sensing the patient's own rhythm and knows it doesn't need to fire.
3. Since the patient has a temporary pacemaker in place and therefore has the pulse generator at the bedside in easy reach, **we can use the pacemaker to overdrive this rhythm and slow the heart rate.**
4. The rhythm is **atrial fibrillation, heart rate mean is 40, range is 19 to 71.**
5. **The pacemaker is doing nothing.** It's set at a rate of 60 so it shouldn't let the heart rate drop below that.
6. There is indeed a pacer malfunction–it's **failure to fire.**
7. **The battery may need to be changed or the pacer wire or cable may need to be changed.**

8. With the first rhythm, the **heart rate is very rapid, causing decreased time for the ventricles to fill with blood.** Less blood goes in, so less blood is pumped out to the body. With the second rhythm the **heart rate is very slow. Unless the heart is able to compensate for the decreased heart rate by increasing the amount of blood pumped out with each beat, cardiac output will fall.** Both rhythms can therefore result in Mr. Johnson's low blood pressure and feeling of faintness.

   After corrective measures, the pacemaker now works properly and Mr. Johnson is in paced rhythm with a good blood pressure. He feels much better.

Chapter Seventeen

Practice Quiz

1. Digitalis is classified as a **cardiac glycoside.**
2. Class I antiarrhythmic medications **affect phase 0 of the action potential by blocking the influx of sodium into the cardiac cell.**
3. Atropine **increases the heart rate.**
4. Vasoconstriction **causes the blood pressure to increase.**
5. **True.** The AED is meant for use by the lay public.
6. Class III antiarrhythmic medications **affect phase 3 of the action potential. They interfere with the movement of potassium into the cardiac cell during repolarization.**
7. **False.** Cardioversion, not defibrillation, involves synchronizing.
8. **False.** Epinephrine is not a cardiac glycoside. It is an unclassified antiarrhythmic medication.
9. Cardioversion differs from defibrillation in that **cardioversion is synchronized with the cardiac cycle; defibrillation is not synchronized.**
10. Isoproterenol is used nowadays to **treat symptomatic bradycardias unresponsive to atropine and epinephrine.**

Critical Thinking Exercises

1. Atrial fibrillation would require **cardioversion.**
2. V-tach with a pulse would require **cardioversion.**
3. V-fib would require **defibrillation.**
4. V-tach without a pulse would require **defibrillation.**
5. SVT would require **cardioversion.**

Chapter Eighteen

Practice Quiz

1. The type of monitor worn for 24 hours to uncover any arrhythmias or ST segment changes that might be causing the patient's symptoms is the **Holter monitor.**
2. Indications for stress testing are the following (choose any three): **to determine the presence or absence of CAD, for post-CABG and**

post-PTCA evaluation, for diagnosis and treatment of exercise-induced arrhythmias, as follow-up to cardiac rehab, and **to evaluate individuals with a family history of heart disease.**

3. Bayes' theorem says that **the validity of a test result depends not only on the test accuracy, but also on the probability that the patient in question would have the disease.**
4. ST segment elevation of 5 mm is **indicative of a positive stress test.** ST elevation that high indicates an infarction beginning.
5. **True.** Patients on beta-blockers and nitrates might be advised to avoid taking these medications for a period of time before the stress test.
6. Target heart rate is **220 minus the patient's age.**
7. Event monitoring differs from Holter monitoring in that **event monitoring can be worn or used over a prolonged period,** whereas Holter monitoring is typically used only for 24 hours. Also, Holter monitoring involves continuous recording of the rhythm, whereas **event monitoring records only abnormalities or rhythms present when activated by the patient.**
8. The most commonly used protocol for treadmill stress testing is the **Bruce protocol.**
9. The protocol used most often for post-MI patients just before or following hospital discharge is the **Naughton protocol.**
10. A MET is a **metabolic equivalent, a measurement of oxygen consumption, where 1 MET is the resting oxygen consumption of a seated adult.**

Critical Thinking Exercises

1. Of only slight concern on this EKG is the sinus tachycardia that is present at rest. Mr. Cameron is overweight and a smoker, and is probably nervous about the test, so it is not surprising that his heart rate is a little elevated.
2. Mr. Cameron is overweight and a smoker, so his getting short of breath early on is not of too much concern.
3. The test should continue as these changes are normal and expected.
4. The rhythm is a bradycardia with bigeminal PVCs, then ventricular fibrillation.
5. The appropriate course of action is to get Mr. Cameron off the treadmill and to defibrillate him immediately.
6. What you should have done differently was paid more attention to Mr. Cameron's alarming change in blood pressure and his symptoms–cool clammy skin, dizziness, pallor, fatigue. He was in distress and the test should have been terminated.

Glossary

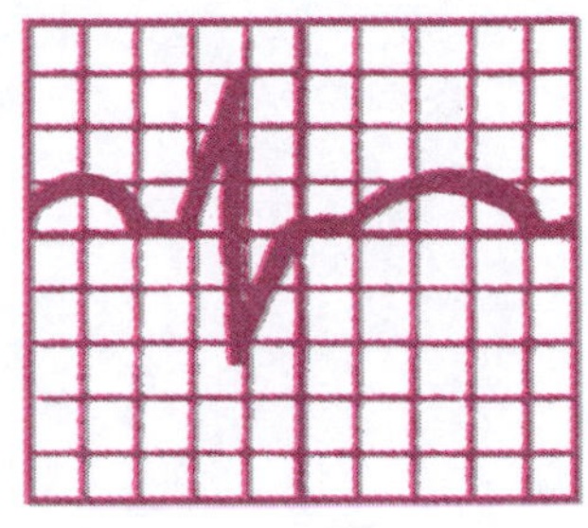

Acetylcholine: A hormone released as a result of parasympathetic stimulation.

Actin: A contractile protein found in cardiac cells.

Action potential: The depolarization and repolarization events that take place at the cell membrane. Also refers to the diagram associated with these polarity events.

Adrenergic: Referring to the sympathetic nervous system fibers that release norepinephrine.

AED: a defibrillator meant for use by the lay public.

Agonal rhythm: A ventricular rhythm characterized by very slow, irregular QRS complexes and absent P waves. Also called *dying heart.*

AICD: an implanted device that shocks the heart out of certain dangerous rhythms.

Algorithm: A flowchart.

Alpha receptors: Receptors that affect vasoconstriction.

Amplitude: The height of the waves and complexes on the EKG.

Anaerobic: Without oxygen.

Angina: Chest pain caused by a decrease in myocardial blood flow.

Angiogram: An invasive procedure in which dye is injected into blood vessels in order to determine their patency (openness).

Angioplasty: An invasive procedure in which a small balloon is used to open narrowed arteries.

Antegrade: In a forward direction.

Anterior: The front side.

Antiarrhythmic: Also called antidysrhythmic. Medications used to treat or prevent arrhythmias/dysrhythmias.

Aorta: Largest artery in the body; into which the left ventricle empties.

Aortic sinuses of Valsalva: The location of the openings to the coronary arteries. Located at the base of the aorta.

Apex: The pointy part of the heart where it rests on the diaphragm.

Arrhythmia: Often used interchangeably with dysrhythmia, which means abnormal heart rhythm.

Arteriole: A very small artery that empties into a capillary bed.

Artery: A blood vessel that carries blood away from the heart to the tissues or the lungs.

Artifact: Unwanted jitter or interference on the EKG tracing.

Asystole: No heart beat. Characterized by a flat line on the EKG.

Atrial kick: The phase of ventricular diastole in which the atria contract to propel their blood into the ventricles.

Atrium: The upper, thin-walled receiving chambers of the heart.

Augment: Increase.

Automaticity: The ability of cardiac cells to initiate an impulse without outside stimulation.

Autonomic nervous system: The nervous system controlling involuntary biological functions.

AV block (atrioventricular block): A disturbance in conduction in which some or all impulses from the sinus node are either delayed on their trip to the ventricles or do not reach the ventricle at all.

AV dissociation (atrioventricular dissociation): A condition in which the atria and ventricles depolarize and contract independently of each other.

AV node: The group of specialized cells in the conduction system that slows impulse transmission to allow atrial contraction to occur.

Axillary: Referring to the armpit.

Axis: The mean direction of the heart's current flow.

Base: The top of the heart; the area from which the great vessels emerge.

Baseline: The line from which the EKG waves and complexes take off. Also called the *isoelectric line.*

Bayes's theorem: The theorem that states that the predictive value of a test is based not only on the accuracy of the test itself but on the patient's probability of disease, as determined by a risk assessment done prior to the testing.

Beta receptors: Receptors that affect heart rate, contractility, and airway size.

Bigeminy: Every other beat is an abnormal beat.

Bipolar: Having a positive and a negative pole.

Blood pressure: The pressure exerted on the arterial walls by the circulating blood.

Bradycardia: Slow heart rate, usually less than 60.

Bundle branches: Conduction pathways extending from the bundle of His in the lower right atrium to the Purkinje fibers in the ventricles. There is a right and a left bundle branch.

Bundle of His: A confluence of conduction fibers between the AV node and the bundle branches.

Calibration: A method of verifying the correct performance of an EKG machine.

Capillaries: The smallest blood vessels in the body; where nutrient and gas exchange takes place.

Capture: The depolarization of the atrium and/or ventricle as a result of a pacemaker's firing. Determined by the presence of a P wave and/or QRS after the pacemaker spike.

Cardiac arrest: An emergency in which the heart stops beating.

Cardiac output: The amount of blood expelled by the heart each minute. Measured as heart rate times stoke volume.

Cardioversion: Synchronized electrical shock to the heart to convert an abnormal rhythm to sinus.

Cholinergic: Pertaining to acetylcholine, or to the parasympathetic nervous system.

Chordae tendineae: Tendinous cords that attach to the AV valves and prevent them from everting.

Conduction system: A network of specialized cells whose job is to create and conduct the electrical impulses that control the cardiac cycle.

Conductivity: The ability of a cardiac cell to pass an impulse along to neighboring cells.

Congestive heart failure (CHF): Fluid buildup in the lungs as a result of the heart's inability to pump adequately.

Contractility: The ability of a cardiac cell to contract and do work.

Contraindications: Reasons to avoid doing a test or procedure.

Couplet: A pair of beats.

Critical rate: The rate at which a bundle branch block appears or disappears.

Defibrillation: Asynchronous electrical shock to the heart, used to treat ventricular fibrillation and pulseless v-tach.

Depolarization: The wave of electrical current that changes the resting negatively charged cardiac cell to a positively charged one.

Diaphoresis: Sweating.

Diastasis: The phase in diastole in which the atrial and ventricular pressures are equalizing.

Diastole: The phase of the cardiac cycle in which the ventricles fill with blood.

Dissociation: The lack of relationship between two pacemaker sites in the heart.

Dysrhythmia: Abnormal heart rhythm.

Ectopy: Beats that arise from a pacemaker other than the sinus node. Understood to mean ventricular beats if the kind of ectopy is not specified.

Einthoven's triangle: The triangle formed by joining leads I, II, and III at the ends.

Electrocardiogram: A printout of the electrical signals generated by the heart.

Electrocardiograph: The EKG machine.

Electrodes: Adhesive patches attached to the skin to receive the electrical signals from the heart.

Electrolytes: Blood chemicals.

Embolus: Blood clot that has broken off and is traveling through a blood vessel.

Endocardium: The innermost layer of the heart.

Epicardium: Layer of the heart that is the same as the visceral pericardium.

Ergometer: An arm bicycle used in stress testing.

Escape: A safety mechanism in which a lower pacemaker fires at its slower inherent rate when the faster, predominant pacemaker fails.

Excitability: The ability of a cardiac cell to depolarize when stimulated.

Fascicle: A branch of the left bundle branch.

Fibrillation: The wiggling or twitching of the atrium or ventricle.

Firing: The pacemaker's generation of an electrical impulse.

Focus: Location.

Frontal leads: Limb leads I, II, III, aVR, aVL, and aVF.

Galvanometer: A component of an EKG machine that transforms electrical energy into mechanical energy, allowing the EKG to be printed out.

Heart rate: The number of times the heart beats in one minute.

Hexiaxial diagram: A diagram of the six frontal leads intersecting at the center; serves as the basis for the axis circle.

Holter monitor: A device used for 24-hour cardiac monitoring to check for arrhythmias or ST segment abnormalities.

Hypercalcemia: Elevated blood calcium level.

Hyperkalemia: Elevated blood potassium level.

Hypertension: Elevated blood pressure.

Hypertrophy: Overgrowth of myocardial tissue.

Hypocalcemia: Low blood calcium level.

Hypokalemia: Low blood potassium level.

Hypotension: Low blood pressure.

Hypoxia: Low blood oxygen level.

Indications: Reasons to perform a test or procedure.

Indicative changes: EKG changes that indicate the presence of an MI.

Infarction: Death of tissue. A myocardial infarction (MI) is a heart attack.

Injury: Damage to tissue.

Interatrial tracts: The pathways that carry the electrical impulse from the sinus node through the atrial tissue to the AV node. Also called *internodal tracts.*

Intercostal: Between the ribs.

Intervals: Measurements of time between EKG waves and complexes.

Ischemia: Oxygen deprivation in the tissues.

Isoelectric line: The flat line between the EKG waves and complexes. Also called the baseline.

Isovolumetric: Maintaining the same volume.

J point: The point where the QRS complex and ST segment join together.

Kent bundle: The accessory pathway in WPW.

Lead: An electrocardiographic picture of the heart.

Macroshock: A large electrical shock caused by improper or faulty grounding of electrical equipment.

Mean arterial pressure: The average pressure in the aorta during the cardiac cycle.

Mediastinum: The cavity between the lungs, in which the heart is located.

MET: Metabolic equivalent, a measurement of oxygen consumption.

Microshock: A small electrical shock made possible by a conduit, such as a pacemaker, directly in the heart.

Multifocal: Coming from more than one location.

Myocardial infarction: Heart attack.

Myocardium: The muscular layer of the heart.

Myosin: A contractile protein found in cardiac cells.

Neuropathy: Condition that causes a decrease in sensation, especially pain, in susceptible individuals.

Oxygen: An element inhaled from the atmosphere that is necessary for body function.

Pacemaker: The intrinsic or artificial focus that propagates or initiates the cardiac impulse.

Papillary muscle: The muscle to which the chordae tendineae are attached at the bottom.

Paroxysmal: Occurring suddenly and stopping just as suddenly.

Perfusion: The supplying of blood and nutrients to tissues.

Pericarditis: An inflammation of the pericardium.

Pericardium: The sac that encloses the heart.

Purkinje fibers: Fibers at the terminal ends of the bundle branches. Responsible for transmitting the impulses into the ventricular myocardium.

Perpendicular: At a right angle to.

Polarized: Possessing an electrical charge.

Preexcitation: Depolarizing tissue earlier than normal.

Protodiastole: The phase of systole in which ventricular, pulmonary artery, and aortic pressures equalize.

P wave: The EKG wave reflecting atrial depolarization.

Quadrant: One-fourth of a circle.

QRS complex: The EKG complex representing ventricular depolarization.

Refractory: Resistant to.

Reperfusion: Supplying blood and oxygen to tissues that have been deprived for a period of time.

Repolarization: The wave of electrical current that returns the cardiac cell to its resting, electrically negative state.

Resuscitation: Returning a lifeless person to consciousness.

Retrograde: In a backward direction.

R-R interval: The distance (interval) between consecutive QRS complexes. Usually measured at the peaks of the R waves.

Segment: The flat line between EKG waves and complexes.

Semilunar: Half-moon-shaped. Refers to the aortic and pulmonic valves.

Sensing: The ability of an artificial pacemaker to "see" the intrinsic rhythm in order to determine whether the pacemaker needs to fire.

Sensitivity: The ability of a test to pick out the people who are truly diseased.

Septum: The fibrous tissue that separates the heart into right and left sides.

Sinus node: The normal pacemaker of the heart.

Somatic: Referring to the body.

Specificity: The ability of a test to exclude those who are not diseased.

Standardization: Calibration of an EKG machine.

Sternum: Breastbone.

Stroke volume: The volume of blood expelled by the heart with each beat.

Stylus: The pen on the EKG machine.

Subclavian: Beneath the clavicle (collarbone).

Subendocardial: Referring to the myocardial layer just beneath the endocardium.

Supraventricular: Originating in a pacemaker above the ventricle.

Syncope: Fainting spell.

Systemic vascular resistance: The pressure the heart must overcome in order to expel its blood.

Systole: The phase of the cardiac cycle in which the heart contacts and expels its blood.

Tachycardia: Fast heart rate, greater than 100.

Telemetry: A method of monitoring a patient's rhythm remotely. The patient carries a small transmitter that relays his or her cardiac rhythm to a receiver located at another location.

Thoracic: Referring to the chest cavity.

Thrombolysis: The act of dissolving a blood clot.

Thyrotoxicosis: Also called *thyroid storm.* A condition in which the thyroid gland so overproduces thyroid hormones that the body's metabolic rate is accelerated to a catastrophic degree. The body temperature, heart rate, and blood pressure rise to extreme levels.

Transcutaneous: By way of the skin.

Transmembrane potential: The electrical charge at the cell membrane.

Transmural: Through the full thickness of the wall at that location.

Transvenous: By way of a vein.

Transverse: A plane of dissection that slices the body horizontally into top and bottom.

Triaxial diagram: The diagram of leads I, II, and III joined at the center or of aVR, aVL, and aVF joined at the center.

Tricuspid: Having three cusps.

Trifascicular: Referring to a block of three fascicles of the bundle branch system or to a block of two fascicles of the bundle branch system plus a first-degree AV block.

Trigeminy: Every third beat is abnormal.

T wave: The EKG wave that represents ventricular repolarization.

Unifocal: Coming from one location.

Unipolar: A lead consisting of only a positive pole.

Usurpation: The act of a lower pacemaker stealing control from the predominant pacemaker; results in a faster heart rate than before.

U wave: A small wave sometimes seen on the EKG. It follows the T wave and reflects late repolarization.

Vagus nerve: The nerve that is part of the parasympathetic nervous system. Causes the heart rate to slow when stimulated.

Valve: A structure in the heart that prevents backflow of blood.

Vasoconstrict: To make a blood vessel's walls squeeze down, narrowing the vessel's lumen.

Vasodilate: To make the blood vessel's walls relax, thus widening the blood vessel.

Vector: An arrow depicting the direction of electrical current flow in the heart.

Vein: A blood vessel that transports deoxygenated blood away from the tissues.

Vena cava: The largest vein in the body, returns deoxygenated blood to the heart.

Ventricles: The lower pumping chambers of the heart.

Venule: A very small vein that drains blood away from a capillary bed.

Glossary of Abbreviations

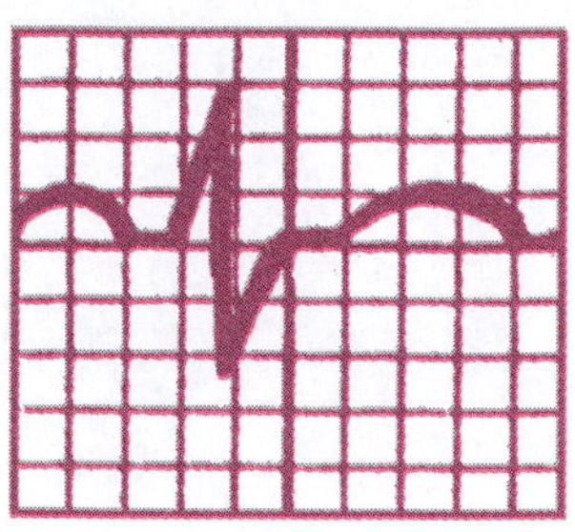

AED: automated external defibrillator.
AICD: automated internal cardioverter-defibrillator
AV: atrioventricular.
AVB: atrioventricular block.
BBB: bundle branch block.
BP: blood pressure.
CAD: coronary artery disease.
CHF: congestive heart failure.
DDD: a type of dual-chamber pacemaker
EKG: electrocardiogram.
LAD: left axis deviation or left anterior descending coronary artery
LBBB: left bundle branch block.
LVH: left ventricular hypertrophy.
MI: myocardial infarction.
MmHg: millimeters of mercury, a unit of measurement of blood pressure.
PR interval: interval of time between the P wave and QRS complex.
P wave: EKG wave representing atrial depolarization.
P-P interval: the interval between consecutive P waves.
PVC: premature ventricular complex.
QRS: the EKG wave representing ventricular depolarization.
QT interval: the interval of time between the beginning of the QRS complex and the end of the T wave.
R-R interval: the interval between consecutive QRS complexes.
RAD: right axis deviation.
RBBB: right bundle branch block.
RCA: right coronary artery.
RVH: right ventricular hypertrophy.
SA: sino-atrial.
ST segment: segment joining the QRS complex and T waves.
T wave: the EKG wave representing ventricular repolarization.
U wave: the EKG wave sometimes seen following the T wave.
VVI: a type of single-chamber pacemaker.

Index

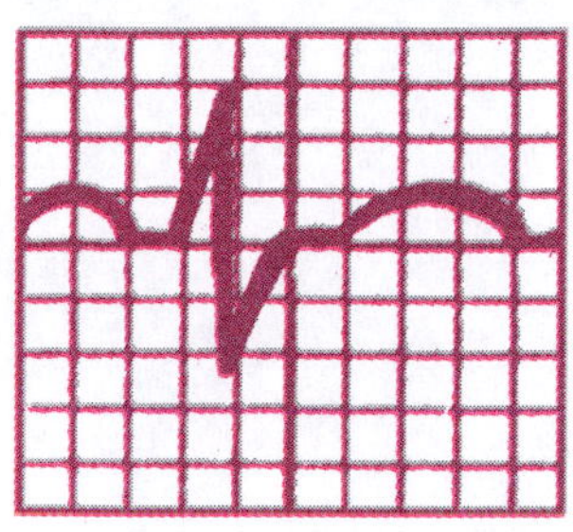

B

C

D

E

F

G

H

I

J

K

L

M

N

O

P

Q

R

S

T

U

V

W